MEDICAL DARK AGES CIRCA 1984

or

CANCER ALTERNATIVE THERAPIES' CURE RATES

by Ralph R. Hovnanian,
Member of Laity, 20th Century Serf, Curator of Cure Rates

COPYRIGHT:

(Second Edition starts on p.147.)

PUBLISHER:

Published by Author (Ralph Hovnanian; forwarding address from mailing depot of: 2128 Prospect Ave., Evanston, Ill. 60201; please write "Please Forward" on envelopes, since personnel at that facility are not involved in any way in this work).

PRINTED: in USA. (Typeset by Author.) **EDITION:** Second. **REVISION:** First.

LIBRARY NUMBERS: Library of Congress Catalog Card #: 81-90082 (1st Ed.); 84-90695 (2nd Ed.).
International Standard Book Number: ISBN 0-9607774-0-7.

LIBRARY CLASSIFICATION: (Suggested for Convenience of Cataloguer)

NLM(National Library of Medicine):	Library of Congress:	Dewey Decimal:
Main Entry:	Main Entry:	Main Entry:
QZ 266 Neoplasms, Treatment.	RC 261 Cancer, Research	616.992 Neoplasms
Added Entries:	Added Entries:	Added Entries:
(QZ 206) Neoplasms, Research.	Cancer, Nutritional Aspects.	(615.8) Physical & Other Therapies
(400) Diet Therapy.	Hygiene.	(615.537) Eclectic & Botanic Medicine
(W 50) Medical Profession, Medical Ethics.	Medical Ethics.	(612.3) Nutrition & Metabolism
(WB 300) Practice of Medicine, Therapeutics.	Medical Economics.	(610.696) Medical Relationships
	Immunology.	

DISCLAIMER: (Continued on p.147.)

"Life is short, the art long, opportunity fleeting, experience treacherous, judgement difficult." - Hippocrates.

"Every man his own doctor." - 1830's US slogan.

Please take responsibility for yourself. Patients, do choose the best treatments, confirm it with a wide range of health experts, & under their periodic guidance or care, get well! God bless us all!

CAUTION: The Author / Publisher / Printer is not responsible for damages or other liabilities. He cannot guarantee accuracy of data herein, nor its safety, effectiveness, etc. Nothing herein is intended to offend anyone or group, or to imply/infer breaking any laws or agency fiats (including "practicing medicine without a license", "cancer laws", "advertising", "labeling", "(mail) fraud", (see "... Quotations...", Q.5.2); "libel", etc.). For critical injuries & some acute diseases, Orthodox Therapy is much more effective; (see "...Quotations.", Q.4.2).

SUMMARY:

Condensed for convenience in the "Table/Matrix" herein, are over 20 categories & over 300 experiments (or clinical trials) of Alternative (Unorthodox, "Unproven") Cancer Therapies. The overwhelming majority of these Alternative Therapies are MUCH LESS EXPENSIVE, LESS HARMFUL (in "side effects"), & shown herein to be equal to, or usually MORE EFFECTIVE than, the Orthodox ("Proven") Therapies (of Surgery, Radiation, & Chemotherapy).

Most of these experiments in Alternatives appear relatively valid, yet with room for further verification. The Researchers are on the whole highly qualified.

It might be of interest to some, that 90-99% of these Alternatives are ILLEGAL in treating cancer, even by (AMA union) licensed physicians, (except by FDA permission, a virtual impossibility).

For perspective in appraising these Alternatives, a "Cancer Quotations Collage" of over 600 concise excerpts from a panorama of sources is juxtaposed.

CONCLUSION:

The abundance of valid experiments showing the effectivity of Alternative Therapies of Cancer has surprised even this Author. Most of over 20 categories of Alternatives proved their potential, with some excellent experiments in each category.

Since cancer is reversible, though with difficulty, then logically, the elimination of any initiator or promoter of cancer, becomes, however slightly, a therapy of cancer. Also. experimentally, the % of synthetic chemicals that cause cancer, is roughly equal to the % of plants that, however slightly, treat cancer; (10-25%; see "...Quotations...": "Note" in "Table...for... Quot'ns"; Q.3.1, 5th sub-section; Q.7.3, 8th sub.; Q.9.2, 10th sub.; & "Table...": 13.1; 14.4). One might wonder whether there are as many therapies, however slight, of cancer, as there are causes!

Although many of these therapies might only have a weak effect, combinations of them might be potent cures of cancer. Synergistic combinations (where the whole is greater than the sum of its parts) have been shown effective as Alternative Therapy of Cancer; (see "Table...": 6.4; 10.19.2; 18.3; A.6.1.1). If one of a patient's responses against cancer is not already saturated, & if the several treatments stimulating that response are not antagonistic (cancelling each other), then combination of the treatments has synergistic promise.

The odds that an individual researcher will be capable of surmounting the most intricate complexities, both natural & societal, is guaranteeing lack of progress in the spread of Alternative Therapies. Researchers, few in number, individualistic, as well in political affiliation, are shy of amalgamation into politically viable pressure groups. The overwhelming forces of various origin impeding implementation of Alternative Therapies are illustrated in the "...Quotations..." & referenced throughout, herein. Aroused members of the lay public & legistlatures have joined in, legalizing one Alternative, Laetrile, in 24 states. They have yet to close ranks with environmentalists, small farmers, hunger fighters, consumerists, & other reformers in: mass media, judiciary, multi-lateral disarmament, sexism, minorities, etc. While there are many legal & Constitutional avenues to explore further, events have readily convinced some that the most lasting & effective measure would be an explicit Constitutional Amendment for "Medical Freedom of Choice".

ABOUT the AUTHOR:

(See p.240-241.)

He believes one's background & stature ought not weigh too heavily in evaluating the worthiness of what he states, but yet be of value. He has a BSE, PRINCETON U. (Cum Laude; Princeton Club of Chicago Award); an MS, STANFORD U. (Ford Found'n Fellow; INCO Fellow; Teaching Ass't. in Invention & Discovery; passing 3/4 of PhD written exams); & an Amer. Chemical Soc. Award. He placed 99%-ile in the Engineering GRE(Grad. Rec. Exam); & was accepted for PhD study at Harvard U., MIT, UC Berkeley, & Stanford U. He has been employed 7 years as a Quality Assurance & Reliability Engineer; in the space shuttle, energy (auto, solar), biology, nuclear accelerator, & semiconductor fields; in 5 Fortune 200 Co.'s, & a National Lab. He is a Member of over 130 Public Interest Health (& Environment & Auto) Groups. He took 2 grad. courses in CANCER: at U. Wisconsin Med., & McCardle Labs, (from the Chairman, NCAB(National Cancer Advisory Board)). He has read over 80,000 pages on the overlap areas of HEALTH / POLITICS / ALTERNATIVE THERAPY. He fancies himself a technical GENERALIST, specializing in INVENTION & DISCOVERY.

FUNDING & FURTHERING; DONATIONS:

This work was wholly funded by its Author. No material support was received from anyone else. Author hopes some generous, ample donations will result from this initiative, to enable continuing the distribution of this book worldwide, & writing other books fulltime (see "Scope"). If only a part time level of effort is affordable, it would take too long for this Author to complete future books, making them out-dated or pre-empted by time of completion. Author is President, (with sole responsibility & authority), of Medical Dark Ages, a tax-deductible Charity, as determined by US IRS, under Internal Revenue Code (Sect.: 501(c)(3); & 509(a)(1); & 170(b)(1)(A)(vi)), (Employer ID #: 36-3225824). CONTRIBUTIONS ARE INVITED. (See "Donations", p.147.)

As a valuable alternative to financial contribution, a generous effort is needed in personally presenting the information herein to decision makers (politicians, bureaucrats, researchers, clinicians, patients, relatives, friends), in various fields: mass media (equal time to Orthodoxy), medical conventions (un-"screened" audience questions), medical schools (curricula), universities, libraries, hospitals, institutes, government (lobbying), insurance / corporations / unions (lower cost of treatment covered).

Employment in these fields would be heartily greeted by this Author, now available for a full time job (see "About the Author"), to apply the knowledge herein.

SCOPE:

For the writing & reading of this folio to be manageable & timely, the following much needed aspects were excluded, from the:

S.1 "Table / Matrix":

S.1.1 CRITICISMS & FAILURES of Alternative Therapies of Cancer.

S.1.2 Those Alternative Therapies of Cancer, with Human (/Statistical) Results, UNKNOWN TO the AUTHOR (who mainly relied on the literature, of the past few years, available from Public Interest Health Groups of the US). Perhaps there are many other therapies; some, like SPIRITUAL / RELIGIOUS are the most effective, yet no statistical data was available to the Author.

S.1.3 Recent Experiments in ALTERNATIVE Therapies of Cancer, AFTER they have received ORTHODOX RECOGNITION (e.g.: Immunotherapy, Hyperthermia, Vitamin A). (The earlier, broader, or more innovative experiments in these therapies are still reviewed herein.)

S.1.4 ORTHODOX Therapies of Cancer.

S.1.5 (deleted)

S.1.6 Alternative Therapy & Diagnosis of OTHER Chronic Degenerative Disease,(except p.288).

S.1.7 PREVENTION of Cancer & other Chronic Degenerative Disease.

S.1.8 (deleted)

S.2 "Discussion":

S.2.1 UNIFIED THEORIES & PRACTICES of Alternative Therapies of Cancer, as a simplified, organized, comprehensive, presentable PRIMER for quick learning by the busy health professional & patient.

Some of these aspects are highlighted in the "Cancer Quotations Collage" herein. The Author will hopefully pursue aspects #   , S.1.6,   , & S.2.1, later; (see "Funding").

TABLE of CONTENTS, GENERAL:

(Continued on p.147.)

FOREWORD:

"Eternal vigilance is the price of freedom." - Thomas Jefferson; or Wendell Phillips, Massachusetts Anti-slavery Society, 1852.

"Since 1945 ... human beings are infuriated by a fellow creature who does strive officiously to keep the human race alive in spite of being told he need not. What business has one man to stay sane when the fashion is to be mad?" - Arnold Toynbee, writing about Bertland Russell, (in London Sunday Telegraph, Feb. 8, 1970; in Keki Sidhwa, Medical Drugs on Trial? Verdict Guilty!, p.177).

DEDICATION:

"If I have seen further, it is by standing upon the shoulders of Giants." - Sir Isaac Newton.

PREFACE:

"There is a principle which is a bar against all information, which is proof against all argument, & which cannot fail to keep a man in everlasting ignorance. That principle is condemnation without investigation." - Herbert Spencer.

"The mind of the bigot is like the pupil of the eye. The more light you pour upon it, the more it will contract." - Oliver Wendell Holmes, Jr.

"Beware of prejudice; light is good in whatsoever lamp it is burning; a rose is beautiful in whatever garden it may bloom." - Abdul Baha.

ACKNOWLEDGEMENT:

"There are a thousand hacking at the branches of evil to one who is striking at the root." - Henry David Thoreau.

INTRODUCTION:

"If any man can convince me & bring home to me that I do not think or act aright, gladly will I change; for I search after truth, by which man never yet was harmed. But he is harmed who abideth on still in his deception & ignorance." - Marcus Aurelius Antoninus, (in Bernard Jensen, The Science & Practice of Iridology).

PROLOGUE:

The most frequent criticism of Alternative, Unorthodox, "Unproven", Therapies of Cancer is that they are based on anecdotal evidence, rather than double blind controlled clinical trials, with stastical confidence. This treatise is intended to calm that criticism, by harvesting from the literature sundry & such statistics, & standardizing them into an assimilatable "Table / Matrix" herein. (Continued on p.148.)

DISCUSSION of EXPERIMENTS, GENERAL:

Treated vs. Controls:

An acceptable experiment by modern standards, very roughly speaking, follows. Identify 2 groups of "matched" subjects; both groups with the same "disease severity", if any; each group having a "statistically significant" number of subjects, to make "random" the individual variations ("noise"). Both groups are handled identically, except one group is "treated", & the other is not & so becomes a "control". Then the health of both groups are "identically" measured. Any difference in "measure of benefit" between "treated" & "controls" is due to "treatment"; unless, differences can be attributed to unforseen, "extraneous" conditions that are actually input (independent) variables, affecting health output (dependent) variables.

Repeatability Affected by the Supposed "Extraneous":

Experiments "should" be repeatable. But rarely are all "extraneous" conditions identical. What we consider "extraneous" might have a considerable effect on the results. Even if "extraneous" variables are held as constant "background" throughout a controlled experiment, their set value might vary from one experiment(or) to another. As an example, up to a limit, the more carrot juice one drinks, the healthier he assumedly is, if organic fertilizer (the supposed "extraneous" fixed factor) was used on the carrots. However, if (a constant "background" of) synthetic (Aluminum & Fluorine) fertilizer was used, the more carrot juice one drinks, the less healthy he is. So the experimentor(s) can get two opposite results. Just because a "treatment" will not work sometimes, that does not mean it will never work, & vice versa. The trick is to find in what situations a treatment will work!

A paradigm of modern science, "repeatability by any experimentor", ignores the mental & spiritual aspects of the animate, in biomedicine.

List of Factors Affecting Results:

Supposedly "extraneous" factors actually having affect abound.

For animals: Gnawing on (trace) metals of cage; Bacteria in rubber nipples for drink; Contact with animals from another group (physical, psychological, absorbing / eating excrement).

For humans & animals: Environmental factors of "Table...";
(e.g. Electro-Magnetic radiation: high voltage power lines; house wiring (interacts with metal in cages, frame & springs of bed); electric blankets; telephone earpiece; remote control; (CB) radio; microwave (broadcasting, ovens); X-ray (TV, displays, fluorescent bulbs, medicine/dentistry, high altitude flight); radar; etc.).
(also: Negative Air Ions decreased by metal ducts in ventilation; Toxic Vapors from painted walls, lab insecticides; Water pollution; Washing cage; etc.).

Bias in Handling & Observing; Altitude & Weather; Disease Vectors (quarantine, vermin).

Administration of Treatment:
- Dosage;
- Preparation prior (chemical vehicle);
- Timing (Chrono-biology; duration);
- Route into body:
  - Nasal inhalation;
  - Oral ingestion;
  - Topical application; Skin absorption;
  - Injection:
    - Intra-dermal;
    - Sub-cutaneous;
    - Intra-muscular;
    - Intra-vascular;
    - Intra-venous;
    - Intra-peritoneal;
    - Intra-organ;
    - Intra-tumoral.

Administration of Control:
- Placebo (sugar, salt, synthetic chemicals, injections).

Variations in Subjects tested:
- Species;
- Genetic:
  - Mixed gene pool of populace; rare genes not represented in a small sample;
  - Inbred (strain, sub-species);
  - Isolated tribes (Anthropo-biology);
  - (Sub-)Culture, Ethnic;
  - Geography of ancestors;
  - Race.
- Sex;
- Age;
- Previous Environment (pre-/post natal).

Species Specific:

To prove a cancer therapy's effectivity on humans, the best trial subjects are humans, then down the animal hierarchy in vivo, & then even less conclusively, in vitro (organ, tissue, & cell cultures). The ethics, of depriving human controls of the benefits of a "therapy", are precluded by comparing the "treated" to the NCI Cancer Patient Survival Report #5, as "controls"; (see "Table...", 1.4).

Disease Severity:

For cancer, spontaneous occuring tumors are closer to the human plight than transplanted tumors, (unless considering Vaccination; see "Table...", 17.0, esp. 17.19).

Cancer treatment effectivity can be overshadowed by "extraneous" factors, just as an overwhelming "background" of carcinogens, spontaneous cancer, & premature death, can overshadow carcinogen testing. Severe ("days left to live") cancer precludes lengthy treatments (e.g. Laetrile) or delayed reactions (e.g. Immunity). Prior treatment, with immune suppressive Orthodox Therapy, can frustrate treatments requiring an immune response; (see "Table...", 1.2, 9.6.2, 17.1).

Anecdotal Evidence:

"Anecdotal Evidence", on rare occasion, can be more revealing than "double blind controlled, statistical" studies; (see "Prologue"). Incredible benefits to a very few patients might be "averaged out" by mediocre effects on the vast remainder of the "treated" group. On discovering how those few patients' supposed "extraneous" background differs from the rest of the "treated" group, the Researcher can identify new uses ("indications") for the "therapy". Also, ethically, can we deny a "therapy" to any individual, even if the vast majority do not benefit from it, (& even if the "therapy" is "non-toxic", both immediate & long-term)?!

Closely observing a single patient's smallest response (e.g. tumor shrinking) to yet the slightest change in "treatment" or supposed "extraneous" variables, can lead to discoveries missed by the busy modern MD with little time for each patient.

Similarly, time keeps this Author from finding: Are there any "double blind, controlled, statistically valid, clinical trials" of Surgery & Radiation Therapy of cancer? The more "side effects" to a "treatment", the more the patient tries to get better, to make the sacrifice "worth it"; (i.e. cognitive dissonance). Are there harmless ways to involve the patient?

Registry for Data Collection:

"5 year survival statistics" shows the % of patients with a certain kind of cancer (i.e. Primary Site, Histological Type, Grade, Stage), who are alive after 5 years from initial date of diagnosis. This procedure for "acceptable proof" is explained & given free on request via any of:

ACS, The Hospital Cancer Registry.
NCI, Biometry Branch, The 1976 SEER Code Manual.
American College of Surgeons, Cancer Registry Manual.

Using these above 3 to gather the data, the final presentation can be as in:
NCI, Biometry Branch, Cancer Patient Survival, Report #5.

Also, using as a supplement:
ACS, Clinical Oncology for Medical Students & Physicians, A Multidisciplinary Approach.

Patients, who have already been diagnosed by Orthodoxy (e.g. harmful biopsy) can be screened into an acceptable study; that, will serve as a common channel for communication between impartial Orthodox & Alternative Therapists.

Security:

Added security measures to convince auditors of the validity of fantastic experimental results, & to preclude tamperings, include:

Identification of test subjects: Humans by fingerprint; Animals by branding (foot, ear - can be chewed off);
Seals over lab entrances, allowing access to experiment only when witnesses present;
Evaluations (e.g. diagnosis) before & after therapy, independent of therapist.

Statistics:

The exact (?) statistics are too complex for accurate discussion within the scope of this book.... The possibility for random fluctuations causing error in evaluation increases with larger populations (e.g. all cancers of a type) from which smaller samples are taken, & with less random choice of samples.

If results of evaluation are binary, (e.g. healthy/unhealthy, survive/demise), then typically, a performance of 2 out of 30 in one group, in contrast to 0 out of 30 in the other group, (or 28 of 30 in one group, vs. 30 of 30 in the other) has differences with statistical significance (at the required confidence level). But to get the same statistical significance, if one group performs in the mid-range, 15 out of 30, then the other needs a greater distance from it (e.g. ±7 instead of the ±2 in the previous example), hence: 8 of 30, vs. 15 of 30, (or 22 of 30, vs. 15 of 30).

In the "Table...", each fraction (e.g. subjects surviving / total initial sample size) is converted to a "Benefited, %" for comparison with other studies, minding the "Treated, total #" for statistical significance.

If instead of the binary evaluation above, a quantitative number (from measurement) is assigned to each subject, then typically, averages (standard deviations, etc.) are calculated for each group, & compared. The difference between the two averages has more statistical significance, the larger the number of subjects, & the less the spread (standard deviation; noise, random fluctuation), within each group.

In the interest of brevity, the Author declines from further discussion, even though imminently needed, in this monograph. See: "Glossary", "Guide / Key...", "...Quotations ..." (: Q.10, all; "Note" in "Table...for...Quotations"; Q.3.1, 7th & 8th sub-sections; Q.3.2, 7th sub.; Q.3.3, 1st & 3rd; Q.4.3, 9th; Q.5.1, 23rd; Q.6.1, 6th; Q.7.2, 1st; Q.7.3, 1st; Q.8.1, 11th).

****
* NOTE: Readers unfamiliar with technical information in cancer therapy, might prefer to read the "...Quotations..." first (e.g. starting on p.65), & next, the "Treatment (Mode, Theory)" column (on left side) of the "Table / Matrix" (e.g. starting on p.20). *
****

Note: PHOTOS: of Nature, are on p.7, 17, 123, 282, & Auto-biographical, are on p.129, 150, 234, 235, 256, 282.

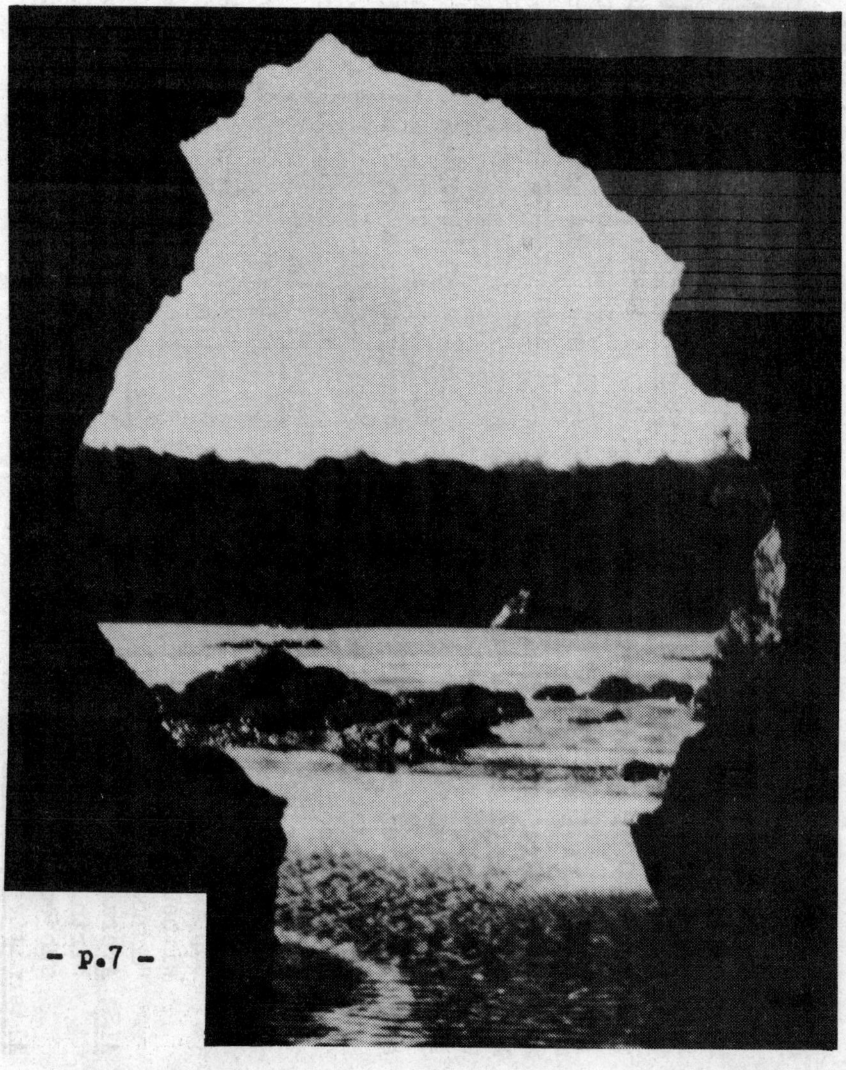

Oregon coast,
(cave on ocean).
"Preview".
(Photo by R.H.)

GLOSSARY:

Abridged; for context of this book only; over-simplified in parts for expediency, (i.e. very "fast & loose" definitions); see "...Quotations...",Q.8.3; "Discussion"; "Guide /Key ...". Very common words herein are Underlined & Capitalized; moderately used, are Capitalized only; less common, are in small case. Words in quotes if defined elsewhere in "Glossary".

air curtain: letting in un-filtered, natural sunlight, by separating cold outdoors air from warm indoors air, by an upward stream of hot air.

Allopathy: treatment of disease by suppressing its outward symptoms without heed to underlying cause; "Orthodox Therapy" of 20th Century US.

ALS: Average Life Span, measured from birth, of group of experimental subjects.

Alternative Therapy: "Unorthodox...", "Unproven Therapy"; complement to "Orthodox Therapy".

an-aerobic: without air.

Anecdotal Evidence: euphemism for patient case histories of varying clinical documentation, in support of a therapy.

angina pectoris: a form of heart attack.

Anti-Coagulant: prevents blood clots (& "Metastases"?).

antigens: enter body & are attacked by immune system.

ascites: abnormal pile-up of fluid between digestive tract & outer lining of abdominal cavity.

atheroma plaque: an atherosclerosis "plaque".

Auto-lysis: self-digestion; in fasting, body digests its own fat,& parts of liver, kidney,(storing poisons), & some un-encapsulated "Neoplasms".

Benign Tumor: only quantitatively different than its complement, "Malignant Tumor"; "Metastases" much less expected; fatal, if obstructing intestines, blood vessels, (to) vital organs, unless treated successfully; a Benign "Neoplasm".

benzidene: a chemical carcinogen.

benzpyrene: a chemical carcinogen.

Bio-cide: killing life (e.g. Pesticide, Insecti-cide, Herbi-cide).

Biopsy: tissue removed from living patient, to evaluate by microscope for cancer cells; on cutting into tumor (to get tissue), the cancer can be spread.

Cachexia: severe malnutrition in "Terminal" stage of "Cancer"; main, direct cause of death from "Cancer", in addition to obstructions of even a "Benign Tumor".

Cancer: "Malignant Neoplasm/Tumor"; with a degree of autonomous growth, "Hyper-plasia", disorganized orientation of cells, changes in cell's DNA-RNA made, lowly differentiation (specialization) of cells, fast growth, invasion into adjacent tissue, "Metastases",& finally "Cachexia".

cancer mix: variety of cancers found in a therapist's practice.

Carcinogen: a cancer causer, e.g. some chemicals.

Carcinogenesis: cancer causation.

cervical: neck, or neck of an organ; e.g. cervix of uterus.

Carcinoma: "Cancer" of tissues from embryo's ecto- or endo-derm (outer & inner 'skins' of body; e.g. mucous membranes, digestive tract, pharynx, respiratory tract, bladder, etc.); complement to "Sarcoma".

Chemo-therapy: treatment by chemicals; arbitrarily limited to poisonous chemicals, synthesized, or isolated/refined from natural sources (excluding the balancing, de-toxifying effect of the whole natural source); & excluding nutrients & others not lending to patent, license, monopoly, & profit; part of "Orthodox Therapy".

collagen: holds cells together, in animals.

Control: (1.) experimental subjects receiving no treatment, used as comparison to "Treated" group, its complement. (2.) strict adherence to treatment protocol. (3.) disease/patient is stable, not getting worse or better.

coronary thrombosis: clump/clot of blood platelets & fibrin, blocking flow of blood in coronary arteries (that bring oxygen to heart muscle).

cps: cycles per second.

Cure Rate: survival fraction; % of original # of patients, surviving for a period of time after diagnosis or therapy.

Double Blind: both patient & therapist (in contact with patient) not knowing whether patient received therapy or "Placebo" (as "Control").

Eclectic: using whatever therapy is effective, (& safe).

epithelioma: a "Carcinoma".

Faraday cage: electro-static shield of wire mesh, grounded.

fecal flora & fauna: bacteria & lowly plants & animals; grow on, & help digest, food in intestines; & give B-vitamins & anti-biotics to the host; or harm host. Prevalent species depends on food eaten, & antibiotics (in food & medicine) taken.

fibrin: main part of blood clot.

fibro-cystic breast lumps: a "Benign Tumor".

gamma globulin: an immuno-globulin, part of body's immune system.

gauss: a unit of magnetism.

glyco-: prefix for sugar.

<u>Grade</u>: severity of "Cancer", per "Histological" exam, at worst location; I=mild, IV=worst.

herpes simplex: disease caused by herpes virus, only virus implicated in human cancer.

Histo-: prefix for tissue.

<u>Histo-logy</u>: microscopic study of tissue, cells.

Hodgkins disease: of lymphatics, supposedly a "Cancer".

Homeopathy, Homo-eopathy: like cures like, (as in "fight fire with fire, & water with water"). For symptoms of poisoning from a substance, give patient an infinitesimal (e.g. 10^{-24}) serially diluted solution of the substance (electronic orientation of solvent carries away poison?-Ed.). Or, for symptoms of mineral deficiency, give mineral in dilute (e.g. 10^{-9}) solution, to absorb easily into body. Too much, or too little, of a mineral in the body shows same symptoms.

hyper-baric: high pressure.

hyper-plasia: high number of cells.

Iatro-genic: disease caused by physician.

<u>ILS</u>: Increased <u>L</u>ife <u>S</u>pan; % extra life-time of "Treated" group, over 100% for "Control" group; measured from time of cancer (detection/treatment), if available, or from birth.

indole: by product of decomposition of protein in intestines, often harmful.

infarct: dead tissue from blockage of artery to it.

interferon: a part of immune system, messenger between cells, alerting of attack by virus.

ion: an atom that has lost or gained an electron, the atom no longer being electrically neutral.

Iridology: detection of disease in body from iris (of eye), topologically connected (by nerves/(fiber optics & imaging? -Ed.)) to rest of body. (0-5% error rate on 600 patients, by Drs. Velkover & Romashov at Lumumba U. in Moscow.)

lactic: of milk.

laparatomy: incision in abdomen (e.g. for exploratory surgery for "Malignant Tumors").

<u>Leukemia</u>: "Cancer" of blood forming organs, bone marrow, blood, etc.

leukoplakia: white lesions inside mouth, increasing chance of "Cancer" there, (pre-cancerous).

ligation: surgically, to tie with a suture.

lipid: of fat.

lympho-cytes: a part of immune system, & white blood cells, travelling in vessels, fighting disease.

(-)<u>lysis</u>, (-)<u>lytic</u>: splitting/killing, of bio-molecules/cells.

macro-phages: a part of immune system, & white blood cells, moving to site of inflammation to scavenge dead cells.

<u>Malignant Tumor</u>: "Cancer", Malignant "Neoplasm", complement of "Benign Tumor".

mammary: of breast.

melanoma: a severe type of skin "Cancer".

menses: flow of blood in menstruation.

<u>Metabolic</u>: of metabolism, i.e. material processes of life; part of "Wholistic", complement to "Holistic".

<u>Metastasis</u>, <u>-es</u>: "Secondary Cancer(s)"; "Cancer" growth remote (unconnected visually, but related) to "Primary Tumor (Site)"; "Orthodox Therapy" has no cure for it, except managment by palliation (i.e. make patient feel better in decline).

Mo: molybdenum, a metal element, mineral in soil for some plants to produce Vitamin C.

mycosis fungoids: a severe "Cancer", of skin, & later of lymph nodes.

Naturo-pathy: therapy using protocols commonly occuring naturally, that humans have genetically adapted to over enough generations.

<u>Neoplasm</u>, <u>Neoplasia</u>: a non-inflamed form of "Tumor", "Benign" or "Malignant".

neuro-blast-oma: "Sarcoma" of nerves, occuring in babies.

Noso-comial Disease: caused by hospital.

oat cell carcinoma: a severe type of lung "Cancer".

occlusion: blockage (of artery, etc.)

-oma: (in US), suffix for: (1) "Benign Tumor" (i.e. name of tissue site, followed by "-oma"); (2) except: lymphoma, myeloma, melanoma, hepatoma, etc., are "Malignant Tumors", as are the more general "Carcinoma" & "Sarcoma".

<u>Oncology</u>: study of "Tumors".

Organic: (1) bio matter exclusively (in agriculture fertilizer, food, environment, etc.). (2) molecules containing carbon (in chemistry). (3) of an organ of the body.

Orthodox Therapy of Cancer: Surgery, Radiation, Chemotherapy, Hormonal Therapy. Creed of cult, in control of healing, in a culture; the norm.

osteo-genic sarcoma: a type of bone "Cancer".

papilloma: a "Benign Tumor" of epithelium (outer surface & inner interfaces (of vessels, organs, joints, & cavities)), containing "collagen".

Patho-: prefix for disease.

peritoneum: abdominal lining enclosing organs.

Placebo: a fake, supposedly inert pill or procedure, (mimicking the therapy trial), administered to the "Control" group of experimental subjects.

plaque: an athero-sclerosis deposit on the inner wall of a blood vessel, (for cardio-vascular).

pleo-morph: having many forms, (e.g. bacteria to virus & back).

pleural: linings between lungs & rib cage.

ppm: parts per million, 0.0001%.

Primary Tumor (Site): (location of) first "Neoplasm" occuring in patient.

Proteo-: prefix for protein.

Radiation Therapy: treatment by E&M (electro-magnetic) rays; arbitrarily limited to cancer causing wavelengths (of x-ray, cobalt, gamma, etc.); excluding other effective wavelengths found naturally; part of "Orthodox Therapy".

Recovery: patient is better.

Recurrence: cancer returns.

Regression: cancer goes away partially, symptoms less severe.

Remission: "Regression".

resonance cavity: a box whose dimensions are equal to certain wavelengths, thus reinforcing those wavelengths.

Response, Positive: effect of therapy has aided patient noticeably.

saline: salty.

salmonella: a microbe group causing typhoid, other diseases of intestines, food poisoning, etc.

Sarcoma: "Cancer" of tissues from embryo's meso-derm or mes-enchyme (bulk between outer & inner 'skins'; e.g. connective tissue; bone, cartilage, etc.); complement to "Carcinoma".

Secondary Cancer: "Metastases".

Seebeck effect: electro-magnetic field due to electron motion due to thermal differences.

sepsis: contamination of body by microbes.

Spontaneous: no known external cause.

squamous: scale or plate-like.

stabilized: "Control" #3.

Stage: severity of invasive & extensive spread of "Cancer" into patient; 0=in situ(least), II=regional spread, III=distant "Metastases".

Suppression of cancer: "Regression".

Survival: alive, for a time period after date of cancer (causation, detection, or treatment).

synergy: an enhanced effectivity, from a combination of treatments, over each treatment separately (or sometimes additively).

Terminal: impending death from "Cancer" if only "Orthodox Therapy" or no therapy is used; in-operable, incurable, hopeless, "Cancer".

thoracic: of chest.

thrombo-embolism: blocking of blood vessel by clot, etc., travelling from another region there.

Treated: experimental subjects on which a treatment is evaluated, in comparison to "Control" group, its complement.

trypanosome: harmful parasites in humans.

Tumor: (1) any inflammation, lump, or bump. (2) a "Neoplasm", "Benign" or "Malignant".

ultra-sound: frequencies of sound above maximum ability of human hearing.

Unorthodox Therapy: treatment not in vogue or fashion in a certain time, place, & (sub-)culture; a heresy to the prevailing sect of treatment; complement to "Orthodox Therapy".

Unproven Therapy: euphemism for "Unorthodox Therapy".

Wholistic, Holistic: Whole/Holy therapy/prevention, of disease; a generalist's approach to health, rather than a specialist's; a mental/spiritual approach to health, rather than only physical/Metabolic.

Cancer Classification:

- tumor
  - neoplasm
    - benign
    - malignant =cancer
      - carcinoma
      - sarcoma
      - leukemia
  - other swelling

- Dorland's Illustrated Medical Dictionary; & H.C.Pitot, Chmn., NCAB (National Cancer Advisory Board), Intro. of Experimental Oncology, 1976, Chapter #2; (used for audit of "Glossary").

Br'er Panda: So, it's "Social Darwinism", or "Blame the Victim"! A disease is genetic in origin, so don't search for culprit co-factors; or: Dis-ease is caused by the lifestyle you choose, not your environment polluted by decision-makers; (auto-immune disease, or smog?).

Br'er Dinosaur: Maybe for a million years, the fittest humans were sifted thru our natural, untampered, environment, by genetic adaptation. But, since the advent of technology (fire...), man has altered his environment (cooking...) faster than he can adapt to it in an optimum fashion. Thus, anything man-made is suspect until proven innocent.

Br'er Buffalo: Agreed! Health Insurance (/) Providers refuse to cover natural therapies, used for 1000's of years, billing them as "experimental" (like "Acts of God" elsewhere), yet they cover "hi-tech" (radiation, gas war) Medical Management of "terminally" ill. (O'Hare Airport, Ill. was for military. & look at the profit of its sails.)

Br'er Alligator Wallet: Ah! A "materialist" society misleads on occassion by fixating on "consuming something" to get well.

Br'er Elephant Tusk: Ditto, you rat! (Food & other (rat poison (fluoride)) allergies are nothing to sneeze at.

Br'er Pre-Med.(itator): Yes, Less Is More, when its toxics, toxins, or aggressive therapy (on un-assertives).

Br'er Rabbit (a.k.a. Wabbit): The patient public is expecting support from the miasma of malpractice morass, that actually adds fuel to the flame of sky-rocketing prices, (defensive medicine, while major league schools of thought play through). Law & Justice are not Partners in Crime.

Br'er Busy Bee: So, the Economic Safety Net can become a cob web (of Red tape).

Br'er Beaver (aside): Dam power to the animals. De-Lighted! More power to you!

Br'er Dolphin: The net can be for tuna, catching the "extra ingredient" us, with the 3rd largest brain (after runner up human (#2), & whale (#1)).

Br'er Wabbit (continues): Meanwhile, pioneers flee civilized medicine's trappings of "side effects, complications, noso-comia, & iatro-genesis". Carrying the torch of health wisdom from the past, they avoid relinquishing it to the titled class, with "unconscious bias, group-think, & conflicts of interest" in their channels: "Green($)Curtain" of economic censors. Lighting the way to public awareness, from the Medical Dark Ages, but without a cloak of arrogance, they shudder at the wanton disregard for "Freedom of Choice in Medicine" (& environmental prevention) with a merciless usurpation of the rights of the frail patient, over-worked practitioner, & mis-educated pedestrian (go at green $, beware of drunks / "Bull-ish" on stock).

Br'er Bear (a.k.a. B'ar): This, with maybe 70% of our legistlators being lawyers. Can candidates be legally held accountable for their campaign promises if they are elected? Are they practicing tactics of "Bait & Switch" (sorry, out of sale item, but we have...) or "Tom & Jerry" (one "wicked" & one "chummy" interrogator)? Saying: A democracy assures the majority get the government they deserve.

Br'er Hippo(crates/critical): Constitutional (body Politik) Rights as "Pursuit of Happiness" (via health), "Right to Contract" (between patient & practitioner), "Freedom of Speech & Press" (unlicensed health advice), & "Freedom of Religion" (herbs, grapes, fasting, enemas), are Purged away to make room for "The Media Is The Message" or "Argument Ad Hominum" (& ad nauseum) hurled at reformers. This, to discredit reform of "Spit in the Soup" or "Feed at the Taxpayers' Trough".

Br'er Giraffe: At the Pork Barrel, servers (serfs only gave 10% of income in taxes, individuals give 40+% in US, 1980), some activists for "Freedom of Choice in Medicine", "Patients' Bill of of Rights", or "Access by the Poor", have yet to "(W)Holistically" amalgamate to escort out freeloaders in the serving line. Are the same Elephants & Donkeys getting a Lion's share, to the dismay of "Environmentalists"?

Br'er Swan: Without stepping on any hooves, let's have ambi-dextrous (both Right & Left Wing) unity amongst all opposed to the "shot", be it bullet, vaccine, or "highway highball".

Br'er Whale: Can "World Hunger" activists learn from "Natural Hygienists" how to break a fast. Can Hygienists learn from Hunger-ists how to finally get mass media attention...after 7 decades of trying?

Br'er Invertebrate: No animal with any spine will survive a nuclear war; but mutation will make us gigantic! Yeah!

"Taboo Therapy Tribute
or
Animal Pharm, 1984-2001, AD(After Dollars)"
by
Ralph Hovnanian
under cover letter.

Br'er Wolf: Pass the Buck!...(sic)err ...book. Aaoohh!

Br'er Bookworm: This inflated greeting card (munch!)/book (yum!) brings cheer from the (Ill.) Land of Corn, (not Hollywood on the Potomac, either).

Br'er Hare: Why, its a work of generalist breadth & scope, not specialist depth. It applies impressionist pointillism, or mozaic art, onto non-fiction, resulting in a "Quotations Collage", the whole being greater than the sum or its parts.

Br'er Flamingo: You mean Calories don't count, People do; not Nutrition by the Numbers; nor painted desserts.

Br'er Opossum: Sorta. The restraint of narrative between quotations is to avoid interjecting invectives. It approaches a compilation / textbook of source documents for medical (ethics) historians / students. A resulting (very edited) documentary / chronicle, hopefully challenges the Reader to find his/her own revelations. This, to inspire Reader's action.

Br'er Owl: Oh! Deleting ingredients on food labels is like turning back the odo-meter (to sell a used car), or would you buy a used "Proven" therapy from this man/woman (m/f)?

Br'er Hippo(crates): Yup! Fat City, or obesity!! To attract the busy body healers' awareness of the extent of hard data available in alternative therapies, the "Table / Matrix" style of scientific data presentation is used herein.

Br'er Mammoth: Don't get bogged down in these "Tables"; (try the left-hand column ("Treatment") first).

Br'er Mongoose: It's chock full of chakras (body energies); from pewter (lead vessels) to computer (when the "chips" are down, Uncle Sam's Auntie Missile has outlaws for inlaws).

Br'er Bald Eagle: So hair fallout can be from radio fallout? .... Food sure is emotional: God, Motherhood, Apple Pie, & the 4th of July. Wait, do I deserve a brake/break (on my energy level / in my chromosomes) today?

Br'er Parrot: You see, in your talons is an attempted overview of the over-looked accounts, to balance out the proclamations produced by trillions of $'s spent on suppressing health.

Br'er Camel: I'll drink to that! Water (hic).... Nah, it's got 3 "ines" (chlorine, fluorine, & your-ine).

Br'er Pre-Med.(itated): Circumcision Circus Circumvented! Oops! Docs originally opposed to socialized medicine (sin?) reaped rapid rewards from it. Welfare for the rich! Everyone gets ice; the poor get theirs in winter!

Br'er Arctic Hare: Oh, to bridge the gap between polarized camps ("flat-world" lemmings vs. socially caring picas & "time machinists")! Enter the "double blind, controlled, statistically valid, clinical trials, with independent diagnosis for cancer". Spanning the stream of incredulity, it delivers its provisioning of hard data.

Br'er Desert Fox: Moreover, some references herein relate to anecdotal accounts of direct experimental empirical observations; yes, of alternative therapies of cancer even, the similarity in detail not due to bias, because of the variety of affiliations across lands & times, independently!

Br'er Road Runner: The Reader is invited to skim the whole book briefly to choose which section is personally most suitable for exploring first, ...

Br'er Rabbit Ears: I thought freedom of choice was between graffiti in the mass media. Wait, aren't "cure rates" like "batting averages" in baseball? Diamonds in the rough; some swing at it.

Br'er Trojan Horse: Sure! Recall & heed: Socio-Econo-Politico-Anthropo-"logical" forces infiltrate what is to be approved as "medical science", or ignored & persecuted as "quack, fad, unproven, unscientific", taboo therapies. What is the clout from the profit margin in medical self care/help using "low-tech."? (What are rejection rates of (grafts/) grants to, or publications of, alternative vs. orthodox therapies?) Aye, that is the rub: to offer the poor cancer patient the same treatment afforded a Shah!

Br'er Fish: Non-prophet, & non-($)denominational, eh? Sqabbling for deck-chairs on the Titanic. Or, drawing straws, for which drowning persons will grasp at....

Inscriptions & Thank You Notes to Choose from, to Meet Your Personal Tastes, or, Caringly Cultivated Kudos Culled

It is a privilege to present you with this book. May it help you in any way.
Note: Any one or more of the following entries might apply to you & your group. (Respect for our mutual time pleads for this format.)

1. May this be a concise survey, for quick learning, saving you considerable effort to amass widely dispersed literature.
2. Please use extra copies as loaners/ gifts to the involved or needy, (friends, colleagues...). PLEASE DO NOT TRASH THIS BOOK/ COPY! THANKS, for my resources are hard (not hardly!) earned & meager. Rather, kindly reseal/return/mail (in its same container), this book to me, via this Library Rate, & I'll gladly pay its postage.
3. I can provide further information, freely/gratis/pro-bono, by grant or contract, loan, or as an employee; for teaching, consulting, litigation, media (print, electronic...); for competition: PhD (medical: ethics, history, science; fulfilling thesis writing requirement), grant (IRS exemption letter available!), or award!
4. You are invited to contact me, for I would appreciate your views highly, & any clinical cancer alternative therapy results, you would like included in a possible 3rd. edition.
5. Will you review this book in (your) media (print ((library...) journal, book, (distribution) catalogue...), electronic (talk show, interview, ...))? Will you list it in your bibliography, booklist, computer data file/base, ...? Will you promote it by publicity (referral system, clearing house, ...), ads (direct mail, ...), ...? Will you write scripts, both fiction & non-fiction, based on the contents herein? Will you lobby, legistlate, & litigate with it? Thanks!
6. Will you inform your group's officers, & global, national, & local: members, visitors, & therapists / physicians, of this book, & or, its contents, please? Would its price be low enough to offer this book as an inducement for new or renewed membership in your group?
7. To all whose work was, is, or will be, in caring for humanity, deep gratitude! This was written partially with you in mind as the audience. Special recognition, if your work is relied on for solid evidence, herein, embellishing & honoring, by your inciseful analysis & assimilatable format! Your admirable & prized works are a fit reflection of your well placed thoughts & genuine spirit. Your contageous interests are an influential inspiration. This, considering the more glamorous & "acceptable" diversions enticing others of notable distinction. You have risked your position while standing up (in "musical chairs" to see "the emperor's (invisible) new clothes"). I am of many who are privileged to sincerely admire your work, & bravery in perseverance, against encroachments on our health freedom. You deserve every continued success & reward for your magnanamous efforts on behalf of the public. Congratulations!
8. Will you perform some of the beneficial activities implicit herein? Thanks!
9. Hello, "New Aquisitions Librarian": Please accept this free book into your collection. For, you, your patrons, (tuition, tax, patient, premium) payers, & other decision-makers (trustees, board members, executives) would appreciate options from a variety of sources. Thanks go notably to "one Dewey among a thousand catalogers, or one leader among as many sheep, (who) can sometimes bring about miraculous changes" (Bill Katz, (Author, Mag's for Libraries, (Bowker); Ed.: J. Ed. Librarianship; RQ (ALA Ref.); "Mag." column, Lib. J.), "Statistical Wailing Wall...", Library Journal, June 1, 1968; in Eric Moon, (Editor, Library Journal), Book Selection & Censorship in the Sixties, (Bowker, 1969), Ch.14, p.114).
10. Thanks again to all above, & Greetings to all.

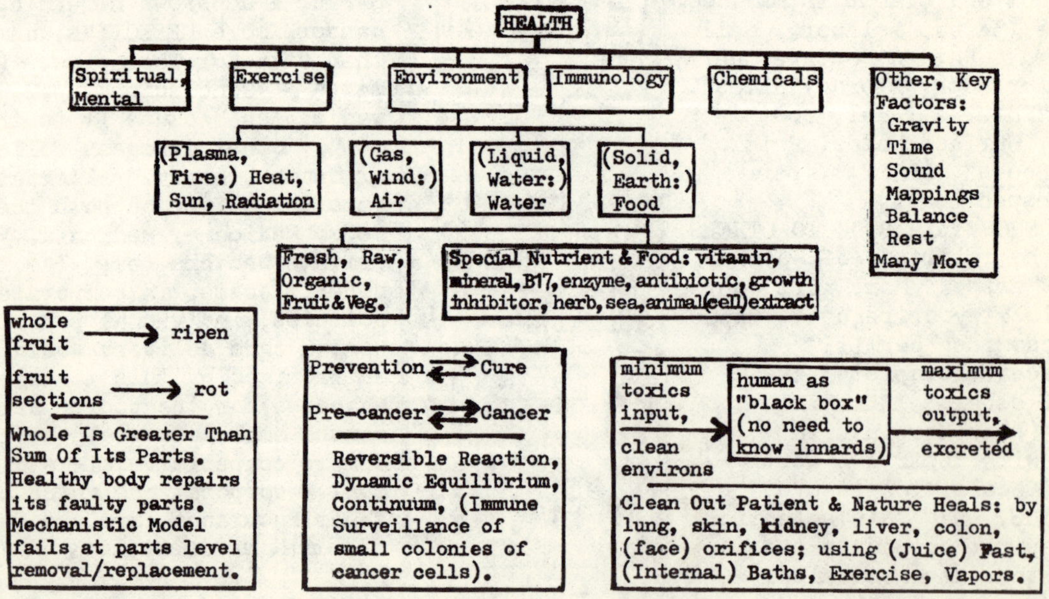

From: Ralph Hovnanian

Ralph R. Hovnanian
Medical Dark Ages (C. 1984)
c/o: 2128 Prospect Ave.
Evanston, IL 60201 USA

Tel.: (312)-869-4346

To: Gary Gordon, MD

GARRY F. GORDON, M.D.
PREVENTIVE MEDICAL CLINIC
1816 Tribute Road
Sacramento, CA 95815

Medical Dark Ages (Circa 1984) is a "non-profit charity" (by special letter from IRS; under IR Code 501(c)(3)); DONATIONS ARE TAX-DEDUCTBLE; (& mail to or fro this "publisher or distributor" of "printed matter...to further the ...interests of...herbariums", qualify for Library Rates (DMM:725).

(please see p.ii too)

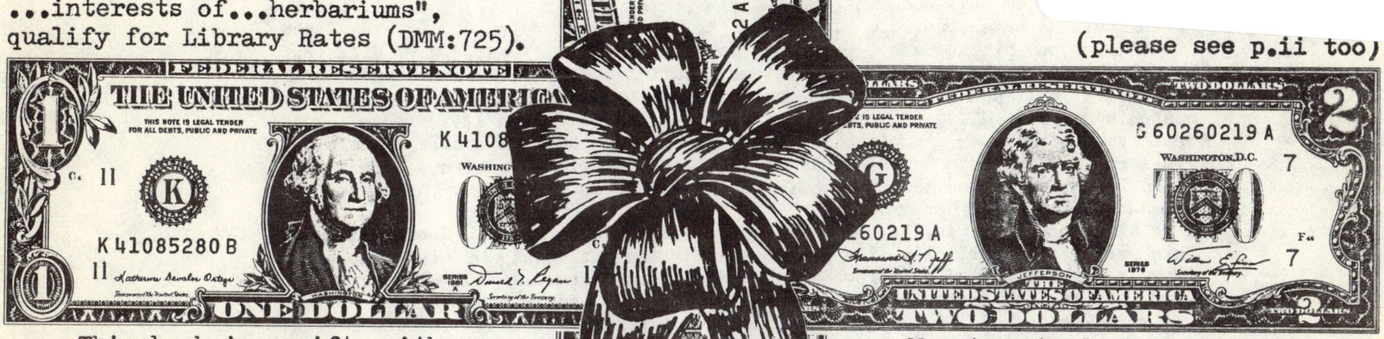

This book is a gift, with greetings, & garlands of gratitude for your generosity to generations, actual or anticipated.

You are invited, if opportune, to raise donations or grants,(f)or to reprint this book (per free release on Copyright, p.1),& (f)or to distribute (or sell) it. To avoid overlap of effort, please coordinate with me. Donations are as efficiently used as the space in this book: objective evidence.... ((Detail: 2nd printing costs were only $1.30/ copy. (Retail, its "Priceless", since "front-end" labor is immense.) Package is 13¢ ea. & labor. Mail is "Forward & Return Postage Guaranteed", for both "Library Rates" (US); or "International, Postal Union, AO, Surface Rates, Printed Matter - Books", ("Gift", per Customs inspection).))

Retail Value: $9

Please SHOW this BOOK TO OTHERS, to realize the multitude of options, as occasions arise. More gift copies are available at your request, apportioned as resources permit.

May cancer therapists take advantage of others' TREATMENT modalities, (some herein), in COMBINATION with their own worthy clinical protocols, to get even BETTER RESULTS. May this eclectic, self-less, spirit spread to the healing of other diseases also.

May true healers & patients have defense from persecution, using the collective information as needed. May we all unite into a politically viable effort to remove institutionalized prejudice, with a vigorous Constitutional guarantee of FREEDOM OF CHOICE IN HEALTH.

We can slash bloated health budgets, hidden costs & suffering, with 1 stroke (of the scalpel at that Gordian knot), via legalizing, & covering by insurance, ALTERNATIVE THERAPIES. Such taboo therapies are already widely accepted as much CHEAPER, much SAFER, & as shown herein against cancer, more EFFECTIVE, on the whole, than Orthodox Therapies. (See "Summary" & "Conclusion", p.2.) Cancer was chosen because it is the "toughest". Other diseases follow suit... or domino theory. Alternatives can ease the burden on both the Public (e.g. Medicare, Medicaid, VA) & Private Sectors (e.g. labor fringe benefit costs, in corporate group policies; individual policies). Health care delivery would not be compromised, by this taxpayer relief, & access for the poor. Rather, citizens & employees would be healthier & & more competitive, in aiding government & corporations which convince their insurance carriers to cover alternative therapies.

ABBREVIATIONS for TABLE / MATRIX (mainly):

(Continued on p.149.)

Abbreviations often used herein, are underlined in this "Glossary".

Å: Angstrom
AAAS: American Association for the Advancement of Science
AAOAC: American Association of Official Analytical Chemists
ACS: American Cancer Society. (American College of Surgeons, & American Chemical Society, are not so abbreviated herein.) (See ICRF, MAD, NRC.)
ADA: American Dental Association
AIS: Average Life Span
AMA: American Medical Association
ANL: Argonne National Laboratory
Abst.: Abstract
Acad.: Academy, Academic
Advis.: Advisory, Advisor
Agr.: Agriculture
Am., Amer.: American
Anat.: Anatomy
Ann.: Annals, Annual
Anon.: Anonymous
App.: Appendix
Art.: Article
Ass., Ass'n., Assoc'n.: Association
BCG: Bacille Calmette Guerin
BSRF: Borderland Science Research Foundation
Biol.: Biological, Biology
Brd.: Board
Bull.: Bulletin
cc: cubic centimeter
CDC: Center for Disease Control
CML: Chronic Myelogenous Leukemia
CO: carbon monoxide
cps: cycles per second
Ca.: Cancer
Cert.: Certificate, Certified
Ch.: Chapter
Chem.: Chemical, Chemistry
Chemo.: Chemotherapy
Clin.: Clinical
Co., Cty.: County
Col.: College
Com.: Committee, Commission
Ctr. Center
Cumb.: Cumberland
DC: Doctor of Chiropractic
DMBA: di-methyl-benz-anthracene
DNA-RNA: de-oxy-ribo-nucleic acid
" - " "
DO: Doctor of Osteopathy
DPM: Doctor of Preventive Medicine
DVM: Doctor of Veterinary Medicine
Dept.: Department
Derm.: Dermatology
Dev't.: Development
Dipl.: Diplomate, Diploma
Dir.: Director
Dis.: Disease
Div.: Division
E&M: Electro-Magnetic
EPA: Environmental Protection Agency
Ed.: Editor, Editorial, Education
Elect.: Electrical
Eng.: English
Ent.: Enterological
Environ.: Environmental
Exec.: Executive
Exp.: Experimental
Experim.: "
F.: Factor, as in Glucose Tolerance Factor
FACS: Fellow, American College of of Surgeons
FACT: Foundation for Alternative Cancer Therapies
FCC: Federal Communications Commission
FDA: Food & Drug Administration
FICS: Fellow, International College of Surgeons
FRCS: Fellow, Royal College of Surgeons
FTC: Federal Trade Commission
Fac.: Faculty
Facil.: Facility
Farma.: Pharmacology
Fed.: Federation, Federal
Found.: Foundation
Ger.: German
Gyn.: Gynecology
H: hydrogen
HBO: Hyper-baric Oxygen
HEW: Dept. of Health, Education, & Welfare (replaced by HHS)
HHS: Dept. of Health & Human Services
HRD: Human Resources Division, of USGAO
Histol.: Histological
Hosp.: Hospital
Hyg.: Hygiene
IACVF: International Association of Cancer Victims & Friends
ICRF: Independent Citizens' Research Foundation. (Imperial Cancer Research Fund, rarer, herein.)
IHC: International Health Council
ILS: Increased Life Span
iu: International Units
IUAC: International Union Against Cancer
IgG: Immunoglobulin G
Infect.: Infectious
Inocul.: Inoculation
Inst.: Institute
Instr.: Instructor
Int.: Internal
Int'l, Intern'l, Internat'l: International

Intro.: Introduction
Investig.: Investigator

J.: Journal
JAMA: Journal, American Medical Association
JNCI: Journal, National Cancer Institute
Jap.: Japan, Japanese

K: potassium
k: thousand

Leuk.: Leukemia
Lib., Libr.: Library

M: million
MAD: Medical Affairs Department of ACS; (Mutually Assured Destruction, in nuclear war, not used herein)
MC: Marine Corps
mm: milli meters
mv: milli volts
MWO: Multiple Wave Oscillator
mx: methyl xanthine
Med.: Medical, Medicine
Mem.: Memorial
Metab.: Metabolism
Metabiol.: Metabiology
Microb.: Microbiology
min.: minimum
Mo: molybdenum
Monog.: Monograph
mos.: months
Mtg.: Meeting

n.: number
NAS: National Academy of Science
NASA: National Aeronautics & Space Administration
NCI: National Cancer Institute
NCP: National Cancer Program/Plan
ND: Doctor of Naturopathy
NEJM: New England Journal of Medicine

NHAC: National Health Action Committee
NHF: National Health Federation
NIH: National Institutes of Health
NRC: National Research Council. (Nuclear Regulatory Commission not abbreviated herein.)
NYU: New York University
Na: sodium
Nat.: National
No.: North
Nuc.: Nuclear
Nutr.: Nutrition

Ob.: Obstetrics
Onc.: Oncology
Org.: Organic
Org'n.: Organization
oz.: ounce

p.: page
pH: acidity - alkalinity
ppb: parts per billion
ppm: " " million
psia: pounds per square inch absolute
psig: " " " " gage
Path.: Pathology
Pharm.: Pharmacology
Phys.: Physiology, Physics
Polytech.: Polytechnical
Prev.: Preventive
Proc.: Proceedings
Procto.: Proctology
Prof.: Professor
Prolif.: Proliferative

R/C: resistance ÷ capacitance
RCAF: Royal Canadian Air Force
RES: reticulo-endothelial system
Rad.: Radiation
Rec.: Record
ref.: referenced, referencing
reg.: regression, regress
Rep.: Represented
Res.: Research

Rev.: Review
rt.: rate

SKI: Sloan-Kettering Institute
SRI: Southern Research Institute; (Stanford Research Institute not referenced herein)
SUNY: State University of New York
Sch.: School
Sci.: Science, Scientific
Sect.: Section
Serv.: Service
So.: Southern
Soc.: Society
Spont.: Spontaneous
St.: State
Surg.: Surgery, Surgeon

Tel.: Telephone
Trans.: Transactions
Treat.: Treatment

U.: University
UCLA: University of California, Los Angeles
UCSF: University of California, San Francisco
USC: Univ. of Southern California
USDA: Dept. of Agriculture, US
USDHEW: see HEW
USEPA: Environmental Protection Agency
USGAO: General Accounting Office, US
USGPO: Government Printing Office
USPHS: Public Health Service, US
USPO, USPS: Post(al) Office (Service), US
uv: ultra-violet

v.: volume
VA: Veterans Administration
Veg.: vegetable
Vit.: Vitamin

WHO: World Health Organization
Webst.: Webster
wks.: weeks

x.: times

(Continued on p.149.)

(Note: This very complex "Guide" may be unnecessary; omit for now.)

TREATMENT (Mode, Theory)	BENEFITED, % of total, or #	TREATED, total #	MEASURE of BENEFIT	DISEASE SEVERITY	RESEARCHER, Credentials	REFERENCE, Publication
GUIDE / KEY for TABLE / MATRIX: (Examples / Explanation)						
00.0 SUPER TOPIC 00.1 TOPIC: EXPLANATION 00.1.1 Sub Topic. MATERIAL, METHOD (Modality, Procedure) for TREATMENT (THERAPY). Brief outline of particulars of experiment & results. THEORIES (Hypothesis?) of how therapy works. Choice of what experiments to enter here is based on: (a) Relevance to Curing Humans of Cancer, (vs. Preventing Animals from Other Disease); (b) Valid Statistics, high Confidence Level; (c) Effectivity, high Cure Rate; (d) Stature of Researchers, etc. (NOTES: NUMBERING order of (Super /Sub) Topics is based on similarity of Materials & Methods. Related (Sub) Topics under other Super Topics are referenced in parenthesis; i.e. (see...). IMPORTANT Therapies & Concepts are in capitals, the first time they appear in this "Table...".)	!*!*!* !*!*!: FINAL RESULT, if Binary (Alive /Dead) Measure of Benefit. % who Benefited, of Total # Treated. Or, # who Benefited, if Total # Treated is not handy. See: "Table", 1.4, reference;	PATIENTS, (Human): Sex, Age, Land, Era. ANIMALS: Species, (Inbred) Strain, Sex, Age. TREATED (by Procedure of (Sub) Topic): # of Beings. CONTROLS (handled identically to treated beings, except for (Sub) Topic Treatment): # of Beings.	Criteria to Evaluate Patient's Improvement over cancer OBJECTIVE: SURVIVAL; AIS; IIS over controls (see "Glossary") REGRESSION, REMISSION of cancer (i.e. patient is better); Free of Cancer (cells; gross); SHRINK tumor (by _%, for _% all tumors). SUBJECTIVE: Pain relief; Appetite; Weight gain; Energy.	CANCER: Location of Primary Tumor; (Leukemias, Myeloma,...); Histo-Pathology, Biopsy; Grade; Stage; Size of tumors; Meta-stases; estimated remaining lifetime. Cancer Mix (various cancers in Therapist's practice). Stress of Orthodox Therapy.	RESEARCHER A, Degree, Medical School; Degree, University; Fellow of a Society; Job, Department, Institution; Award; Honor; # of Articles, Books, published; Country, if other than US. (For more biography, see Subtopic ( ).) Researcher B, worked directly on experiment with Researcher A. (Researcher C, did related but not identical experiment, or free of Researchers A & B; in parenthesis.) (Persons of stature & credibility, who witnessed / supported trusted / praised Researcher A & B; in parenthesis.)	AUTHOR (name deleted if same as Researcher), "Title of Article", Name of Journal J., Volume v._, Number n. , Page p. , Month, Day, Year. (Article, related, but not directly to experimental results, in parenthesis.) (Related Article 1, referenced in Article 2.) (Article 3 referring to related Article 4.)
00.1.2 Average "Measure of Benefit" of "Treated" group is compared to "Controls"'s. Rather than showing what fraction of a group passed a test (see 00.1.1), this shows the whole group's average.	&"...Quotations ...",Q.8.1 Averaged	Treated Controls	!*!*!*!*!*!: FINAL RESULT, if Averages of Quantity Evaluation. high average low average	Cancer, caused by STRESS (by cancer cells injected into animal; carcinogen)	(Note: Horizontal lines (except in 00.1) have relevance beyond columns in which drawn, e.g. in 00.1.2, the line between "Treated" & "Control" links "high average" & "p.1" with "Treated". Rarely, vertical lines are erased to extend "Notes".) Researcher D.	Author, Book 1, p.1, p.10.
00.2 TOPIC: EXAMPLES 00.2.1 Management of patient. Statistically valid. 2½ times (i.e. 2½ x) as many "Treated" survive for 5 years as "Controls".	50% 20%	Patients: Treated: 30 Control: 30	Survival, 5 years	Cancer: Advanced, Terminal, Hopeless, Inoperable.	3 PhD's & 4 MD's (7 Researchers total)	Article 5

TREATMENT (Mode, Theory)	BENEFITED, % of total, or #	TREATED, total #	MEASURE of BENEFIT	DISEASE SEVERITY	RESEARCHER, Credentials	REFERENCE, Publication
00.2.2 If NCI 5 year survival rate for this cancer is 1%, then Researcher had to find 2000 rare patients, for chance survivals.	20 in # (can't compute %)	Patients: Treated: (# not available)	Survival, 5 years	Cancer, Incurable Site, Rare	(continued: "Guide/Key for Table/Matrix") Researcher E	Lecture (Same Lecture(r) refers to 00.2.2 & 00.2.3, so no horizontal line in this column; but, separate Researchers did experiments.)
00.2.3 "Treated" lived 2x as long as "Controls". Or, 100% Increased Life Span (ILS), measured from birth.	averaged	Mice: Treated:50 Control:50	Average Life Span: 2 years (ALS): 1 year	Any cause of death.	Researcher F; (same Researcher for 00.2.3 & 00.2.4, but separate References).	
00.2.4 ILS computed from diagnosis at 11 months age. "Treated" (surviving 13 mos.) had 1200% ILS over "Control" (surviving 1 mo.). If no diagnosis, ILS is from birth; (see 00.2.3)	averaged	Animals: Treated:29 Control:27	Average Life Span: 2 years 1 year (1200% ILS over Control)	Leukemia		Symposium 1, referenced in Book 2.
00.3 TOPIC: EXAMPLES, MORE COMPLEX		Patients:		Cancer:	(Note: Within a column, horizontal line is cut short, between 2 similar row entries; e.g.: 00.2.3 & 00.2.4 are "averaged" & "ALS"; 00.3.1&00.3.2&00.3.3 are "Patients"; 00.3.4&00.3.5 are "Rats" & "Subjective Improv.")	
00.3.1 Therapy was more effective, when Primary Site of Cancer was at Organ 1, than 2; (considering absolute & relative aid).	80% 40% 60% 45%	Treated Control Treated Control	Survival, 5 years	Organ 1 Organ 2	Researcher A; (see 00.1.1 for more data on this Researcher).	Book 3, referring to Symposium 2.
00.3.2 Therapy was more effective, for survival, than shrinking tumor; (both are "Objective" criteria).	70% 35% 45% 40%	Treated Control Treated Control	1 yr. after diagnosis: survival tumor volume shrink by $\frac{1}{3}$	Ca.: Grade I, Stage I, no spread (local).	Researcher G ", & Researcher H; (who measured tumor volume).	TV, Network, Local Station, Show Title, Speaker, Date. (Note: "Ca." is Abbreviation for "Cancer".)
00.3.3 Therapy A & Therapy B: Therapy A only : Only Therapy B: No therapy:	80% 35% 15% 10%	Treated:50 200 100 Control:80	tumor radius shrink by $\frac{1}{2}$, in 90% of tumors/patient	Ca.: Grade IV, Stage IV, meta-stases (spread far)	(Note: Therapy A is more effective than B, but their combination is even more effective, i.e. synergistic. By itself, each Therapy is a "Control" to their combination.)	
00.3.4 Therapy was effective at high dose, but not low. High dose: Low dose: No dose:	65% 40% 40%	Rats: Treated Control	Subjective Improvement: weight gain	Chronic Degenerative Disease	Researcher J	Newspaper
00.3.5 Therapy was more effective against cancer caused by low stress, than high.	75% 15% 20% 10%	Treated:20 Control:20 Treated:30 Control:30	able to work (treadmill) 1 month after stress	Stress: low high	Researcher K, interpreting govt. records.	(Note: Horizontal lines have rare zigzags if extra space is needed.) Government documents.
00.3.6 Since few Treated, 100% cure rate may be partially due to random error.	100%	Patients: Treated: very small #	Cure; cancer free (e.g. no cancer left)	Ca., spread to lymph, regional	(Note: Probability of Spontaneous Cure of cancer is 1/100,000 or 0.001%, of all cancer patients, (see "Table...", 1.1).)	
00.3.7 Changes to populace before (& causing ?) a drop in cancer incidence by $\frac{1}{2}$.	0.160% 0.080%	Populace, Region: before after	Prevented 50% of previous cancers	Cancer Incidence, rate/year	(Note: A "Treatment" number in an Appendix relates directly to the same number, if any, in another Appendix or basic Table; e.g. B.99.1 would relate to an A.99.1 or 99.1, if any.)	
00.3.8 No statistics on Patients/Cure/Cancer; but, other bases makes Therapy worthy of entry here.	averaged	Animals	Prevention	other disease		
(End: "Guide/Key for Table/Matrix")					See "Discussion..." & "Glossary".	

TABLE of CONTENTS for TABLE / MATRIX:

(Continued on p.149.)

Publicized Researchers' names are entered (in parenthesis), if aiding to identify a therapy.

13.0 GROWTH INHIBITORS, PLANTS
13.1 Plants, General
13.2 Berries of Mountain Ash;(Garb)
13.3 Asparagus;(Vensel)
13.4 Garlic

14.0 NUTRITION, HERBS
14.1 Herbs & Potassium Iodide;(Hoxsey)
14.2 Mistletoe;(Steiner)
14.3 Poison Ivy
14.4 KC-555;(Sarkisian & McQueen-Williams)
14.5 Essiac;(Caisse)
14.6 Creosote
14.7-8 Root of Puccoon; Zinc Chloride; (Fell; Pattison)
14.9 Herbs;(Evans)
14.10 " ; Statistics
14.11 " ;(Kloss)
14.12 " ;(Lin Xiang)
14.13 Bamboo
14.14 Eleutherococcus
14.15-16 BF-70& 69;(Head Shrinkers)
14.17 Cocaine
14.18 Inner Bark, "Pau Arco"

15.0 SEA
15.1 Plants, Seaweed, Tekarina, etc.
15.2 Animals
15.2.1 Mercenene, Clams;(Schmeer)
15.2.2 Sponge
15.2.3 Sea Urchin, Starfish
15.2.4 Mollusk

16.0 ANIMAL (CELLULAR) EXTRACTS INJECTED
16.1 Cellular Therapy;(Niehans)
16.2 Eclectic;(Issels)
16.3 Carcin:(" & Pawlotzki)
16.4 Adrenal;(Coffey)
16.5 Pituitary;(Wachtel)
16.6 5; GOD; Simplicity;(Gibson)
16.7 Testicle, Ovary;(Alecce)
16.8 Parathyroid Growth Inhibitor; (Thompson; Ollerenshaw)
16.9 Anti-Neoplaston;(Burzynski)

17.0 IMMUNOLOGY, FEVER
17.1 De-Blockers;(Burton; Friedman)
17.2 Krebiozen;(Ivy)
17.2.1 Carcalon "
17.3 Goat Intestine;(Bonifacio)
17.4 Anti-Biotics;(Gregory)
17.5 M-P Virus;(Molomut; Padnes)
17.6 Vaccine, Novocaine;(Fonti)
17.7 Interferon
17.8 Bacteriophage Virus;(Lincoln)
17.9 Pleomorph;(Glover; Crofton)
17.10 Progenitor Cryptocydes (Livingston; Alexander-Jackson)
17.11 Universal Vaccine;(Sawyer)
17.12 Tubercle, Human;(Maruyama)
17.13 BCG
17.14 Bacillus Cereus;(Hadley)
17.15 IgG Coated Cancer Cells;(Rand)
17.16 Toxins & Bacteria;(Coley)
17.17-18 Fever
17.19 Vaccination Causes Cancer
17.20 Thymosin: Hormone for Immunity
17.21 Imexon: Drug " "

18.0 CHEMICALS
18.1 Free Radicals, Carbonyl;(Koch)
18.2 Fossil
18.2.1 Clay
18.2.2 Charcoal
18.2.3 Petroleum;(Ganner)
18.3 DMSO
18.4 Hydrazine Sulfate;(Gold)
18.5 Aspirin
18.6 Balloons
18.7 Hypotonic Injection of Water

19.0 GRAVITY

20.0 TIME, CHRONO-BIOLOGY

21.0 MUSIC, SOUND, NOISE

22.0 MAPPINGS OF BODY

APPENDIX A (of TABLE / MATRIX)

A.2.0 SPIRITUAL, MENTAL
A.2.0.1 Spiritual Healing
A.2.1.1 Skin Contact
A.2.1.2 Massage
A.2.5.3 Hypnosis: Immunity
A.2.8.1.3 Loss of Loved One
A.2.9 Psyche
A.2.10 Meditation
A.2.11 Personal Effort
A.2.12 Psychic Breathing

A.3.0 EXERCISE
A.3.1 Light Exercise
A.3.2 Chiropractic, Osteopathic

A.5.0 ELECTROMAGNETIC RADIATION
A.5.1.4 Sunshine
A.5.1.5 Anti-Oxidants: Vit. A
A.5.1.6 Artificial Light
A.5.4.1 Underground Radiation, Water Crossing, harms
A.5.5.1.1 Damp Soil, harms
A.5.7.1 Short Wave;(Samuels)

A.6.0 AIR
A.6.1.1 Negative Air Ions
A.6.3.3 Hyperbaric Oxygen
A.6.5.1 Hydrogen Peroxide
A.6.8 Oxygenate with B Vitamins

A.7.0-1 WATER, Drinking
A.7.1.1 Fluoridation

A.8.0-1 FASTING, Human

A.9.0 NUTRITION, GENERAL
A.9.1.1.1 (Senator George McGovern)
A.9.5.8 Vegetable Juices;(Breuss)
A.9.6.1 Vit. C;(Robinson)
A.9.6.5 " ;(Klenner; Stone)
A.9.7.5 Crocetin
A.9.9.2 Vit. E
A.9.10.6 Macrobiotic;(Ohsawa; Kushi; Sattilaro)
A.9.10.7 Selenium

A.10.0 <u>NUTRITION, LAETRILE</u>
A.10.5 Laetrile;(Richardson, cont'd)
A.10.13 " ;(Soto, ")
A.10.21 " ;(Rubin)
A.10.22 " ;(Jones)
A.10.23 " ;(NCI)

A.11.0 <u>NUTRITION, ENZYMES</u>
A.11.7 Enzymes & Minerals;(Nicolini)
A.11.8 Lysozyme;(Alexander Fleming)

A.12.0 <u>NUTRITION, ANTIBIOTIC</u>
A.12.1.5 Yeast, Glucan;(DiLuzio; Mansell)
A.12.2.1.4 "Devil's" Mushroom
A.12.2.4 <u>Fungi</u>
A.12.2.4.1 Rootlets: Soil to Sap
A.12.2.4.2 Chaga;(A. Solzhenitsyn)
A.12.2.4.3 "Tree Ears"

A.14.0 <u>NUTRITION, HERBS</u>
A.14.4.1 Egyptian

A.16.0 <u>ANIMAL EXTRACTS</u>
A.16.1 Cellular Therapy

A.17.0 <u>IMMUNOLOGY</u>
A.17.1 (Burton; Friedman; cont'd)
A.17.3 **Cells made by villi (cont'd);(Morishita)**
A.17.6.1 (Hartman)
A.17.10 (Livingston; cont'd)
A.17.16 (Coley; cont'd)

A.18.0 <u>CHEMICALS</u>
A.18.2.3 Petroleum (cont'd)
A.18.3 DMSO
A.18.4 Hydrazine Sulfate

<u>APPENDIX B</u> (of TABLE / MATRIX)

B.2.0 <u>SPIRITUAL, MENTAL</u>
B.2.0.1 Spiritual Healing, Prayer
B.2.1 Contact, Social & Physical

B.3.0 <u>EXERCISE</u>
B.3.3-4 Exercise Wheel
B.3.5 Extra-Cellular Fluid;(Gruner)

B.4.0 <u>HEAT</u>

B.5.0 <u>ELECTROMAGNETIC RADIATION</u>

B.6.0 <u>AIR</u>
B.6.1 <u>WEATHER, ALTITUDE, LATITUDE</u>

B.8.0 <u>FASTING</u>

B.9.0 <u>NUTRITION, GENERAL</u>
B.9.1 Diet Advise from non-MD's
B.9.3.7 Low Protein
B.9.6.3 Vit. C;(Murata, Morishige)
B.9.7.6-7 Carrot, Juice
B.9.7.8 Vit. A
B.9.7.9 Carotene
B.9.10.4-6 Refined Sugar
B.9.15 Folic Acid;(Butterworth)
B.9.16 Calcium
B.9.17 Glutathione
B.9.18 Anti-oxidants
B.9.19 Chlorophyll, Sprouts

B.10.0 <u>NUTRITION, LAETRILE</u>
B.10.15 Laetrile;(Gibson)
B.10.20.7.1 Apricot Kernels

B.11.0 <u>NUTRITION, ENZYMES</u>
B.11.1 Raw Soybeans

B.14.0 <u>NUTRITION, HERBS</u>
B.14.2 Mistletoe
B.14.4 General Effectivity
B.14.17 Coca
B.14.18 Tree, Tajibo
B.14.19 Evergreen, Plumyew
B.14.20 Easter Lily

(Continued on p.149.)

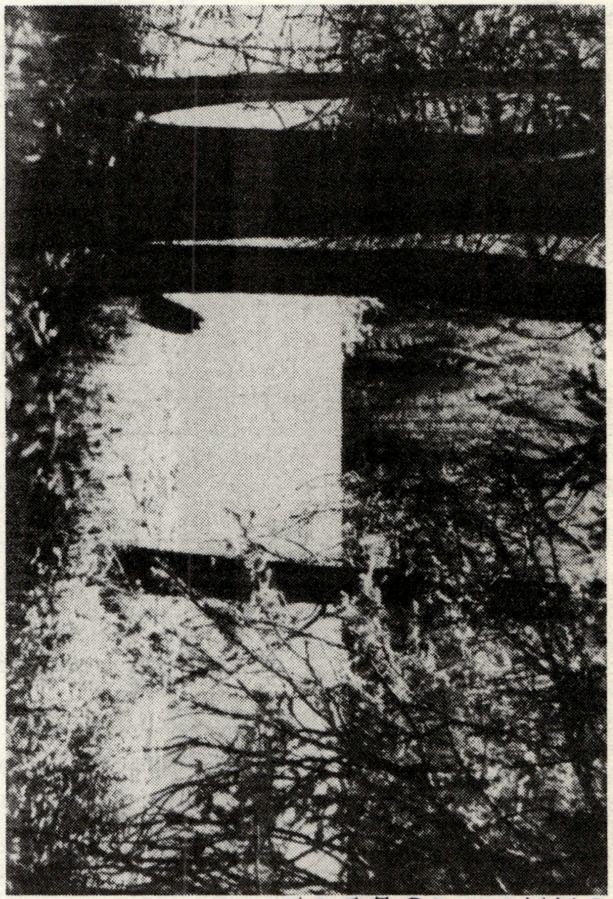

Olympic National Park, (river from glacier). Clean, mineralized water. (Photo by R.H.)

TABLE / MATRIX:

(Continued on p.151.)

TREATMENT (Mode, Theory)	BENEFITED, % of total, or #	TREATED, total #	MEASURE of BENEFIT	DISEASE SEVERITY	RESEARCHER, Credentials	REFERENCE, Publication
1.0 CONTROLS for COMPARISON 1.1 SPONTANEOUS REGRESSION/REMISSION		**TABLE / MATRIX**				**TABLE / MATRIX**
1.1.1 No known external cause for cancer symptoms shrinking.	.001%	all patients	spontaneous remission	cancer	E.F.Bashford	G.L.Rodenburg, J. Cancer Research, v.3,p.193, 1918.
1.1.2 Biological/internal causes of "spontaneous" remission may be as many as causes of original cancer. (Study excluded epithelioma of skin, leukemia, lymphoma, retino-blastoma, and melanoma of choroid.)	patients: 1000	in literature	partial or full regression of primary or metastatic tumor	ca., no biopsy	Tilden C. Everson, MD, PhD, FACS, Prof. Surg.	"Spontaneous Regress. of Cancer" Ann. N.Y. Acad. Sci., v.114,p.721,Apr.2,1964.
	119	" this century		ca. mix		
	176	"		biopsy required for primary tumor only	"& Warren Cole,MD,FACS, FRCS,Emeritus Prof.Surg, both at U.Ill. Med.,Chi.. ACS grant.	Spont. Regress. of Ca.1966.
	92	"	over 2 yrs.			"Spont. Reg. Ca." Ann. NY Acad. Sci., v.230, p.111, Mar. 18, 1974.
1.1.3	16%	44 patients	spontaneous cure	neuro-blast-oma	C.E.Coop	"Neuroblastoma in Childhood" Surg.,v.38,p.272.
1.1.4	500 patients	all in lit. this cent.	spontaneous remission	ca. mix		Cancer News J., v.13,n.3, p.3, Aug.-Sept., 1978.
1.1.5(EARLIER cancer liklier to **spont. regress**, & to be treated. "Cure" of therapy is spont. reg.)	8%	cancerous mice	"	spontaneous breast cancer	W.H.Woglom	"The Regress. of Spont. Mammary Carcinoma... Mouse" J.Ca.Res.,v.7,p.379,1942.
1.1.6 Spontaneous CONTROL. 15% of women had positive Pap test, but only 0.37% die of cervical ca. 100%x(1-(.37/15))=97.5%	97.5%	large # of U.S. women	not killed by cancer	**cervical** ca., ass-u-me if + Pap. test	Linus Pauling, Nobel Prize winner twice, & Ewan Cameron,MD,U.of Glascow, FRCS(see 9.6.2)	Cancer and Vitamin C,p.93. (See 1.2.2.)(Solomon Garb, Cure for Cancer, A National Goal,p.38.)
1.2 ORTHODOX THERAPY "SIDE EFFECTS" **1.2.1** Surgery causes cancer. See Stress,2.8. (Anasthesia is immune suppressive & carcinogenic -Thomas H. Corbet,MD, in Cancer & Chemicals, p.173-94.)	100%	50 rats	ca. free at: 20 weeks	inoculated with 50 cells of highly malignant cancer	Bernard & Edwin R.Fisher, Dept. Surg., U. Pittsburg Med., Penn.	"Experimental...Dormant... Tumor..." Science, v.130, n.3380,p.918, Oct.9,1959.(Lecture, H.C.Pitot, Directer, McCardle (Cancer)Lab., U. Wisconsin.)
	0%		20 wks. after 3 surgical laparatomies			
1.2.2 IATRO-GENESIS/NOSO-COMIAL (Physician/Hospital Induced) Disease. Orthodox Therapy (Surgery, Radiation, Chemo-therapy) are TOXIC, IMMUNO-SUPPRESSIVE, & CARCINO-GENIC.-Linus Pauling & E.Cameron in Cancer & Vit. C.	53%	200 child patients	free of 2nd. ca. CAUSED by radiation THERAPY	primary cancer (assumed independent of secondary ca.)	Anna T.Meadows,MD,Children's Hosp.,Phila.(Statistics of 13 hosp. in Phila.)(Dean Burk,PhD Biochem., U.C.Berkeley;U. London;Kaiser Willhelm Inst. Bio.;See 7.1.1&18.4)	Ed."Radiation,Chemotherapy Linked to Higher Incidence of Cancer in Future" Public Scrutiny, v.3,n.4,p.11, June, 1980. (Letter from D.Burk in Cancer Control J.,v.1,n.3,p.3-6.)(See1.1.6 & 9.6.2)
	24%	& genetic prone				
	171xa%	patients	chemo-THERAPY CAUSED 171x more 2nd. ca.			
	a% (of 2nd. ca.)	general populace				
1.2.3 INTENSIVE Radiation & Chemo-Therapy caused 29x increase in Secondary cancers (assumed independent of Primary ca.).	29xa%	35 patients	THERAPY CAUSED 29x more 2nd ca.	Hodgkins disease	Vincent T.DeVita,Director,NCI; James Arseneau, G.Canellos,NCI. R.Sherins	"Recently Recognized Complications of Ca. Chemo." Ann.NY Acad. Sci., v.230, p.481(p.485),Mar., 18,1974.
	a% (of 2nd. ca.)	general populace				
1.2.4 Anasthesia: ether 75%; carbon tet.300%	75%,300%	animals	Caused more ca.	tumors	W. Cole & G.O.McDonald,MD's	Ralph Moss,Cancer Syndrome,p.48.

TREATMENT (Mode, Theory)	BENEFITED, % of total, or #	TREATED, total #	MEASURE of BENEFIT	DISEASE SEVERITY	RESEARCHER, Credentials	REFERENCE, Publication
1.3 NO THERAPY vs. ORTHODOX THERAPY						
1.3.1 No known Orthodox Therapy: survived 4x longer than Orthodox Therapy: (of Surg., Rad., Chemo., & Hormonal)	aver-age	23 yrs.' study of cancer statistics	survival: 12.5 years 3 years	cancer mix	Dr. Hardin B. Jones, Prof. Dept. Med. Phys., U. of Cal. Davis; Lecturer, ACS 11th Annual Sci. Writers Conf., Mar. 7, '69	"Demographic...Cancer...", Trans. NY Acad. Sci., s.2, v.18, n.3, p.298, Jan. 1956. Ca. Control J., v.5, n.3-6, p.147 (p. 61-150).
1.3.2 Surgery, Mid-19th Century. 1.3.2.1 Deaths in 1st. 6yrs. discarded.		patients: 2,781	survival; after surgery: 17 months	cancer mix	Dr. Leroy d'Etoilles, info. from 174 physicians published in French Academy of Sci.	W.H. Walshe, The Anatomy, Phys. Path. & Treatment of Cancer, ref. in Nat Morris, The Cancer Blackout Amended, p.35-7.
1.3.2.2 No Therapy patient survival is 48% above Surg./Caustics	48% more in #	1,837	6 yrs. after diagnosis			
1.3.3 No Radiation Therapy patient survival is 10% above Radiation Therapy's.	10% more in #	8 of 10 groups of patients	survival	breast cancer	Dr. Jan Stjersward, Ludwig Inst. for Cancer Research, Switz.	Cancer, v.39, n.6, p.2846, (Tables 16-18), June 1977, Suppl. (NCI, ACS, White House.)
1.4 ORTHODOX THERAPY, SURVIVAL RATES			survival,			
1.4.1 ALL CANCERS; white patients; both sexes; in Conn., Cal. (L.A. & S.F.), & 2 teaching hosp. (N.O. & Iowa)	64%	patients: 450,000 total	years: 1	average mix all Grades & Stages ca.	SEER, End Results Sect., Biometry Branch, Div. of Cancer Cause & Prevention, NCI (National Cancer Institute, of NIH, PHS, DHEW, USA).	Cancer Patient Survival, Report # 5, 1976,
	47%		3			
	41%		5			p.1
1.4.2 TERMINAL Ca., DISTANT METASTASES				terminal ca.:		
1.4.2.1 Colon (common location of Primary tumor)	32%	1,000's	1	colon		" P.76
	8%		5			
1.4.2.2 Lung (")	13%	1,000's	1	lung		p.153
	2%		3			
	1%		5			
1.4.2.3 Breast (")	50%	1,000's	1	breast		" p.160
	9%		5			
1.4.2.4 Liver (rare location of Primary tumor)	7%	100's	1	liver		" p.126
	2%		3			
1.4.2.5 Pancreas (")	7%	100's	1	pancreas		" p.132
	1%		3			
1.4.3 PERMANENT CURE Rate for cancer, world wide, is 1.5%.	1.5%	world-wide	permanent cure	cancer (no skin ca.)	WHO (World Health Organization)	Cancer Victory Bull., v.6, n.10, p.3, Oct. 1980.
ALTERNATIVE / ECLECTIC / UNORTHODOX / WHOLISTIC / METABOLIC / NATURAL / ENVIRONMENTAL: CURE / THERAPY of HUMANS (supplemented by statistics on PREVENTION, ANIMALS, & OTHER DISEASES as warranted).						
2.0 SPIRITUAL, MENTAL, EMOTIONAL, PSYCHOLOGICAL, STRESS REDUCTION, PLACEBO.						
2.1 TENDER LOVING CARE. Cuddling visits, 4x daily. Prevention in Animals of Other Diseases.	on average	rabbits	50% less severity/animal	athero-sclerosis	Fred Cornhill, MD, Prof. Surg., College of Med., Ohio St. U.	Awake, June 22, 1980, p.28.
2.2 EMOTIONS Related to INTESTINAL BACTERIA. "Anger-Stress of host...produced greatest difference...in Fecal Flora of...individuals in same population."	indi-viduals	in same population	greatest difference in fecal flora	anger, stress	W.E.C. Moore & L.V. Holdeman, Virginia Polytech. Inst.	"Discussion of... Bacterio... Flora, Diet... Cancer." Cancer Research, v.35, p. 3419, Nov., 1975.

TREATMENT (Mode, Theory)	BENEFITED, % of total, or #	TREATED, total #	MEASURE of BENEFIT	DISEASE SEVERITY	RESEARCHER, Credentials	REFERENCE, Publication
2.2.1 (Gut germs make/use Vitamin B/toxins, reacting with brain)	1	1	feeling well headache	germs/oz. feces: 6 bill. 120 billion	Battle Creek Sanitarium tests on Upton Sinclair	U. Sinclair, Fasting Cure, p.17.
2.3 INFORMED, COOPERATIVE patient. (Nontoxic therapy, glyco-lytic, proteo-lytic enzymes to de-shield tumor.) (See 16.2 & 16.6)	averaged	all his cancer patients (100's)	250% higher cure rate 220% higher 18 mo. cure rt.	cancer mix	Hans Nieper, MD, Pres., Int. Acad. of Prev. Med.; Dir., German Soc. for Medical Tumor Treat.; correlated high elect. R/C with low immunity; authored 200 articles; (see 9.11 & 10.10)	Cancer News J., v.13, n.1, p.5, May, 1978; & v.15, n.3, p.18, Fall, 1980.
Hospital stay worse than at home. (Better food, LOVING CARE, & a FLEXIBLE SCHEDULE at home.)	18% 45%		18 month cure rate (survival)	incurable ca.: in hospital out of hosp.		
2.4 IMAGERY. Imagine body systems (immune, excretion, regeneration) mastering over cancer. Aid seen, grouping patients by ATTITUDE:	75%	patients: 134	survived 2+ years	Stage IV cancer	Carl Simonton, MD, Chief, Radiology, Travis AFB; Oncology Assoc., Ft. Worth. (Eugene Pendergrass, MD, Pres. ACS: "mind...can...inhibit...progress of cancer.") (See C.2.4) (Dr. Bruno Klopfer, UCLA)	Cancer Victory Bull., v.4, n.9, p.4, Sept., 1978. Psychic, July/Aug. 1973, p.21. (Simontons, Getting Well Again) (C.C. Elwell II, "The Image of Cancer", Human Behavior, Aug. 1975, p.41.)
		152 tot.:	dramatic improvement			
Fully Cooperative, Very Enthused:	100%	9				
Cooperative, Mildly Enthused:	100%	42	improvement			
Sometimes Cooperative:	50%	66	"			
Un-Cooperative:	6%	35	"			
2.5 HYPNOSIS. 2.5.1 Empathy with patient.	85%	patients of 23,000 treatments	permanently cured	various serious diseases	Prof. J.O. Crone (& Prof. Weltmer) (7 US Senators as patients.)	Crone, The Magnetic Healers Guide, p.81, 99.
2.5.2 Hypno- & PSYCHO-THERAPY	47%	21 patients	full remission	ca., no other therapy for over 6 months	Bernauer W. Newton, PhD, Newton Ctr., L.A.	Judith Glassman, "Alternate Cancer Therapy", Ca. News J., v.15, n.3, p.14, Fall, 1980.
2.6 PLACEBO 2.6.1 PILLS, fake, mimick oral medication (drugs), nutritionals. (Double blind CONTROLS: neither physician nor patient knows.)	39% 21%	patients: 288 57	half or more of pain relieved	cancer mix, mild / moderate pain	Mayo Clinic, Minn. "	John Richardson, Laetrile Case Histories, p. XX. The Medicine Show, Consumers Union, p.21-2.
Other diseases: (Pill color affects ca. pain relief; 30%)	40%		regularly help	angina pectoris	Evans & Hoyle	Evan Shute (see 9.9.1) in Herbert Bailey, Vit. E, p.178.
2.6.2 SHAM SURGERY 2.6.2.1 Shallow incision on skin (Sham Operation) mimicks surgical ligation ("therapy"). Sham (Placebo) group can exercise more, & needs less medicine for heart pains.	averaged " " "	patients: 8 ligated 9 placebo 8 ligated 9 placebo	endurance: +15% +36% medicine need: -34% -42%	"	L.A. Cobb, MD, & 4 MD's, all Prof./Instr. in Med./Surg., U.Wash., Sch. of Med., Seattle. NIH grant.	"An Evaluation of Internal Mammary Artery Ligation by a Double Blind Technic", NEJM, v.260, n.22, p.1115, May 28, 1959. Ref. in Marcia Millman, The Unkindest Cut, p.222.
2.6.2.2 Sham Operation (Placebo) better than ligation ("therapy") of mammary artery.	77% 100%	13 ligated 5 placebo	benefit, cure	"	E.G. Dimond, MD, FACC. C.F. Kittle, MD. J.F. Crockett, MD. Depts. Med. & Surg., U. of Kansas Med.	"Comparison of...Ligation & Sham Operation for Angina Pectoris", Amer. J. Cardiology, v.5, p.483, Apr. 1960.

TREATMENT (Mode, Theory)	BENEFITED, % of total, or #	TREATED, total #	MEASURE of BENEFIT	DISEASE SEVERITY	RESEARCHER, Credentials	REFERENCE, Publication
2.7 PSYCHIC SURGERY 2.7.1 Cut blood vessels, stop blood flow by verbal command. No anti-sepsis, no anti-biotics, but no infection.		300 patients/ day; tot.: 100,000's	none testified against him	many diseases	Jose Arigo (patient: J. Kubitshek, MD, Sorbonne U. Pres. of Brazil, founder of Brazilia; (see D.2.7.1))	John Fuller, Arigo: Surgeon of the Rusty Knife. (Movies with bright lights inches from the surgery.)
2.7.2 Religion, Sham Operation (or no incision), Theatrics.	93% 95%	111 patients: 30,000	not quackery improvement	many diseases including cancer	Tony Agpaoa & 30 others in Philip-pines. (Dr. Nelson Decker)	ACS, MAD, "Antonio Agpaoa". Tom Valentine, Psychic Surgery; & Newsreel, n.1, May 1977. H. Sherman, Wonder Healers.
2.8 STRESS 2.8.1 Causes cancer in humans. 2.8.1.1 Recent LOSS of SOMEONE DEAR (for 62% of ca. patients).	possi-bly the: 62%	of the ca. patients: 250	could be pre-ventable by attitude on loss	ca. mix & recent: lost one	Herbert Snow, London Cancer Hosp.	L. LeShan, PhD, "Psychological States as Factors in Devel-opment of Malignant Dis-ease", JNCI, v.22, n.1, p.1-18, Jan. 1959.
2.8.1.2 Marriage Ending (for 35% of ca. patients, over 2x controls).	35% 16%	184 controls		marriage ending	D.P. Murphy, published by Harvard U. Press	
2.8.2 Causes cancer in animals. 2.8.2 Electric shock. None: One Escapable shock : Many In-escapable shocks: Few In- " " : One In- " shock :	best each a bit worse worst	controls 90 mice total	symptoms: (tumor area; time of: onset, survival)	injected with tumor cells	Lawrence Sklar, & Hymie Anisman, Dept. of Psych., Carleton U., Ottawa, Can-ada.	"Stress & Coping Factors Influence Tumor Growth", Science, v.205, p.513, Aug. 3, 1979.
3.0 EXERCISE (See Heat 4., Air 6.; & 7.2.1, 8., 16.2)						
3.1 Exercise (wheel in cages for mice) aids oxidation, metab. (See 8.1, 16.2). Prevention; (see for cure).	37% 7%	mice: exercised controls	cancer free	benzidine given (ca. causer)	Labor Science Research Institute, Japan	George Berkley, PhD, Cancer, How to Prevent It, & Help Your Doctor Fight It, p.217.
ENVIRONMENT: 4 Phases of Matter (Plasma, Gas, Liquid, Solid) viewed as- Radiation, Air, Water, Food. (& Temperature, Pressure).						
4.0 HEAT (See Emotion 2., Exercise 3., Electro-magnetism 5., Fever 17.) 4.1 Cancer cells killed at lower temperature than normal cells. Patient circulation & excretion aided. Head: 104°F, Body: 107°F, Tumor: 111°F, 30 minutes each of 6 times total over 2 months.	76%	50 patients under age 40	return to normal living	cancer mix	Dr. Manfred von Ardenne, Founder, Ardenne Inst., Dresden. Founder, Lichter-felder Inst., Berlin. (See 6.4, & 10.20.5) Dr. R. Kir-sch, Acad. of Med., Dresden.	R. Adler, "Top European Sci-entist Reveals 111.2°F Su-per Heat Treatment Kills 99% of Cancer Cells", Pag-eant, Jan. 1966, p.76. ACS, Unproven Methods..., p.93.
4.2 Blood going to extremities is heated to 107°F. HYPER-THERMIA	36%	22 patients	complete dis-appearance of ca., 2yrs. well	cancer in limbs	Dr. Charles Heidelberger, a Chairman, McCardle (ca.) Labs, U. Wisc.; U. Rome.	ACS Seminar for Science Writers on April 2, 1969. Chicago Today.
4.3 Perfusion into limb, TOURNI-QUET, blood: 110°F, muscle: 104°F. Chemo-, & Immuno-therapy (BCG); more lympho-cytes against pa-tient's cancer. EXERCISE (See 3.) FAMILY OVERNIGHT (See 2.3). Diet.	74% 20% 98.8%	patients: 30 heated 27 controls 165	survival, 5 yrs. survival	melanoma in limbs, Stage IIIA, regional meta-stasis side-effect of therapy	John S. Stehlin, Jr., MD, M.D. Anderson Hosp. & Tumor Inst.; Stehlin Found., Hou-ston. & 4 Drs. (& Vincent DeVita, Dir., NCI, on ABC TV, "Good Morning America"	"Results of 11 Yrs.' Exper-ience...", Ca. Res., v.39, n.6, Part II, "Hyper-thermia", p.2255, June 1979. JAMA, v.241, n.13, p.1321, Mar. 30, 1979.

TREATMENT (Mode, Theory)	BENEFITED, % of total, or #	TREATED, total #	MEASURE of BENEFIT	DISEASE SEVERITY	RESEARCHER, Credentials	REFERENCE, Publication
4.4 Body core: 108°F, for 2 hrs. General anasthesia. No patients with heart or liver disease. Body FLUID REPLACED. Longer blood coagulation time temporarily, (see Anti-Coagulant, 11.)	43% 27% 93.5%	patients: 78, total 22, lung 78	objective response, regression survival	far advanced ca., no response to orthodox therapy side-effect of therapy	James M. Larkin, MD, U. New Mexico Med., V.A. Hosp., Lovelace Med. Found'n, Albuq. (Testing at 40 "Establishment" med. ctrs. -JAMA, v.245, p.1109.)	"A Clinical Investigation of Total-Body Hyperthermia as Cancer Therapy", Cancer Res., v.39, n.6, p.2252. (Cancer, v.40, p.3155, 1977; &v.20, n.9, p.1351, Sep. 1967)
4.5 Hyper-Thermia, (107.5°F), (of whole body, can suppress immunity).	50%	175 patients	remission, 2 yrs. (see B.4.5)	cancer mix	Donald Cole, MD, Temple U., Am. Brd. Surg.; Floral Pk., NY	Gary Null, Ca. News J., v.14, n.4, p.15-6, Dec. 1979.
4.6 Hot BATHS, Water Jackets, 109° F. (See Hydro-therapy, 7.1.1)	100%	28 patients	alive 2-3 years	advanced cancer	Dr. Rolf Harzmann, U. of Tubingen, Germany	New York Times News Service.
4.7 ULTRA-SOUND HEAT (Heat simulates body's normal defense mechanism of fever; see 17.)	54%	21 patients	objective response of tumor	shallow ca., no response to orthodox therapy	Marmor, et. al.	"Clinical Trial of Ultrasound Induced Hyperthermia" Proc. 14th. Ann. Mtg., Am. Soc. Clin. Onc., v.19, p.330, 1978.
5.0 ELECTRO-MAGNETIC RADIATION (E & M)						
5.1 NATURAL SUNLIGHT						
5.1.1 UNFILTERED to eyes (no "glasses, contacts") or skin (no panes). Stay outdoors, NO ARTIFICIAL light (bulbs, TV). HELIO-THERAPY.	100%	14 patients	cancer under control	cancer mix	John N. Ott, Grand Honors Award, National Eye Inst. &: Dr. Jane C. Wright, Bellvue Med. Ctr., NYC.	Ott, Health and Light, p.71 (Ott: Ann. NY Acad. Sci., v.117, Art.1, p.624, Sept. 10, 1964. Ann. Dentistry, v.27, n.1, Mar. 1968. Optom. Wkly, Sept. 5, 1968. Total; 42 papers at: AAAS, National Geographic, Oxford, Dartmouth, U. Mich., U. Wisc. 1000 lectures.)
5.1.2 AIR CURTAIN healthier than cool white fluorescent. Activates Vit. B_2, D, Calcium, etc., by skin, retina blood, pineal, etc.	on average	hamsters	50% ILS (Increased Life Span, from ca. date)	transplant tumor, slow acting	Dr. Edward Scanlon, Pres., ACS; Chief of Surg. Evanston Hosp., Ill.	p.100
5.1.3 DAYLIGHT, even thru glass, is healthier than pink fluorescent. (Low sun: less % harmful UVrays.)		C3H strain mice: 3,000 " : 3 & 30	9 months ILS 3 " ILS	spontaneous tumor	Dr. Sam Lee Gabby, Sherman Hosp., Elgin, Ill.	p.97 p.72
5.2 ORGONE ENERGY						
5.2.1 E&M resonates in Zinc lined box, size of patient's body. As a RESONANCE CAVITY, it selects body wavelengths, & zinc energy. FARADAY CAGE. Causes mild fever. Replaces SEX ENERGY. Animals.	100% 31%	13 patients	tumor softened living over 2 years	terminal cancer, advanced cachexia	Willhelm Reich, MD, U. of Vienna, assoc. of Sigmund Freud. Science: Reich's "work in psychoanalysis generally accepted by (analysts) as ... important". Author of 11 bks.	Reich, The Cancer Biopathy, p.332 (Science, Oct. 1954, referred by ACS. p.317 "Social Orgonomy", NYU Course, Sp. 1970. p.302-6 R.M. Eisberg, Fundamentals of Modern Physics, p.220, 251. ACS, Unproven Methods..., p.175.)
5.2.2 Animals. Orgone charged red blood cells injected into cancerous mice, prolonging life.		mice: 36 treated 101 " 27 controls	ALS (Ave. Life Span), wks.: 11.1 9.1 3.9	cancer mix	& Michael Silvert, MD.	
5.3 MAGNETIC Field. NORTH pole slows cancer & extends life. (South pole does opposite.) Stationary magnet.	90% on average	patients animals, small	improvement 50% longer total life	cancer mortality, "normal"	Dr. Albert Roy Davis, U. Fla., many honor. degrees, Director Res. Lab, Green Cove Sp., Fla. Kim in-Su, MD, Carnegie Med.	"Biomagnetics... Disease Control", Newsreal, n.1, p.47, May, 1977. (Many scientific papers, 370 general science courses.)

TREATMENT (Mode, Theory)	BENEFITED, % of total, or #	TREATED, total #	MEASURE of BENEFIT	DISEASE SEVERITY	RESEARCHER, Credentials	REFERENCE, Publication
5.4 TELLURIC Radiation, crossing at GEO-PATHO-GENIC point, promotes cancer (in animals. Prevent) Neutral zone is safe. Controls: Underground crossing of water-veins.	0% on average	25,000 mice, 15 years' study	survival, at 40 days normal coats & behavior	carcinogen inoculated	E.Hartman, MD, Heidelberg U., W.Germany. Blanch Merz, PhD, Internat'l Ctr. Biol. Res., & Inst. Geo-biol. Res., Switz.	Herald of Health, v.84, n.3, p.7, March 1979. (Geo. Crile, Sr., founder, Cleveland Clinic, "Phen. Life: Radio-Elec...", Am. Col. Surg., Cong. 1933)
5.5 LAKHOVSKY. 5.5.1 SOIL's SECONDARY RADIATION & E&M Currents cause cancer. Prevention.	% ca. occur.: .05-.10 .14-.33	sample: French population	incidence of cancer, annual %	soil conductivity: low high	Georges Lakhovsky, Engineer, author of 8 books, paper to French Academy of Science.	The Secret of Life (intro. by Prof. D'Arsonval), Ch.IX,
5.5.2 MULTI WAVE OSCILLATOR. Resonance with cell's DNA-RNA open coiled spirals, & membrane capacitances. Use: a) E&M wave generator (.75-3 billion cps), or b) OPEN SPIRAL (1 turn, metal wire) influencing natural radiation, coiled around patient.	100%	patients: 5	shrinkage of tumor	ca., 3 with metastasis	Prof. S. Attilj, Cong. Radiol., Flor., Italy, May, 1928	", p. 154. (DLaw, A Guide to Alternative Med., p.150)
	100%	4	total remission of tumor	ca., 3 biopsied	7 Drs. (&Andrevont & Shereshevsky, Harvard. Dr.H. Ehrenwald, Vienna Neuro.)	Mark Clement, Waves That Heal, p.32-40.
		300	cure, greatly improved	some ca.& arthritis, anemia, ulcer	Dr. Raul Araujo, Prophyl. Inst., Montev., Uruguay	", p.18 — BSRF, The Lakhovsky MWO; & The Koch Remedy..., III.
		100's			Anonymous, FACS, Urology Brooklyn	", p.54 — Dr. Bruce Copen's books.
5.6 DOTTO RING. Electro-motive Force, induced by thermal differences in metals, act on DNA in cells. Seebeck Effect simulates cosmos. 10 gauss, 1.8M cps modulated at 100K cps, at 45mv, suffices to correct orientation of base pairs in DNA repair; no harm to spin of H bonds.	92%	12 mice, inbred CFW: treated	survival at 21 days with no cancer cells in ascite fluid	cells of sarcoma 37 injected into mice	Giovini A. Dotto, PhD's in Physics, & Mech.E.; Elect. E.; head, Alpha Romeo racing div.; direct descendent of Galileo. Italy.	Bio-Physics Res. Found., Pittsburgh, Pa.
	0%	12 CFW mice, : controls				
	46%	mice, AKR: 13	alive, no ca. trace left	leukemia	Gerald Willis, Prof. Biol. U.Dayton; Robert Zipf, PhD, Coroner, Montgomery Co.; Clayton B. Conover, MD, Sidney; Ohio.	Dotto, personal letter, on June 12, 1973, to Richard Ericson, GE-PS Ca. Mem.
	100%	treated	survived			
5.6.1 PYRO-PIEZO-ELECTRIC Effect.	0%	11, controls	"			
5.7 SHORT WAVE RADIO E&M, 13M cps, longest by FCC for med. Electrodes to skin, tumor in between heats to 46°C+, & is killed. Blood flow (heat transfer) thru tumor is 1-15% of normal. For solid tumor only, not leukemia.	100%	patients: 21 (& 16 later)	destroys tumor, much regression, relieves pain	advanced solid tumors (7 lung carc., 7 head /neck squamous cell carcinoma)	Dr. Harry LeVeen, Chief, Surg. Serv., VA Hosp., SUNY, Brooklyn; So. Carolina Med.; & 3 MD's. Lauded by Dr. M. Parrott, Pres., AMA, as a: "Revolution in...cancer treatment".	"Tumor Eradication by Radio-Frequency Therapy", JAMA, v.235, n.20, p.2198, May 17, 1976.
5.8 Radio Inductive Heat, 27.12M cps heat, & X-ray:	78%	patients: 14	complete disappearance of cancer, 18 mos.	cancer: mycosis fungoides	J.H.Kim & E.W.Hahn, Dept. Rad. Therapy, Mem. Sloan Kettering Ca.Ctr., NY, NY	"Clinical...Localize Hyper-Thermia", Cancer Research, v.39, n.6, p.2258.
only " :	16%	12				
" heat, & " :	86%	22	" , 9 mos.	melanoma		
only " :	26%	19		"		
5.9 E&M emissions, half-wave of human size, onto patient. Cures other dis-eases. (Other wavelengths can be un-safe.)	76%	patients:	cure	joint disease	Thomas Colson, BS, LLB, DO, Editor, J. Electronic Medicine; 28 other doctor's reports in book.	Molecular Radiation, p.145. (E. Raab, Internationaler Radio-longen Kongress, v.II, p.501, Zurich.) (Note: see D.5.9)
	91%	5000	great improve.			
	90%	total	cure	lumbago, acute rheum.		

TREATMENT (Mode, Theory)	BENEFITED, % of total, or #	TREATED, total #	MEASURE of BENEFIT	DISEASE SEVERITY	RESEARCHER, Credentials	REFERENCE, Publication
5.10 E&M waves (9.4 billion cps, modulated by 17 million cps), in magnetic field (1000 gauss), & 17 other E&M radiations.	100%	rats: 24 treated	no trace of ca., many mos.	cancer, T8 uterine, grafted under skin	Antoine PRIORÉ, PhD requirements met, U. Bordeaux. Prof. Robert Courrier, Secretaire Perpétuel, Academie de Science, France. Profs. André Lwoff, Nobel Laureate, & Director, & Marcel Rivière, & Maurice Guérin, all of Inst. for Cancer Research, Villejuif.	David Rorvick, "Do the French Have a Cure for Cancer?", Esquire, v.84, n.1, p.110, July 1975.
	0%	24 controls	survived 1 mo.			
Animal tests repeated, supervised by Courier's aide. (Prevention in animals, cured of ca., by	100%	4 treated (2 hrs./day)	excellent health			(Note: Louis Kervran, Member, NY Acad. Sci., in Biological Transmutations, (lauded by Prof. Tanon, V. Pres., Acad. Med., Paris), shows elements (of matter) changing in living cells (in sealed ampoules). (Ed.: (?) Structure of (sub-) cell concentrates cosmic rays onto a focal atom, changes atom's nucleus; e.g. diffraction).)
rejecting new ca. grafts; immune)	0%	10 controls	survived			
Prevention of other diseases in animals.	100%	mice: treated	survived 12 days	trypanosome (parasite) injected		
Auspices of committee of 10	0%	controls				
science profs., & a General, a	97%	30 treat.	survived		Prof. Raymond Pautrizel, Dept. head, U. Bordeaux. French DGRSI (science agency). World Health Org'n grant. J. Chaban-Delmas, French Premiere.	
Dean, a Prefect, etc.	13%	30 cont.	", few days			
Trypanosomiasis prevented, immunity enhanced.		mice, rats, rabbits: 10's	specific immunity, 2 yrs.			
Prevents lipid rise in blood of rabbits on high cholesterol diet.		rabbits: 6 treated	lipid level: normal	high cholesterol diet		
		6 control	200% increase			
5.11 ELECTRIFY. 100 small shocks each time. 1000 experiments. Cures. (See 2.8.2)	tried, effective	patients	cure	malignant ulcer	John Wesley, Oxford U.; Founder, Methodist Church ...Dr. De Haen.	Wesley, Primitive Remedies, n.266.
5.12 MAGNETIZED sugar FED. Prevents death in animals.	on average	house-flies	86-130 day ILS	mortality	L.K. Komarov, Inst. of General Genetics, USSR.	New York Times News Service.
5.13 Electrically UN-GROUNDED cages. AIR ION effect. Cures cancer in animals. (See 5.2.1)	100%	6 mice	regression, many mos. ILS	ca. cells injected into mice	Tchijewsky, Russia	Fred Soyka, The Ion Effect, p.77.
6.0 AIR						
6.1 NEGATIVE AIR IONS. More oxygen to blood. Prevents ca. in animals.	93%	mice: 30 treated	prevented	lung cancer	American College of Chest Physicians	"Negative Ions", EIS, POB 928, Capitola, CA. (5000 articles on air ions' biol.)
	26%	30 controls				
6.2 FRESH COLD Air. (Siberian, -20 to -50°F, FURS on patients.) Cures other diseases. (°F shifts ratio of gases in air.)	high %	patients: many of army	even weakest recovered	typhoid & typhus	Officers, White Russian Army.	Paul Kourennoff, Secrets of Oriental Physicians, p.104.
6.3 HYPER-BARIC OXYGEN (HBO). 6.3.1 Oxygen added to air, 45 psia (in pressure chamber), 1 hr., 15times. Increases plasma oxygen 20x. If done (hrs.-1wk.) after stroke, cures paralysis & amnesia. Cures other diseases. Pressure affects chemistry.		patients	cures/aids: IQ up, burns heal faster, cosmetic, vision, less bone inflammation	senility, ulcers, gangrene, anemia, CO poison, cardiovascular ills	Dr. Edgar End, Med. College of Wisc. Edwin Levine, MD, Ravenswood Hosp., Chi. Edward L. Carl, ND, HMD, Port of Health, Guadalahara, Mexico.	National Tattler, May 18, 1975. Cancer News J., v.12, n.1, p.7, 1977.

TREATMENT (Mode, Theory)	BENEFITED, % of total, or #	TREATED, total #	MEASURE of BENEFIT	DISEASE SEVERITY	RESEARCHER, Credentials	REFERENCE, Publication
6.3.2 (mixed results; try no rays) HBO(45psig) & cobalt rays:	45%	patients: 50,treated	alive & free of disease	carcinoma of cervix, Stage III,IV	R. J. R. Johnson, MB, DMRT, Manitoba Cancer Treat.& Research Facil., Canada.	"Preliminary... Hyperbaric ...", NCI Monograph n.24, p.83, Nov., 1965 (Feb., 1967).
Only cobalt rays:	20%	50,control				
6.4 High % Oxygen in air & B Vit.	90%		prevents cancer spread	meta-stasis	M. Von Ardenne, Member of Research & Sci. Councils, &(E.)German Acad. Sci. (See 4.1, 10.20.5; A.6.4.1).	"Selective Multiphase Ca. Therapy... Hyper-acidity..."
Only B Vitamins (B-2,3,15, oxygenate):	71%	patients				
Neither:	0%	controls				
6.5 SALINE OXYGEN's osmotic pressure forces oxygen into cancer cells (which thrive on ferments, not oxygen); kills cells & germs. Radio-, chemo-therapy, antibiotics lower saline oxygen level.	100%	12 patients		cancer	Stanley L. Jamison, DVM, ND. (Mallams, MD, Prof., Baylor U. John B. Score ND, Wimborne, England.) (Otto Warburg, Nobel Laureate, 2x; W.Koch, see 18.1.)	Jamison, personal letter, on April 16, 1973, p.3 to R. Ericson, GE-PS Ca. Mem. (WARNING: Choice, v.6, n.3, p.22) (Score, Natural Immunity.)
	Enema (1.5% sea salt, 0.5% hydrogen peroxide, in distilled water) every 3rd day. Eat CRANBERRY, pineapple, VIOLET LEAVES.					
6.6 SMOKING continued precludes cancer cure. Tobacco has: nickel, arsenic, & mercury pesticides; radioactive wastes; sugar; etc.	0%	patients: 1000's	survival, if continue smoking	cancer mix & not stop smoking	Jason Winters, adventurer, Cal.	Winters, Killing Cancer, p.65. NHF Bull., v.26, n.1, p.15, Jan., 1980. William Dufty, Sugar Blues, p.190-9
6.7 FRESH AIR, Nature Cure: Homeo-pathy:	best	patients: 6800 tot., to 1 of 3 treatments	lasting results	dis-ease mix	Karl Saller, MD; Director R. Bosch Hosp., Stuttgart; Prof. & Director, Anthro. Inst., U. Munich, Germany.	Dr. A. Keller, lecture, referred in: Geo. S. Weger, MD, Dietetic Disappointments & Failures, p.33.
Allo-pathy: (More % Oxygen per cooler air.)	less					
7.0 WATER 7.1 DRINKING 7.1.1 FLUORIDATION CAUSES CANCER. Poisons most body enzymes. Causes mongolism, goitre. Worsens tooth decay after an initial delay from childhood. ("Don't drink fluorid. water."-Charles Heyd, MD, President, AMA.)	# of extra ca. deaths /year: 10,000 to 35,000	USA populace	annual excess cancer death due to drinking water: fluoridation	cancer mix	John Yiamouyiannis, PhD, Editor, Chem. Abstracts; Sci. Director, NHF; Exec. Dir. & Co-Founder, NHAC... Dean Burk, co-founder NCI, Head Cyto-chem. Div., co-auther 3 bks. & 100's of papers on ca. (See 1.2.2, 18.4)	"Fluoridation & Cancer", for US House of Reps., Subcom. on Intergov. ..., Sept. 21, 1977; Fluoride, v.10, p.101, 1977; both referred in Cancer Control J., v.5, n.1&2, p.38-42, Win., 1977.
7.1.2 CHLORINATION CAUSES CANCER Chlorine is Vitamin E ANTAGONIST. (To drink/swim: Air Irradiate by uv light, 1500-2000Å; charges water negative, destroys virus, bacteria, larva.) Chloroform in 95% of water EPA tested; Mean: 3 ppb, Max.: 55 ppb. To PURIFY drink: (a.) Reverse Osmosis/Distil (Solar, Sterile), (b.) Boil/Solarize/Aerate, (c.) Add: Friendly Bacteria/Organic Minerals (drops of ocean/fresh water, sea veg., fruit & veg. juice.)	60,000		chlorination			
	63%	3446 ca. deaths in upstate NY	ca. deaths prevented if no chlorination	cancer of digestive & urinary tracts	Dr. Michael Alvanja, Columbia U. School of Public Health; USEPA grant	Environmental Defense Fund, & R. H. Boyle, Malignant Neglect, p.98-9.
	23%		ca. incidence prevented if (100 ppb) chloroform ended	bladder	Dr. Michael Hogan, National Inst. Environ. Health Sci.	" (National Exchange, v.2, n.9, p.12, Apr. 1978.)
	4-6%			colon & rectum	Dr. Kenneth Cantor, NCI.	" (US EPA, Prelim. Asses. of Suspected Carcinogens in Drink. Water, p.12)
	33% to 50%	1000's of ca. deaths in Wisc., Ill., La., N. Carolina	ca. deaths prevented if no chlorination.	digestive tract	Dr. Robert Harris, Council on Environmental Quality, Exec. Office of President of USA.	Chicago Tribune, Oct. 17, 1980 referred in Public Scrutiny, Jan. 1981, p.16. (Samuel Epstein, The Politics of Cancer.)

TREATMENT (Mode, Theory)	BENEFITTED, % of total, or #	TREATED, total #	MEASURE of BENEFIT	DISEASE SEVERITY	RESEARCHER, Credentials	REFERENCE, Publication
7.1.3 CHLORINATION CAUSES ATHEROSCLEROSIS. High chlorin. water:	5%	male chicks: 50	plaque free at 7 months of drinking	atheroma plaque in aorta	Joseph M. Price, MD. (Dr. Herbert Schwartz, Prof. Org. Chem., Cumb. Co. Col., N.J.)	Coronaries, Cholesterol, Chlorine, p.64-70. (Spotlight, Dec. 15, 1980, p.29.)
Controls, drank distilled " :	100%	50				
7.2 OCEAN 7.2.1 HYDROTHERAPY (Ocean, Shower-cold). EXERCISE (10x/day; See 3.) ENCOURAGEMENT. ORGANIC: wheat bread MOLD, honey, fruits (grape, lemon), vegetables (legume).	100%	patients: 100	not lost a single case	cancer	Nathan D. Mininberg, ND, Chernegow Hosp. diploma, Kiev U. Med., student of Father Sebastian Kneipp (Offered to donate his $100,000 facility to ACS)	"Steve Allen Show" (tv), Oct. 26, 1956; Herald of Health, May, 1961; referred in ACS, Med. Affairs Dept., Statement, Aug. 22, 1962.
7.2.2 TRACE ELEMENTS in Sea Water. For deficiencies in any of 92 naturally occurring elements.	100% 1,000's in #	patients	not lost cured	cancer, 90% have 1 of 2 germs	Drs. Kellans & Stovall hospital in Richmond, Va. (1900-48 AD)	Arlin Brown, March of Truth on Cancer, p.56.
7.2.3 SEA WATER drops added to drinking water. Different from Fresh Water in BACTERIA, yielding organic complexed minerals.	100%	mice	prevented cancer	tumor prone strain	Prof. Macginitie, Dept. Biology, Cal. Inst. of Tech., Pasadena.	(Winter, 1946)
8.0 FASTING (See Juice Fasting 9.2) 8.1 HUMAN. No: food. Yes: drink pure water, ENEMAS, bathing, fresh air, sun shine, light exercise,	100% 84%	patients: 5 38	improved or remedied	ca. mix benign tumor	James McEachen, MD, Case Western Med.; Santa Monica, Cal.	Arnold DeVries, Therapeutic Fasting, p.18.
MASSAGE, low stress. Fast's AUTO-LYSIS digests tumor; & frees organs (liver, pancreas) from digestion, for cleansing body.	78% 96%	18	recovered improved	" "	Robert Gross, PhD, DC, Pauling Health Manor, Hyde Park, NY.	" , p.20. (A. Ehret, Mucos-less Diet Healing System)
Water cleanses body of tumor toxins released by auto-lysis, into blood. Fresh air, exercise, & massage: move/excrete toxins.	1,000's in #	patients	auto-lysis, body digests tumor	cancer mix	Dr. Herbert Shelton, supervisor of 30,000 fasts.	"Physiological Rest" & "Auto-lysis", Hygienic System, v.3, ch.5.
BREAK FAST: juicy fruits (orange, grape); if bowels not move, eat cooked starch-less veg. (spinach); NEVER: meat, sugary fruit (date), nor starchy veg. (potato)	1,000's in #	patients	"	"	many	Hannah Allen, Are You A Candidate For Cancer?, p.23
8.2 ANIMALS. Total Life Span Increase of 19 to 37x,	averaged	worms	1,900 to 3,700% ILS		Julian Huxley	Prof. Hilton Hotema, Live Longer, ch.10, p.53.
& 50x. Periodic fasting for longevity. Prevention in animals.		insects, 15 yrs. study	5,000% ILS		Prof. C.M. Child, U. of Chicago, Ill.	H. Shelton, Fasting Can Save Your Life, p.82.
9.0 NUTRITION, GENERAL 9.1 OVERVIEW 9.1.1 Nutrition Therapy reverses CACHEXIA (malnutrition, emaciation). Increases Life Span after detection of cancer, by 10 times.	averaged	patients, USA: treated controls	1,000% ILS; survive: 6 yrs. " : 6 mos.	terminal cancer, cachexia	Dr. Gio Gori, NCI Deputy Director of Cancer Cause & Prevention: Diet, Nutrition, & Cancer	J. Nutritional Academy, v.1, n.2, p.48, Fall, 1978. (E. Cheraskin, MD, et. al., Diet & Disease, p.225, 229.)

TREATMENT (Mode, Theory)	BENEFITTED, % of total, or #	TREATED, total #	MEASURE of BENEFIT	DISEASE SEVERITY	RESEARCHER, Credentials	REFERENCE, Publication
9.1.2 Diet related to 50% of cancer deaths.	50%	patients, USA	diet related	cancer deaths	Dr. Arthur Upton, Director, NCI (National Ca. Inst.)	Choice, v.4, n.6, p.13-4, July, 1978.
9.1.3 Cachexia causes 50% of terminal cancer deaths.	50%		cachexia caused	terminal ca. deaths		Cancer News J., v.14, n.4, p.14, Dec., 1979.
9.1.4 Nutritional, METABOLIC, Alternative Therapy increases % patient survival 10x over Orthodox Therapy controls:	100% 98% 69% 6.4%	patients: 25 87 59 173	survival	pre cancer advanced " terminal " mixed "	Walter Ermer, Exec. Dir., International Health Council, Berea, Oh.	A Program for Prevention and Detection of Pre-Cancer, p.43.
9.2 FRUIT & VEGETABLE, Calf Liver, Juices (FRESH, RAW, ORGANIC, WHOLE). PAPAYA, CARROTS, DARK GREEN LEAFY veg. high in potassium/sodium ratio. Potassium Iodide, Niacin. Peppermint. Coffee ENEMA. JUICE FASTING of 25 lbs. fruit & veg./day. Juicer needs air access, to prevent static electric discharge's ruin of oxidizing enzymes. NO: spices, coffee, tea, chocolate, cola, high protein, aluminum, salt, hair dye.	90% 40-50% 25% all 30% 99%	patients: 100's 10,000 450	remission " (Note: See: A.3.1; C.9.2.1) cure "	cancer: early to intermed. advanced terminal, mostly early hopeless mix	Max GERSON, MD, & daughter Charlotte Straus. Lauded by Dr. Albert Schweitzer as: "one of the most eminent geniuses in the history of medicine". Author, 4 bks. & 51 articles: Exp. Med. Surg., v.7, n.4, p.299, Nov. 1949; Med. Klin., Jan. 29, & Jun. 25, 1954. NY & Germany. Ferdinand Sauerbruch, MD, Nobel Laureate, world's first heart surg. win	Cancer News J., v.12, n.4, p.3, Oct.-Nov., 1977; & v.14, n.4, p.10, Dec., 1979. (Ca. Res. Hearings, US Senate, S.1875, July 1-3, 1946, p.98.) Walter Ermer, "The Truth About the ACS". (Rev. Gastroent., v.12, n.6, p.419, Nov. '45.) George Berkley, PhD, Cancer How To...Help Your Doctor Fight It, p.7, 9. (Gerson, A Cancer Therapy, Results of 50 Cases) " , p.74.
9.3 Confirmation of GERSON (9.2). 9.3.1 IODINE, oxidizer, fights an-aerobic cancer cells.	100%	10	positive response	breast dysplasia	Dr. Bernhard Eskin, Chief, Gyn. Endocrin., Albert Einstein Med., Phila.	(Surg., v.59, n.2, p.278, Feb. 1966. Lancet, April 24, 1976, p.890.)
9.3.2 POTASSIUM 9.3.2.1 Deficiency causes ammonium excretion, body protein breakdown, cachexia. (See 9.1.)	averaged	10, obese	potassium deficiency causes half of rise	rise in ammonium excreta in starvation	D. G. Sapir, Nancy Chambers, J. W. Ryan, MD's, Johns Hopkins & Ft. Howard VA Hosp., Md.	Metabolism, v.25, n.2, p.33, Feb. 1974. (Exp. Med. Surg., v.4, p.69; Blut, v.39, p.398; J. Nuc. Med., v.11, n.7, p.426.)
9.3.2.2 Potassium replaced sodium in all prescriptions. Prevention.	100%	14 yrs. of patients	prevented	cancer	Dr. F. W. Forbes Ross, London, Eng. (1912)	Health Res., Is Ca. Curable?, p.38. (Ross, Ca., It's Genesis....
9.3.3 NIACIN (Vit. B3), oxidizer, prevents 80% of ketosis on fasting too long (like cachexia, see 9.1)	averaged	rats: 12	decreased ketosis by 80%	fasting ketosis	Yu Yan Yeh, St. Jude's Res. Hosp. & U. Tenn. Ctr. Health Sci., Memphis	Life Sciences, v.18, n.1, p.33. (Biochemistry, v.11, n.3, p.393, 1972.)
9.3.4 PEPPERMINT (See 10.1.1, 12.2, 12.2.3.3, 14.) treated: controls:	78% 0%	chick egg embryo: 74 " 26	survival	Herpes Simplex virus injected	Ernest C. Herrmann, & Louis S. Kucera, Mayo Clinic; NIH grant.	"Anti-viral...in... Mint (Labiata)", Proc. Soc. Exp. Biol. Med., v.124, p.874.
9.3.5 ALUMINUM. (In baking powder, synthetic fertilizer, drink water, cookware.) Causes cancer, recurrence in humans, & in animals. Injures kidney, blood cells, spleen, lymph glands, nerves, brain (senile dementia), digestive tract lining.	3 in # averaged	patients mice	Alum. caused ca. to return 4,300% more ca. with Alum.	cured of cancer spontaneous cancer	Dr. Guyon Richards A. L. Tchijivsky (10 MD's as U. Prof.s) S.E. Levick, MD, Yale Med.	Health Research, The Story of Aluminum Poisoning, p.19. Edward M. Averill, Examiner, FTC, 90 page summary, in 1926, of Docket #540.) NEJM, v.303, n.3, p.164, July 17, 1980. (Science, v.208, p.297, 1980; Br. Med. J., 2, p1610, 1978.)

TREATMENT (Mode, Theory)	BENEFITED, % of total, or #	TREATED, total #	MEASURE of BENEFIT	DISEASE SEVERITY	RESEARCHER, Credentials	REFERENCE, Publication
9.3.6 COFFEE, TEA, CHOCOLATE, COLA. Have methyl-xanthine(m-x; i.e. caffeine, theo-bromine, & theo-phylline). Causes benign, fibrocystic breast tumors.	65% / 80% / 4%	patients, women: 20 / 27	tumor gone after 6 mos. of: no m-x & no smoking / controls	benign fibro-cystic breast tumor, menses independent	John Minton, MD, PhD, Dept. Surg., Ohio St. U. Med. Many MD's confirmed.	JAMA, v.244, n.10, p.1078, Sep. 5, 1980. Eden Ranch, v.59, n.41, Oct. 9, 1979. Nutrition Action, v.7, n.8, p.3, Aug. 1980.
9.4 BIO-CHEMICAL INDIVIDUALITY 9.4.1 Wide variations in nutritional needs, intestinal flora, anatomy, physiology, etc., among clinically healthy humans.		humans: 18 male / 15	difference between individuals: 10x / 4x	high intake Vitamin A measured in sera / Vit. C, measured in sera	Roger J. Williams, PhD, discoverer, Vit. B-5; pioneer, folic acid; President, Amer. Chem. Soc.; Member, National Research Council; Prof. Emeritus, U. Texas.	Biochemical Individuality, p.145, p.64. (Nutrition Today, Sep./Oct., 1974, p.4)
9.4.2 Taylored diet, based on URINE-SALIVA test (of pH, sugar, albumin, ammonia, & salt). LEMON Juice, Distilled water, or CRANBERRY. Avoid pork, soap (removes skin's Vit. C). Leuk.: misuse Vit. A.	99.9% / 95% / 100%	patients: 10,000	respond, survive 1 yr. / success	cancer: terminal / breast / leukemia	Carey Reams, PhD, WWII brain injured veteran, cured by Kathryn Kuhlman. Nord Davis, 10 yrs. at IBM. R. L. Preston, D.N., author, sold 500,000 copies.	Salem Kirban, Health Guide for Survival, p.53, 107, p.161, p.121. (Reams, Choose Life or Death. R.L. Preston, Health-ology.) (Note: See: C&D: 9.4.2)
9.5 NO CONCENTRATED VITAMIN/MINERAL SUPPLEMENTS. 9.5.1 ORGANICALLY home grown food. Synthetic (bio-cide, fertilizer) causes cancer, & recurrence.	100%	patients: 5	cured, no sign of ca. in autopsy yrs. later	extensive malignancy biopsied	Donald C. Collins, MD, FIAP, Hollywood, Cal.	"Anti-Malignancy... in Organically Grown Food", Am. J. Procto., v.12, n.1, p.36, Feb. 1961; in Cancer Control J., v.3, n.1-2, p.12, 1975, & p.26, referring to:
9.5.2 Fruits, Vegetables, & Protein Powder (low in tyrosine, phenylalanine, needed by melanoma).	100%	8	stopped, reduced, or cleared, at 9 mos. max.	melanoma (deadly skin ca.)	Dr. Harry Demopoulos, Prof. Pathology, USC, Cal. (Gobind Behari Lal, Science Editor Emeritus, Hearst.)	Lal, "Special Diet for Melanoma Cancer", L.A. Herald Examiner, Oct. 12, 1965.
9.5.3 Fruit, Veg., Nut, & Seed	25 in #		alive 2-5 years	cancer mix	Dr. Alec Burton, DO, DC, ND; Amer. Natural Hyg. S.	Hannah Allen, Are You A Candidate For Cancer?, p.8.
9.5.4 Fruit, Veg., NO Nut/Seed; low protein, high alkaline diet.	77%	13	favorable, fall in # of blast cells in bone marrow	leukemia	Dr. B. Kalikowski	"Low Protein & Purine Free Diet... Leukemia...", Polish Med. J., v.5, n.3, p.558, 1966; in Kulvinskas, Survival..., p.27.
9.5.5 Fruit, Veg.: fresh, organic, whole.	78%	225 in last 4 yrs.	survival	cancer mix	A. H. Grimmer, MD	Cyril Scott, Cancer Prevention Fallacies & Some Re-
9.5.6 " " " " ", & no salt.	100 in #		cure		Anon. female, MD, degrees from 3 British Univ.'s	Assuring Facts, p.11 & 19.
9.5.7 Fresh, 100% Raw, Organic, Whole - Fruit, Veg., Nut, Seed. Ocean Bath, Fresh Air, Sun.	over 5 in # / 99%	patients / 4,000	total remission / recovery	diabetes	Kristine Nolfi, MD, Humlegaarden, Denmark. / 3 MD's & 5 Chemists, USA	My Experience With Living Food, p.14-17.
9.6 VITAMIN C 9.6.1 Fresh Fruit & Veg., Vit. C (2.5 % of food). Prevents in animals, 97% of a "spontaneous" cancer.	97% pre-vented	mice, hairless: 50 & controls	(Note: see A9.6.1) suppression, of lesions/mice, by 35x	skin ca. (squamous, spontaneous)	Art Robinson, BS, Cal. Tech.; PhD & Prof., UCSD; Co-Founder, Linus Pauling Inst. (R. Yonemoto, Dir. Oncol. Surg., City of Hope (ACS), LA, Cal.)	National Health Federation convention, Summer 1979, San Francisco, Cal.

TREATMENT (Mode, Theory)	BENEFITED, % of total, or #	TREATED, total #	MEASURE of BENEFIT	DISEASE SEVERITY	RESEARCHER, Credentials	REFERENCE, Publication
9.6.2 VITAMIN C (Calcium Ascorbate bests Sodium or Acid forms). Stimulates IMMUNITY (6 ways). Surg., Rad'n, & Chemo-therapies lower body supply of Vit. C. Dosage limited by diarrhea; higher dose in "sicker". De-toxifies digestive tract, body (see 18.1). Used up by Stress (see 2.8). Stored in nerves, adrenals (see 16.4). Aids making collagen, prevents bleeding in leukemia (see 17.11; 18.3).	averaged 22% 0.4%	patients: match by age, sex, & primary ca. site – 100 treated matched to 1,000 controls	ILS over matched controls: 400% 700% (later tally) survival, 1 year	advanced cancer, un-treatable	Linus PAULING, Presidential Medal for Merit, National Medal of Science, funding advised by National Ca. Advis. Board. Ewan Cameron, Civil. Consult. Gen. Surgery to Royal Navy, Sr. Consult Surg. at Vale of Leven Hosp. (See 1.1.6 & 1.2.2) (Pauling: Lenin Prize; Gold Medal, Acad. Sci., USSR.)	Proc. National Acad. Sci., v.73, n.10, p.3685, Oct., 1976. (Oncology, v.27, p.181, 1973. Cancer & Vit. C.) Caveat Emptor, v.10, n.10, p.15, Oct., 1980. (Speech, Intern'l Soc. Preventive Oncology, London, July, 1980.) (I. Stone, "Megascorbic Therapy of...Leukemia", Ca. Control J., v.2, n.1, p.1, Jan.-Feb., 1974 (1967).
9.6.3 Vit. C. High dose (min.: 5g/day; ave.: 29g/day): Low dose (max.: 4g/day): (Vit. B-12 in food is not lost if no pernicious anemia.)	51% 7%	patients: 55 44	survival, 100 days	terminal cancer	Drs. P. Morishige & A. Murata, Fukuoka Tarikia Hosp., Japan.	"Prolongation of Survival Times in Terminal Human Cancer by...Ascorbate", J. Intern'l Acad. Preventive Med., v.5, p.47.
9.6.4 Vit. C increases INTERFERON in body (see 17.8). (Prevent acid/base kidney stones by best cat-ion for ascorb. Monitor.)	averaged	mouse L-cell in vitro	interferon up 100-200% with Vit. C, over without	virus attack	B. V. Siegel, MD, Prof. Dept. Path., Div. Immun., U Oregon, Portland J. I. Morton, MD, " , " .	"Vit. C, Interferon, & the Immune Response", Intern'l J. Vit. & Nutr. Res., v.47, p.245, 1977.
9.7 VITAMIN A 9.7.1 Beets (fresh, organic, whole) 9.7.2 Vit. A (300,000iu/day, 6 mos, Vit. C (prevents Vit. A toxicity; Monitor liver.)	95% averaged	patients: 22 218	improvement regressed or stationary	inoperable cancer	A. Ferenczi, Nobel Laureate H. Reinhold	Nutr. Abst. Rev., v.30, p.274, 1960, in Adelle Davis, Let's Get Well, p.298-9: Nutr. Abst. Rev., v.31, p.601, 1961. (Brit. Med. J., v.281, p.957, 1980.)
9.7.3 Vit. A (emulsion) & Radiation: 9.7.3.1 Only Radiation: Vit. A, a 100% ILS over controls.	36% 9%	50 treated 82 controls	survival, 1 year	lung ca. (bronco-genic carcinoma)	Wolfgang Scheef, MD, Med. Director, Janker Clinic (staff of 140), Bonn, W. Germany. Dr. Karl Ransberger, Head, Med. Enzyme Research Inst., Munich. Max Wolf, MD.	The Janker Clinic, p.18-21, by Patrick McGrady, Jr. (of Yale, Paris Inst., Newsweek chief bureau in Moscow, 200 visits on national tv & radio).
9.7.3.2 Vit. A only. (Emulsion, "A-Mulsin", by-passes liver, less toxicity, approx. 1,000,000iu/day, for months. See 10.13, 10.19.)	100%	20	no failures, many total remissions	cancer of head, neck, tongue		
9.7.3.3 Clinic record totals. (Vit. A increases by 100x the anti-cancer effect of BCG, see 17.15)	70%	76,000	partial remission (shrink tumor 50%, 1 mo)	cancer, mostly terminal	Hans Hoefer-Janker, MD, Director, Janker Clinic. (See 11.1)	" & Cancer News J., v.14, n.2, p.30, Feb.-Mar., 1979. (ACS, MAD, "Unproven Methods")
9.7.4 Vit. A: (a) is immune stimulant; (b) is hormone (see 17.10); (c) aids patient's digestion of ca. cells by lysosomal splitting; (d) affects tumor metabolism; (e) raises DNA & Mitosis of ca. cells.	40%	animals	prevented 40% by diet high in Carrots	lung ca.	Dr. Richard Doll, Pres., Brit. Assoc. Ca. Res. (Oxford/Radcliff & Brit. United Provident Assoc.)	Public Scrutiny, April 1981, p.20, (Can. Med. Assoc. J., v.122, n.7, p.757. JNCI, v.54, n.6, p.1489. Science, v.189, n.4206, p.886.)
9.8 HYPER-NUTRITION & Radiation: (See 9.7.3.1 & 14.2) Only Radiation:	97% 63%	27 treated 27 controls	response	cervical cancer	U. Alabama Med. Ctr.	George Berkley, Cancer, How to...Fight It, p.XI.

TREATMENT (Mode, Theory)	BENEFITED, % of total, or #	TREATED, total #	MEASURE of BENEFIT	DISEASE SEVERITY	RESEARCHER, Credentials	REFERENCE, Publication
9.9 <u>VITAMIN E</u> 9.9.1 Vit.E. Oxygenates. Anti-coagulant(see 11.1.3), yet aids healing wounds. Dilates, & aids growth of new, blood vessels(see 5.7). Dissolves plaque. Protects heme in red blood cells. Removes excess scars. Saves an estrogen from oxidation. Not used in high blood pressure, & chronic rheumatic heart. Dose minimum: 600iu/day, 3 months, (all 4) natural tocopherols. Lost from refining & exposure in milling grains, inorganic iron, (see 7.1.2).	38%	patients: 26 women, age 23-40	regression, tremendous improvement	non-cancerous lumpy breast (2-18 x greater cancer risk)	Robert S. London, MD, Asst. Prof. Johns Hopkins Med. Dept. Director Sinai Hosp. Baltimore; & 2 MD's & 2 PhD.'s; ACS grant.	"Vit. E Relieves Most Cystic Breast Disease", <u>JAMA</u>, v.<u>244</u>, n.10, p.1077, Sept. 5, 1980, (report at Endocrine Society mtg.)
	84%		"/ fair responder			
	80%	20 women	moderate/ complete relief of symptoms	(found in 50% of menstral women)	Archie Abrams, MD, Chief of Obstetrics, Boston U. Med.	"Use of Vit. E in Chronic Cystic Mastitis", <u>NEJM</u>, v. <u>272</u>, n.20, p.1080, May 20, 1965. (<u>Breast</u>, v.<u>4</u>, p.19, 1978.)
	significant %'s	180 MD's as patients 20,000 by Shutes 60,000 in world	excellent results	diagnosis by others in 90% of cases: cardio-vasc., diabetes...	Evan & Wilfrid Shute, MD; Evan, genius, entered U. Toronto at age 14, Dipl. Am. Brd. Ob. Gyn., FRCS, 120 articles. 28% of 800 MD's in Toronto.	122 favorable articles (90 not by Shutes up to 1963) referenced in Herbert Bailey, <u>Vit. E...</u>, App.B. (1,000's by 1970 in:) W. Shute, <u>Vit. E...</u>
		patients		thrombo-embolism	Michael DeBakey & Alton Ochsner, world famous heart surgeons	<u>JAMA</u>, v.<u>144</u>, n.10, p.831, Nov 4, 1950.
9.10 REFINED vs. WHOLE; BULK; CARBO-HYDRATES						
9.10.1 WHOLE wheat bread(60x more Vit.B-6 than 80% extraction refined flour. Whole rice cures beri-beri. Vit.B-6 deficiency in cancer patients.)	averaged	80,000 Brit. soldiers	health improved so much	obstructions in abdomen	(Raymond Brown, PhD, Prof.; Carol Potera, MS; D.P.Rose, MD, PhD; Wisc. Clin. Ca. Ctr; Paul Carbone, Dir., (& Acting Clin. Dir., NCI).)	Sylvester Graham, <u>Treatises on Bread & Breadmaking</u>, p. 52-3, & 64-5, publ. 1837. (<u>Am. J. Clin. Nutr.</u>, v.<u>30</u>, p. 1677, Oct. 1977.)
	100%	patients: 100's	difficulty disappeared	costiveness of bowels		
9.10.2 LOW CARBO-HYDRATE fruits & vegetables(NO: grains, potato, carrot, cauliflower).	100's in #		drugs taken 40 yrs. prior are expelled		Prof. Arnold Ehret, Cal. (See 8.1, 9.13.3)	<u>Mucos-less Diet...</u>, p.28.
9.10.3 CRUCIFERS (Cabbage, Brussels Sprouts, Broccoli, Cauliflower) de-toxify carcinogens, via indoles. Prevents 71% of colon cancer.	averaged	patients: 257	hi crucifers prevents 71% of incidence in low crucifers in diet	colon cancer	Dr. Saxon Graham, SUNY, Buffalo. Dr. Wm. Haenszel, Public Health, & Dr. Wm. Loub, U. Ill. Dr. Curtiss Metlin, & Dr. Fred Bock, Roswell Park Mem. Inst. Dr. J. Lyon, U. Utah Med.	("Need to Pursue New Leads ...", <u>JNCI</u>, v.<u>63</u>, n.4, p.879, Oct. 1979.) <u>Organic Consumer Report</u>, v.<u>60</u>, n.23, June 3, 1980. (<u>Ca. Res.</u>, v.<u>35</u>, n.11, part 2, p.3326, Nov. 1975)
9.10.4 NO refined sugar/preservatives (in ice cream & sodas). No intestinal putre-faction. Prevents <u>90%</u> of polio, (& some ca.)	90% less	all of state in 1948-9	incidence prevented	polio	Dr. Benjamin Sandler, Oteens VA Hosp., Asheville NC. (Dr. Otto Meyerhof, Nobel Laureate, U. Penn. Med)	Hannah Allen, <u>Don't Get Stuck</u>, p.82. (See 12.2.3.2; 13.4.6) (Raymond Bernard, PhD, <u>The Revolt Against Chemicals</u>, p.14.)
9.10.5 CHROMIUM, 94% lost in sugar refining from whole cane. Prevention, animals	averaged	rats	doubled lifetime to 2 years	mortality	Dr. Henry Shroeder, Director, Trace Minerals Lab, Dartmouth Med., N.H.	George Berkley, <u>Cancer, How to...</u>, p.79. (Note: See C.9.24.1)

TREATMENT (Mode, Theory)	BENEFITED, % of total, or #	TREATED, total #	MEASURE of BENEFIT	DISEASE SEVERITY	RESEARCHER, Credentials	REFERENCE, Publication
9.11 POTASSIUM MAGNESIUM ASPARTATE (& OROTATE fights cancer).	84%	patients: 7yrs.' study	decreased death rate	cardiac infarct	Hans Nieper, Member: Ger. Ca. Soc.; Ger. Soc. Circulation Res.; AAAS. (See 2.3 & 10.10)	Mineral Transporters, p.49.
Magnesium Orotate; ion carrier across cell membranes.	94%	1.5 " "	success rate	arterio-sclerosis		
9.12 Vit. E, Egg yolk(Vit. B's), red WINE(capillary dilator), CITRUS juice, fruit & veg.(fresh, whole, org.)	42%	patients: 64	cure	cancer, over 2 mos. left	Cornelius Moerman, MD,	A Solution to the Cancer Problem, p.98,
Vegetarian diet rationed to Dutch in WWar II. Prevention.	0.178% 0.125%	pop. of The Hague: 1942 " : 1945	rate drop due to Veg. diet	ca. incidence rate /year	W. Romjin, dept. of Welfare & Health, Netherlands	" , p.39. (Hippocrates, June 15, 1956.)
9.13 FLESH FOODS/WORMS						
9.13.1 No animal flesh for long time. Prevention.	only 4 got ca.	vegetarians, 1000's	over 99% prevented	cancer	John H. Kellog, Physician in Chief, Battle Creek Sanit.	Mathew Bokmiller, The Principal Causes of Cancer, in Blanche Leonard, Check That Chick, p.7, 38. (Eloise Allison, Unveiled Myst.)
9.13.2 Trichina worms possibly cause 80% of disease mortality. (Worms block arteries.) Prevent.	80%	USA population	mimick "cancer, coronary, stroke"	death from worms	Neil Norton, MD.	
9.13.3 Worms & ENCRUSTED FECES, decades old, 5-10 lbs. average, 60 lbs. max. Prevention.	60%	patients: 1,000's	removed by fasting, found at autopsy	worms & old feces	Prof. A. Ehret(see 8.1; 9.10.2) Dr. Norman Walker Eloise Allison, ND, BA.	Robert L. Preston, Healthology..., p.133, ref. Ehret, Mucusless, p.35.
9.14 SPROUT (Wheat, Mung, Lentil) extract has approx. 50x Vit. B-17 of seed. Prevention.	99%	liver cells, in vitro	sprouts prevent mutation	Ames test, known carcinogen	Charles R. Shaw, MD, Prof. Biol., U. Texas Cancer Ctr., Houston; & 2 PhD's.	The Soil & Health News, v.8, n.6, p.6, May 1979. (V. Kulvinskas, Nutr. Eval. Sprouts, p.30)
10.0 NUTRITION, LAETRILE						
10.1 Laetrile, Amygdalin, Vit. B-17, contains cyanide(like Vit. B-12, cyano-cobal-amine). Preferred release at tumor, because more beta-glucosidase (releases cyanide), & less rhodanase (neutralizes cyanide) there, than in normal cells. (APRICOT etc. SEED, sprout, GRASS, BEAN, BERRY, MILLET.)	15%	treated (Laetrile)	survival, 5 years (large #'s of patients)	cancer: advanced, terminal	Ernst T. KREBS Sr. & Jr. co-discoverors of Vit. B-17 & B-15. Jr.: BS Bact., U. Ill.; grad. study at Hahnemann Med., U. Cal. U. Miss.; many Honorary PhD's; Sci. Director, John Beard Mem. Found. Sr.: MD, grad. Pharm., RE-DISCOVERED ANTI-BIOTICS in US on 1918.	G. Edward Griffin, World Without Cancer, p.233; J. Applied Nutrition, v.22, n.3&4, p.74, 1970. (For Vit. B-15: Acad. of Sci.; & Sci. Advis. Comm.; USSR.) (J. Beard, "Embryo....Carcinoma", Lancet, June 21, 1902.)
	0.1%	controls (Orthodox Therapy)				
	80%	treated		moderate		
	28%	controls				
	100%	treated		presently healthy		
	81%	controls				
10.1.1 Anti-Biotic: root of Leptotaenia Dissecta used by Washoe Indians. Kills Pr-8 flu virus in egg embryo, 100's of microbes. Cure of other diseases. (See 12.2)	100%	patients: 100's	survival	influenza of 1918 in USA, millions killed	(Carlson & Douglass, Western Reserve U., Cleveland. Others at U. Utah School of Med. Dan. E. Johnson, PhD, UCLA; USC)	" , p.99; ref. to Carlson & Douglass, J. Bacteriol., v.55, n.5, p.615, May 1948; & Antibiotics & Chemotherapy, v.3, n.4, p.393, April 1953.
10.2 Laetrile, only. More effective in cancer of lung, pancreas, prostate, stomach, lymphomas.	4%	1000's	remission: total	cancer: advanced, terminal	Ernesto Contreras, MD, post-doc. at Harvard, Chief Path. & Prof. Histology at Mexican Army Hosp. & Med. School. & 30 MD's.	Cancer Control J., v.4, n.3/4, p.27, May-Aug., 1976. (Gary Null, Ca. News J., v.14, n.4, p.15, Dec. 1979.) (Anti ca. use, 2800BC China, in: Ralph Moss, Ca. Syndrome, p.105.)
	40%		" : partial, 25% smaller			
Less effect in ca. of ovary, lung (spread to liver). Inject intravenously, approx. 10g/day.	66%		subjective improvement			
("Amygatrile" brand.) (See A.10.13)	3 in #		survival, 5yrs	lung (oat cell)		

TREATMENT (Mode, Theory)	BENEFITED, % of total, or #	TREATED, total #	MEASURE of BENEFIT	DISEASE SEVERITY	RESEARCHER, Credentials	REFERENCE, Publication
10.3 Laetrile & DE-TOXIFICATION & METABOLIC. Vitamins, Minerals, Enzymes, Enemas. (See 8. & 9.)	67%	patients: 5,000	positive response (50% recurrence)	cancer:	Contreras (see 10.2). (1,000 physicians using Laetrile) (See C.10.2.1)	Michael Culbert, Freedom From Cancer, p.119.
10.4 "	90%	89	controlled/ reversed	terminal	Maurice Kowan, MD, U. Cal. Irvine Med.	"The National Health Fed., Do We Need It?" II, NHF.
10.5 " & Vit. E & B-15. INJECT INTO TUMOR: enzymes & B-17. (Little Orthodox Therapy prior.)	60 to 75%	50	alive & well 6-7 years	terminal, ¼-1 years left	John Richardson, MD, U. Rochester Med.; Fellow, Kaiser Hosp.; & Pat Griffin, RN	Richardson Newsletter, v.1, n.7, p.3, 1979. (Laetrile Case Histories.) (See A.10.5)
10.6 Laetrile & PANCREATIC/PROTEOLYTIC ENZYMES (Enzymes digest cancer cell surface, so immunity can attack cell; need maintenance dose.) & Vit. B-15 (Pangamic Acid, Oxygenates, aids Blood Circulation, see 5.7)	15% 85% 90% 96%	324 many 1,000	remission: permanent temporary recovery survival, up to 10 years	mix hopeless mix	Howard H. Beard, Sc.D., PhD, Yale; Prof. Biochem./Med. at: Western Res. & Louisianna St. & Chicago Med.; Biochemist at 3 institutes; author of 150 articles & 3 books.	Cancer News J., 1976 Bicent., p.21. (Enzymologia ACTA Biocatalyta, XVIII, 31-7, 1957, Fasc. 5, p.293.) New Approach..., ch.2, p.16. Arlin Brown, March of Truth on Cancer, p.56.
10.7 " & FRESH, ORGANIC, WHOLE CASSAVA (high in Vit. B-17); chiesa SEED; TROPICAL PLANTS.	60 to 70%	2,000	positive response	terminal, mostly	Manuel Navarro, MD, FPCP, Prof. Biochem., Faculty of Med., U. Santo Tomas; Member, 10 med. groups; author 130 articles; Philippines	Choice, v.6, n.1, p.20, Spring 1980. (Note: See D.10.6.3) (2 Monographs by Dr. Navarro.)
10.8 "	all	6,000	relieved	mix	Dr. Goenawan, Indonesia.	Dore Deverell, How I Healed My Cancer Holistically, p.23.
10.9 "	average 38%	501 175	shrink tumor "/gain body wt., progress	breast carcinoma	Dr. Simandjuntak, Cisarua Health Resort, Bogor, Indonesia.	Richardson, Laetrile Case Histories, p.30.
10.10 Laetrile & De-toxification & Metabolic. (As co-developer of cyclo-phosphamide & cobalt-60 for ca. therapy, Nieper says Laerile is superior, especially for CML leukemia.)	almost all some 100%	70 3	general improvement regression ", shrink spleen -70%	some histol. confirmed metastasis leukemia (CML)	Hans Nieper, MD, Head, Aschaffenburg Hosp. Lab. Dir. Med., Silbersee Hosp., Hanover, Germany. In Who's Who in World Sci. (See 2.3, 9.11, C.9.23.4)	Cancer News J., v.6, n.1-4, p.19, Jan.-Apr. 1971.
10.11 BENZ-ALDEHYDE, from FIGS - Bible, II Kings, Ch.20, V.1-7. Part of Laetrile molecule, harmless; regresses squamous cell & adeno-carcinoma. Studies at 5 hosp. Prevention in animals. (For Laetrile: Prof. Joseph Maisin, Director, Inst. Cancer, U. Louvain; President, IUAC, see 18.1; A. McNaughton is son of: Commander of Canadian Armed Forces in WWar II, Pres. UN Security Council, National Research Council of Canada, see 10.13)	50% 5% 100% 74%	200 83 mice, breed: 25 treated 25 control	positive response complete recovery prevention, cancer free	terminal, most mix papilloma, (caused by NQO)	Matsuyuki Kochi, MD, Tokyo U.; Inst. Infectious Dis.; Ichijo-Kai Hosp.; Kochi Tumor Ctr.; Prof. Bact., Yokohama Med. Dr. Heiichi Yano. Speech, Jap. Ca. Assoc., 38-th. Ann. Mtg., 1979 Proceed.	Choice, v.5, n.3, p.8, May-June 1979, (& v.6, n.1, p.22, Spring, 1980. Intern'l Union Against Cancer (IUAC) 12th Int'l Ca. Congress, Buenos Aires, 1978. NCI, Cancer Treatment Reports)
	30%	patients: 100	recovery	lung, myel., leuk., lymph.	Dr. Kenji Sakaguchi, Jap. (Dr. Andrew A. Benson, Scripps Inst., La Jolla, Cal.)	Choice, v.5, n.1, p.10, Feb. 1979.

TREATMENT (Mode, Theory)	BENEFITED, % of total, or #	TREATED, total #	MEASURE of BENEFIT	DISEASE SEVERITY	RESEARCHER, Credentials	REFERENCE, Publication
10.12 LAETRILE & VIT. A (emulsion) & ENZYMES (Wobe-Mogus, from: LENTIL,	82%	patients: 227	survival, 2 years	cancer: terminal (97% given 3-6 mos. to live)	Marco Brown, MD, Ditmar Schildwaechter, MD, Dr. Flynn, Dr. Wedel, of Fairfield Medical Ctr., Montego Bay, Jamaica.	Cancer News J., v. 13, n. 4, p. 17, Oct.-Nov. 1978.
PEA, calf Thymus, beef Pancreas, Papayotin, Mannitol; see 11.).	54%		remission: partial			
TROPICAL Vegetarian diet, ozone,	17%		complete			
fresh air, SCENIC RESORT, mind-	85%		improve			Choice, v. 6, n. 3, p. 21, Fall 1980.
body, Cellular Therapy (see 16.1),	78%		well; over 1 yr.			
Chelation (see 10.14).	52%		" , " 5 "			
10.13 Laetrile, Vit. A, C, Enzymes.	55%	180	response	diagnosed ca.	Dr. Mario Soto, 20th de Nov. Hosp.; Med. Dir., Clinica Cydel, Tijuana, Mexico.	M. Culbert, Freedom From Ca. p. 123. Moss, Ca. Syndrome, p. 142.
(McNaughton: on Court of Royal	46%		ca. shrink 40%			
Soc. Med.; Board of Inst. Nutr. Res.; Chief Test Pilot, RCAF; see 10.11.)	30 to 50%	1,000 (approx.)	regress & stabilize	terminal, mostly	Andrew R.L. McNaughton, Canada	Gary Null, "Alternative Cancer Therapies", in Cancer News J., v. 14, n. 4, p. 15, Dec. 1979; p. 12;
10.14 Laetrile, Vit. A, C, Enzymes, Herbs, Vegeterian diet, Minerals;	50%	6,500 total	success	ca.: no Orthodox Therapy prior Ortho. Therapy	Ray Evers, MD, Vanderbilt U.; BS Biochem. & Biol., Auburn U.; awards from many internat'l nutr./metab. groups; Knight, Order of Malta.	
CHELATION ((EDTA) removes heavy metals from body, but also good	25 to 40%					
minerals (zinc), replenished by nutrition). Slow chelation pre-	35%	400	remission, complete	terminal, mostly		Choice, v. 5, n. 3, p. 12-3, May-June, 1979.
vents fatally overloading kidneys. Therapy of other diseases.	75%	10,000	recovery, complete	cardio-vascular		
10.15 Laetrile, Vit., Min., Enzymes, Vegetarian.	68%	2,000 less terminal	positive results	ca., non-terminal	Robert Gibson, MD, U. Okla. Med., Ponca City, Ok.	", p. 12;
10.16 " & Chelation.	25%		recovery	terminal	Glen Green, MD, Prince Albert, Saskatch., Canada	", p. 13;
10.17 " " .	30%	600 total, ca. mix	regression	lung	Jack Slingluff, MD, Canton, Ohio	", p. 13;
	90%		improve	cachexia & malnutrition		
10.18 " & Heat (see 4.5)	54%		remission	terminal, 80% of patients	B. Briggs, MD; Art Davis, MD; Don Cole, MD; Amer. Internat'l Hosp., Zion, Ill.; Dr. H. Manner	", p. 16. (See 10.19)
" & Attitude (see 2.) Intensive 21 day program. (Mendelsohn, Assoc. Prof., U. Ill. Med.; Chair., Ill. Med. License Comm.)	80 to 90%	patients in 1 yr. of practice	success (med., energy, vitality, lab test)	ca. mix	Brian E. Briggs, MD; Dr. Ann Clague; (Advis. Brd.: Robert Mendelsohn, MD, U. Chicago Med.; Dr. Lendon Smith.)	Choice, v. 6, n. 3, p. 16, Fall 1980. (Mendelsohn, Confessions of a Medical Heretic. L. Smith, Feed Your Kids Right.)
10.19 Laetrile & Vit. A & Enzymes.		patients:				
10.19.1 COMBINATION (of all 3) is a SYNERGY (multiplicative) aid.	68%	145 total	improve	ca. mix	Harold Manner, MA & PhD, Northwestern U.; Chair., Dept. Biol., Loyola U., Chi.; author 50 sci. articles & 5 textbooks; grants/scolarships, Arthritis & Rheum. Found., NIH, NSF, etc. 160 MD's, Metab. Res. Found.	Manner, "Metabolic Therapy Statistics" (unpublished); (The Death of Cancer)
	69%	16		lung ca.		
	80%	10		brain ca.		
	170 in #	women	lumps gone	breast, biopsy		Ca. News J., v. 14, n. 1, p. 9, Jan. 1979.
10.19.2 Cure in animals (to end of 10.)						
10.19.2.1 Laetrile & Vit. A & Enzymes. (Laetrile injected into muscle,	89%	mice, C3H strain:	regression: complete	spontaneous mammary tumor		NHF Bull., v. 23, n. 10, p. 1, Nov. 1977.
for blood vessels too small.)	100%	84	partial			Manner, "Laetrile Therapy, a New Approach" (unpublished).

TREATMENT (Mode, Theory)	BENEFITED, % of total, or #	TREATED, total #	MEASURE of BENEFIT	DISEASE SEVERITY	RESEARCHER, Credentials	REFERENCE, Publication
10.19.2.2 Laetrile & Vit.A & Enzymes (all 3): Enzymes alone or with either Laetrile or Vit.A, but not both: Laetrile or Vit.A alone; or controls:	76% 52-54% 0-4%	mice, C3H/HeJ strain: 550 total, 11 groups	total regression at 30 days	spontaneous mammary tumors, larger	Dr. Harold Manner (Continued).	"Amygdalin...Regression of...Adeno-carcinoma", J. Manipulative & Physiol. Therapy, v.1, n.4, p.246, Dec. 1978.
10.19.2.3 (All 3,) Laetrile & Vit.A & Enzymes: Laetrile & Enz.(only 2:) Vit.A & Enz.(only 2:) Laetrile or Vit.A or Enz.(only 1:)	averaged	mice, BDF1 strain: 100	ILS over controls: 100% 45% 30% 10-20%	lung ca. cells (L1210), injected in newborn mice	Mark Paulik, student, Marquette High School, Michigan City, Ind.	Public Scrutiny, v.3, n.6, p.6, June 1980. (Manner, "The Non-Toxicity of Amygdalin...", Science of Biology J., v.3, p.347, May-June 1977.)
10.20 Laetrile (Alone)						
10.20.1 Laetrile, treated: Controls:		rats: 200 200	80%	cancer	Bioresearch Labs Ltd., Canada	Cancer News J., v.6, n.1-4, p.19, Jan.-Apr. 1971.
10.20.2 Laetrile, treated: Controls:		200 200	80%	Walker 256 carcinoma	Scind Lab., UCSF, Calif.	Wynn Westover, See the Patients Die or Let the Patients Live, p.25-6, 1974.
10.20.3 Laetrile, treated:	majority	mice, BDF strain: 280	++%	Lewis lung ca.	Southern Research Inst., Birmingham, Alab.	
10.20.4 Laetrile, treated: Controls:	averaged	mice: 20 20	100%	human ca. into mice	Dr. T. Metiano, Pasteur Inst. & Ministry Agr., Paris	Ralph Moss, The Cancer Syndrome, p.114.
10.20.5 Laetrile (Note: Von Ardenne is: Member, Acad. of Science, & of both Research & Science Councils, & Pres., Soc. Biomed. Tech., E. Germany)	33% 66% 34%	rats: 6 treated, 5 controls	total regression " or inhibition no effect	DS-carcinosarcoma (very lethal)	M. Von Ardenne, pioneer of TV, Electron Micr., multi-step cancer therapy, blood-nerve barrier, (see 4.1. & 6.4) & P.G. Reitnauer	"Tumor Regression Thru... Amygdalin Infusion & Intra-Tumoral...Beta-Glucosidase", Cancer Control J., v.2, n.5, p.9, 1974.
10.20.6 Laetrile (Testing model is not responsive to Orthodox Chemotherapy. Use Laetrile longer.)	averaged	mice: 30 30	ILS over controls: 41% 44%	Lewis lung cancer cells injected sub-cutaneously	NCI & Southern Research Inst. (SRI). (Statistics by Dr. W. Edward Deming, USA, top Japanese Deming Award for 25 years.)	Dean Burk (see 7.1.1, & 18.4), Cancer Control J., v.1, n.3, p.6, Sep. 1973. (Walter Ermer, IHC News Release # 61, on SRI Test # 34 & 4.)
10.20.7 Laetrile 10.20.7.1 " (ABSCISSIC ACID, a Vit. A; & anti-cancer GROWTH REGULATOR; as Dormans in seeds; is lost in refining out Laetrile.)	40% 60%	mice: Swiss Webster: 5	regression: total " or partial	mammary tumors, small	Dr. Kanematsu Sugiura, Crocker Lab., Columbia U.; Sloan-Kettering Inst. (SKI), NY; author, 200 cancer articles; Order of Sacred Treasure, Japan; NYAS; (see C.12.1.5.2).	"A Summary...Amygdalin Upon Spontaneous Mammary Tumors in Mice", SKI report at Baden Baden, Germany, June 13, 1973, in Griffin, World W/O Ca., p.62.
10.20.7.2 Laetrile gave "70% total inhibition of such metastases"	82% 22%	treated: 23 control: 23	prevent metastasis	"		M. Culbert, Freedom From Cancer, p.39-42.
10.20.7.3 Laetrile "anti-tumor effect significant at the .04 level of probability".	69% 0% averaged	treated control mice	" " to lung ILS: 50%	"	" & Franz A. Schmid, DVM; SKI.	" . (Science, v.198, p.1231, Dec. 23, 1977.) Cancer Control J., v.4, n.3/4, p.29, May-Aug. 1976.
10.20.8 Laetrile & PINEAPPLE Enzymes (Bromelain). 20 positive Laetrile experiments total by SKI. Laetrile & Enzymes.	50% 100%	animals mice: few	total tumor regression cure	cancer	Dr. Lloyd Schloen & Dr. Elizabeth Stockert, SKI, NY.	Gary Null & Robert Houston, "The Cancer Fraud", Penthouse, Sept. 1979, p.278. Moss, Ca. Syndrome, p.139, 149.

TREATMENT (Mode, Theory)	BENEFITED, % of total, or #	TREATED, total #	MEASURE of BENEFIT	DISEASE SEVERITY	RESEARCHER, Credentials	REFERENCE, Publication
11.0 NUTRITION, ENZYMES 11.1 Enzymes("Wobe-Mogus") INJECTED 11.1.1 IN TUMOR (see 10.6 & 10.12; & other parts of diet, see 9. thru 16.)	40%	patients	positive regression	tumors	H. Hoefer-Janker. (See 9.7.3) K. Ransberger. W. Scheef (son of Anton Scheef, Founder, Catholic Mission Inst., China). Max Wolfe, MD, re-discoveror of enzyme therapy.	"The Importance of Vit. A & Proteo-lytic Enzymes in Ca. Therapy", Mtg., Bayerische Rontgen Gesell., Apr. 4, '71.
11.1.2 " & Vit. A (A-Mulsin). Enzymes are FIBRINO-LYTIC, ANTI-COAGULANT; dissolve micro-throm-	50%		cancer disappeared	ca.: abdomen lining, chest cavity		National Enquirer, June 12, 1973. (Ärztl. Praxis, v.21, n.93, 1969; v.23, p.(1221 & 2805), 1971.)
11.1.3 Enzymes. bi of cancer cells covered by fibrin; prevent spread of meta-stasis thru blood.	70% 5%	rats: treated: 120 control: 120	survival	Yoshida sarcoma cell, inoculate		"Proteo-lytic Enzymes... in Ca. Therapy", Mexican Ca. Cong., Mex. City, Sept. 30, 1971, p.4.
11.1.4 " Enzymes lower fatality from cancer by 87.5%	0.2%	patients: treated: 540	fatality, 1/8 x % in controls'	ca. mix	L. Michaels, MD, PhD, MRCP, FRCP; Manitoba Clin.; Winn. Gen. Hosp.	"Effects of Proteol. Enzymes ... Upon Growth of Tumor... Metastatic", Med. Enzym. e.v. Munich; 10th Int'l Ca. Cong., 1970, Houston; Lancet, n.7364, p.832, Oct. 17, 1964.
11.1.5 " . Enzymes lower recurrence rt. of primary tumor by ½. i.e. 100%-91% = ½(100%-82%)	91% 82%	treated: 2278 control	free of primary tumor return	fem. genital ca., Stage II, III	H. Ludwig	
11.1.6 ENZYMES INJECTED INTO META-STASIS of chest cavity, stops their oozing.	47% 19%	treated: 119 control: 236	effusion (oozing) all gone	exudative pleural carcinosis	R. Titscher, O. Kokron, K. Letnansky, Cancer Res. Inst., U. Vienna.	"To the Local Therapy...", Wiener klin. Wockenschrift, v.85, n.18, p.338, 1973.
11.2 Pineapple, BROMELAIN: Anti-Coagulant; prevents anti-immunity & raises tissue permeability (see 10.20).	60% 0%	mice, hairless strain: treated: 20 control: 20	free of skin cancer	ultra-violet radiation	Dr. Steven J. Taussig, Lab. Director, Dole Co. Norman Goldstein, MD, Kuakini Research Ctr.; Honolulu	German Society for Tumor Therapy, Baden-Baden.
11.3 MULTIPLE Proteo-lytic Enzyme Therapy. CHYMO-TRYPSIN alone, then with TRYPSIN, (DE(S)-OXY)/RIBO-NUCLE-ASE, PEPSIN-OGEN injected intra-venously, LIP-ASE, AMYL-ASE orally. Tumors/Meta-stasis gone in 3 days, but returned (because patient not detoxified). (Trypsin removes altered antigens from cancer cell surface. Lipase, (deoxy)/ribonuclease inhibit cancer. Proteolytics penetrate inflamation, & normalize.)	averaged most 12 in #	patients: 193 (in hospital over 10 years)	liquefying ca. tissue at will; tumor gone increase # of white blood cells alive	far advanced cancer, proof by pathology should have passed on	Frank Shively Sr., MD, Northwestern U. Med.; Cert. of Distinction, both Miami Valley Hosp. & Ohio St. Med. Assoc.; on Board of Directors, Red Cross; Pres., Dayton Brd. of Ed.; therapy under Miami Val. Hosp. Brd.; 28 MD's refer patients to Shively. (Miles H. Robinson, MD, Prof. Physiol. & Pharm., Vanderbilt & U. Penn. Med; (see 17.2.))	U.S. Senator Edward Long, "Is the FDA Hamstringing Cancer Research", Congressional Record, v.112, Part 19, p.25187, Oct. 5, 1966. Shively, Multiple Enzyme Therapy. John Beard, DSc, The Enzyme Treatment of Ca., 1911. (Dr. Franz Bergel, (Dean, Chester Beatty Cancer Res. Inst., Royal Ca. Hosp.; Prof. Chem., U. London,) Chem. of Enzymes in Ca.) Brown, March of Truth on Cancer, p.94.
11.4 Chymo-trypsin	many	patients: 40	tumor melts, smaller/gone	advanced cancer	Dr. C. J. Michet, Med. Dir., Ca. Res., Holy Cross Hosp., Chi.	", p.99. Sen. Long, Cong. Rec., v.112, part 20, p.26913, Oct. 14, 1966.
11.5 Pancreatic Enzymes, HCl. TIMED DAILY INTAKE; NEURO-STIMULATE pancreas. No hi/animal protein. Eat ALMOND; CARROT & CELERY juice fast; lemon. RINSE NOSE.	99.5% 20%	3,000 20,000 tot.	alive, if early diagnosis recover	cancer mix ca., 1 month left	Wm. Donald Kelley, DDS, BA, BS, Baylor U.; post grad., Wash. U., U. Alab., U. W. Va.; Fellow, Royal Soc. Health; Council Nutr. Res.	One Answer to Cancer, p.62-3. (Note: See C.11.5.1) Public Scrutiny, Mar. 1981, p.24.

TREATMENT (Mode, Theory)	BENEFITED, % of total, or #	TREATED, total #	MEASURE of BENEFIT	DISEASE SEVERITY	RESEARCHER, Credentials	REFERENCE, Publication
11.6 BEE: HONEY(enzymes), POLLEN (rare minerals), ROYAL JELLY(vit. B5), PROPOULIS(tumor healer). 11.6.1 BEEKEEPERS;200x less ca. death.	0.1% 20–25%	1,000 beekeepers controls	prevention of cancer mortality	% from ca., of all deaths	Alin Caillas, Grand Medal of Gold, French Acad. of Agr.; Knight, Legion of Honor.	George Berkley, Cancer, How to...Fight It, p.98–103 & 213.
11.6.2 " ;more common among centenarians;(ca. immune from sting?)	hi % bee keepers	150 Russians	lived over 100 years		Prof. Nicolai Tsitsin, Russia.	" ref. The Bee J., Apr. 1946.
11.6.3 Pollen prevents inflammation from radiation therapy, raises Vit. E & red cell count in blood by 36 & 4%; radiation alone lowers same by 43 & 12%.		patients: 15, pollen & rad. controls: 10, only radiate	prevent inflammation of bladder by ½, & rectum by 2/3.	advanced, inoperable cancer of cervix	Peter Hernuss, MD, & 6 MD's, U. Vienna.	" ref. Strahlentherapie, v.150, n.5, 1975.
11.6.4 Pollen prevents cancer.		animals	inhibited	breast ca.	U.S. Dept. Agriculture.	" ref. Let's Live, Jan. 1977.
11.6.5 Honey			antiseptic	ulcers, burns	Robert Blomfeld, MD.	" ref. JAMA Letters, May 7, 1973.
12.0 NUTRITION, ANTI-BIOTIC, ANTI-VIRAL 12.1 CULTURES 12.1.1 YOGURT	18 in #	patients	cure	cancer	I. Bogdanov & P. Prophriotov, Lecture at Interna'l Symp. of Anti-Cancer Anti-Biotics (Oct. '58, Moscow) & Cong. of Anti-Biotics (May '59 Prague), of Bulgaria. J. Gordon Roberts, developer of Vit. D (from cod liver oil) added to milk, to rid rickets. (Elie Metchnikoff, von Baer Prize; Prof.: U. Odessa, U. St. Petersburg, Pasteur Inst.; Nobel Laureate; 6 of his books translated in Eng.	Inside book cover in:... "The Anti Cancer Action of Antibioticum Bulgaricum on Crocker Sarcoma" in Roberts, Cancer, How...It May Be Wiped Out, p. 253-7. (Note: See C.12.1.1.1) (Metchnikoff, Revue Scientifique, v.2, p.103, 1904; & Scientifically Soured Milk ...Arresting Intestinal Putrefaction.)
12.1.1.1 Strain: Lacto-bacterium Bulgarium-51, anaerobically cultivated on sterilized, water extract of soybean. Injected intra-peritone-ally, 1cc. daily). Causes tumor to shrink, be softer, change color (pink to black), dry, fall off, replaced by healed tissue. Internal tumors & meta-stasis reorganized by connective tissue. Yogurt has B Vitamins, (esp. B-2, -6, -12); (see 9.3.3, 9.10.1, & 10.6.). Vit. B-6 balances Na/K (see 9.3.2.)	30% 64% 0% 100%	mice, white: treated: 455 control: 119 104	complete recovery, no meta-stasis for 220 days " &/or tumor dissolves so quick, fatally poisons. survival (none by 45 days) immunity, no new tumor	Crocker Sarcoma 180 implanted (histo-logically proven) " re-implant after 1st ca. cured		
12.1.1.2 Yogurt in drinking water. Prevention in animals. (For humans, also in enema, poultice, douche.)	28%	mice	inhibits ca. cell proliferation	infected with cancer cells	U. Nebraska (Calvary Hosp., Bronx)	JNCI ref. in Cancer Control J., v.1, n.4, p.20, Nov. 1973; ref. JAMA Letters, Dec. 8, 1969.
12.1.1.3 Lacto-Bacillus extract. (Anti-biotics can also kill friendly gut flora: Vit. B loss.)	50%	mice	prevented, & immune in future	cancer	3 MD's in New York	G. Berkley, Cancer, How To...Fight It, p.92, ref. to J. Amer. Geriatric Soc.
12.1.2 LACTIC ACID FERMENTED: milk, wheat, maize, mistletoe (see 14.2). Solution (¼ – 3%), externally & orally. Mold makes Vitamins (CHOLINE for liver), hormones, enzymes, CELL ACTIVATORS & REGULATORS, ANTI-BIOTICS. Inhibits fermention of tumor. Pre-digests unhealthy items in food.	1,000 in # over 15 in #	patients	successful tumor gone, normal	cancer mix mostly terminal	Johannes Kuhl, MD, PhD, Prof., Nuclear Res. Inst., Rome. (W. Zabel, MD, Prof.)	E. L. David, FISPh, An Experiment in Treating Cancer With Lactic Acid. (Kuhl, Fantasy & Truth in the Cancer Sphere.)

TREATMENT (Mode, Theory)	BENEFITED, % of total, or #	TREATED, total #	MEASURE of BENEFIT	DISEASE SEVERITY	RESEARCHER, Credentials	REFERENCE, Publication
12.1.3 Mucorhicin: liquid exudate of MOLD grown on whole wheat, yeast, & distilled water; treats 70 diseases. (See 7.2.1)	90%	patients: 3,000	subjective improvement before death		Lilian Lazenby & Phil Drosness. Paul A. Murray, MD, top med. stud., U. Pittsburgh.	N. Morris, Ca. Blackout, p.119. (Congressional Record, v. 99, part 12, p.A-5352, Aug. 3, 1953.)
	80%	2,000	pain relief	terminal ca.	Joseph Wilson, MD	A. Brown, March of Truth..., p.94.
12.1.4 Whole wheat/growth medium of bacteria, but not bacteria itself (Aerobacter, from fermented dried egg-white.) Trace organic chem. made by a species affects other species via culture medium.	90%	mice, random bred; (inbred unaffected by diet). treated	survival	typhoid salmonella injected; non-virulent before virulent by 1-2 days.	Howard Schneider, Rockefeller Inst., & Inst. for Biomed. Research of AMA & NIH.	"Ecological Ectocrines in Experimental Epidemiology", Science, v.158, p.597, Nov. 3, 1967. (C.E. Lucas, Biol. Rev. Cambridge Phil. Soc., v.22, p. 270, 1947.)
Semi-synthetic diet:	10%	controls				
12.1.5 YEAST (uni-cell fungi; see 12.2; A.12.2) 12.1.5.1 Yeasts cure many diseases. Rich in Vit. B-2, B-3, Selenium (oxidizers); & Vit. B-12, & Chromium.					Egyptian physicians. (Also treated with: beer (un-refined), soil (fungi), excretions (urine; see 16.8; 16.9; 17.10), etc.)	Papyrus Eberrs, circa. 3000-1500 BC
12.1.5.2 BREWER'S Yeast (SACCHROMYCES CERVISIAE): injected into tumor.	averaged	mice	ILS over controls: 30%	adeno-carcinoma	W. Joechle, Schering AG, Berlin	Cancer News J., v.10, n.5, p. 14, 1975.
12.1.5.3 " :in drinking water.		cats	2-3 months	tumors	Dr. Triebel, Clinic for Tumorous Disease, Municipal Hosp., Braunschweig, Germany	
12.1.5.4 Yeasts extracts (ZYMOSAN & HYDRO-GLUCAN) injected intravenously; (avoid toxic-ity).	94%	mice: 300,	regression at 60 days	Sarcoma 37	Dr. Irene C. Diller, NCI grant. Z. T. Mankowski, Dept. Microbio., Rutgers. Mary Fisher.	"The Effect of Yeast...on Mouse Tumors", Cancer Research, v.23, p.201, Feb. 1963.
	91%	treated, 200		" 180		
	12%	controls				
12.2 PLANTS (See 9.3.4, 10.1.1) 12.2.1 MUSHROOM (FUNGI; see 12.1.5) 12.2.1.1 Boletus Edulis	averaged	mice	sharply inhibiting	induced tumor	Sloan Kettering Inst.	George Berkley, Cancer, How To...Fight It, p.91.
12.2.1.2 Of 332 species, 213 destroy harmful bacteria.					Dr. William J. Robbins, N.Y. Botanical Gardens	
12.2.1.3 PS-K extract of mushroom (kawaradake), common in Japan. Taken orally. Immune stimulant.		patients: 40	survival, years:	terminal ca.	Chikao Yoshikumi.	
	45%	includes: 21		", stomach	Ichiji Itoh, Chief of Surg.,	
		" :14	4	", intestine	Tokyo City Med. Ctr.	
(Mushrooms are plant on plant PARASITES (see 14.2).)	67%	total: 100	2	terminal ca.	Yoshio Sakurai, Director, Japanese Found. for Cancer Research.	
	82%	includes: 11		", lung		
	42%	" :72		", stomach		
12.2.2 MAYTANSINE, Anti-biotic from Maytenus Ovatus plant of E. Africa.	averaged	mice	ILS over controls: 100%	leukemia	S. Morris Kupchan, (& G. Howie, Prof. Chem.; & S. Remillard & L. Rebhun, Prof. Bio. U. Va., Charlottsville.)	(Vincent DeVita, Dir. NCI, et al, "New Directions...NCI ...", in ACS, Metast. & Dissem. Ca., p.182. Science, v.189, p. 1002, Sep. 19, 1975.)

TREATMENT (Mode, Theory)	BENEFITED, % of total, or #	TREATED, total #	MEASURE of BENEFIT	DISEASE SEVERITY	RESEARCHER, Credentials	REFERENCE, Publication
12.2.3 GRAPES. "I am the true 12.2.3.1 Vine."-Jesus, Bible. MONO-DIET: 1 species/meal, (MODIFIED) or 1/day(s). Only grapes/weeks, & grape: poultice, internal rinse.	100%	patients: 5	cured	hopeless cancer	Johanna Brandt. Prof. Dr. Martin Zeller, Munich, Germany. Dr. Herman Rieder. Dr. Lambe (early 1800's in England).	R. C. Williams, Grandma the Life Saver, p.3-4.
	200 in #		saved no failures reported	cancer		A. Brown, March of Truth Cancer, p.3. (J. Brandt, The Grape Cure.)
12.2.3.2 Herpes simplex virus 1 (2 implicated in human ca.) is 99% inactivated by grape (skin). High in Chromium (glucose tolerance f.), IRON (heme, oxygen), Potassium (see 9.3.2; 9.10.5).	99% 99.9% 0%	cell culture: treated controls	virus inactivated, as % input	Herpes Simplex 1 virus polio-virus	J. Konowalchuck & Joan I. Spears, Bur. Microbiol. Hazards, Health & Welfare Agency, Ottawa, Canada	"Virus Inactivation by Grapes & Wines", Applied & Environmental Microbiology v.32, n.6, p.757, Dec. 1976. (See 9.10.4, 13.4.6.)
13.0 GROWTH INHIBITORS (ALLELOPATHY), PLANTS (for animals, see Mercenene 15.2.1, Carcalon 17.3.1).						
13.1 PLANTS. Of 498 species tested, 4.5% INHIBITED RC-dba animal ca. test system, & 10% inhibited C3H-egg " , & 2.5% " both systems. (See 14.0, 14.4.)	40% 50%	mice, dba strain egg	inhibited cancer, by over a pre-set % criteria (i.e. 40 or 50%)	transplant, mammary: adeno-carcinoma, RC carcinoma of C3H mice	George F. McKenna. Alfred Taylor, Biochem., U. Texas, & Clayton Found. Betty S. Gibson. C. C. Albers, Prof. Pharmacognosy, U. Texas, Austin	"Screening Plant Extracts for Anti-Cancer Activity", & "Extracts of Plants in Cancer Chemo." & "Essential... Plant...Ca. Chemo." Texas Rep. on Bio. & Med., v.20, n.2, p.214, Sum. 1962; & v.18, n.2, p.233, Sum. 1960; & v.19, n.2, p.321, Sum. 1964; ref. in Garb, Cure for Cancer: A National Goal, p.150; referencing T. B. Heaton, J. Pathol. Bacter., v.32, p.565, 1929.
13.2 BERRIES of MOUNTAIN ASH; Parasorbic acid. (Also, germs in soil excrete chemicals absorbed by roots.) (Also, COMPANIONATE GARDENING) (Is growth inhibit. of plants like CONTACT INHIBITION of non ca. cells in animals?-Ed.)		rats	complete cure	Jensen sarcoma	Solomon Garb, MD, FACP, Prof. Pharm. U. Missouri Med; Sci. Dir. Amer. Med. Ctr., Denver; Co-Chairman Citizens Comm. Conquest of Cancer (with Sidney Farber, MD, as in Ca. Ctr.).	
13.3 ASPARAGUS. Histones control cell growth. Do cook (to wreck cholinerase & asparagin); (do not use with mustard gas). Grass; see 10.1.	60 in #	patients	completely recovered	cancer mix	Richard R. Vensel, DDS, Pittsburgh.	Arlin Brown, "Asparagus Therapy". ("Substances in Fescue Inhibit Other Plants", Bio-Dynamics, n.136, p.45, Fall, 1980)
13.4 GARLIC (Anti-biotic, see 12.2) 13.4.1 Garlic (& Onions PREVENT (bad) BLOOD CLOTS & CHOLESTEROL (see 11.1.2). Has Selenium (see 9.10.7).	93%	patients: 194	complete healing	leukoplakia (often pre-cancer), etc.	D. M. Sergaiev & L. D. Lenov, District Oncological Dispensary, Kirovograd, USSR.	Garlic, Health Research, p. 57. Nutr. Rev., v.34, n.2, p.43, Feb. 1976.
13.4.2 Garlic (eat & juiced); has growth inhibitor, & SULFER (Oxygenates; in body heparin, see 11.1.3).	averaged	guinea pigs	inhibited	cancer	Cancerology Inst., Heidelberg U., Germany	Spotlight, Apr. 21, 1980, p.18. (Codex Ebers, circa 1500 BC)
13.4.3 Inject into mice, viable cancer cells, then garlic.		mice:	delayed onset of cancer		A. S. Weisberger & J. Pensky, Western Reserve U., Ohio	Garlic, Health Research, p. 77, "Exper. With Garlic & Ca.", referring to Science v.126, p.1112, Nov. 29, 1957.
13.4.4 If first soaked in garlic, cancer cells injected into mice are prevented from causing ca.: No garlic soak, controls; (Allicin reacts with sulfhydryl of tumor; see 18.1.)		treated controls	cancer: prevented for 6 months death in ½ month	ca. cells injected into mice		

TREATMENT (Mode, Theory)	BENEFITED, % of total, or #	TREATED, total #	MEASURE of BENEFIT	DISEASE SEVERITY	RESEARCHER, Credentials	REFERENCE, Publication
13.4.5 If first soaked in garlic (raw; 2x; 7 days apart), ca. cells injected into mice IMMUNIZE 100% against same ca. cell line (non-garlic-ed) injected 14 days after.	100% 0%	mice, DDD strain: treated: 20 controls: 20	prevention of cancer(/death) for 100 days	Ehrlich ascites injected in mouse peritoneum	Motonori Fujiwara & Toshikazu Natatu, Dept. Hygiene, Faculty Medicine, Kyoto U., Japan (See 17.2)	"Induction of Tumour Immunity with Tumour Cells Treated with Extract of Garlic", Nature, v.216, n.5110, p.83, Oct.7, 1967.
13.4.6 Garlic kills bad germs whose toxins spread from transverse colon to spine, paralyzing. (See 9.10.4) Prevent other disease.	100.0% 99.47%	children: treated: 1,204 controls: 12,625	prevention (incidence drop from 0.53% to 0.0%)	polio	Dr. Ragnor Huss, burough med. officer, Malmo, Sweden (Dr. Mayerhofer, Germany) (See 12.2.3.2)	Garlic, Health Research, p.57, referencing R. Huss, Svenska Lakartidningen, v.35, p.216.
14.0 NUTRITION, HERBS (i.e. Land Plant, Traditionally Eaten, in Small Quantities. See 9.3.4, 10.1.1, 12.2, 13, 15.1)						
14.1 Potassium Iodide (see 9.3), & HOXSEY HERBS: licorice, cascara RED CLOVER, ROOT (of burdock, stillinga, barberis, poke), BARK (of prickly ash, buckthorn), (& Aromatic USP 14) in combinations, Internally. Externally, either: 1) arsenic sulfide, sulfer, talc; 2) antimony trichloride, zinc chloride, bloodroot; 3) trichloro-acetic acid.	89%	patients: 27	alive over 2 years	ca., biopsied, some very bad breast	Harry Hoxsey Dr. Sam Scothorn, Pres., Amer. Osteopathic Assoc.	H. Hoxsey, You Don't Have to Die, p.198,
	100's in #		successfully treated, some symptom free 24 years	pathology proven ca.	10 MD's nation-wide, independently observed therapy (& 6 Drs.: Louis Heimer, MD, Head, Amer. Stomach Hosp.)	" , p.58-9,
	averaged	80	owe lives to treatment	terminal cancer	80 patients sworn in court	" , p.166,
Internal treatment:	77%	mice: 13	survival: 12 weeks		Clarence Little, MD, Head, Jackson Mem. Lab., Bar Harbor, Maine; a Director, Amer. Soc. for Control of Cancer,	" , p.176, (Congressional Record, v.99, part 12, p.A5350, Aug.3, 1953.)
External " :	46%	13	(fertile)			
" :	60%	100	4 weeks	cancer ridden		" , p.177.
controls:	0%	100				
	80%	patients: 1,000's	got well	cancer	Mildred Nelson, RN, & 6MD's	Public Scrutiny, Nov. 1980, p.14; & Dec. 1980, p.16.
14.2 Iscador, from MISTLETOE, Viscum Album, PARASITE (see 12.1.2, 12.2.1)	averaged	1,000's	survival rate doubled over Orthodox Therapy	cancer of breast, uterus	Dr. Rudolph Steiner, Founder, Soc. for Cancer Research, Switzerland, & 200 MD's & Lucas Klinic	W. Kaelin, Hippocrates, v.4, p.325, 1933. ACS, Unproven Methods of Cancer Management, p.115.
Iscador & Radiation, treated:	87%	women: 45	survival, 5 years	cervix: Stage II	Prof. W. Bickenbach, MD, Director, 1st Gynecological Unit, Munich U. Hosp., Germany. Profs. Ries & Breitner.	K. E. Fellmer, "A Clinical Trial of Iscador," Brit. Homeopathic J.", v.52, n.1, p.44, Jan. 1968, (transl. from Medizin. Klinik, v.62, n.1, p.44, Feb 1967.
Only Radiation, controls:	77%	334				
(See 9.7.3.1, & 9.8) treated:	70%	27		Stage III		
controls:	56%	283				
Statistical Signif. of P=.015						
Iscador	averaged	patients: 4 studies	" " (5 yr. mortality 30-40% less)	ca. & Surg. Radiation Therapy	(Pliny the Elder, Roman Empire)	A. Leroi, MD, "Rudolph Steiner's...Ca." transl. from Die Drei, n.1, Jan. 1961, Stuttgart.
14.3 POISON IVY (Immune Stimulant, see 17.); to ear, 2x, before test sarcoma into loin, then ivy daily.	26% 0%	mice, Balb-C treated: 19 controls: 10	survival, days: 60 39	transplanted sarcoma, pleomorphic	Dr. Richard Leneghan	Poison Ivy Research", Ca. Forum, v.5, n.1, p.6.

TREATMENT (Mode, Theory)	BENEFITED, % of total, or #	TREATED, total #	MEASURE of BENEFIT	DISEASE SEVERITY	RESEARCHER, Credentials	REFERENCE, Publication
14.4 KC-555 (Extract of Asiatic plants: Aloes, Cinchona bark, Gentian, Rhubarb, Zedoary, Agaric, Columba, Galangal, Bryona, Myrrh, Calamus, Angelica, Chamomile, Peppermint; "Greenlife"; Spiritus Frumentus as preservative; Cedar Cones from Iran, Pini Stroebus, (Fiery Pine).) (See 13.1) Also: About 3,100 plants have compounds of some anti-cancer activity; &10% of "old wives" tales on herbal medicine have some truth to them.-James A. Duke, head Economic Botany Lab., USDA, & NCI contract; (see 14.4.2) ; ref. in Natural Food & Farming, v.27, n.9, p.8, Mar. 1981.)	most	patients: 100's, over 12 years	survival, some 12 years	terminal ca., mostly	Kegan Sarkisian, Amer. U. of Beirut; U. New Hampshire; Pres., Inst. of Natural Science; JFK Medical Research Award; MD, PhD. Morovith McQueen-Williams, MD, Surg. Thesis Prize, Yale; Phi Beta Kappa, Gold Medal PhD, U. of Cal.; Faculty of Johns Hopkins, Case Western, Seton Hall; Med. Dir. "MD" Magazine: Fellowships: AAAS, AA Geriatrics, Acad. Med. of NJ; Board Cert. Radiol.; PhD.	Hearings, National Cancer Attack Act of 1971, Part 2, U.S. Congress, SN 92-41, p. 534-548. Papers at 2nd & 3rd International Cancer Congresses, 1959 & 1960, Antwerp & Lyon.
	36 in #	treated: n	remission	terminal ca.		
	0	control: n	survival, 1 month			
	80%	treated	successfully effective	terminal ca., many		Tests by Dr. Chaltikian, U. Yerevan, Armenia.
		mice, strain of: Lethal Yellow	prevented cancer in 9 generations	hereditary cancer expected		(Note: Dr. Lewis Terman, Stanford U., "founder of Silicon Valley", rated Dr. McQueen-Williams as most brilliant of a group of geniuses. -CCS, Ca. Control J., v.6, n.1, p.117, Jan. 1978, 1982.)
		chickens	lumps disappeared	diagnosed leukosis		
		wild cell	inhibited proliferation	first 3 cleavages	Dr. Clement Markert, head of Biol., Johns Hopkins & Yale.	
		normal cell	non-toxic			
14.5 ESSIAC. Ancient Canadian Indian herbal remedy. (Proponents: Dr. F. Banting, insulin co-discoveror; Dr. B. Guyatt, Anatomy Dept., U. Toronto; Dr. P. Merker, SKI; M. Hepburn, Premier, Ontario; in: Ca. Victory Bull., v.7 (n.8, Aug.; n.9, Sep.) 1981.)	aver-aged	patients: 30	(Note: See C.14.5) ILS: $1\frac{1}{2}$ years; broke tumor to normal	terminal cancer	Nurse Renee Caisse & 5 MD's at Northwestern U. Hosp., Chicago. (Dr. Charles Brusch, Founder, Brusch Med. Ctr., Cambridge, Mass.; 8 Canad. MD's.)	Choice, v.4, n.6, p.22, July 1978. Fort Lauderdale News, Nov. 6, 1977, Sec. C, p.1. ("Essiac", Cancer Forum, v.4, n.3, p.8.) (Jethro Kloss, Back to Eden.)
	380 in #	patients	cured	cancer mix		
14.6 Chaparrel Tea from CREOSOTE bush (Larrea divaricatu).	majority	patients: 34	stimulated, some regress		Charles R. Smart, MD, Assoc. Prof. Surg., & Hugh Hogle, MD, U. Utah Med., Salt Lake City. Dean C. Fletcher, PhD, Chair. Biochem. Dept., U. Nevada	Cancer Chemotherapy Rep., Part 1, v.53, p.147, 1969; & speech at Amer. College of Surg., Utah Ch., in ACS, Unproven Methods..., p.55.
	4 in # (2 in #)	patients	regress (", by 75-95%)	terminal cancer		
14.7 Root of Puccoon (used by Lake Superior Indians), & ZINC CHLORIDE.	aver-aged	patients: 25	tumor removed (enucleate, granulate, & scar)	cancer mix	Dr. J. Weldon Fell, a Founder, NY Acad. Med.; Faculty Member, NYU, New York. 100 London MD's witness.	Endorsement report by Board of Middlesex Hosp., London, in Nat Morris, The Cancer Blackout, p.29,
14.8 " & diet (no salt) & resinous alkaloids.		4,000	sloughed off tumor		Dr. John Pattison, NYU, New York, & London	" , p.33,
14.9 Herbs (Welsh). Extract applied externally until cancer's roots are out, leaving a crater treated by another solution, leaving a scar.		total: 16 (15 confirmed diagnosis)	cured:	cancer: (10 hopeless, 6 mix cases)	Dr. Rees Evans, London; Presbyterian Hosp., Newark, NJ.	" , p.126. (London Picture Post, Sept. 23, 1950.)
	56%		complete			
	72%		"/partial			
	40%	100	no ca. return over 5 years	mix		Is Cancer Curable?, Health Research, p.14.
	98%		non-failure			

TREATMENT (Mode, Theory)	BENEFITED, % of total, or #	TREATED, total #	MEASURE of BENEFIT	DISEASE SEVERITY	RESEARCHER, Credentials	REFERENCE, Publication
14.10 Herbs. 60 Combinations, from 160 herbs. Other diseases. Anti-Ca.: Chaparral, Red Clover, Comfrey, Ginseng, Celandine, ROOT of: Burdock, Echinacea, Golden Seal, Blood; as base. Other: Poke, Blue Violet, Parsely, Licorice, Garlic, Dandelion, Cayenne, Prickly Ash, Cleavers, Gotu Cola, Periwinkle, Sassafras, Agrimony, Ground Ivy.	94% average	patients: total: 281	effective; cure	120 ailments	F. Joseph Montagna. (Lendon Smith, MD, FAAP. Harold Manner, (see 10.19) Dr. John R. Christopher, MH, ND. 3 DC's.)	"Statistical Data Analysis Report on 60 Traditional Herbal Formulas", J. Alternative Med. Assoc., v.1, n.1, p.12. Herbal Formula Testimonial, p.1.
	89% 2 in #	patients	prevention cure	cancer		
14.11 Herbs. Wisconsin Indian therapies, (& see 14.5 & 14.10).	over 4 in #	patients	cure	cancer	Jethro Kloss	Back to Eden, 5th ed., p.342, & 452-477.
14.12 Herb Combination, traditional Chinese, "Anti-Tumor-B3". Lowers an endemic cancer's incidence (due to hyperplasia) from 7% to 1.5%.	98.5%	patients: treated: 72	prevention of cancer resulting	hyperplasia, severe, of esophagus (low Mo soil)	Chinese Cancer Research Inst., Peking.	TV: NOVA, "The Cancer Detectives of Lin Xian", WGBH, Boston, Oct. 1980. (Barefoot Doctor's Manual, p.406, 477.)
	93%	control: 70,000 pop.				
14.13 Bamfolin, extract from leaf of BAMBOO grass (Yakusa) of alpine country.	10%	patients: 69	successfully normal by ½ yr.	incurarable, inoperable, cancer	Dr. Misanobu Oshima, Pres., Japanese Contra Cancer Council.	Bunte Illustrierte, n.20, p.20, Aug.1, 1964; referenced in ACS, Unproven Methods, p.29.
	47%		survival ½ yr.			
14.14 Eleutherococcus Senticosus Maxim., common in NE Asia.		patients	reduced changes	ca. metastasis	Petrov Oncological Inst., Leningrad	Natural Food & Farming, v.27, n.9, p.9, Mar. 1981.
Root extract in drinking water. Animals.	51%	mice: treated	survival, 70 days (after transplanted tumor in)	carcinosarcoma, Walker 256	K.V. Yaremenko. N.B. Lazarev, MD, & I.I. Brekhman, MD, Inst. Biol. Active Substance, Acad. of Sci., Vladivostok, USSR.	"Influence of Preparations of Eleuth. ... on Neoplastic Disease", Cancer News J., v.10, n.4, p.21, 1975.
	23%	controls				
Lowers incidence of a cancer from 13% down to 2%, in animals.	98%	rats: treated: 56	prevention of leukosis, for 15 months	indole injection	A. N. Stukov, "	
	87%	controls: 67				
14.15 BF 70 & 69, isolated from species of plant family (Aristolochia), one of 33 plants for head shrinking by Jivaro Indians of Amazon.	73%	patients: 85	positive response	cancer mix	Dr. Rao Nulu, U. Calif.; U. Texas.	Choice, v.5, n.5, p.16, Fall 1979;
			effective	lab analysis	U. Kansas, M.D. Anderson, NCI, WARF, SRI, U. Miami.	
14.16 " , 6 of 33 plants. (Other Researchers: Wm. P. Aikin, MD, Northwestern U. Med. Charles Fletcher, PhD, Plant Physiol., Johns Hopkins. & 3 MD's, Los Angeles Co. Hosp.)		patients	regressed considerably	cancer	Dr. Wilburn H. Ferguson, Chief Anasth., all Ecuad. Hosp. Señ. Galo Plaza, President of Ecuador.	K. O. Gilmore, & H. Simons, "Secrets of the Headhunters", Sat. Eve. Post, v.231, p.34, Nov. 22, 1958; referenced in ACS, Unproven Methods..., p.113, 1972.
		animals	some degree of success	tumors & leukemias	Bruce W. Halstead, MD, Asso. Prof., Loma Linda U. Med.; Dir. World Life Research Inst.	
14.17 COCAINE, alkaloid from coca leaf; poultice/tumor inject. Aids Carbohyd. metab. (See 17.6)	74%	patients: 239	cured, tumors gone, healing rapid	cancer mix	Frank Psota, MD.	Arlin Brown, March of Truth on Cancer, p.81.

TREATMENT (Mode, Theory)	BENEFITED, % of total, or #	TREATED, total #	MEASURE of BENEFIT	DISEASE SEVERITY	RESEARCHER, Credentials	REFERENCE, Publication
14.18 Inner BARK of Trees, Tabebuia Avellanedae/Altissima, (red "pau d'arco"), RESISTS FUNGUS. Found in South America, (as is Avelos, a tumor tearer). (Has Carbonyl; see 18.1)	many	patients: many at hospital	cures: pain in hours, other symptoms in days	cancer mix (terminal, leukemia); ulcers; diabetes; anemia; rheumatism; osteomyelitis	Dr. Orlando dei Santi, Prof. Dr. Walter Accorsi, Dr. Octaviano Gaiarsa, & other MD's, Municipal Hosp.; & City Council, Santa Andre, Brazil. Colonel Amatea.	Alec de Montmorency, "Exotic Medicine...", Spotlight, Jan. 5&12, 1981, p.10, (& July 14, 1980, p.10); references O Cruzerio, Mar. 18 & 25, 1967.
15.0 SEA, 15.1 PLANTS (See 7.2) 15.1.1 SEAWEED, Tekarina; extract injected. Brings Iron (heme, oxygen) to blood. Induces fever. Natural hormone. Restores cell permeability. (See 12.2.3.2 &17.)	80%	patients: 5,000	cure	cancer mix, except liver.	Guiseppe Lo Monaco, Tecate, Mexico, & 2 MD's (If poor quality Tekarina & no cleansing diet, patient detoxify too fast & die.)	Arlin Brown, "Natural Cancer Treatment". Cancer Victory Bull., v.3, n.7, p.4, July 1977.
15.1.2 Seaweed, red, extract. " . (This virus suspect in human ca.)			blocks virus	Herpes Simplex II virus	E. Fran Deig, Virologist, & D. Ehresmann, U. Calif.	G. Berkley, Cancer: How to..., p.103, 213; ref. Time, June 21, 1976.
15.2 ANIMALS 15.2.1 MERCENENE, extract of common CLAM, Mercenaria Merc., most anti-cancerous of mollusks, (& anti-viral). Invertebrates have no spontaneous cancer. Clams & mushrooms (see 12.2.1) are rich in RETINE (natural retarder of cell division, see 13.), & poor in PROMINE (promoter, cell div.). Eating RAW, UN-POLLUTED, WHOLE Clams Increased Life Span (remaining) by 10x, in some cancer patients. PAOLIN, a MUCO-PROTEIN, anti-viral to Herpes Simplex (see 12.2.3.2), is high in clams (& calf thymus & snow peas, see 10.12).	some	patients	ILS: 1,000%	cancer	Sister M. Rosarii (Arline C.) Schmeer, OP, PhD, U. Colo.; Detroit President's Cabinet Medal; ACS grant; Chair. Biol., Coll. St. Mary's, Columbus, Oh.; Prof. Biomed., Amer. Med. Ctr., Denver; Sr. Investig., Marine Bio. Lab., Woods Hole, Mass.	ACS, MAD, "Anti-Ca. ...Clams."
	80% 0%	mice: treated control	good health, 6 months survival, 1 mo.	Sarcoma 180 cells inject into mice		Solomon Garb, Cure For Cancer, A National Goal, p.248 (Science, v.149, p.34, 1965)
	90%	animals	regress, complete; & inhibit	Krebs-2 carcinoma		Schmeer, "Mercenene: An Anti-Neoplastic...", NCI Monog. n.31, p.581, '69
	70% 27%	hamsters: treated: 10 controls: 11	prevention of tumor resulting	Adenovirus type 12	Albert Szent-Gyorki, MD, PhD, Nobel Laureate.	Li & Prescott, "Common Clam Extracts Show Anti-Tumor Act." JAMA, Feb. 15, 1965.
	averaged	mice	ILS: 100%	leukemic spleen	Dr. Andrew Hegyeli, Chief, Biomed. Br., US Marine Bio. R&D Lab., Md. Dr. D. Clark, SKI. Dr. C. P. Li, Sr. Virologist; & Dr. Ben. Prescott, Div. Bio. Standards; NIH.	J. R. Judge, "Inhibition... Leukem. ...by Mercenaria...", Proc. Soc. Exp. Biol. & Med., v.123, p.299, 1966. (Last 3 articles ref. in: ACS, Med. Affairs Dept., "Anti-Cancer...Clams."
15.2.2 SPONGE, rare, Caribbean, extract from. (US Senator Magnuson's bill to estab. National Inst. of Marine Med. & Pharm.)	50% 48%		controlled symptoms	leukemia	NCI. Dr. Seymour S. Cohen, U. Penn. Med. Dr. Joseph Burchenal, V. Pres., SKI, NY.	Ted Morello, "Opening the Ocean's Medicine Chest", World Book Encyclopedia.
15.2.3 SEA URCHIN, STARFISH (Echinoderms). Holothurin extract.	range	mice	ILS: 10 days thru 18 mos.	tumor	Battelle Mem. Inst. (Dr. R. Nigrelli, Osborne Labs.)	
15.2.4 MOLLUSK (meat powder, "Neptone"). (Also, Sea Cucumbers.)	100%	patients: 3	remission, cancer free	terminal cancer	Dr. Echevirra, Sup., Public Health Hosp., San Jose, Costa Rica.	Cancer Victory Bull., v.6, n.7, p.2, July 1980.

TREATMENT (Mode, Theory)	BENEFITED, % of total, or #	TREATED, total #	MEASURE of BENEFIT	DISEASE SEVERITY	RESEARCHER, Credentials	REFERENCE, Publication
16.0 ANIMAL (CELLULAR) EXTRACTS INJECTED (See Enzymes 11, Immunology 17)						
16.1 CELLULAR THERAPY. 16.1.1 CELLS FROM ORGANS OF ANIMAL EMBRYO INJECTED INTO	99%	patients: 2,000	prevented for 35 years	spontaneous cancer	Prof. Paul Niehans, 3 Doctorates: Sci., Med., & Philo.; nephew of Emperor Wilhelm II; Papal Appointee to Chair vacated by Sir Alexander Fleming. (Alexis Carrel, Rockefeller Inst.; Nobel Laureate. 50,000 MD's.)	Fredrico Ramos O., Treatment of Cancer by Means of Cellular Therapy, p.48. " , p.45. (Niehans, Cellular Therapy. 900 sientific publications. Ivan Popop, Stay Young, p.211. A. Brown, March of Truth on Ca., p.84.)
16.1.2 HUMAN. PREVENTION of cancer in 99% of humans using sheep embryo, & 93% using cow & pig embryo. (Cancer incidence in sheep is 1/1000 that in dogs, cats, mice, rats, hens.) (See 16.4; 17.3.)	88% 0%	animals: treated: 40+ control: 40+	survival, 220 days / no cancer	benzpyrene & Walker ca. cells injected		
16.1.3 Fresh splenic cells from other rats activated by other tumors, into host rats.	33% 3%	rats: treated: 40 controls	survival: 253 days	benzpyrene under skin causes ca. in host rats.	Prof. Dr. Hermann Hoepke, Heidelberg, & Fluhr.	"Cellular Therapy in Tumors", in F. Schmid & J. Stein, Cell Research & Cellular Therapy, p.488,
16.1.4 Fresh thymus cells from 4 wk. old rabbits, & fetal sheep, into host rats.	84% 0%	treated controls	tumor free, 220 days			
16.1.5 Lypholized splenic cells from 4 wk. old pigs. Umbelical cord cells & heparin A into tumor. (Heparin is an anti-coagulant, see 11.1.2)	52% 100% 0%	treated controls	at 183 days: complete regression " /inhibition survival		Dr. A. Landsberger, Heidelberg.	" , p.491, "Results of... Malignant Cells with Body's Own Tumor Defense".
16.1.6 Umbelical cord cells & heparin & dextran. (Dextran causes mast cells to pour out heparin.)	35% 50% 0% 25%	treated: 20 controls: 20 same group, treated: 20	at 179 days: cancer free survival at 790 days: cancer free		"	" , p.498.
					(Notes: "Cellular" is like EMBRYO THERAPY - to eat FERTILIZED EGGS (animal) & SPROUTS (plant). Also, diet of Fresh, Organic, Whole, Fruits & Vegetables. EMBRYO TISSUE MATCHED TO PATIENT'S DISEASE.)	
16.1.7 " , & increased cellular therapy.	70% 0%	treated: 20 control: 20	at 198 days: survival			
16.2 ECLECTIC: use best method for each case. CELLULAR Therapy. Fever Therapy. Oxygen/Ozone infusion or treated blood.	16.6%	patients: 252	totally free of cancer, 5 years	terminal ca., independent: histology, diagnosis	Joseph Issels, MD; Member: Bavarian Ca. Soc., German Nat. Ca. Soc., Royal Med. Soc. (Scot.); Lecturer: Oxford U., Sloan Kettering Inst., Swedish Med. Assoc. for Biol. Med.; Chief, Ringberg Clinic, Germany. & 4 MD's. Dr. Arie Audier, Leiden U. Holland. Dr. H. Weiler, Pres., Bavarian Med. Assoc. Dr. P. Kretz, Editor, Aus-	Issels, Cancer: A Second Opinion. "Immuno-...", Clin. Trials J., Lond. 7, p.357, 1970. Audier, Die Medizinische, Oct. 3, 1959. BBC-TV, "Go Climb A Mountain", Nov. 3, 1970. Gordon Thomas, Dr. Issels..., Ref. in (Penthouse, Aug. 1980), Cancer News J., v.15, n.3, p.2, Fall 1980, & v.9, n.4, p.16, 1974. Ericson, Cancer Treatment, p.A16. A. Brown, March of
Mental: COMMUNICATION, BEAUTIFUL SCENERY, OPEN VISITS Exercise: MOUNTAIN CLIMBING, JOGGING. (See: 2.3, 3, 6, 17.) Eliminate low grade, chronic, local infections (in tonsils, teeth).	87%	370	well, no relapse, no detectable metastasis	cancer mix; after surgery & radiation		
		8,000				
LACTIC ACID FERMENTED Foods (see 12.1.2). CH-23 (plant toxins). CARCIN.	50%		cured	hopeless cancer		

(continued)

TREATMENT (Mode, Theory)	BENEFITED, % of total, or #	TREATED, total #	MEASURE of BENEFIT	DISEASE SEVERITY	RESEARCHER, Credentials	REFERENCE, Publication
16.2 (continued)					trian Ca. Soc. J. Dr. John Anderson, WHO Adviser; Prof. Med., King's College Hosp., London; Rockefeller Research Fellow.	Truth on Cancer, p. 48.
16.3 Carcin & Neo-Carcin. Mixed extracts from animal GLANDS, plants, poly-peptides, in-organics.	70% 100,000 in #	patients	efficacious cure	serious ca.	J. Issels " . Dr. Jacob Pawlotzki, MD, U. Bern, Dipl. in Chem., Switzerland.	ACS, Unproven Methods of Cancer Management, p.47.
16.4 Sheep ADRENAL Cortex extract. (See 16.1.2. Goats make 330x human RDA of Vit. C; stored in adrenals.)	10%	patients: 1,040	survival, over 4 years	inoperable, hopeless, terminal ca.	Walter Coffey, MD, Chief Surg. & Dir., So. Pacific R.R. Hosp. Dr. Eaton, Urol.	Nat Morris, Cancer Blackout, p.60. (L. Pauling (see 9.6) in Ericson, Cancer Treat..., p.197.)
16.5 Anti-neol. PITUITARY, posterior lobe, of cattle; extract (by acetone).	75%	300 minus losses of 1st. month	marked improvement, return to work	metastasis & extreme cachexia	Henry Wachtel, MD, U. Vienna; Dir., Ca. Res. Council, & Dept.; Prof. Physiol., Fordham U.	N. Morris, Cancer Blackout, p.152.
16.6 FAITH IN GOD, SIMPLE NATURAL LIFE, (see 2.), & 5: Anti-neol, Carzodelan (like Trypsin), Krebiozen, Mucorhicin, Laetrile.	70%	patients	cure	cancer mix	Donald Gibson, MD, Yale Med.	(Cancer, v.11, p.232, 1961, & v.14, p.40, 1964, in:) ACS, Unproven Methods..., p.77,
16.7 CNT. Water solution of: TESTICLE & OVARY, nucleinate, adenine, mertiolate.	25 in #		improved well being & general health		Dr. Antonio Alecce, Pres. Inst. Farma. Ital., Rome. & 78 Italian MD's.	", p.59.
16.8 Peptide extract from a normal human's urine injected into patient. "H-11" has Sulphonic acid, Phenolics, & PARA-THYROID GROWTH INHIBITOR (excreted in URINE).	15% 53%	patients: 32	survival, over: 1½ years " 1 "	advanced cancer	James Thompson, BS, London U. lecturer. Dr. G. J. W. Ollerenshaw, MA, BM, BCh, Oxford U.; Fellow, Roy. Soc. Med. Sir Geo. Mitcheson, Member of Parliament.	Brit. Med. J., v.2, p.835, 1948 & 5 other articles. "H-11...", Clin. Med., v.55, p.149, 1948. ACS, Unproven Methods...", p.87.
	65%	3,885	pain relief	cancer mix		
16.9 ANTI-NEO-PLASTON (in urine)	86% 19%	41	clinical improvement total remission	advanced cancer	Stan. Burzynski, MD, PhD; M. Curie Med., Poland; NCI Grant; Baylor Med.; MD. Anderson	Gary Null, Ca. News J., v.14, n.4, p.2, Dec. 1979, (from Penthouse; & Our Town; 1979)
17.0 IMMUNOLOGY (Injections), FEVER (see Heat 4.)						
17.1 Re-inject (into patient) "DE-BLOCKERS" isolated from same patient's drawn blood. "De-blockers" fight "blockers"; tumor produces "blockers" against immunity. "Blockers" in discarded blood.	16% 44%	patients: 186	survival, over: 2 years " 1 "	hopeless, terminal ca. immunity damaged by radiation & chemotherapy	Lawrence Burton, & Frank Friedman, both: PhD & NYU & Cal. Tech.; grants from USPHS, Damon Runyan, & 3 Found'n; Oncologists, St. Vincent's Hosp., NY; Directors, Immun. Res. Found., NY. Burton: Dir., Immun. Res. Ctr., Freeport, Bahamas. US Congressman Larry McDonald, MD Florida St. Legislature Majority.	CBS-TV, 60 Minutes, May, 1980. Trans. NY Acad. Sci., v.25, p. 29, Nov. 1962. Allan Anderson, "The Politics of Cancer: How...Medical Establishment to Listen", New York, v.7, n. 30, p.42, July 29, 1974. US House of Rep., Bill HR7936, "To Exempt Certain Blood Fractions...". Ericson, Ca. Treatment..., p.109. National Enquirer, Sep. 13, 1977, p. 26. Midnight/Globe, Aug. 9, 1977, p.3.
BETTER RESULTS IF NO RADIATION OR CHEMOTHERAPY (see 1.2.2). (Dr. Sidney Farber, Children's Hosp., Boston (see 13.2): "You're ten years ahead....") (Pat McGrady, Sr. (see 18.3): "He'd make the (mouse) tumors disappear while you watched." - Ca. Syndrome, p.190.)	most	mice	shrink tumors to ½ size, in 1 hour (Note: See: A, C, & D, 17.1)	skin ca.		

TREATMENT (Mode, Theory)	BENEFITED, % of total	TREATED, total #	MEASURE of BENEFIT	DISEASE SEVERITY	RESEARCHER, Credentials	REFERENCE, Publication
17.2 KREBIOZEN. Inject into patient an extract from serum of horse, after horse injected with Actinomyces Bovis (extract of benign, "Lumpy Jaw" tumor in cattle). Horse's RES (Reticulo-Endothelial System) was stimulated to produce Krebiozen, a growth regulator.	73%	patients: 159	decrease or arrest of tumor size	ca.:95% of patients-advanced, hopeless; 40-55%-terminal (bed)	Andrew C. Ivy, MD, PhD, Rush & U. of Chicago; Director, ACS; Exec. Dir., National Advisory Ca. Council; AMA Counc.; Dir., Naval Med. Res. Inst.; Head, Med. School, & V.Pres, U. Illinois; President (Soc. Int. Med.; Am. Physiol. Soc.; Am. Gastro-Ent. Assn.; Chi. Inst. Med.); Ed., Soc. Exptl. Biol.; Council, Am. Assn. U. Profs.; Ed. Gastroent.; most referenced in Sci Citation Index; 1500 papers published; world's top gastroent., per Who's Who; rep. Allied govts. in medical ethics at Nurenberg; DSc; LLD; FACP.	Ivy, Observations on Krebiozen in the Management of Cancer, p.19, 84, & Fig.1.
	12%	189	survival, over 4 years			
	10%	500	free of ca., 3-8 years	hopeless, terminal ca.		Congressional Record, v.105, part 7, p.8608, May 20, 1959. (Nat Morris, Cancer Blackout, p.156.)
Research auspices of: Dr. Ivy:	70%	250	beneficial (& non-toxic for 100%)	terminal ca.		
Lankenau Ca. Research Ctr:		40				
3 independent groups:		1,500				
300 MD's (US & 29 countries:		1,200				
(6 large University clinics & 2 world fame med. centers)	10%	2,000	survival, 4-12 years	", 90% under ½ yr. left		Congress. Rec., v.108, part 11, p.14286, July 20, 1962.
Of patients, 80% observed for first 3 months, & 20 % for up to 12 years.	61;77%	65	tumor size: smaller; arrest % ; %	brain		(Arlin Brown, March of Truth on Cancer, p.63; & Cancer Victory Bull., v.4, n.10, p.4, Oct. 1978.)
	70;88%	113		" metast.		
	30;91%	62		liver		
(Sponsors: J. Roscoe Miller, MD; Dean, Med. School & President, Northwestern U. Board of Trustees, U. Ill. Ill. State Legistlature. 17 US Senators: Paul Douglas, William Langer, William Proxmire. 37 US Congress-persons. Howard Shuman, Pres., Oxford Union, Oxford U. Dr. Miles Robinson, MD, U. Penn. Med.; & Faculty, Vanderbilt U. Med., (see 11.3). Dr. Stanley P. Reimann, Dir., Lankenau Cancer Inst.)	23;94%	177		pancreas		
	29;91%	286		stomach	Stevan Durovic, MD, Asst. Prof. Med., U. Belgrade; Chief, Dist. Public Health Service; Yugoslavia.	(Congress. Rec., v.109, part 10, p.12914, July 18, 1963.)
	22;81%	115		melanoma		
	75;75%	22		myeloma		
	27;75%	340		lung		
	" as %	4,000		cancer mix	225 MD's in USA. 3,000 MD's in world	
	36%	5,000	objective improvement	hopeless, terminal, cancer	John Pick, MD, Ass't. Prof. Surg., U. Ill.; Head, Dept. Plastic Surg., Columbus Hosp., Chicago; Honor, John Howard Org.	Congress. Rec., v.109, part 11, p.14498, Aug. 7, 1963.
	54%		arrest of tumor growth			(Congress. Rec., v.109, part 18, p.23611, Dec. 6, 1963.)
	10%		no gain or worsening		Louis Krasno, MD, Ill. St. & AMA Awards; Dir. Med. Res., United Airlines.	
	64%	mice, C3H: treated: 100	free of tumor, 8 weeks	breast ca., spontaneous	WFP Phillips, MD, St. Francis Hosp., Evanston, Ill.	Ivy, Observ. on Kreb..., Fig.1.
	45%	control: 100				
17.2.1 CARCALON. Naturally found in all cells (esp. RES). Inhibits cancer, & multiplication of repaired cells. (See 13., & 15.2.1)	5%	mice	tumor: vanish	cancer		Ivy Cancer News, v.10, n.3, p.3, Dec. 1972; & v.11, n.4, p.1, May 1975.
	32%		smaller/ "			
	82%		stop/ " / "			
	averaged		ILS: 100% over controls			

TREATMENT (Mode, Theory)	BENEFITED, % of total, or #	TREATED, total #	MEASURE of BENEFIT	DISEASE SEVERITY	RESEARCHER, Credentials	REFERENCE, Publication
17.3 GOAT Serum, Anti-Cancer. Inject into patient protein extracted from intestinal villi of goats. (See 16.1.1, 16.4.) Species resistance to potent carcinogen.	11 in #	patients	successfully treated	cancer mix	Dr. Liborio Bonifacio & 6 MD's (with 1 Prof.), Italy. Commission appointed by Minister of Health (found cancer arrested in 31% of patients).	G. Grazzini, "Why Have Goats Conquered Cancer?", Epoca, v.72, p.46, 1969. "(In... Rome, 3 ill people...inoculated; 2 improved)", Nazime, Dec. 7, 1969. Referenced in ACS, Unproven Methods..., p.39.
	31%	patients: 16	cancer arrested			
	100%	goats: 50	resistance to severe ca. causer	benz-pyrene applied for 40 days		
17.4 ANTI-BIOTICS. Inject into patient: "Anti-vin" & "Grego-mycin" (from white MOLD of Streptomyces), against "cancer causing" bacteria/virus (which have time to develop resistant strains). Diet: Fruit; NO: meat, fat.	20%	patients: 100	entire regression, continued good health	far advanced cancer	John E. Gregory, MD, Loma Linda Med., Pasadena, Cal. (Spent $250,000 & 20,000 hrs. on ca. research, including Electron Microscope).	Nat Morris, The Cancer Blackout, p.100.
	80%		subjective improvement			
17.5 M-P VIRUS. Inject into patient (lympho-cyto-penic) virus isolated from (Ehrlich ascite) carcinoma. Causes "VIRAL INTERFERENCE" & stimulates immunity; destroys cancer (evidenced in pathology/histology studies of humans); does not kill normal cells.	averaged	patients: 22	remission, 17 months	terminal cancer	Norman Molomut, PhD, Bact., Columbia U. (Assoc. Bacteriologist, Dept. Med.); Pasteur Inst.; Dir., Biol. Lab., NY; Dir. Res., Waldemar Med. Res. Found., NY; Major, US Air Force; NCI grant. Morton Padnes, PhD, Protozo., NYU; Lab. Officer, US Army; Protozo. Res. Collabor., NY Aquarium; Dir. Dev't., Protista Res. Lab. Dr. H. E. Webb, St. Thomas Hosp., London. A. Gale Borden, MD. (Frank Rauscher, Dir., NCI: In "mouse leukemias... there is evidence that an oncolytic virus can trigger an animal to produce INTERFERON (see 9.6.4 & 17.7), which attacks tumor produced by oncogenic virus".)	JNCI, v.34, n.3, p.403, Mar. 1965. Lancet, 1, p.366, Feb. 13, 1965. "Virus... Fighting Ca.", Medical World News, v.10, p.19, Sept. 26, 1969. "Inhibition of a Transplantable Murine Leukemia by a Lympho-cytopenic Virus", Nature, v.204, n.4962, p.1004, Dec. 5, 1964. ("Viral Inhibition of Mouse Leukemia", Lancet, v.1, n.7381, p.366, Feb. 13, 1965.)
	6 in #	patients	tumor shrinks	cancer mix		
		mice, Balb/C strain:		lymphoid leukemia injected: 500 cells		
M-P Virus (1 day after low dose leukemia), treated:	55%	9	survival, free of leukemia cells			
No M-P Virus, control:	0%	56				
No leukemia injection, control:	0%	15				
M-P Virus (hi dose leukemia); no survival; treated:	averaged	60	ILS: 37%	500-5 million cells		
M-P Virus (same time as ca. inject.; (hi dose: worse)); treated:	90%	10	survival, free of cancer cells	Ehrlich Ascites inj.: 500-5000 cells		
No M-P Virus, control:	25%	12				
M-P Virus (12 days after transplant cancer in), treated:	averaged	mice, C3H strain: 120	tumors 43% smaller than control's	mammary carcinoma transplant		"Inhibition of...Tumors by the M-P Virus", Nature, v.208, n.5014, p.648, Dec. 4, 1965. All referenced in: ACS, Unproven Methods..., p.155.
No M-P Virus, control:		100				
M-P Virus (intra-peritoneal, at 6 mos. age), treated:	100%	mice, female, AKR strain: 21	survival, (suppress leukemia)	leukemia, spontaneous		
No M-P Virus, control:	39%	28				
17.6 VACCINE from cancer to cure cancers. Proteo-lytic & lactic ferments. Potassium. NOVOCAIN (Pro-caine; see 2., & 14.17).	100%	human: 1 (MD experiment on her-self)	cured ((continued))	no cancer 1st; gave self baso-cell. epithel-	Dr. Clara Jolles Fonti, Italy, Pres./V. Pres./Dir. of 6 internat. med. assoc., honor. of 3 med.	Fonti, "Neue Forsch...", Med. Klin., v.49, p.180, 1954; & Ezio-patogenesi del Ca.,... Giornale d'Italia, Jan. 1951.

TREATMENT (Mode, Theory)	BENEFITED, % of total, or #	TREATED, total #	MEASURE of BENEFIT	DISEASE SEVERITY	RESEARCHER, Credentials	REFERENCE, Publication
"Micro-colorer after Fonti", sold by Bayer. VIRAL cause of cancer.		(continued)		-ioma, (3 independent biopsies)	Prof. Avv. Mario Palladini. Prof. Kukowka, E. Germany.	Referenced in ACS, Med. Affairs Dept., May 20, 1963. (Herbert Bailey, <u>GH3....</u>)
17.7 INTERFERON, made by cell infected by virus, travels to other cells, preventing their infection by same or unrelated virus. (See 9.6.4, 17.5)	31%	patients: 16	remission, partial	breast ca.& metastases	ACS, & 10 Med. Centers in USA	"The Big IF in Cancer", <u>Time</u>, March 31, 1980, p.60.
	50% 25%	treated: 44 controls	survival, 5 year	osteogenic sarcoma & Surgery	Hans Strander, Karolinska Inst., Stockholm	
(Lympho-blast-oid Interferon contains cancer causing virus.)	50% 41% 60% 55%	total: 38 17 10 11	positive results	advanced ca.: breast myeloma lymphoma	Dr. Jordan Gutterman, MD Anderson Tumor Inst. Houston	(Robert Mendelsohn, (see 10.18) "Update on Interferon", <u>Public Scrutiny</u>, v.<u>3</u>, n.7, p.12, Aug. 1980.)
17.8 LINCOLN. Inject(/oral/nasal spray) into patient (each 2 days) BACTERIO-PHAGE virus causing fever. Each virus specifically seeks & destroys a different strain of Staph. Aurius (bacteria that destroy patient's tissue, including red blood cells, causing emboli). (Chronic swollen membranes protect bacteria from viral attack.) US License #299. Staphage Lysate.	95%	patients: 65	completely relieved, apparent cures	chronic degenerative disease (some ca.)	Robert E. Lincoln, MD, Boston U., inventor, mech. heart pump, Harvard U. A. Ernest Mills, MD, Tufts U. Stuart Mudd, MD, PhD, Pres. Int'l Assoc. of Microb. Sci.	Nat Morris, <u>Cancer Blackout</u>, p.103. (<u>Mills</u>, "Present... Lincoln...", <u>NEJM</u>, v.<u>253</u>, n.24, p.1090, Dec. 15, 1955.) R. Erickson, <u>Cancer Treatment....</u>, p.54. (<u>Is Cancer Cureable?</u> Health Research, p.80. ACS, <u>Unproven Methods...</u>, p.195. <u>Congressional Record</u>, v.<u>97</u>, part 5, p.6486, June 13, 1951; & Feb. 11, 1952; & v.<u>99</u>, part 12, p.A5350, Aug. 3, 1953)
		25 million doses	safety of treatment	disease mix	Dr. Edna Follensby, Dept. Bact., Boston U. Med. W. G. Workman, Chief, Lab. Biol. Cont., NMI, NIH. (Dr. Matthews, McGill U. Med. Isaac N. Frost, MD) US Senator Chas. Tobey.	
17.9 GLOVER. Inject into patient serum from blood of horses injected with a PLEO-MORPH micro-organism. Pleomorph isolated as a bacilli, yet in virus phase, is in each cancer cell nucleus; co-cause of cancer. (Similar to Dr. William M. CROFTON's "microbial antigens" taken from patient's blood/urine & killed & injected back into patient to stimulate anti-bodies.- 7th International Cancer Congress, July 1958.)	majority	patients: 237	responded favorably, significant rate of recovery,	cancer mix, 200 cases: biopsy confirmed (100 biopsies at National Stomach Hospital)	Dr. Thomas J. Glover, <u>Studies</u> approved by Comm. of US Surgeon Gen. & National Advisory Council; St. Michael's Hosp., Toronto, Canada. Dr. George McCoy, Director, Hygiene Lab., USPHS, Bethesda, Md. Michael J. Scott, MD, Creighton U., FACS. J. L. Engle, MD, NIH. Tom Deaken. J. E. White, MD. (Wm. M. Crofton, MD, MB, BCh, BAO, all with Gold Medal, Catholic U.; FRSM; Lect., Path., U. College; Steeven's Hosp.; Dublin)	Glover (& Engle), <u>Studies in Malignancy</u>. Phila <u>No. Amer.</u>, June 4, 1924. Phila. Clinical Soc., speech, "The Etiol. of Cancer... Serum". 4 articles by/on Glover in <u>Canada Lancet & Practice</u>. <u>J. of Cancer</u>, (<u>Dublin</u>), v.<u>3</u>, p.18. <u>Public Health Report</u>, v.<u>48</u>, p.319, Mar. 31, 1933. (<u>Crofton</u>, <u>Therapeutic Immunization.</u>) Referenced in: N. Morris, <u>Cancer Blackout</u>, p.66; Dick Ericson, <u>Cancer Treatment...</u>, p.99, 107, A-11; ACS, <u>Unproven Methods...</u>, p.67, &79.
		50	" , 14 year follow up			
(Florence Nightingale: "Diseases are not... in classes (species)... but... growing out of one another." Pasteur found microbial species to undergo many transformations, per his co-worker, Dr. Dulaux. Both in Hannah Allen, <u>Don't Get Stuck</u>, p.14, 18.)						

TREATMENT (Mode, Theory)	BENEFITED, % of total, or #	TREATED, total #	MEASURE of BENEFIT	DISEASE SEVERITY	RESEARCHER, Credentials	REFERENCE, Publication
17.10 LIVINGSTON. Inject into patient killed germs grown from same patient's own urine. Germs are PROGENITOR CRYPTO-CYDES, a PLEO-MORPH changing form & size from virus like to bacteria & back. Germs are in Actino-mycetales order, as are: Actino-myces bovis used for Krebiozen (see 17.2), & TB & leprosy germs. Immune Stimulant. Prog. Crypto. found in: Rous sarcoma ("filter-passing" bacteria, as Rous said; lacking a cell wall), & cardio-vascular disease. Its spores only die at auto-clave for 3 days. Detected in blood by dark-field microscope; (J. Franklin Inst., v.237, n.2, p.103 (esp. p. 120-1)). Grows on copper, sugar, in diet. Creates Human(like) Chorionic Gonado-tropin. Countered by Enzymes, Acid (Ascorbic, HYDRO-CHLORIC (stomach...)), Vit.A (ABSCISSIC Acid, Dormans in plants, a Growth Inhibitor (of germ), in Sprouts, Whole Grains, Nuts, Seeds); (see: 10.6; 11.; 9.6; 9.7; 9.14; 9.5.3; 9.5.7).	60%	patients	remission, complete	cancer mix	Virginia Werthele-Caspe LIVINGSTON Wheeler, MD, NYU; BA, Vassar; 1st woman Resident, infect. dis., NYC; Assoc. Prof. Biol., Rutgers U.; Director, Lab. Prolif. Dis., Newark; Battelle Mem. Inst.; San Diego State U.; Grants from ACS, 9 others. Afton Livingston, MD, U. Penn.; Mormon Missionary; Manhat. Eye & Ear Hosp.; Kaiser. (See A.17.10) Eleanor Alexander-Jackson, PhD, NYU; BA, Wellesley; MA, Columbia; Res. Fellow, Cornell; Cancer Res. Lab., Newark; Columbia U. Med.; U. Cal. San Diego; NY Acad of Sci. Prize; 20 papers; 5 Internat'l Cong. Roy M. Allen, PhD. 8 MD/PhD's Work confirmed by Harvard U.; Herman Cohen & Alice Strampp, Princeton U. Lab.; Samuel Koide, MD, PhD, Rockefeller Inst.	Cancer News J., v.11, n.6, p. 5 (& n.5, p.14; & v.7, n.5, p. 22; & v.10, n.2, p.2). Globe ("Treatment of Neoplastic Disease: Determination of Actino-mycin (Urine, Culture) ...Aid to Diagnosis / Prognosis", J. Amer. Med. Women's Assoc., v.20, n.9, p.858, 1965; & v.11, n.4, p.120, Apr. 1956, by 4 MD's & 2 PhD's; & "Myco-bacterial Forms in Myocardial Vascular Dis.", v.20, n.5, p.449, 1965. "Progenitor Cryptocides, The Specific Pleomorphic Micro-organism Isolated from Cancer", J. Intnat'l Acad. Metabiol., v.5, p.31, Mar. 1976. Cancer Res., v. 27, p.1402, 1967. Amer. J. Path., v.27, p.736, 1951. Am. J. Med. Sci., v.220, p.638, 1950. Science, v.99, p.307, 1944; & v.101, p.563, 1945. Growth, v.18, p.37, 1954. ICRF Newsl., June 1980. Ericson, Ca. Treat...., p.97, A13.
	80%		helps			
	80%	mice: 1,200	protected	implanted tumor		
	82%	patients: treated: 62 (randomly chosen from 10,000 patients)	success (for 1-24 years after treatment start)	cancer, diagnosis by other pathologists, 17 terminal		
	(Note: ref. in: V. Livingston, The Conquest of Cancer, (Intro. by Alsoph Corwin, PhD, DSc, Prof. Chem., Emeritus, Johns Hopkins U.), p.15-18, 120.)					
		(US Senator Melcher, Nutrition & Cancer Research, Hearings, Subcomm. on Nutrition, Comm. on Agri., Nutr., & Forestry, June 12&13, 1978, p.55.)				
17.11 Universal vaccine of bacterial isolate from human breast cancer. Prevention in animals. (Also, Vit.C aids collagen; see 9.6.2)	100% / 0-8%	chickens: treated: 25 / control: 25	survival	Fowl Leukosis & Mareck's Disease	Dr. James Sawyer, Princeton U.	V. Livingston, "Treatment of ...Ca. & Collagen Disease", speech, An Int'l Symposium Conq. Ca., SD, Cal., June 14, 1980
Human Chorionic Gonado-tropin causes cancer.					Dr. Richard Lerner, Scripps Inst.	" , ref. National Acad. Sci. publ'n in press.
17.12 MARUYAMA. Inject into patient extract (protein free), from human tubercle bacilli. Non-toxic, unlike BCG (see 17.14). (Shown to stimulate interferon (see 17.7) in mice, & lymphocytes in humans, against cancer cells.)	50%	patients: tot: 108,000	positive response	terminal cancer, almost all	Dr. Chisato Maruyama, Prof.; President, Nippon Med. School; Director, Research Inst. of Vaccine Therapy for Tumors & Infect. Dis. Keishiro Fujita, MD. Tohoku U. Med. Japan.	Choice, v.5, n.3, p.6, May, 1979; & v.6, n.1, p.19, Spring, 1980. " , & 16 reports in Jap. Cancer Therapy Cong., 1979. Maruyama, at An Int'l Symp. Conq. Ca., SD, Cal., June 14, 1980.
	50%	16,306				
	50%	1,408	" , treated 3-14 years			
	10.4%	23,647	survival, 5 year	advanced cancer		
			(continued)			

TREATMENT (Mode, Theory)	BENEFITED, % of total, or #	TREATED, total #	MEASURE of BENEFIT	DISEASE SEVERITY	RESEARCHER, Credentials	REFERENCE, Publication
	16% 47%	patients: 2,474	tumor vanish "/ survival, 3 years	terminal cancer	Maruyama (continued)	XI Internat'l Cancer Congress, Oct. 1974, Florence, Abstracts, v.1, p.307-8, 311; ref. in Cancer Victory Bull., v.1, n.4, p.1, April 1975.
	100%	10	rapid improvement	cancer, non-terminal	Dr. Chariton Tylliankis, Govt. Insur. Clin., Athens, Greece.	
	33% 35% 50%	24	objective regression respond: effectively very " / "	terminal cancer	Arthur Sakamoto, MD, Englew, Colo. John B. O'Keefe, MD, Glendive, Mt.	"Clinical Exper.-Maruyama Vac.," Proc. Amer. Soc. Clin. Oncology 1976, Abstract, #C-251; ref. in Ericson, Cancer Treatment, p.113.
17.13 BCG (bacille Calmette Guerin) injected into patient's tumor. BCG: dried, live strain of Mycobacterium tuberculosis variant Bovis; potent immune stimulant; (caution- can promote ca.; rare?)	91% 55% 25% 58%	patients: treated controls treated	regress initialy survival, 3½ years benefit	melanoma	Dr. Don. Morton, UCLA Med. (Dr. Sol Roy Rosenthal; Pasteur Inst.; Prof. Preventive Med., U. Ill.; IIT Research Inst., Chicago.)	Rosenthal, speech at An Internat'l Symposium, Conquest of Cancer, Livingston Wheeler Found., San Diego, Cal., June 14, 1980. J. Glassman, The Ca. Survivors, p.213.
17.14 HADLEY. Inject under skin of patient, an antigen extract from killed Bacillus Cereus/ Mycoides cultured from a human cancer. Causes immune reaction, except in far advanced cancer & leprosy. PREVENTS 75% of cancer deaths, 6 years after injection, compared to 1 year after.	50% 0.17% 0.68% 0.00%	humans: 8,354 4,001 treated "control" 15,000	prevention, in death rate years after injection: 5-6 yrs. 0-1 yrs. (prevents 75%) 1-15 yrs. (prevents 90+%)	disease mix deaths per year from: cancer leukemia	Henry G. Hadley, MD, Geo. Wash. U.; Cert. Amer. Brd. Internal Med.; Director, Res. Found.	"Causality & Cancer Res.", & "Statement" to US Congress, Comm. on Interstate & For. Commerce, July 28, 1965, in Pacific Med. & Surg., v. 73, p.371, Nov. 1965. 69 sources cited by Hadley ACS, Unproven Methods..., p.91.
17.15 RAND. Inject into patient, cancer cells (removed from same patient), after coating ca. cells (in vitro), with rabbit gamma globulin, glued on by benzidene. Patient's body is stimulated to make anti-bodies against cancer's haptens. To make one vaccine effective for all ca. patients, pooled ca. cells from many ca. patients. (Other supporters: US Senators Stephen Young, & Henry Jackson.) (Note: See C.17.15)	35% 65% 87% 94% 93%	patients: 600 15 16 14	improvement: objective (x-ray, blood) " / subjective remission, 1-29 months benefits, ½-11 months swift immunity to own tumor	terminal cancer leukemia cancer mix	Dr. Norbet Czajkowski, Wayne St. U., Detroit. H. James Rand, 3 yrs. U. Vienna Med.; Hon. PhD, U. Berlin; Pres. Rand Dev't Corp.; invented/donated defibrillator (re-starts heart); holds 100 patents; elected Outstanding Young Man, Cleveland; son of founder of Remington Rand Inc. Dr. J. Ernest Ayre, co-developer, Pap Test; Dir., National Cancer Cytology Ctr. 75-200 MD's in 35 clinics.	Len Guttridge, "How the US Govt. is Blocking a Cancer Cure", IACVF. A. Brown, March of Truth..., p.103. (Pageant, Dec. 1966, & Jan. 1967) Sergio De Carvalho, "Prelim. ...Neoplastic... IgG", Cancer, v.16, p.306, 1963. N. Czajkowski, Lancet, Oct. 28, 1967. ("Medical Scandal Blocking Cancer Cure" Saga, May 1968. "New Vaccine for Ca", Drug News Weekly, Dec. 26, 1966. ACS, Unproven Methods..., p.183.)

TREATMENT (Mode, Theory)	BENEFITTED, % of total, or #	TREATED, total #	MEASURE of BENEFIT	DISEASE SEVERITY	RESEARCHER, Credentials	REFERENCE, Publication
17.16 COLEY. Inject into patient killed bacteria & their TOXINS. Bacteria: (Rehleisen's) Streptococcus Pyro-genes, " " Erysipelatus, Bacillus Prodigiosis, Serratia Marcescens. Best results if: patient gets FEVER over 104°F, & used often for 6 months. Causes erysipelas. Danger in "new bone forming" cancer.	22%	patients: 1,200	regression, complete	cancer mix	William Bradley Coley, MD, Harvard Med. (Honors); BA, Yale; Prof. Clin. Surg., Cornell; Attending Surg., NY Cancer Hosp.; FACS; Acad. of Med., NY St. Med. Assoc.; NY Surg. & Path. Soc.; Fel., Am. Surg. Ass'n.; Honorary FRCS. (See: A.17.16; C.17.16.) Bradley L. Coley, MD.	Nauts, Swift, & B.L. Coley, "A Review...", Acta Medica Scandin., v.145, Supll.1-103, 1953, (& Cancer Res., v.6, p.205, 1946.) Amer. J. Surg., v.4, n.2, p.188. Chandler et.al., Amer. Surg., v.31, p.443, 1965.
	20 in #	patients	survival: over 20 years	inoperable, confirmed diagnosis		
	10 in #		1-20 "			
	237 in #		cures			
	22%	170 (some Surg. & Radio-Therapy)	well, 5-30 years	sarcoma of long bone		W. B. Coley, Archives of Surgery, v.13, n.6, p.780-836; Dec. 1926; & v.14, n.1, p.63-141, Jan. 1927.
(Ca. Res. Inst.'s Sci. Advis. Council: (Med. Dir.:) Lloyd Old, MD, V. Pres., SKI. Robert Good, MD, PhD, Pres., SKI. Geo. Klein, MD, DSc, Head, Inst. Tumor., Karolinska Inst., Sweden. Geo. Mathé, MD, Dir., Inst. Ca. & Immuno., Villejuif, France. R. T. Prehn, MD, Dir., Jackson Lab., Maine. M. G. P. Stoker, MD, FRS, Dir. Res., ICRF Lab., London. Otto Westphal, MD, DSc, Head, Max Planck Inst. Immun., W. Germany. 39 MD/PhD/DSc's total. Mary Lasker.)	47%	896	survival, 5-80 years	majority hopeless, all histol. proven	Helen Coley Nauts, found. & Exec. Dir., Cancer Res. Inst.; compiled 385 sci. articles by others.	R. Ericson, Cancer Treatment..., p.53. N. Morris, Cancer Blackout, p.57. ACS, Unproven Methods..., p.61.
	100's in #	patients	cured	hopeless cancer	(Predecessors: William Busch, MD, Bonn; & Dr. Tuffier, France.) Dr. Edward Hazer, Harvard Med. Dr. Moses Tendler, Yeshiva U. Alois Nowotny, PhD, Temple U.	Cancer News J., v.13, n.2, p.4. June 1978.
	26%	34	objective benefit	cancer		Johnston, "Clinical Effects of Coley's Toxins", Cancer Chemo. Reports, v.21, p.19-68, 1962. (Cancer, v.27, p.524, 1971.)
	21%		less pain			
	50-80%	mice	tumors gone	cancer		NY Ca. Res. Inst. booklet.
17.17 FEVER. Prevents ca. No cancer near malaria infested Pontine Swamps in Rome, until swamps drained; then cancer rose to average incidence.		populace of Pontine Swamps	prevents cancer 100%	malaria infested	Paavo Airola, PhD, ND.	Cancer: Causes, Prevention, & Treatment; The Total Approach, p.24.
			ca. incidence rose to average	swamps drained		
17.18 FEVER. Prevents ca. Pneumonia, typhoid, (acute), prevent ca.; TB, Syph., Immuniz., (chronic) cause ca.		patients	95% never had fever, (acute), disease	cancer	Percy, ref. by: O. Cameron Gruner, MD, Leeds Inst.; McGill U., Montreal.	Gruner, An Interpretation of Cancer, p.10, & 22.
17.19 Vaccination causes cancer, (by introducing filth, & precluding fever). ("Cancer (is on) vaccinated arms exactly where the poison was applied." -Dr. E. J. Post, in Health Research, Is Cancer Curable, p.10.)		patients: 200 (circa 1909)	100% were vaccined for other disease	cancer	W. B. Clark, MD. (Robert Bell, MD, Brit. Ca. Hosp. Forbes Laurie, MD, Med. Dir., Metro. Ca. Hosp., London.	Eleanor McBean, The Poisoned Needle, p.41, ref. NY Press Jan 26, 1909. (Hannah Allen, Don't Get Stuck, p.67, ref.
	80%	patients	caused by vaccin./inocul.	cancer deaths	Herbert Snow, MD, Surg., London Ca. Hosp.	J. W. Hodge, MD, The Vaccination Superstition.)
17.20 THYMUSIN. HORMONE stimulating patient's IMMUNE System (Thymus).	28%	patients: 21	survival, free of ca., 2 years	lung ca., small cell	NCI	Healthwise, v.4, n.3, p.2, Mar. 1981, ref. to Science 81, v.2, p.73, 1981.
	average		ILS: 87%			
17.21 Imexon, drug stimulating patient's Immune System.	60%	60	survival, 1 year	terminal ca., $\frac{1}{4}$-$\frac{1}{2}$ yr. left	Dr. Michael Micksche, Inst. Ca. Res., U. Vienna	Ericson, Ca. Treatment..., p.42. NY Times News Service.

TREATMENT (Mode, Theory)	BENEFITED, % of total, or #	TREATED, total #	MEASURE of BENEFIT	DISEASE SEVERITY	RESEARCHER, Credentials	REFERENCE, Publication
18.0 CHEMICALS 18.1 Active FREE RADICALS in non-isolated arranging of CARBONYL to ETHYLENE BONDS. Of carbon compounds: open chain (GLY-OXYLIDE, di-form-aldehyde PEROXIDE), or cyclic (PARA-BENZO-QUINONE, Benz-aldehyde), Vit. C, Anti-biotics, (see 9.6; 10.11; 17.4). Functional Carbonyl Group's (=C=O) DOUBLE BOND MOBILE ELECTRONS are a catalyst, to: Oxidize & DE-POLYMERIZE (by chain reaction), pathogenic/parasitic GERMS, breaking them into good germs. Germs' firmly bound amine groups block Carbonyls. Carbonyl's activity depends on molecule it is in. More active Carbonyls are used in more dilute (10^{-12}) distilled water solution, clinically, to avoid cancer breaking down faster than body can eliminate it. Carbonyl is found in Pau d'Arco (see 14.18). Patient's cure is cyclic. Symptoms from action of germs as they polymerize (grow), show now in reverse order, ending in fever of initial acute stage, as germs de-polymerize (break). HOMEO-PATHIC dose & response. Patient's DIET- EAT: Fresh, Organic, Whole, Fruit (banana, apple, sugar cane, watermelon), Veg. (Green Leafy, carrot, beet, cabbage), Grain, some Legume, all washed well. Juice Fast & Enema (1% sea salt) to first remove germs in crypts & diverticulae of bowels. Dandelion, Camomile, Potassium Iodide, to deter Sulfhydryls (which bind & block Free Radicals, Iodine, Selenium, Vit. A (in retina)).	0.097% 0.068%	populace of Detroit: circa. 1920 " 1923	rate change (many treated) 20% drop	cancer death rate, annual	William Frederick Koch, MD; PhD, Prof. Chem. & Histol., U. Mich. Med.; Prof. Physiol., Wayne St. U.; Pathologist, Women's Hosp., Detroit; lauded in JAMA editorial for sparing para-thyroid from surgical removal (caused tetany); nephew to Robert Koch, Nobel Laureate in Med.	W. F. Koch, The Survival Factor in Neoplastic & Viral Disease, p.27-34, 209-211, & 255-256. (Koch, Medical Record of NY, Oct. 30, 1920. Congressional Record, v.94, part 6, p.7232, June 7, 1948)
	0.097% 0.131%	Los Angeles: circa. 1920 " 1923	(controls) 30% rise			
	75%	patients: 12	cured, 4 officially witnessed	advanced cancer, biopsied		Koch, Neoplastic & Viral Parasitism, p.36.
	46% 72%	patients of other MD's	cured	non-terminal		Koch, The Survival..., p.210. (Koch, Cancer J. (Phila), Oct. 1924)
	99%	patients: 100	non-failure	disease (ca., polio)	Federal Court testimony in Detroit.	Cancer News J., v.14, n.3, p.4, April 1979.
	29%	72	survival, up to 14 years since start treatment	ca., many hopeless	Dr. J. W. Kannel, Surg., Ft. Wayne, Ind.; testimony at Cancer Comm. of Ontario. (& Dr. H. M. Candlish)	Newsreal, n.4, p.20. (Suzanne Caum, Cancer Cures Crucified.)
	to: 80%		recovery 20 yrs., some	advanced cancer	(4,000 MD's in USA used Koch's. 600 world MD's offered testimony for Koch, 60 called to witness stand.)	J. Amer. Med. Soc., Editorial, Sept. 27, 1913, ref. in:
	500,000 in #		complete	ca. /fatal allergies		
	87%	400+, in Belgian Congo	successfully treated in 2 months	leprosy	Dr. J. Maisin, (see 10.11), praised: "Koch's formula (as) a very important step in medicine... likely to change the whole picture of medicine & pathology". (US Senator William Langer.) (Chas. Mayo, MD, of Mayo Clinic, sent a hopeless ca. patient to Koch.)	The Koch Remedy for Cancer, Borderland Science Res. Found.
	100%	10	cured in 3 days	polio, acute		Koch, The Survival..., p.29. (Detroit Times, Feb. 6 to Mar. 12, 1943; & Detroit Free Press, Feb. 10 to Mar. 19, 1943; both praise Koch cure. A. Fitz Roy Anderson, The Koch Trial,... Argument for Investigation Into Organized Medicine.)
	100%	2	" in 18 mos. (leg 1½" longer)	" , chronic		
	80%	10	cured in: 36 weeks	syphilis, chronic		
	100%	20	6 weeks	rheumatic fever		
	82%	144	27 weeks	arthritis, hypertrophic		
	97% 52%	mice: treated: 50 control: 40	prevention up to 147th day	benzpyrene induced cancer	Intern'l Cancer Res. Inst.; Louvain U., Belgium. ((continued))	Koch, The Survival..., p.255.

TREATMENT (Mode, Theory)	BENEFITED, % of total, or #	TREATED, total #	MEASURE of BENEFIT	DISEASE SEVERITY	RESEARCHER, Credentials	REFERENCE, Publication
18.1 (continued) Eat NO: Animal protein (except yogurt); NO: Peanuts (high argnine), Yeasts (high di-amine), Grapes (tartaric acid robs body of Minerals, esp. Calcium), Citrus, Asparagus (high methyl-mercaptan), Spices, Pepper, Coffee, Tea, cooking in Aluminum (see 9.3.5; 9.3.6; 9.12; 12.1.5; 12.2.3; 13.3). Although Sulfhydryl & Amines, from high protein in colon, block Free Radicals, this can be averted by Cyanide, (see 10.12). NO polluted water, (Fluorides, Sulfides, Selenium see 7.1.1; 9.10.7). Guess 30% of patients break diet. Stop bad emotions, since Sympathetic nerves & Adrenals constrict capillaries, lowering Oxygen from blood. Free Radical dilution to 10^{-30}; affected by least impurities, e.g. air pollution (gas stove; see 6.). Clean old local infections in: tonsils, appendix, fallopian tubes, teeth roots. Cancer grows with no Oxygen, but is reversed with PARA-MAGNETIC OXYGEN & PER-OXIDE; Soil, Magnetic Storms, Sun (spots) & rotation period of 27 days, affect it, (see 5.&6.). Unless ca. returns (periodicity 16½ or 33 wks.), SOLO INJECTION suffices.	89%	mice: (Exp't I-B) treated: 9	cancer free, 190 days	breast cancer, C57, transplant	Jackson Mem. Lab, Bar Harbor, Me. Dr. Stanley Bandeen, Louisville, Ky. (Koch lauded as "so far ahead of the thinking of his profession" by Dr. W. Dow, Pres. Dow Chem.; & "Modern Pasteur" by Dr. Hale, Dow's VP & Chief Chemist.) Koch was taught at U. Mich. by Dr. Moses Gomberg, discoveror of Free Radicals, (at U. Berlin). (Koch lauded by Dr. A.R. Mitchell, Chairman, Brd. of Trustees, AMA.)	Koch, The Survival..., p.30-4. (Petition from 25 Michigan State Legistlators to US Congress to investigate Federal Court Injunction on Koch.) (Note: Role of Free Radical ("lone electron"), in cancer was offered 40 years after Koch's thesis, by A. Szent-Gyorki, discoverer of Vit. C & P, (see 15.2.1).) (Jayme Treiger: A Folia Medica, v.44, n.1, p.9, 1962; & 2nd. Ann. Brazil. Congress on Ca., 1961.)
	averaged	control: 5	survival, 17 days			
	100%	(Exp't II-B) treated: 5	cancer free, 135 days	"		
	averaged	control: 5	survival, 16 days			
	66%	(Exp't II-C) treated: 6	cancer free, 164 days	"		
	100%	(Exp't IV-C) treated: 4	cancer free, 184 days	Sarcoma 37, inoculated		
	averaged	control: 4	survival, 34 days			
	95%	cows: 100's in Canada	cure	acetonemia	Dr. David Arnot. K.C. MacDonald, Minister of Agr.	Koch, The Survival..., p.211.
	80-90%			mastitis	Many DVM's, labs, & ranchers. U. of BC, Br. Columbia, Canada.	
	max. 96%	30,000				
	appr. 100%	10,000 in France			(Robert C. Olney, MD, FICS; Providence Hosp., Lincoln, Neb.)	Albert L. Wahl, MD, A Least Common Denominator in Anti-biotics, p.27. (Olney, Blocked Oxidation)
	20%	control				
	96%	horses: treated	recovery	swamp fever	Dr. J. J. Reid, Texas	(Wahl, Medical Forum, v.15, n.4, p.68, Mar. 1, 1947.)
	0%	control				
	84%	cattle, zebu: treated: 13		rabies (from a vaccine; 40 already died of it)	(Prof. R. de S. Lopez, Med. U., Brazil.)	Koch, Neoplastic..., p.25,
	0%	control: 7				
	80-90%	dog: treated: 200	", of total function	paralytic distemper	Army Hosp. for small animals, Rio de Janeiro.	", p.28. (Colombo & Carneiro, Veterinaria, v.4, n.1, p.21, 1950; & v.5, n.1, p.75, 1951.)
	0%	control	survival			
18.2 FOSSIL 18.2.1 CLAY (Minerals, Antibiotic; see 7.2; 9.3; 9.10; 9.11; 12.). Volcanic Ash solution to: drink, enema, douche, & external pack. (Clay ABSORBS TOXINS; has OXIDASES, Enzymes; kills Staph A, Strep, E. Coli.)	97%	British Army, treated	survival	cholera	(US Testing Co., Hoboken, NJ; antibiotic test; Dr. Howard E. Lind)	Hanna Kroeger, Old Time Remedies for Modern Ailment, p.18.
	40%	control				
	many	patients	cured	cancer	La Granja Health Ranch, (PO Box 92), Puerto Cabezas, Nicaragua	(Michel Abehsera, The Healing Clay, p.18, 21, 31.)
18.2.2 CHARCOAL. Absorbs Toxins.	"	"	"	"	"	

TREATMENT (Mode, Theory)	BENEFITED, % of total, or #	TREATED, total #	MEASURE of BENEFIT	DISEASE SEVERITY	RESEARCHER, Credentials	REFERENCE, Publication
18.2.3 PETROLEUM, distilled, boiling point under 150°C; best from Poland. Special process. (Most of Modern drugs are from Petro-chemicals)	20,000 in #	patients	grateful correspondents	cancer, many diseases	Paula Ganner, Voels, Tyrol, Austria; (see C.18.2.3)	Gero Haupt, 3 articles in 7 Tage magazine, 1961(?), ref. in ACS, Med. Affars Dept., Statement, Feb. 25, 1972.
Crude Oil: (See A.18.2.3).	all	patients	cured	ca., not too far gone	William A. Rockefeller, (& sons)	Griffin, World Without Cancer, p.329.
18.3 DMSO (DI-METHYL SULF-OXIDE). Solvent, crosses body membranes easily (carrying other chemicals). Local analgesic, relieves pain & inflammation, dilates blood vessels. DMSO is to plants, as Vit. C is to (collagen of) animals, holding cells together.	aver-age	mice	ILS: 100%	at least 7 different ca. models	Dr. Charlotte Maddock & Dr. Morris Green, Children's Ca. Res. Found., Bos.	Pat McGrady, Sr., The Persecuted Drug: The Story of DMSO, p.54-5, & 287, ref. to: G. E. Moore, Lancet, v.1, n.7971, p. 1238, June 5, 1976. (CBS-TV, 60 Minutes, Mar. 23, 1980.)
		patients, few	completely destroyed meta-stases	solid tumor metastases	George E. Moore, MD, PhD, U. Minn.; head of Roswell Park Mem. Inst., Buffalo.	(McGrady Sr.: ACS Science Editor, & Science Writers' Seminar originator; author, The Savage Cell.)
(Sponsors: US Senator James McClure; US Congress-persons Mary Rose Oaker, Steve Symms, Larry J Hopkins, Robert B. Duncan, Claude Pepper: "70% of...veterinarians ...used(DMSO), 95% of(whom) claimed(it) was effective".) (Note: G. E. Moore used DMSO & DNCB.)					Stanley JACOB, MD, cum laude, FACS, Harvard Med, Prof. Surg., Phi Beta Kappa, Markle Schol., Kemper Schol. of Amer. Coll. Surg., U. Oregon Med. Dr. Harold Brown, Pres., Aerospace Med. Assoc. (See A.18.3) (M. von Ardenne (see 4.1; 10.20.5)) Dept. Surg., U. Colo.	4 international symposia (auspices: NY Acad. Sci.; U. Vienna); 1000 articles on DMSO. (If Horses Can- Why Can't You?, ICRF, Aug. 1980.) (M. v. Ardenne, "Selektive Krebs...", Arch. für Geschwulst. Band 33, Heft 4, p. 331, 1969.)
Inject into patient DMSO & a dye (Haematoxylon, "H"); both transported into tumor, killing its inner cells. SYNERGY with Orthodox therapy.	70% 38% 6%	patients: (Orthodox &DMSO&H): 37 (DMSO&H): 37 (Orthodox): 37	improvement	cancer mix, pre-terminal	Eli J. Tucker, MD, Tulane U., USA. A. Carrizo, MD, Dir., National Cancer Control & Ca. Ctr., Panama.	"Haema...DMSO...Neoplasm", Internat'l Surg., v.49, n.6, p.516, June 1968. ACS, Ca-A..., v.21, p.386, 1971.
18.4 HYDRAZINE SULFATE. Orally taken. Inhibits patient's wasting (of energy & muscle) in Gluconeo-genesis. (Gluconeogenesis is patient's response to Lactic acid from tumor Glyco-lysis; this Lactic acid, bad for heart (slows it), can be reduced by Lactic acid in diet (see 12.1.2), or Vit. B-1, (& B-6, for pain, weakness in limbs). Benefits in hours, for some patients.	50-75% 65% 12% 44% 2%	patients: 2,500 225	good results reversal of cachexia regression, max. shrink: ½ "/ tumor stable, 3-6 mos. minor side effects	cancer mix " ", late stage	Joseph Gold, MD, Dir., Syracuse Cancer Res. Inst., NY. Dean Burk; Harvard U.; USDA; Prof., Cornell U.; Domagk prize for Cancer Res.; Knight (Mark Twain; & Command. Med. Order of Bethlehem); (see 1.2.2; 7.1.1).	(Oncology, v.22, p.185, 1968; v.24, p.291, 1970; v.27, p.69, 1973.) National Enquirer, Feb. 3, 1974. Spotlight, July 2, 1979, p.6. (German Soc. Med. Tumor Therapy, Baden-Baden, Nov. 3, 1973.) (Harris, Vitamins in Theory & Practice, p.65; ref. in Lee Found., Reprint #6.)
Effective in a very deadly tumor model, in animals. (See A.18.4).	aver-age	rats	ILS: 133% tumor shrink in size by: 98%	Walker 256 Ascites Carcino-Sarcoma	Dr. Michael L. Gershanovich, a Director, Petrov Res. Inst. of Oncology, Leningrad, USSR	"Cancer Cachexia & Gluconeo-genesis", Ann. NY Acad. Sci., v.230, part 1, p.103, Mar. 18, 1974.

TREATMENT (Mode, Theory)	BENEFITED, % of total, or #	TREATED, total #	MEASURE of BENEFIT	DISEASE SEVERITY	RESEARCHER, Credentials	REFERENCE, Publication
18.5 Aspirin, Anti-Coagulant, in high dose. Prevents implanting of circulating cancer cells, in animals. (Side-effects: inhibit Interferon; deplete Vit. C; bleed stomach (if ulcers); thicken new-born's arterioles; Reye's Syndrome)	60%	mice: treated: 10	free of cancer spread to lungs	breast cancer cells inoculated into host mice	Dr. Gabriel Gasic, U. Penn. Med.	(See 11.1.2)
	10%	control: 10			Dr. James Kolenich, Cleveland Metro. Gen. Hosp. (Interferon- Duke U.)	((Interferon), Proc. NAS, v.77, p.5437, 1980.) ("Reyes...", Chicago Tribune, Jan. 4, 1981, p.1.)
18.6 Balloons, sterilized, inserted in bladder, filled with salt water, pinching blood vessels to tumor for 7 hours, killing tumor.	55%	patients: 20	excellent results, tumor pieces urinated out	bladder cancer	Dr. Robin Glashan, Royal Infirmary, Huddersfield, England.	
18.7 HYPO-TONIC INJECTION of sterile, DISTILLED WATER, intra-muscular, at varying sites away from spine. Causes cells to burst from osmotic pressure, releasing contents.			cure?	cancer	John T. Stephens. (O. Cameron Gruner; see B.3.5; D.16.4; book lists 152 HOMOEOPATHIC, (of 252 tot.), ca. therapies).	Arlin Brown, March of Truth on Cancer, p.20; (p.113; ref. to: Gruner, A Selected Materia ... Therap. ... Inoperable Ca.)
19.0 GRAVITY (See Exercise 3., Heat 4.1, (& 5.7)						
19.1 Relieves congestion & pressure of body fluids in higher part of body (e.g. lungs, in congestive heart failure), & supplies blood to lower (as in Heat, see 4.). Need blood to brain in shock. Slant board/bed, reclining rocker.	91.7%	patients: treated: 81 (armchair)	survival, 2 weeks (prevented 40% of deaths)	acute coronary thrombosis	Samuel A. Levine, MD; Harvard U. Med.; Peter Bent Brigham Hosp., Boston.	"The Myth of Strict Bed Rest in the Treatment of Heart Disease", Amer. Heart J., v.42, n.3, p.406, Sept. 1951.
	86.2%	control: 138 (bed)			" & Bernard Lown, MD. USPHS Grant.	"'Armchair' Treatment of Acute Coronary Thrombo.", JAMA, v.148, n.16, p.1365, Apr. 19, '52.
20.0 TIME, CHRONO-BIOLOGY						
20.1 Body varies with daily (diurnal, circadian), monthly (lunar), yearly (solar; see 5.) cycles. Affects body's reaction to therapy. (ASTRO-LOGY)					Emanual Revici, MD, Sci. Dir., Inst. Applied Biol., NY.	Leading Edge Bull., v.1, n.6, p.2, Dec. 1980.
					C. Pittendrigh, Stanford U. Chas. Ehret, Argonne (ANL) Wm. Hrusheski, Masonic Ca. Ctr., U. Minn.	Let's Live, Feb. 1981, p.113.
21.0 MUSIC, SOUND, NOISE						
21.1 Infra-sonics, very low frequency (below 20 cps) sounds, cause stress (see 2.8; 4.7).		Chicago	cause auto accidents, absenteeism	heavy infra-sonics	Dr. Floyd Dunn, U. Illinois. (John Green, Bell Tel.) (NASA)	E. Cheraskin, MD, & W. M. Ringsdorf, DMD, Psycho-dietetics, p.133.
22.0 MAPPINGS OF BODY						
22.1 ACUPUNCTURE. Enhances Immunity. Normalizes Glands. (A System of body maps (1 to 1, onto (?)) another System.	100%	patients: 4	improvement	ca.: terminal	(Young S. Kim, PhD; Physics Dept., Ohio St. U.) (William A. Tiller, PhD; Chairman, Materials Sci. Dept., Stanford U; Guggenheim Fellow, Oxford; 100 articles.)	Amer. J. Chinese Med.: v.3, n.3, p.302, 1975; "A Summary of Research... Effects of Acupuncture", v.3, n.4, p.377, 1975. (B. Jensen, The Sci. ... Iridology.) Amer. J. of Acupuncture, v.4, n.1, Jan. 1976.
		1	some success	lung		
		1		bowel		
To detect: (e.g. IRIDOLOGY: Iris links to retina by nerves; then to brain, body).		1		womb		
	50%	2	positive response	post surgery		
To treat: Polarity, Zone Therapy, Reflexology, Acupressure, Moxibustion; see 2.1)	1 in #	1	remission, 4 yrs.	esoph. & metas.		

TREATMENT (Mode, Theory)	BENEFITTED, % of total, or #	TREATED, total #	MEASURE of BENEFIT	DISEASE SEVERITY	RESEARCHER, Credentials	REFERENCE, Publication
APPENDIX A APPENDIX A A.2.0 SPIRITUAL, MENTAL, etc. A.2.0.1 SPIRITUAL HEALING			APPENDIX A		APPENDIX A RELIGIOUS MESSENGERS TO WORLD	APPENDIX A Bible, Koran, Religion Texts Everywhere.
A.2.1.1 SKIN CONTACT. Pre-mature babies gained $\frac{1}{2}$ oz./day more lying on sheepskin (see 6.2) than on synthetic fiber.	averaged	patients:	weight gain: $\frac{1}{2}$ oz./day over controls	pre-mature babies	(Ashley Montagu; Chair, Anthro. Dept., Rutgers U.; Prof. Anthro., Princeton U.)	TV
A.2.1.2 MASSAGE. Avoid tumor.						
A.2.5.3 Hypnosis alters immunity: Delayed Hyper-sensitivity: Immediate Hyper-sensitivity: (See 17.)					Stephen A. Levine, MD, PhD, article in Price-Pottenger Nutrition Found. Bull., v.5, n.4, p.25, 1980.	Brit. Med. J., v.6, p.1649, 1963. Jap. J. Med. Prog., v.50, p.451, 1963. Folia Psychiatr. Neurol. Jap., v.17, p.16, 1963.
A.2.8.1.3 Loss. Depresses immune surveillance. 7.2x as much loss (of central relation, up to 8 years prior), in cancer patients, than others in psycho-therapy.	72% 10%	patients: 400 control	preventable by attitude on loss: 62% (=72%-10%) ?	loss, despair, before: ca. mix psycho-therapy	Lawrence Le Shan, PhD, Chief..., Psycho.... Ca., Trafalgar Hosp.; Res. Assoc., McDonnell Found.	Edit., "Cancer... Mind:... Connected?", Science, v.200, p.1363, June 23, 1978.
A.2.9 PSYCHE assessed, 3 months after surg.; ca. not yet biol. affect psyche(?). Denial of ca., Fighting Spirit: Stoic Acceptance: Helpless, Hopeless: Fighters had 2x survival of Stoics.	 75% 37% 20%	patients: fem., 69 tot. 20 32 5 57 tot.	survival, no recurrence, 5 years (after surg.)	breast ca., Stage I & II, & simple mastectomy & x-ray (25 treated)	S. Greer, Dept. Psycho. Med.; T. Morris & K. Pettingale; Human Studies in Cancer, King's College Hosp., London	"Psychological Response to Breast Cancer: Effect on Outcome", Lancet, v.2, n.8146, p.785, Oct. 13, 1979.
A.2.10 MEDITATION. Complete Commitment. 3 months, at 2 hours /day.	100%?	patient: 1	can eat, exercise; relieve pain	carcinoma, 2 breasts, path. proof, meta-stasis	Ainslie Meares, MD, DPM; author, Relief Without Drugs; Melbourne, Australia.	"Regression of Cancer After Intensive Meditation", The Med. J. of Australia, v.2, n.5, p.184, July 31, 1976.
A.2.11 PERSONAL EFFORT to change LIFESTYLES to defeat cancer, only 10-25% of patients are ready to make.	10-25%	patients	ready for personal effort to defeat ca.	cancer mix	Jean Kohler, Prof. of Music, Indiana	
A.2.12 PSYCHIC BREATHING. Pranayama. (See 3.; 6.)	100%?	patient: self	cure	cancer of spine	Dr. Patel, FRCS, Dean, Fac. Med., Nagpur U., India	
A.3.0 EXERCISE A.3.1 Only Light Exercise, even 8 months after (Gerson, see 9.2) therapy started. Heavy exercise causes return of cancer.					Charlotte Gerson Straus (see: 9.2; C.9.2)	IACVF, "Midwest Health Seminar", Chicago, May 2, 1981. (Ca. Res., v.35, n.11, part 2, p.3339, Nov. 1975)
A.3.2 CHIRO-PRACTIC / OSTEO-PATHIC. (See 2.1; A.2.1). Adjust posture to aid flow to/fro organs, through nerves/vessels (pinched between vertebrae/ribs/joints).	many	patients: women	relieved by un-pinching vein	breast swelling	Albert T. Hunt, DO	"&...It Isn't Cancer", Health Res., Is Ca. Curable?, p.103.

TREATMENT (Mode, Theory)	BENEFITED, % of total, or #	TREATED, total #	MEASURE of BENEFIT	DISEASE SEVERITY	RESEARCHER, Credentials	REFERENCE, Publication
A.5.0 ELECTRO-MAGNETIC RADIATION (E&M) A.5.1.4 SUNSHINE prevents internal cancer, but causes skin ca. Co-factors: Fresh Ocean Spray & Breezes, vs. Navy food & chemicals.	.0116%, .0133%, ann. int. ca. deaths	US Navy matched populace	prevented internal ca., by: 12.7%	cancer (no skin, lip) annual deaths	Sigismund Peller, MD; Dept. Biol., School of Hyg. & Public Health, Johns Hopkins U.; & its Chas. S. Stephenson, Commander, MC; Bur. Med. & Surg., US Navy.	Amer. J. Med. Sci., v.194, n.3, p.326, Sept. 1937.
A.5.1.5 Prevent skin cancer from sun, by diet: high in Anti-oxidants (Vit. A, C, E, Selenium), & low in oil, so ca. causing free radicals are not formed from oil; (no: suntan lotions) (See 9.6.1; 9.7.3; 11.2; A.9.6.1)	47% 20%	mice, hairless, albino treated: 61 control: 56	(prevention by B-CAROTENE); free of skin ca. over (4mm)^3	artificial light, ultraviolet, cause: skin ca. (squamous)	John H. Epstein, Clin. Prof. Derm., U. Cal. Med., San Francisco. NIH Grant.	Zane R. Kime, MD, MS, Sunlight Could Save Your Life; ref. to Photochem. & Photobiol., v.25, n.2, p.211, Feb. 1977.
A.5.1.6 ARTIFICIAL LIGHT A.5.1.6.1 Lamps, (light cut-off at 3100Å & shorter), therapy. (Note: Sunshine is best at: high altitudes, morning & evening.)	90% 55% 92% 64%	rabbit: treated: 10 control: 9 treated: 12 control: 11	survival	cancer inoculate bone metastasis	Louise Pierce, MD, & C. M. Van Allen, MD, Rockefeller Inst. & Dr. Wade Brown	"Influence of Light on... a Transplantable Neoplasm...", J. Exp. Med., v.45: n.3, p.483, Mar. 1927; & n.4, p.727, April 1927.
A.5.1.6.2 Lamp, UV, therapy. (Sun prevents non-skin cancer by raising: Blood Oxygen, Stress Tolerance, Sex Hormones, etc.-Z.R. Kime; see A.5.1.5)	59% 20%	mice, breeding female: treated: 17 control: 15	free of (a non-skin) cancer	breast ca., spontaneous	F. L. Apperly & M. K. Cary, Dept. Path., Med. College Va., Richmond	"The Deterrent...Light Upon ...Cancer...", Brit. J. Exp. Path., v.23, n.3, p.133, June 1942.
A.5.4.1 Underground Radiation, & Water Crossings, cause "Cancer Houses", with more ca. cases than chance. Total # of ca. cases (5348), packed in fewer houses (2108); (190 cases in houses with 10 or more cases each).	99%	city of Stettlin (control?)	found under ca. patients' home	underground radiation & water crossings	Dr. Heger, MD, Germany. (Prof. Dr. F. Sauerbruch, see 9.2). Alexis Carrel, "world's first" successful vascular surg., (see 16.1.2). Ernst Hartman, MD, Pres., German Inst. Geo-biol., 124 articles, (see 5.4). 6 other famous MD's.)	J. Natural Health & Parapsychology, March 1981, p.36.
A.5.5.1.1 Of 10 counties with most stomach ca., 8 counties have damp soil. Of 10 counties with least stomach ca., 8 counties often have dry soil. (See 5.5; 17.17)		English counties: 10 10	stomach ca. rate: highest lowest	% of counties with damp soil: 80% 20%	Dr. G. W. Griffith	Medical Press (Brit.), ref. in: Fry's, Cancer Folio #1.
A.5.7.1 Short wave E&M re-balances pituitary's growth hormones. Thyrotropic: speeds growth, is in Eosinophils, & causes cancer. Gonadotropic: slows growth, is in Basophils, & causes benign tumors.	50% 80%	patients	stop tumor growth, improve patient saved	cancer: advanced, Stage IV distant meta-stasis Stage III	Jules Samuels, MD. Francis P. deCaux, MD. 50 MD's globally. Prof. D. Kobak, Chicago; Chief Editor, Arch. Physical Therapy, X-Rays, & Radium.	Arlin Brown, March of Truth on Cancer, p.68.

TREATMENT (Mode, Theory)	BENEFITED, % of total, or #	TREATED, total #	MEASURE of BENEFIT	DISEASE SEVERITY	RESEARCHER, Credentials	REFERENCE, Publication
A.6.0 AIR A.6.1.1 Negative Air Ions, 6,000/cc, start on day of transplant: " & CALCIUM LACTATE: Only Calcium Lactate: (Ca. cell surface is less negative.)	aver-aged	rats: treated control treated control	tumor size, (at 4 wks; cc): 6.5 12.5 2.7 9.9 10.4	carcinoma transplant (175 G)	W. H. Eddy, et. al., Southern Bio-Research Lab., Fla. So. College, Lakeland, Florida.	"The Effect of Negative Ionization on Transplanted Tumors", Cancer Research, v.11, n.4, p.245, April 1951. (Fred Soyka, The Ion Effect, p.76.)
A.6.3.3 Hyper-Baric Oxygen (HBO). HBO & Radiation: Only Radiation: Only half of patients fit for radiotherapy, were fit for HBO PRESSURES.	 56% 27%	patients: treated: 51 control: 52	survival, 4 years	cancer, head & neck	Dr. J. M. Henk, Royal Marsden Hosp., London; Dr. C. W. Smith; both of South Wales Radiotherapy & Oncology Service, Cardiff, Wales.	"... HBO in... Cancer", Lancet, v.2, n.8029, p.104, July 16, 1977.
A.6.4.1 (continued) High % Oxygen air through tube to nose; 36 hours total, over 12 weeks.				cancer	M. von Ardenne, developer, Soviet A-Bomb, (see 4.1; 6.4; 10.20.5). 50 European Clinics.	J. Natural Health & Parapsychology, Jan. 1981, p.37.
A.6.5.1 Hydrogen Peroxide, 0.3% solution.	aver-aged	mice	cancer gone in 1-2 months	cancer	Dr. Reginald Holman, Cardiff, Wales.	Father Richard Willhelm, "A Progress Report on Cancer Research".
A.6.8 Riboflavin, Niacin, PANTO-THENIC Acid, (Vit. B-2, 3, &5), to bring Oxygen to cancer cells. (See 6.4; 9.3.3; 10.6).		patients?	prevention/cure	cancer	Dr. Otto Warburg, Nobel Laureate twice, in Med.; Dir., Max Planck Inst. for Cell Physiol., Berlin.	
A.7.0 WATER A.7.1 DRINKING A.7.1.1.1 Fluoridation causes ca., (& mongolism, tooth mottling, bone disease, mouth ulcers, enzyme loss, etc.) Rinse for kids.	16% to 27%	49 cities, pop. over 10,000, in Ontario	excess cancer deaths due to drinking water fluoridation, (% of tot. ca. deaths)	cancer	Victor A. Cecilioni, MD, Hamilton, Ontario, Canada (U.S. Congressman James J. Delaney.) (12 Nobel Laureates.)	Voice of Med. Freedom, May 1981, p.6; ref. to Vital Statistics... Ontario. (John Yiamouyiannis, "Lifesavers Guide to Fluor.".
A.7.1.1.2 "Fluorides (F) are general proto-plasmic poisons.... Sources of F intoxication are drinking water...1ppm or more of F,...insecticidals..., superphosphate ... fertilizer."-JAMA.	50% 0%, almost	pop. of a city, age 24-41	any teeth remaining free of caries	1.6 to 4.0 ppm F in drinking water	M. C. Smith & H. V. Smith. (Spotlight, Mar. 7, 1977; (Sep. 28& Oct. 12, p.14; Nov. 16, p.32; Nov. 30, p.27,) 1981.)	JAMA, v.123, n.3, p.150, Sept. 18, 1943. Am. J. Public Health, v.30, p.1050, Sep. 1940; ref. in: J. Amer. Dental Assoc., (v.20, p.1137, July 1933; &) v.31, n.19, p.1360, Oct. 1, 1944.
A.8.0 FASTING A.8.1 HUMAN A.8.1 Fasting followed faithfully.	4 in # averaged	many 1,000's	splendid results	cancer disease	Charles C. Haskell	Upton Sinclair, The Fasting Cure, p.147.
A.9.0 NUTRITION, GENERAL A.9.1 OVERVIEW A.9.1.1.1 Of 91 cancer MD's polled, 34% said Nutrition had a major effect on patient.					USGAO poll at NIH Clin. Ctr., Harvard, U. Penn., M.D. Anderson.	USGAO, HRD-79-46, Enclosure I, p.3, in Report to US Senator George McGovern, Jan. 22, 1979.
A.9.1.5 Nutrition affects immunity.	averaged	mice: strain	doubles total lifetime		Dr. Robert Good, Pres. & Dir., Mem. Sloan Kettering Ca. Ctr.	Nutrition Health Review, Winter 1980, p.8.

TREATMENT (Mode, Theory)	BENEFITED, % of total, or #	TREATED, total #	MEASURE of BENEFIT	DISEASE SEVERITY	RESEARCHER, Credentials	REFERENCE, Publication
A.9.5.8 Vegetable juice (strained thru linen), ¼ to 1 liter/day; savor it. Herbal tea. Sauerkraut juice. No solid food, 42 days. NO ALBUMIN in diet, so body consumes albumin of ca. cells, by Auto-lysis. Auto-suggest.	in #: 1,000	patients	cured	cancer mix	Rudolph Breuss, Bludenz Vorlberg, Austria; (treated 1,000 of the 10,000 total).	Cancer Victory Bull., v.7, n.4, April 1981.
	10,000		regained health	disease mix		
	100%	28	cure, in 6 days, able to work	leukemia (portal vein)		& n.5, p.2, May 1981.
A.9.6.1 (continued) (High Protein nulls benefit of only Fruit, Veg., (& Vit.C) diet.) Vit.C, (9.6% of) "lab food", & no Fruit & Veg.: treated. (Low dose Vit.C oddly increased ca., (due to Mental?; see 2.1, & A.2.1.1)).	prevent 85% of ca.	mice, hairless: treated: 50 (& control) (total: 900)	suppression of lesions/mice, by 35x	skin ca. (squamous), spontaneous, from uv light (see 11.2; A.5.15)	Arthur B. Robinson, (see 9.6.1) (Slightly high cancer at low dose Vit.C due to statistical noise.-Richard Peto, Com. of Biostatistics, IARC; Radcliffe Infirmary, Oxford, Eng.)	Barron's, Sept.3, 1979, p.7. (Linus Pauling Inst. Newsletter, v.1, n.12, Summer 1981; ref. to: Walter Cronkite, Universe, CBS-TV; & Proc. 3rd. Internat'l. Symp. on Vit.C, Sept. 1980.)
A.9.6.5 Vit.C (Note: See C.9.6.5.)					Irwin Stone, PCA, FAIC; pioneer in Vit.C as preservative & leukemia therapy; Member, Sigma Xi, NY Acad. Sci., AAAS, AAOAC, Amer. Inst. Chem.; Sr. Amer. Chem. Soc.; 120 articles.	The Healing Factor, Vit.C Against Disease. 60 scientific articles. "... Ascorbate in the Control of Leukemic...", Ca. Control J., v.2, n.1, p.1, Jan. 1974. 25 US Patents.
A.9.7.5 CROCETIN, of Carotenoids (includes Vit. A). Saturated in solution, injected into (ca.'s) host, & applied topically (on tumor). Diffuses Oxygen. Non-toxic.	averaged	chicks: treated: 9 control: 9	survival, days: 27.1 17.4 (ILS: 55%)	Rous sarcoma injected	J. L. Gainer, PhD; D. A. Wallis; J. R. Jones; U. Va., Charlottesville, Va.	"The Effect of Crocetin on Skin Papillomas & Rous Sarcoma", Oncology, v.33, n.5, p.222, 1976.
	free of ca.: 67% 20%	mice: (Swiss Webst.) treated: 10 control: 10	tumors/mouse, at 40 days: 0.58 5.6	skin papillomas (caused by DMBA)		
A.9.9.2 Vit.E. (Caution: Adriamycin is very toxic.) Vit.E & Adriamycin: (See 1.1.2) Only Adriamycin:	85% 15%	mice: treated control	survival, 1 month	cancer	NCI	Public Scrutiny, v.1, n.2, p.17, March 1, 1978.
A.9.10.6 MACRO-BIOTIC. BALANCE body YANG (from: animal protein, root, cooked, alkaline, compress; cause Sarcoma), & YIN (from: sugar, citrus, fruits, raw, spices, chemicals, acid, expand; cause Carcinoma, Leukemia). Treat by diet of WHOLE Grains (50-70% of tot.), Legumes (10%), Veg. (25-35%), Seaweed (5%; see 15.1); from same climate as home; SPECIALLY COOKED. No animal food. Anti-Yin: more cooking, grains; no nuts/fruit. Anti-Yang: 33% raw veg., few nuts, few fruit (sun dried/cooked), more legumes. Chew well to change pH. Exercise, Climate, Physique. Ginger/Taro Packs on tumor.	over 10 in #	patients	cure	terminal cancer	Georges Ohsawa Michio Kushi Anthony J. Sattilaro, MD, Pres., Methodist Hosp., Phila.	East-West J.: v.7, n.3, Mar. 1977; v.8, n.1, Jan. 1978; v.8, n.7, p.64, July 1978; v.11, n.3, Mar. 1981. East-West Found., A Dietary Approach to Cancer. Naboru Muramoto, Healing Ourselves.

TREATMENT (Mode, Theory)	BENEFITED, % of total, or #	TREATED, total #	MEASURE of BENEFIT	DISEASE SEVERITY	RESEARCHER, Credentials	REFERENCE, Publication
A.9.10.7 SELENIUM. Oxygenates. Affects thrombosis, meta-stasis; prevents ca./death. In Garlic, some Brewer's Yeasts; NOT IN DEPLETED SOILS. (See 11.1.2; 12.1; 13.4)	averaged	patients of 28 countries	prevention (1/1,000 due to chance)	death from ca. of: breast, prostate, intestine, rectum	(Daniel Medina, PhD; Prof., Baylor Med.)	Advances Experim. Med. Biol. v.91, ch.22, p.323, Table 3. (Med. Clin. No. Amer., v.60, n.4, Symp. on Trace Elements, p.745 (p.754-5).)
Excess/inorganic is toxic.	high%'s	animals	prevention	cancer	very many researchers	(Richard Passwater, Amer. Lab., June 1973, p.16)
A.10.0 NUTRITION, LAETRILE A.10.5 (continued) 70% of patients in his book, are alive & well 3½ years after printing book.	70%	patients: treated: 90	alive & well, over 3½ years, to 6 years	terminal cancer mostly	John Richardson, MD & Patricia Griffin, RN, U. Mich.; BS. (Note: see 10.5)	Richardson Newsletter, v.1, n.7, 1979. IACVF, "Midwest Health Seminar", Chicago, May 2, 1981. Laetrile Case Histories.
A.10.13 (continued) Laetrile more effective in ca. of: lung, colon, rectum; than: lymphoma, melanoma.					M. Soto, MD	FACT J, v.2, n.7, p.5. (See 10.2)
A.10.21 Laetrile, 30-70g./24 hr. day, constant, intra-venous. Goat's liver (see 16.1.1; 16.4; 17.3) converts analog of Laetrile in Apricot Leaves.	averaged	patients: treated: 60	significant results, tumor shrinks, skin metastases gone	cancer	David Rubin, MD, Hadassah U.; Israeli Med. Res. Found.; (articles in: Oncology; Path. & Microbiol.)	NHF Bull., v.23, n.11, p.16, Dec. 1977.
A.10.22 Laetrile		patients			S. M. Jones, MS, PhD; MD, Stanford U. Med., Cal.	Nutrition Rudiments in Cancer.
A.10.23 Laetrile (DL, synthetic, degraded), Intravenous, 8g/day:	100%	patients: treated: 6	non-toxic	cancer, beyond hope; & very damaged by Orthodox Therapy	Charles Moertel, MD, & 3 MD's, 2 PhD's, Mayo Clinic. NCI Grants. " & SKI; UCLA; U. Ariz., Tucson.	JAMA, v.245, n.6, p.591, Feb. 13, 1981. (Choice, v.6: n.1, p.1, Spr.; n.2, p.1, Sum.; n.3, p.2, Fall; 1980. Spotlight, May 18, p.8; May 25, p.3; 1981. Public Scrutiny, v.3, n.7, p.2 & 10, July 1980. Choice, v.7, n.2, p.1, 8, Sum., 1981.)
" , Oral, ½g, 3x/day:	100%	" 6				
" " & Raw Almonds:	50%	" 2	nausea			
(No aids to Excrete ca. toxins. Vit. A not emulsified to bypass liver. Vit. C dose 1/100 optimal. Pancreatic, but no Proteolytic Enzymes.)	20%	" 156	survival, 8 months, (low dose Laetrile after 1st. 3 weeks)			
Initial, hi dose, i.v., Laetrile: (70% of patients stable until dose lowered)	70%	" 163	cancer arrest, stable, 3 weeks			AMF, Voice of Med. Freedom, July 1981, p.1; Spotlight, Aug. 17, 1981, p.10.
A.11.0 NUTRITION, ENZYMES A.11.7 Enzymes & Minerals, various pH, injected into patient to normalize blood (pH imbalance precipitates salts from protoplasm, changing colloids, & cell reproductive cycle, (from 8 to 2 phases)).	40% 25% 90%	patients	remission pain relief	cancer: stomach lung mix	Dr. Juan Nicolini Mena. Xavier Farias, MD (UCLA)	Arlin Brown, March of Truth on Cancer, p.72. (LA Times, Oct. 11, 1955.)
A.11.8 LYSOZYME, muco-lytic enzyme, anti-biotic. Found in tears, saliva, nasal mucos, milk. Extracted from egg white. Better ca. cure than Interferon, it was combined with in tests on patients; (see 17.7).		patients: 150			Sir Alexander Fleming, Nobel Laureate, discoveror of penicillin; & lysozyme, to cure cancer. Dr. E. O. Bierman, & O. E. Lobstein, PhD; St. Eliz. Hosp., Lafayette, Ind.	Bierman, JAMA, v.170, n.15, p.1842, Aug. 8, 1959. Ericson, Cancer Treatment, ..., p.116. Spotlight, May 11, 1981, p.26, ref. to Oncology News, Aug. 1980, John Steinbacher, & his Ca. Fed.

TREATMENT (Mode, Theory)	BENEFITED, % of total, or #	TREATED, total #	MEASURE of BENEFIT	DISEASE SEVERITY	RESEARCHER, Credentials	REFERENCE, Publication
A.12.0 NUTRITION, ANTI-BIOTIC A.12.1 CULTURES A.12.1.5 YEAST A.12.1.5.5 Glucan from cell wall of Saccromyces Cervisia yeast; Glucan: (Ca. cause; see 9.2; 9.3.2; 9.5.6), Saline: Glucan: (Ca. cause; see 9.10.4; 9.10.5), Glucose: Glucan: Glucose:	averaged	rats: treated: 42 control: 42 treated: 10 control: 8 treated: 9 control: 7	tumor weight (g) 4.6 10.1 1.0 4.2 .38 1.26	ca. cells implanted: leukemia adeno-carcinoma melanoma	Drs. Nicholas Di Luzio, J. A. Cook, W. Browder, Dept. Physiol., Tulane U. Med. E. O. Hoffman, Dept. Path., LSU Med. P.W.A. Mansell, Dept. Surg., Royal Victoria Hosp., Montreal, Canada. (See: 12.1.5.5).	Ericson, Ca. Treatment, p.86. "Glucan Induced Enhancement in Host Resistance", Progress in Ca. Res. & Therapy, v.2, Control of Neopl. ...Immune..., p.475, Ed. by: Michael Chirigos, PhD, Asst. Lab Chief, Lab RNA Tumor Virus, NCI.
A.12.1.5.6 Glucan injected into tumor; activates Macro-phages within walls of abscess; leaves pus, but no bacteria; non-toxic.	100% 100%	patients: treated: total: 9 3	tumor shrank, much necrosis, in 5 days. ", 100% gone	lung adeno-squam. carc., breast carc., melanoma ", smaller	Mansell & Di Luzio (see A.12.1.5.5). H. Ichinose, R.J. Reed, E.T. Krements, R. McNamee NCI Grant	JNCI, v.54, n.3, p.571, Mar. 1975.
A.12.2 PLANTS A.12.2.1 MUSHROOM (Fungi) A.12.2.1.4 "Devil's" Mushroom, from Pyrenees Mountains. Slows supra-renal gland.	100% averaged averaged	animals: treated control humans: treated: 9	success survival, 20 days immunity stable, remission	Sarco-matose 180 lymph ca., 3 mos. left	Dr. Florencio Segura, U. Cordoba, Buenos Aires, & 4 MD sons.	Fry's, Cancer Folio #1.
A.12.2.4 FUNGI. Anti-cancer Anti-biotics isolated from SOIL Fungi (see 12.1.5.1). Refining active substance may remove others (naturally found at the source), PROTECTIVE against side-effects. 7 isolates used in Chemotherapy, toxic (see 1.2).						
A.12.2.4.1 "Myco-rrhizal Fungi surround rootlets, & stimulate metabolism as a living Fungus Bridge which connects soil & sap."		patients	injured by synthetic fertilizer (& bio-cides)	disease from depleted soils	James A. Shield, MD, Ass't Prof. Neuropsych., Med. College Va., Richmond, Va.	"Farm Practices Influencing the Incidence of Multiple Sclerosis", So. Med. J., v.40, n.1, p.55, Jan. 1947.
A.12.2.4.2 CHAGA, a fungus, "benign tumor" on birch tree; not killing tree. Taken orally as tea.	averaged	patients	improve whole body defense	cancer	Prof. Sergei Sergev, Dir., Getsen Cancer Inst., Moscow	(Alexander Solzhenitsyn, Cancer Ward, p.133-4, 141-2, 227-8.)
A.12.2.4.3 MO-ER, "Tree Ears", is a fungus on trees in China; eaten in Szechwan bean curd. (See 11.1.2)	averaged	patients	slows blood clotting; (& meta-stasis?)		Dr. Dale E. Hammerschmidt, U. Minn. Med.	Organic Consumer Report, v.60, n.52, Dec. 23, 1980.
A.14.0 NUTRITION, HERBS A.14.4.1 Plants, Egyptian. Of 8 Species (from 8 Families), 3 (or 37.5%) had anti-tumor activity.	averaged	mice	anti-cancer activity	Ehrlich ascites carcinoma	M.M. El-Merzaban; et. al.; NCI, Cairo U. Fac. Pharm, Alexandria U. Acad. Sci. Res. & Tech., Egypt	Planta Medica, v.36, n.2, p.150, June 1979, many more, in Lloydia.
A.16.0 ANIMAL EXTRACTS A.16.1 CELLULAR THERAPY; harms in infections, inflammations, toxic-osis, (i.e. contra-indications).	averaged	patients	rehabilitated	damaged: liver, thyroid, bone marrow, plasma	Anthony Schenk, MD, PhD (Dr. Kuettner. Prof. Dyckerhoff.)	Cancer Forum, v.4, n.5, p.5.

TREATMENT (Mode, Theory)	BENEFITED, % of total, or #	TREATED, total #	MEASURE of BENEFIT	DISEASE SEVERITY	RESEARCHER, Credentials	REFERENCE, Publication
A.17.0 IMMUNOLOGY A.17.1 (continued) De-Blockers. (Beaty:"I believe this is...the single best frontier in cancer therapy today.") (Note: See C.& D.: .17.1)	50%	patients: treated:20	regression, shrink tumor	cancer, advanced	Burton & Friedman(cont'd) John Beaty,MD; Prof.,Columbia U.Med. (John J.Harris,MD; Robert Kassel,MD;both,SKI.) (Dr.R.J.Clement,President, Bahamian Med. Assoc.)	Ralph Moss, The Cancer Syndrome,p.194.
A.17.3 (continued) Cancer cells in vivo grow by fusion, not by division (as in vitro). Food, transforms to red blood cells, to white blood cells, to bone marrow & body cells; reversed on fasting (see A.9.10.6).					Kieichi Morishita, MD, & Ass't. Prof. Physiol., Tokyo Med. U.; Technical Chief, Tokyo Red Cross Blood Ctr. (Prof. Halpern, French Acad. of Med. 3 MD's)	The Hidden Truth of Cancer.
A.17.6.1 Inject into patient washed ca. cell sediment, after ca. was taken from another patient & irradiated.	100%	patients: treated:2 female	clinical cure, 3 years	cancer of ovary & metastases	Philippine Hartman, gynecologist & surgeon	Ericson, Cancer Treatment, p.108, (ref. to: 10th Int'l. Ca. Congress; much unpublished)
A.17.10 (continued) Purified antigen (from Progenitor Cryptocides) & Vit.A, & Abscissic Acid (10 mg).	97%	mice	inhibition	tumor	Livingston (continued) (see 17.10)	Natural Food & Farming, v.27,n.15,p.3,Sept. 1981.
A.17.16 (continued) Coley's Toxins. Regeneration of bone. (For effective bacterial virulence, need QUALITY CONTROL of its production.)	79% 87% 65% 100%	patients: treated: 19 38 20 13	survival, 5 years	ca.: bone, giant cell: inoperable operable ca.: breast: inoperable operable	Coley (continued) (see: 17.16; C.17.16)	Ralph Moss, The Cancer Syndrome,p.98;
Double Blind; Coley' Toxins: Fever inducing placebo:	26% 3%	treated: 34 control: 37	tumor shrunk, spread less	cancer	Barbara Johnston,MD,head, med. onc.,St. Vincent's,NY	" ,p.101-2.
A.18.0 CHEMICALS A.18.2.3 (continued) Kerosene, pure, non-African. Kills if taken too long.	some	patients	healings, permanent	ca.: liver, gall bladder, esophagus, stomach	(Dr. Juraj Koerbler, Zagrab, Yugoslavia)	J. of Natural Health & Parapsychology, July 1981, p.48.
A.18.3 (continued) DMSO,& Laetrile,& Vit.C, intravenous & topical. DMSO kills free radicals, forms stable coordination complexes with metals (chelates; see 10.14 to 10.17). DMSO from wood pulp mfg.	100% 100% 100%	patients: 1 1 1	tumor shrink ½ return to normal life	melanoma ca.: tongue, (1 week left) ca.: brain, (hopeless)	MD's, Surgeons (Dr. Charlotte Friend, famous virologist) (Nova U., Ft. Lauderdale) (Dr. Peter Camp, UC San Diego Med.)	Archie Scott, Voice of Medical Freedom, AMF, July 1981, p.4; (Dec.1980,p.13; Jan. 1981, p.3; Mar.1981, p.1; Apr.1981, p.1, 14).
A.18.4 (continued) Hydrazine Sulfate.					(100's of MD's in US)	Ralph Moss, The Cancer Syndrome, p.163-7, (ref. to 25 articles). Joseph Gold, MD, Nutrition & Cancer, Gio B. Gori (Ed.; see 9.1.1), v.1, n.4, p.4.

TREATMENT (Mode, Theory)	BENEFITTED, % of total, or #	TREATED, total #	MEASURE of BENEFIT	DISEASE SEVERITY	RESEARCHER, Credentials	REFERENCE, Publication
APPENDIX B APPENDIX B			APPENDIX B		APPENDIX B	APPENDIX B
B.2.0 SPIRITUAL, MENTAL, etc.						
B.2.0.1 SPIRITUAL HEALING. PRAYER: before:	70%	cows, Holstein:	free of TB for next 20 years	tuberculosis (TB)	Dr. Kelso Glover. (Cows tested by 3 govt. inspectors)	Demos Shakarian, The Happiest People on Earth, p.78.
after:	100.0%	1000				
B.2.1 CONTACT, SOCIAL & PHYSICAL. 50 mice/cage, Crowded:	71%	mice, female, DBA :100	free of cancer	spontaneous breast cancer	O. Muhlbock	Acta IUAC, v.7, p.351, 1951; ref. in Richard LaBarba, PhD, "Experiential & Environmental Factors in Ca.; a Review of Research With Animals", Psychosomatic Med., v.32, n.3, p.261-2, May 1970; ref. to Ca. Research, v.22, p.597, 1962.
1 mouse/pot, Isolated:	16%	100				
B.3.0 EXERCISE						
B.3.3 Exercise wheel, treated:	57%	98				
No " " , control:	33%	103				
B.3.4 Exercise, treated:	several	rats, male, Wistar	total regression	Walker 256 ca. cells injected into rats	SA Hoffman, et. al.	
			tumor weight: 2.3 grams			
Isolated, no " , control:	averaged		66.9 grams			
B.3.5 EXTRA-CELLULAR FLUID carries nutrients & waste between blood, cells, lymph. Tidal; flows by MUSCLE ACTION, water fluid balance (SWEAT, bathing); disease if flow blocked.					O. Cameron Gruner, MD, McGill U., Montreal (see 18.7; & D.16.4)	An Interpretation of Cancer
B.4.0 HEAT B.4.5 (continued) Ca. cells, acidic by lactic acid, so, more sensitive to heat. Heat not fight leukemia.	80%	patients, treated: 245	subjective improvement	cancer (Note: see 4.5)	D. Cole; Cornell Med.; SKI; NCI; Assoc. Prof. Surg., NYU Med.; (see 4.5).	NFA, Natural Food & Farming, v.27, n.16, p.16, Oct. 1981. Public Scrutiny, Nov. 1981, p.12.
B.4.8 Red hot irons.		patients	control	cancer	Ramajama, 2000BC, India. Hippocrates, 400BC, Greece.	The Evanston Review, Dec. 3, 1981, p.100.
B.5.0 ELECTRO-MAGNETIC RADIATION (E & M) B.5.1 Sunlight. Heals skin.					Niels Finson, Nobel Laureate	NFA, Natural Food & Farming, v.27, n.18, p.4, Dec. 1981.
B.6.0 AIR B.6.1 WEATHER. HUMIDITY, PRESSURE, TEMPERATURE; ALTITUDE, LATITUDE. Less air filter of sun, on Equator, & Mountains (less Air Pollution). See 4., & 5. (A, B, & C).					Dr. O. Harflinger, Dir., German Weather Service. Dr S. W. Tromp, Dir., Netherlands Bio-meterological Research Ctr.	Biosocial, J. Behavioral Ecology, v.2, n.9, p.1, 1981. Bernard Jensen, DC, ND, The Science & Practice of Iridology, p.343-5.
B.8.0 FASTING B.8.1 HUMAN. (Used by: Pythagoras, Hippocrates, Celsus, Plutarch, Avicenna, Paracelsus.) (See A.17.3)		patients	aids: bone marrow, spleen, white blood cells	leukemia	S. Morgulis, Prof. Bio-chem., U. Neb. Med. (H.S. Langfield, Harvard U. F.M. Allen, Rockefeller Inst. F.G. Benedict, E. G. Ritzman, Carnegie Inst.)	Arnold De Vries, Therapeutic Fasting, p.5, 24.

TREATMENT (Mode, Theory)	BENEFITED, % of total, or #	TREATED, total #	MEASURE of BENEFIT	DISEASE SEVERITY	RESEARCHER, Credentials	REFERENCE, Publication
B.9.0 NUTRITION, GENERAL						
B.9.1 Diet changes & supplements: Diet changes only: (See A.2.11) Diet advice not used:	21% 4% 20%	patients: 100	non-MD's diet therapy advice	cancer	A.S. Theologides, Prof Med., U. Minn. Med.	Gio Gori, Editor, (see 9.1.1), Nutrition & Cancer, v.2, n.1, p.40, 1980.
B.9.3.7 Low Protein diet, treated: control: " " "	95% 5%	mice, inbred	free of ca. ALS: 500% over control	spontaneous breast ca. " & lung ca.	Germany (Peyton Rous, in 1913; Nobel Laureate)	D.G.Jose, MD, MRACP, FNHMRC, Nutrition Today, Mar. 1973, p.5.
B.9.6.3 Vitamin C. 30g/day max. (orally, fewer mutagens made by colon bacteria; see 2.2;&2.3). (For 9.6.1&9.6.2: Voice of Medical Freedom, v.1, n.12, p.1, Dec. 1981.)	averaged	patients	survival rate: 600% over controls' ILS: 300 days 1,440% 360%	terminal cancer " uterus " mix	Dr. Akira Murata, Saga U. (See 9.6.3) ("); Dr. Morishige / Kozan Hosp., Japan	Medical Tribune, July 22, 1981; (ref. in Today's Living, Jan. 1982, p.6; & Harold Buttram, MD, Okla. Med.; Baylor U.; Public Scrutiny, Dec. 1981, p.11).
B.9.7.6 Carrot Juice to treat ca. (Carrots have: zinc to metabolize Vit. A; Vit. B-13; fructose & an "insulin" for easy energy; Vit. C in tops.)			(Note: B-Vitamins work together; see 6.4)		Bernard Peyrilhe, Prof., Ecole Sante; Prof., Royal Col. Surg., Paris. Acad. of Lyon Prize, 1773.	Ralph Moss, Cancer Syndrome, p.183. (Arthur Snyder, Nature's Way to Health, Juice Fasting.)
B.9.7.7 Carrots have 6 anti-fungal chem.; (see: 9.7; 9.10.2; 12.0; A.12.1.5; A.12.2)					Finland	Eloise Allison, Unveiled Mysteries of Natural Healing, p.73.
B.9.7.8 Vitamin A, supplemental: Vit.A. in blood: Vit.A in diet:	50% 50% 50%	patients smokers men: 16,000 humans: 3000 smokers: 8000	reversed prevented	skin ca. cancer (of lung, stomach intestines, or bladder)	Dr. Peter Elias, UCLA Med. Scandinavia. England. Georgia, USA. Norway	Organic Consumer Report, v.61, n.6, Feb.10, 1981.
B.9.7.9 PRO-Vitamin A (CAROTENE: dark green leafies, carrots, some YELLOW & RED fruits & veg.), much in diet, prevented 85% of lung cancer. Preformed Vit.A (Retinol, from animals) had no effect.	0.4% 2.9% 0.2% 2.7%	men, middle age: 1,954 high Vit.A low Vit.A high Vit.A low Vit.A	prospective epidemiology: incidence (85% prevented) mortality (92% prevented)	lung ca., 19 years after diet evaluated	R.B. Shekelle, PhD, Prof.; & 5; Rush-Presby.-St. Luke's Med. Ctr., Chicago. O. Paul, Harvard Med. Anne Shryock, U. Mich. Nurs. J. Stamler, Northwestern U. Med.	"Dietary Vit.A & Risk of Cancer in the Western Electric Study", Lancet, v.2 for 1981, n.8257, p.1185, Nov. 28, 1981.
B.9.10.4 Refined sugar in diet coincident with (& causes) breast cancer.		populace, female	prevented by low sucrose diet	breast ca.		Brit.J.Ca., v.37, p.974, 1978; Current Concepts in Nutr., v.6, Nutr. & Ca., p.25, 1977; both ref. in: Nutrition & Cancer, v.1, n.3, p.27, Spr. 1979.
B.9.10.5 Diet: 5% fat, 68% carbohydrate, REFINED: Dextrose: (%'s by weight) Sucrose: Wheat Starch:	30% 30% 65%	rats, female, Sprag. Daw: 20 : 20 : 20	free of ca.	" " (adeno-carcin) from DMBA	Susan Hoehn, Dept. Biochem. U. Manitoba. Grant: NCI of Can. Kenneth K. Carroll, Dept. Biochem., U. West. Ontario.	
B.9.10.6 "The appetite of tumors for sugar...."					Dr. Otto Meyerhoff, U. Penn. Med., Nobel Laureate	Raymond Bernard, PhD, The Revolt Against Chemicals, p.14.
B.9.15 FOLIC ACID, (a B Vitamin); 10 mg/day, oral, 3 months. Cures dysplasia (pre-cancer?) caused by oral contraceptives.	4 in #	patients, women: 47, treated & control	regression, complete	cervical dysplasia, moderately severe	Charles E. Butterworth, Chief, Div. Nutr., U. Alab. Med. &3 MD's, (1 of NIH)	"Folate for Oral Contraceptive Users May Reduce Cervical Cancer Risk", JAMA, v.244, n.7, p.633, Aug. 15, 1980.

TREATMENT (Mode, Theory)	BENEFITED, % of total, or #	TREATED, total #	MEASURE of BENEFIT	DISEASE SEVERITY	RESEARCHER, Credentials	REFERENCE, Publication
B.9.16 CALCIUM in ca. cells is 1% of normal's; Oxygenator (see C.9.26).					Keith Brewer, donor of $½ million library; (see C.9.23.1)	Herald of Health, v.87, n.1, p.3, Jan. 1982. (See C.9.23)
B.9.17 GLUTATHIONE. Oxygen carrier non-toxic; found in food; has Sulfer (see 13.4.2, & 18.3). Bind with persistent carcinogens in ca. cells. (Rats' 16 months = 4/5 lifespan.)	81% 0%	rats, female: treated control	cancer gone survival: 4 months after treatment	liver cancer from aflotoxin (at 16 months prior to treatment)	Anna Novi, MD, magna cum laude; Temple U. Med.; USD HHS consultant; head, Dept. Path., U. Dusseldorf, W. Germany; author, 60 articles.	Dr. Lawrence F. McNamee, Spotlight, Oct. 19, 1981, p.30.
B.9.18 ANTI-OXIDANTS, in diet, (%'s by weight): Vit. E (0.2%, synthetic); Vit. C (2%); Gluta-thione (0.1%); BHT (0.5%, toxic). Prevents ca. from short uv light (mercury arc lamp).	100% 76%	mice, hairless strain: treated: 13 control: 21	free of cancer	skin cancer, squamous carcinoma, biopsy	Homer S. Black, Photo-biochem. Lab., VA Hosp.; & Depts. Derm. & Biochem., Baylor Med. Grants: NCI, ACS.	"Effects of Dietary Anti-Oxidants on Actinic Tumor Induction", Res. Comm. in Chem. Path. & Pharm., v.7, n.4, p.783, April 1974.
B.9.19 CHLOROPHYLL. Structure like heme (Oxygenates), except Magnesium instead of Iron in center; (see 5.1; 9.11; 9.14; A.6.8). In green of plants.	85%	cells in vitro (Ames test)	prevents mutation, lowers toxicity	carcinogens needing metabolic activation	Chiu-Nan Lai, Dept. Biol., U. Texas Cancer Ctr., MD Anderson Hosp. & Tumor Inst.	"Chlorophyll: the Active Factor in Wheat Sprout Extract...", Nutrition & Cancer, v.1, n.3, p.19, Spr. 1979, (Figure 1, ▲).
B.10.0 NUTRITION, LAETRILE B.10.15 (continued) Bromelain & Pancreatic Enzyme Enemas & oral.	69%	patients: 1,100	survival, 2 years	ca., mostly terminal	Dr. Bob Gibson, Ponca City, Ok. (See 10.15)	Spotlight, Oct. 29, 1979, p.16.
B.10.20.7.1 Apricot Kernels in diet. (See: 9.10.1; 9.14; 10.1; 17.10.)	90%	mice, inbred	prevention	spontaneous breast ca.	Dr. Vern van Breeman, Salisbury State Col., Md.	Cancer News J., v.12, n.6, p.10, Feb. 1978; ref. to Choice.
B.11.0 NUTRITION, ENZYMES B.11.1 RAW SOYBEANS. Has Proteolytic Enzymes, PROTEASE INHIBITORS.	56% 26%	rats: treated control	free of cancer	breast ca. from X-rays	Dr. Walter Troll	M.G. Schwartz, PhD, The Soil & Health News, R. Rodale, Ed., v.10, n.1, p.2, Feb. 1981.
B.14.0 NUTRITION, HERBS B.14.2 (continued) Mistletoe.	50%	mice	prevention	tumors	Roswell Park Mem. Inst.	R. Moss, Cancer Syndrome, p.106.
B.14.4 Herbs: 50% have genuine medical value. (See 13.1; & 14.4)		patients			Nairobi Res. Ctr. for Traditional Med.	AMF, Voice of Medical Freedom, Nov. 1981, p.2.
B.14.17 COCA (source of refined Cocaine; see 14.17).		patients	treatment	nausea, indigestion	Harvard U. (W.E. Carter, National Inst. Drug Abuse)	Spotlight, Dec. 14, 1981, p.19.
B.14.18 TREE, "tajibo", "lapacho morado", of Andes Mts. Has xyloidin: anti-biotic & anti-viral. (See 14.18) (NCI, Progress Against Ca., 1969, p.74.)	100%	patients: 3	cure, (leukocyte count of 149,000 cut to 6,500)	leukemia, hopeless; cancer mix	Dr. Theodoro Meyer, U. National of Tucuman; Dr. Pratz Ruiz, Concep., " ; Argentina (free supplies to 300 MD's)	Alec de Montmorency, Spotlight, June 8, 1981, p.6; (ref. to: la Razon, Buenos Aires, Nov. 6, 1967; & Prof. C. Burgstaller)
B.14.19 EVERGREEN bush, plumyew. (In 1535 AD, Indian gave white pine (Vit. C) & cured J. Cartier's sailors of scurvy. Europe ignored heathen remedy. J. Lind started lemons in 1747; common by 1795)	averaged	mice	ILS: 300% 200% shrink	leukemia melanoma colon ca.	USDA	NFA, Natural Food & Farming, v.27, n.17, p.7, Nov. 1981; ref. to Dallas Times Herald. (G. Edward Griffin, World Without Cancer, p.48)
	up to 80%	patients	cure, only few months follow up	leukemia	PRC (People's Republic of China)	
B.14.20 EASTER LILY. Immune & Metabolic Stimulant; dissolves tumors; (see (A. & B.) 4.; 17.; A.9.1.5).		patients	body temp. raised to normal 98.6%	ca., 96.8-97.8 °F, body temperature, all	Dr. MacCoy, & Barbara Huntington, St. John's Naturopathic Med. Ctr. Donald Clark, MD.	IACVF, Cancer News J., v.15, n.4, p.16, Win. 1981. (Ancient Chinese)

(Continued on p.151.)

CANCER QUOTATIONS COLLAGE: MEDICAL DARK AGES CIRCA 1984 ; or

P.I.G. / J.O.B. (Prejudice, Ignorance, Greed, / Jealousy, Oligarchy, Bureaucracy)

TABLE of CONTENTS for CANCER QUOTATIONS:

NOTE: Within a section of quotes, i.e. Q.#.#, each sub-section is defined by its separation from the next sub-section by a blank line. (Continued on p.131 & 168.)

CANCER QUOTATIONS COLLAGE:

(Continued on p.131 & 169.)

Q.1.0 HISTORY, CIVICS:
Q.1.1 REMEDIES' HISTORY:

"And God said, Behold, I have given you every herb bearing seed, which is upon the face of all the earth, and every tree, in which is the fruit of a tree yielding seed; to you it shall be for meat." - Genesis 1:29

"There are three things which build and maintain civilization throughout time: pure air, pure water, and pure food. And as a truth eternal I say unto you, that there are three things which bring the end of civilization, even the mightiest that have ever been and shall ever be, from the beginningless beginning to the endless end of all time: impure air, impure water, and impure food." - Zend Avesta, c. 3000 BC, (in Price - Pottenger Nutr. Found. Bull., v.5,n.1,p.25, 1980).

"... for night-blindness in the eyes: liver of ox ... is given against it. Really excellent." - Papyrus Ebers, (c. 3000-1550 BC).

"All the blood of the body is under the control of the heart & flows in a continuous circle & never stops." - Chinese writing, 2697 BC, (by O. Cameron Gruner,MD, in Independent Citizens Research Foundation, Newsletter, April 1979, p.3).

"Exposure to the sun is highly necessary in persons whose health needs restoring." - Herodotus, (484?-425? BC), (in Zane Kime,MD,MS, Sunlight Could Save Your Life, p.260).

"The cure of many diseases remains unknown to the physicians of Hellos (Greece) because they do not study the whole person." - Socrates, (470-399 BC), (in Health Research, Is Cancer Curable?, p.68).

"The great error in the treatment of the human body is that physicians are ignorant of the whole. For the part can never be well unless the whole is well." - Plato, (427?-347? BC).

"It is better not to apply any treatment in cases of occult cancer; for if treated (by surgery), the patients die quickly; but if not treated, they hold for a long time." - (Aphorism, n.38)

"Let food be your medicine, and medicine your food...."

"Natural excretion ... by ... belly, urine, sweat, sputum, mucus, the womb, haemorrhoids, leprosy, tubercles, carcinoma." -(Book on Nutriment)

"At first, do no harm." - Hippocrates, (460-370 BC).

"...an ancient Carthaginian rule (forbade) the drinking of wine by a bridal couple on their wedding night so that defective children would not be conceived." - in Thomas H. Corbett,M.D., Cancer & Chemicals,p.73.

"...Roman.... wrestlers ate only the coarse (whole) wheaten bread in order to preserve the strength of their limbs.... Hippocrates... recommended (it) 'for its salutary effect upon the bowels'." - in Ross Hume Hall,PhD, Food for Nought, p.13, referring to Sylvester Graham, Treatise on Bread & Breadmaking, circa 1837.

(Disease can be transmitted by airborne germs or by physical contact.) - Varro, 100 BC, (National Health Action Comm. Bull., Jan. 1981, p.9).

"The art of medicine is a question of timeliness: wine timely given helps, untimely, harms." - Ovid, (43BC-18AD), Remediorum Amori, 1.131

"...gourd, having a stalk..., fill it with water...,enter your hinder parts (as an enema), that the water may flow through all your bowels..., then let the water run out your body..., see...and smell...all the...uncleanesses which defiled the temple of your body.... Renew your baptism with water on every day of your fast, till...water...out of you is...pure." - Jesus, The Essene Gospel of John.

(- in Viktoras Kulvinskas,MS, Survival Into the 21st Century, p.60).

"It is part of the cure to wish to be cured." -Seneca, (4BC-65AD), Hippolytus 1.249.

(Advanced cancer is) "irritated by treatment; & the more so the more vigorous it is."

"Some have used caustic medicaments, some the cautery, some excision with a scalpel; but no medicament has ever given relief; the parts cauterized are excited immediately to an increase until they cause death."

"After excision, even when a scar has formed, nonetheless the disease has returned, & caused death; while ... the majority of patients, though no violent measures are applied in the attempt to remove the tumor, but only mild applications in order to sooth it, attain to a ripe old age in spite of it." -Celsus, (1st Century AD).

"When (a tumor) is of long standing & large, you should leave it alone. For I myself have never been able to cure any such, nor have I seen anyone else succeed before me." - Abul Qasim, (1013-1106 AD).

"It should be forbidden & severely punished to remove cancer by cutting, burning, cautery, & other fiendish tortures. It is from nature that the disease arises, & from nature comes the cure, not from the physicians." - Paracelsus, (1493-1541 AD)

- (Last 3 above, in Ralph Moss, Cancer Syndrome, p.37-39.)

"411 years lag (between) initial scientific discovery (that) rhythmic inflation of lung with positive pressure provides adequate pulmonary ventilation in animals (by) Vesalius, 1543 AD, (and the) clinical application (of) mouth-to-mouth artificial ventilation." - J.H.Comroe & R.D.Dripps, The Top Ten..., USDHEW Pub.#:(NIH)78-1521.

"Smoke... makes a kitchen also oftentimes in the inward parts of men, soiling and infecting them, with an unctuous and oily kinde of Soote as hath bene found in some great Tobacco takers, that after their death were opened." - James I, A Counter-Blaste To Tobacco, p.32; 1604 AD.

"Sugar...ingendreth...cachexias,...rotteth the teeth, making them look blacke.... And therefore let young people especially beware...." - James Hurt, Doctor, The Family Companion, 1633 AD, in William Dufty, Sugar Blues, p.77.

"...The Hellish & dismal cloud of ... Coal ... perpetually imminent over (London) ... that her inhabitants breathe nothing but impure & thick mist, ... corrupting the lungs & disordering the entire habit of their bodies; so that Catarrhs, ... Cough, & Consumption, range more in this one City, than in the whole Earth besides." - John Evelyn, 1661 AD, (in Ecology Information Group, The Breather's Guide to Invisible Air Pollution, p.1).

"Disease is nothing else but an attempt on the part of the body to rid itself of morbific matter." - Thomas Sydenham, 1624-89, (in Henry G. Bieler, MD; of Tilden - Weger - Bieler Chair of Dietetic Medicine, Columbia U. Hosp.; Food Is Your Best Medicine, p.40.

"Nearly all men die of their medicines, not of their diseases." - Moliere,(1622-72)

"He's the best physician that knows the worthlessness of most medicines."

"God heals, & the Doctor takes the Fee."

"Wouldst thou enjoy a long life, a healthy body, and a vigorous mind, and be acquainted also with the wonderful works of God, labor in the first place to bring thy appetite to reason." - Benjamin Franklin, (1706-90).

"In 1748, Virginia's House of Burgesses, with George Washington & James Madison present, passed a resolution to appoint a committee to test Mary Johnson's 'receipt of curing cancer', which consisted of garden sorrel, celandine, persimmon bark, & spring water. The report of the committee, giving the testimony of many witnesses that this concoction had cured them of cancer, was read to the House of Burgesses, & Mrs. Johnson was ... voted a reward...." - J. Brody & A. Holleb, ACS, You Can Fight Cancer & Win, p.145.

"Water, air, & cleanliness are the chief articles in my pharmacopoeia."

"Take a dose of medicine once, & in all probability you will be obliged to take an additional hundred afterward." - Napoleon Bonaparte, (1769-1821)

"Adulterations .... Addition of substances usually of greatly inferior value.... Addition of colouring matters ... to conceal other forms of adulteration.... possessing ... poisonous properties." - Arthur H. Hassall, MD, Food & Its Adulterations, Analytical Sanitary Commission of "The Lancet", London, 1855, p.A4.

"An enormous mass of experience, both of homeopathic doctors & their patients, is invoked in favor of the efficacy of these remedies & doses. But the regular profession stands firm in its belief that such experience is worthless & that the whole history is one of quackery & delusion." - William James, (1842-1910)

"...You may honestly feel grateful that homeopathy survived the attempts of the allopaths (Orthodoxy) to destroy it."

"The doctor of the future will prescribe no drugs but will interest his patients in the care and nutrition of the human frame and in the cause and prevention of disease." - Mark Twain, (1835-1910).

"Disease can carry its ill effects no farther than mortal mind maps out the way."

"... disease as error ... Truth or Mind can heal." - Mary Baker Eddy, (1821-1910)

"Treat disease through diet, by preference, refraining from the use of drugs, and if you find what is required in a single herb, do not resort to a compounded medicament." - Bahá'u'lláh

"When the science of medicine reaches perfection, treatment will be given by foods, aliments,...fruits, and vegetables, and by various waters hot and cold in temperature." - Abdu'l-Bahá

Q.1.2 UNJUSTLY PERSECUTED / CHARLATANS, HISTORY:

"One may survive the fall of a thunderbolt on one's head, but one cannot expect to escape the fatal effects of medicine prescribed by an ignorant physician."

"It is better for the person who has put on the garb of the physician to quaff the venom of the cobra or to swallow heated iron balls than to extort food, drink, or money from a man who is afflicted with disease and has sought his aid."

"It is better for the quack to offer himself up in the fire than enforce his treatment on the patient." - The Caraka Samhita, (circa 1000-500 BC), Chapter 14, p.364-5, translated by Shree Galabkunverba Ayurvedic Soc., Jamnagar, India in 1949.

"About 9 million people were executed as witches from 1479 to 1735. Most were women. Many were healers and midwives." - Gena Corea, The Hidden Malpractice, p.26.

"To protect herbalists from persecution by the Company of Physicians and Chirurgeons. Company of Surgeons in London, minding their own gain, and doing nothing for the profit or ease of the diseased, have sued, troubled and vexed honest persons (herbalist).... Said persons havé not taken anything for their pains and skill.... Surgeons have small cunning, yet they take great sums of money and do little for it." - Act of Parliament, 1512 AD, Appendix 2, Chapter 2, p.2, (from Walter Ermer, IHC (International Health Council)).

"The Answer of Richard Guy, Surgeon ... to certain insidious Falsehood and Reflections upon his Method of Curing Cancers without Cutting ... London ... 1764 AD. .... 100 Cases Successfully Treated.... Breast.... incipient Cancer... how easily in that State they are remediable by Care and proper Management;....the cancerous Humour is a Virus...the lymphatic vessels are the immediate instruments of its Circulation .... carried & lodged...to those more remote ('glands')." - Richard Guy, Practical Observations, 1762 AD, (in Nat Morris, The Cancer Blackout, p.24-5).

Q.1.3 FREEDOM of CHOICE vs. LEGAL MONOPOLY in HEALTH CARE, US:

"Unless we put medical freedom into the Constitution, the time will come when medicine will organize into an undercover dictatorship.... To restrict the art of healing to one class of men and deny equal privileges to others will constitute the Bastille of medical science. All such laws are un-American and despotic..., and have no place in a republic.... The Constitution of this Republic should make special provisions for medical freedom as well as religious freedom." - Dr. Benjamin Rush, Signer, Declaration of Independence; Member, Continental Congress; B.S., Princeton U.

"Samuel Thomson (1769-1843, herbalist) so upset New Hampshire doctors that they persuaded the state legistlature to pass a law specifically naming him, not for practicing medicine 'illegally' ('the usual term with which to charge non-allopathic practitioners'), but to prevent him (from) healing people without charging them." - Donald Law, A Guide to Alternative Medicine, p.133.

"The entire medical profession of the United States in so far as its organization is concerned, is today at the mercy of one man and a board of trustees that is subservient to him." - Editorial, Illinois Medical J., Dec. 1922, p.478.

"The efforts of the medical profession in the US to control: ... its ... job it proposes to monopolize. It has been carrying on a vigorous campaign all over the country against new methods and schools of healing because it wants the business .... I have watched this medical profession for a long time, & it bears watching." -Clarence Darrow, (1857-1938), (in FACT, Cancer Forum, v.5, n.5, p.10, 1979).

"A conspiracy, not a profession.... Every doctor will allow a colleague to decimate a whole countryside sooner than violate the bond of professional etiquette by giving him away." - George Bernard Shaw, (1856-1950)

"... I was a member of the Health Committee of London Borough Council, & I learned how the credit of vaccination is kept up statistically by diagnosing all the re-vaccinated cases (of smallpox) as 'pustular eczema, varioloid', or what not - except smallpox." - George Bernard Shaw, (in Hannah Allen, Don't Get Stuck!, p.71).

"The right of privacy shall include Freedom of Choice in Health Care.... No person shall be denied access to a therapy merely because of disagreement regarding its effectiveness....The final decision regarding the merits & personal choice of a therapy shall be made, not by the state or medical society, but by the individual or the prescribing physician utilizing such therapy." - Proposed Constitutional Amendment, (by G. Edward Griffin, John Richardson, Michael Culbert, et. al.)

Allow every one, LICENSED or NOT, for pay or not, to use on theirself or others (with their permission), any SAFE, non-toxic, items or methods, to or not to, prevent, diagnose, alleviate, or CURE, ANY DISEASE, health condition, etc. Items or methods may be PROVEN OR NOT. Safe, non-toxic, items or methods, are that which produce no more harm than existing items or methods, legally permitted, with prescription or not. - Proposed Law, (by Arlin Brown, re-worded for brevity by this Editor)

(Allow access of cancer patients to) "unconvential therapies, (i.e.) any method used for the control & cure of cancer which has not been approved by the Federal FDA." - Cancer Therapeutic Research Bill of 1981, State of Florida, (in Spotlight, July 13, 1981, p.26); HB 747 passed by Legistlature, vetoed by Governor, (in Voice, v.1, n.9, p.4, Sept. 1981).

"I do not have a medical license; yet a recent settlement with the Oakland-Piedmont Municipal Court granted me the legal right to continue my health practice under certain conditions. ...I must not provide the services that statutory law reserves to physicians, which are the diagnosis or treatment of disease, ...; I must encourage clients to go to physicians for (that).... ...I must make legal agreements with my clients that define what my responsibilities are as a health practitioner & what responsibilities they have as clients. ....This settlement...does not set a legal precedent.... ...it shows ...how one court chose to deal...." - Dana Ullman,MPH, (in The Holistic Health Handbook, p.395).

Q.2.0 TOP OFFICIALS, RECENT & RESEARCH:
Q.2.1 PRESIDENTS, US, RECENT:

(The AMA is) "just another mean trust." - Harry S. Truman, (in Ruth Harmer, American Medical Avarice, p.9).

"...the right of the individual to elect freely the manner of his care in illness must be preserved." - Dwight D. Eisenhower, (in Susan B. Anthony University Journal, v.1,n.2,p.23, Oct. 1975).

"Presidents ... need to show more interest in what the specific results of research are .... I think the time has come to zero in on the targets — by trying to get our knowledge fully applied .... We must make sure that no life-saving discovery is locked up in the laboratory." - Lyndon B. Johnson, (in Comroe & Dripps, The Top Ten Clinical Advances ..., DHEW Pub. No. (NIH)78-1521; p.5).

" (Doctors) collectively have done more to block adequate medical care for people of this country than any other single group. " - James E. Carter, (in Health Policy Advisory Center, Health PAC Bulletin, n.72, p.12, Sept. 1976).

"I've heard drug experts say they believe if penicillin were discovered today, the FDA wouldn't license it." - Ronald Reagan, (in Spotlight, March 9, 1981, p.29).

Q.2.2 FEDERAL LEGISTLATORS, US, RECENT:

"But the doctors in the past, as the review of the evidence showed, branded Jenner, Semmelweis, Oliver Wendell Holmes,Sr., Pasteur, Lister, Koch, and Keen as charlatans.... Napoleon said that war is too important to be left to the generals. We go on the assumption in the Senate that foreign relations are too important to be left to the diplomats. ...this question (on a novel cancer cure) is too important to leave purely to doctors...." - US Senator Paul Douglas, in Congressional Record, v.109, part 11, p.14501, Aug. 7, 1963.

"It is a terrible thing that we cannot really trust either the FDA or the NCI. We need, therefore, an independent scientific investigation." - Senator P. Douglas, Congressional Record, v.109, part 18, p.23619, Dec. 6, 1963.

"Yet, not only has the FDA done everything it could to discourage (a 'good or better' & 'non-toxic') treatment of human cancer, but also the NCI appears to have been negligent in not pursuing this whole line of investigation." - US Senator Edward V. Long, "Enzyme Treatment of Cancer", Congressional Record, v.112, part 20, p.26913, Oct. 14, 1966.

"Government controlled medical research, which verges on monopoly, may possibly delay medical advances."

"There has been very little emphasis in NCI on relatively non-toxic approaches, some radically different."

"... serious shortcomings in the administrative practices ... of the FDA. ... there is no appeal to the courts in cases involving medical research." - US Senator E. V. Long, "Is the FDA Hamstringing Cancer Research?", Congressional Record, v.112, part 19, p.25187, Oct. 5, 1966.

"The Hearings have revealed police-state tactics ... possibly perjured testimony to gain a conviction, ... intimidation & gross disregard for the Constitutional Rights ...(of) the First, Fourth, Fifth, & Sixth Amendments, (by the FDA)."

"The FDA (is) bent on using snooping gear to pry & invade...." - Sen. Long, Invasion of Privacy, p.835, Hearings, US Senate, 1965.

"... instance after instance of FDA raids on small vitamin & food supplement manufacturers. These small, defenseless businesses were guilty of producing products which FDA officials claimed were unnecessary..." - Sen. Long, (in J. Turner, The Chemical Feast, p.33-34).

"If the FDA would spend a little less time & effort on small manufacturers of vitamins ... & a little more on large manufacturers of ... dangerous drugs ..., the public would be better served." - Sen. Long, Hearings, Subcom. on Administrative Practices & Procedures, 1965, (in O. Garrison, The Dictocrats, p.63).

"(It) could involve the AMA and others in an interstate conspiracy of alarming proportions...."

"Public and private funds have been thrown around like confetti at a country fair, to close up and destroy clinics, hospitals, and scientific research laboratories which do not conform to the viewpoint of medical associations."

"Request (was) made by US Senator Elmer Thomas following an investigation made by the Senate of the Hoxsey Cancer Clinic... & addressed to the Surgeon General (USPHS),... to enlist support ... to make an investigation.... No such investigation was made, in fact, every effort was made to avoid & evade the investigation by the Surgeon General's office."

"The record in the Federal Court discloses that (the NCI) took sides & sought in every way to hinder , suppress & restrict ...(a) treatment of cancer." - Benedict Fitzgerald, Special Counsel to the Senate Interstate & Foreign Commerce Committee, "A Report to the Senate IFCC on the Need for Investigation of Cancer Research Organizations", inserted by US Senator William Langer in the Congressional Record, v.99, part 12, p.A5350, Aug. 3, 1953.

"Cancer: ... Organized Medicine must ... keep an open mind as to any scientific evidence which provides ... the ... answer .... Irrespective of past disputes, what counts at this point are: (a) sound study by the FDA, & (b) sound trial by the NCI, together with other(s) .... By 'sound' I mean - independent, un-biased, scientific, in the highest sense of these terms - so as to get at the truth, whatever it may be ...; frank, impartial, well-qualified judgement, 'letting the chips fall where they may'." - US Senator Hubert H. Humphrey, "... My Own Health Activities", (Code H 6-9-63, in Suzanne Caum, Cancer Cures Crucified, p.361).

"I & many other Members of Congress have received a large volume of mail from individuals ... benefited from Laetrile treatments, ... who believe the Government is party to a conspiracy to suppress an inexpensive, non-toxic, & effective anti-cancer drug. ... public confidence in our Government has not been strengthened by the highly unusual actions of the FDA in first advising ... that clinical studies with Laetrile could be initiated, & then terminating this authorization...."

(There is a) "deeply held conviction of a large number of Americans that they are being forced by their Government to leave the country in order to obtain therapy with a drug that is both safe & effective for the control of cancer.... (A) review should be done by cancer experts who have no conflicting interests & who are able to evaluate the evidence objectively.... In light of the tremendous sums of money that have been spent with relatively little productivity ..., I find it very surprising that the (NCI) has not sought on its own initiative to do further animal testing with this drug which apparently has shown some activity in the tests sponsored by the McNaughton Foundation." - US Congressman L. H. Fountain, (in a letter to HEW Sec'y, in Cancer News Journal, v.6, n.1, p.10, Win. 1971).

"Money appropriated for FDA in 1945 (was) $3 million; in 1968, $66 million. Numbers of employees in 1945, approx. 850; in 1968, 5100. Seizures of foods in 1945, 2504; in 1968, 384. Injunctions for violative foods in 1945, 26; in 1968, 3.... Prosecutions for violative foods, in 1945, 278; in 1968, 70. - US Congressman L. H. Fountain, (in Beatrice T. Hunter, Mirage of Safety, p.298).

"Anyone may logically wonder why this information has not been put into proper investigated format & presented to various medical bodies. The answer is simple. With the powerful alliance of the media, the federal agencies & orthodox medical groups, anyone attempting to present such ... would be destroyed with orchestrated cries of "Quackery". There is ample evidence to document this beyond any question." - US Congressman Larry McDonald,MD, (in Cancer News Journal, v.12, n.6, p.7, Feb. 1978).

"When it was first introduced, the claims for penicillin were also a minority view, & it (penicillin) was suppressed for 11 or 12 years." - Hon. Larry McDonald, (in Steven Fredman,MD, & Robert Burger, Forbidden Cures, p.22).

"No (cancer) cure is in existence today, & anybody who says that any particular system is hocus-pocus is speaking from authority that does not exist...."

"Hundreds of affidavits have been filed in court which the court took no notice of, by people stating they were cured by the Hoxsey (herbal) treatment.... (A) court ... first call(ed) up the dept. of health & then the next day rejected the affidavits."

(Maybe) "a cure for ... cancer will ... be made by someone not within the medical fraternity." - US Congressman Usher L. Burdick, Congressional Record, v.104, part 7, p.9531, May 26, 1958.

"There seems to be a well formed conspiracy between the big chemical companies & the AMA & the FDA to inject these poisonous chemicals into food.... An examination of the records leaves little in doubt as to the facts of this conspiracy." - Hon. Usher Burdick, Congressional Record, v.103, part 3, p.3302, March 7,1957.

"... the influence of the manufacturers of food ... are too strong politically, & Members shy away from raising any protest that might stop the sale ...." - Hon. Usher Burdick, Congressional Record, v.103, part 6, p.7922, May 28, 1957.

"...I acted as vice chairman of the ... commission, duly appointed by the Illinois Legistlature, to conduct an inquiry to determine whether or not there was a conspiracy to prevent freedom of research at ... a tax-supported institution."

"...I will proceed ... to introduce a resolution to investigate those elements that are preventing the carrying out of such a test, on the ground that the public interest demand such action. It is fundamental that a conspiracy to prevent scientific research is in itself within the Congressional prerogative to protect the welfare...."

"I am warning the AMA ... to pay heed to Dr. Ivy's appeal for fair play...." - US Congressman Roland V. Libonati, Congressional Record, v.104, part 15, p.19745, Aug.23, 1958.

"No one seems to care. Certainly, no one in the million dollar fund-raising cancer clinics are excited over the almost miraculous ... record of ... Krebiozen...."(Feb.12,1959).

"Maybe the raising of millions of dollars of funds for charitable projects has become a 'racket', & the longer that they remain in the test-tube stage of development, the longer patronage & job payrollers remain in their soft berths."

"... this charity.... They quibble too much over procedures ... while we seek a cure. They complain too loudly against another who, seemingly, has perfected a work that the public expects its charity dollars to do. Maybe we should investigate the American Cancer Society's operations."(Feb. 16, 1959).

"... Dr. Andrew C. Ivy, (is) the champion of the scientific doctrine of freedom of research, which has suffered in recent years through the falsity of certain politico-physician leaders of the AMA, who faked reports, suppressed honest information, brutally slugged the opposition, both physically & through pressures, used to prevent the truth about Krebiozen reaching the American people."(Mar. 3, 1959).

- US Congressman Roland V. Libonati, Congressional Record, (in S.J.Haught, Has Dr. Max Gerson A True Cancer Cure?, p.139-144). (Ed.: 13 out of 25 entries by Hon. R.V.Libonati in the 86th Congress, 1st Session, are on repression of cancer therapy & Krebiozen. - Congressional Record, v.105, part 16, Index, p.532).

"The FDA and much, but not all, of the orthodox medical profession are actively hostile against vitamins and minerals.... They are out to get the health food industry.... And they are trying to do this out of active hostility and prejudice." - US Senator William Proxmire (in National Health Federation Bulletin, April 1974, cover).

"There should be freedom of scientific basic research into innovative methods of prevention of disease other than those employed by the AMA & supported by the government." - US Senator William Proxmire, The Fleecing of America, (in American Natural Hygiene Society, Health Science, v.4, n.3, p.25, April 1981).

"In a free society men & women should not be prevented by Government from seeking medical remedies which they believe will be effective. ...."

"Despite the fact that a predicted 350,000 persons in the US will die of cancer this year, the cancer bureaucracy keeps a closed mind. ... the basic issue is not the efficacy of Laetrile, but the infringement of freedom in what amounts to a life & death question."

"Freedom of choice must be brought to bear upon US medical practice." - US Congressman Philip M. Crane, Congressional Record, v.121, part 25, p.31903, Oct.6, 1975.

"... we are not pursuing (cancer cures) with as much dilligence & innovativeness as we should ...."

"Why not permit (alternative cancer therapists) to demonstrate their work through the grants (of $ from NCI)?"

"If we are just going to be brokering out these grants on the basis of who has published a paper that passes some peer group as the only criteria, then I dare say we will be fumbling in this morass of inconclusive research forever & ever." - US Senator John Melcher, (p.56).

"This dogged, same track approach (by the NCI) is even more astonishing...."

"This total failure to address the diet/cancer relationship is most disturbing to ... (those) informed...." - US Senator, & Nominee for US President (by Dem. Party), George McGovern, (p.2).

"... we really have a credibility crisis here in terms of the way research allocations are being made at the (NCI), & the suspicion that provoked these hearings in the first place, that we are losing the war on cancer because of mistaken priorities, ... has grown all the stronger ... as I have listened to your testimony ...." - US Senator George McGovern, (p.64).

"The public is very sophisticated, & if we give them the (nutrition) information, they would probably make a fair judgement. But if they don't have it, & you send it to the doctor or some university, I am not certain that is ever going to reach the right people."

"Even though the nutrition research budget has increased 21-fold in the last 4 years, it still remains less than 1% of the total NCI budget ... even though one half of all cancers are diet related.... Does the peer review simply turn into a "buddy" system for awarding grants?" - US Senator Bob Dole, (p.68, 79).

"... the NCI, which has received a $200 million increase in its annual budget since ... 1975, has not made any effort to expand the nutrition research initiative mandated by Congress (in 1974)." - US Senators: George McGovern, Ted Kennedy, Bob Dole, Chuck Percy, Pat Leahy, Henry Bellmon,(p.80).

- all in Nutrition & Cancer Research, Hearings, Subcom. on Nutrition, US Senate, June 12 & 13, 1978, (p.2, 56, 64, 68, 79, 80).

"Eminent nutritionists have traded their independence for the food industry's favors." - US Congressman Benjamin Rosenthal, (in Feingold Association, "I'm A Natural", Jan. 1978, p.3).

"... surgeons, radiologists, chemotherapists,... fear that a major new emphasis in the (NCI) toward the environment will reduce ... funding for other research...."

"... some people in both government & industry ..., feel that 'economic considerations' should be given greater weight, despite clear evidence that additional cancer deaths will result."

"... conclusive proof of (a cancer) link often is ... decades away."

"Failure to heed the early warning signs (have) economic consequences (also): increased medical bills, lost income & productivity,... Medicare,... Social Security..."

- US Congressman David Obey, (Forwarding Samuel S. Epstein,MD, The Politics of Cancer).

"Yet the contrast is startling between the runaway spending for health care & the resistance of most of American business to spending for environmental health protection." - US Congressman Paul Rogers, head, National Coalition for Disease Prevention & Environmental Health, (in Samuel S, Epstein,MD, The Politics of Cancer, p.435).

"Congress has given the highest priority to the search for a cancer cure. At the same time that the government has been searching for a cancer cure, however, government agencies have permitted introduction into the food supply of substances which may themselves cause cancer. .... Animal drugs...are given the benefit of every doubt, & little is done to investigate the risk...." - US Senator Abraham Ribicoff, (in William Robbins, The American Food Scandal, p.227-9).

"No one knows how (the food grain multinational corps.) operate, what their profits are, what they pay in taxes, & what effect they have on our foreign policy - or much of anything else about them." - US Senator Frank Church, (in Spotlight, May 18, 1981, p.25).

"A serious situation involving conflict of interest emerged involving one physician. Then we found at least six other similar conflict situations involving NCI. $1.1 million disappeared from the Eppley Institute, & the money has yet to be recovered."

"... I was shocked to find that the (NCI) director, although fully knowledgeable regarding why Dr. (Marc) Straus was asked to leave Boston (U.), did not order an official inquiry.... Only after the Boston Globe exposed this situation was a formal investigation ordered...." - US Senator Orrin G. Hatch, (in letter on July 3, 1981, to Richard Ericson, GE-PS Cancer Memorial).

"Since the war on cancer was launched, some $9 billion has been committed, but we are demonstrably no closer to a cancer cure than we were 10 years ago." - US Senator Orrin Hatch.

"Practices such as this (NCI handling of Dr. Straus) reveal a gross breach of professional ethics & will not be permitted to continue." - US Senator Paula Hawkins.

"It took 10 days for Boston U. to investigate (Dr.) Straus & demand his resignation, yet 22 months later, you (NCI) are still giving him a grant." - US Congressman Harold L. Volkmer.

- (Last 3 quotations above in National Health Federation, Public Scrutiny, Sept. 1981, p.8-11.)

"The FDA has been accused of...forcing submission to its orders by blacklisting investigators, threatening scientists with unwarranted court action, (&) conviction by press release...." - US Congressman Wendell Wyatt, "DMSO, the Persecuted Drug", Congressional Record, (in Pat McGrady,Sr., The Persecuted Drug: The Story of DMSO, p.132-3).

Hopkins: "They (the FDA) have been dragging their feet...for 15 or 16 years"(on DMSO, which treats cancer, arthritis, brain injury - Ed.).

Donahue: "In the age of...getting government off our backs, (since) this (DMSO) can't hurt anybody, why are we so presumptuous in not allowing people to do...? Its like telling somebody they can't pray to a totem pole...!"

Hopkins: "Exactly!...But Congressmen are very reluctant to tell the FDA what they ought to be...just because we're not scientists."

Donahue: "Do you see any evidence of the drug industry lobby trying to insure that this is not approved...?"

Hopkins: "They say it can be produced for $4 a quart. It would tell me they have no interest in manufacturing it, because they are not going to make any money off of it."

- US Congressman Larry J. Hopkins, on Phil Donahue Show, WGN-TV, Ch.9, Chicago, Nov.5, 1981.

"Badly needed drugs are delayed from joining the fight against disease - not because they are dangerous, but because of the agency's (FDA) own well-deserved inferiority complex about its scientific judgment." - US Senator Edward M. Kennedy, (in Steven Fredman,MD;Robert Burger; Forbidden Cures, p.192).

"... profit making .... motives are at the root of the failure of the health insurance industry ... to assure that the health care system is responsive to America's needs .... The industry would remain a moneychanger taking a percentage of our dollars for a dubious service ...." - US Senator Edward Kennedy, (in Ruth M. Harmer;BA,Barnard; MA,Columbia;PhD,USC; American Medical Avarice, p.243).

Q.2.3 FDA COMMISSIONERS:

"Under the very nose of the President (Taft, they) so controlled the action of the 3 Secretaries.... Not only was every decision of the courts violated by this order, but President Taft's specific directions for labeling were also disregarded. It is very strange that the President himself did not make a protest. ...." - Harvey W. Wiley, MD, 1st Commissioner of the FDA, The History of a Crime Against the Food Law, "The Amazing Story of the National Food & Drugs Law Intended to Protect the Health of the People, Perverted to Protect Adulteration of Foods & Drugs", p.150.

"For centuries, the approved medical theories of one generation have become outmoded in the next. What was accepted medically ... 50 years ago,... would be quackery today." - FDA Commissioner George P. Larrick, (at National Congress on Medical Quackery, Oct. 1961, in Suzanne Caum, Cancer Cures Crucified, p.497).

"Your Attorneys have helped make a mockery of the procedures for getting food standards. There is endless repetition of testimony.... When several industry lawyers are involved, they won't get together.... Everyone has to speak. They'll ask for a recess of weeks to study documents that ... were available in advance.... And appeals to the courts at every stage: you set a hearing date, they ask a postponement, you deny it, they go to court. They seldom win, but everything stops while it is argued." - Winton B. Rankin, Commissioner of the FDA, (in Mark J. Green, The Other Government, The Unseen Power of Washington Lawyers, p.149).

(It is) "not our (FDA) policy to jeopardize the financial interests of the pharmaceutical companies." - Dr. Charles C. Edwards, Commissioner of the FDA, testifying in US House Subcom. on Intergov. Affairs, (in G.E. Griffin, World Without Cancer, p.451).

(The War on Cancer is) "a Medical Vietman". - Donald Kennedy, Commissioner of the FDA; President of Stanford University.

Q.2.4 NCI/FDA/USPHS/ACS/SKI, OFFICIALS, RECENT:

"After careful study of the literature and other information available to it, the ACS does not have evidence that treatment with (each of over 66 alternatives, such as Vitamin A, Hyper-thermia, Immunology, Mental Attitude,...to Orthodox Therapy) results in objective benefit in the treatment of cancer in human beings." - ACS: Unproven Methods of Cancer Management; & Medical Affairs Dept.

"There are only 3 proven ways - & only 3 - to curb cancer: (1) X-ray, (2) radium, (3) & surgery, either singly or in combination..." - ACS, Cancer Facts, 1955, (in Eleanor McBean, The Poisoned Needle, p.45).

"Although claims have been made for the efficacy of various non-toxic substances, NCI investigations to date of all such materials have shown to be without significant value in the treatment of cancer." - NCI, OCC (Office of Cancer Communications), PIS (Public Inquiries Section) Chief, Robert J. Avery, (in letter to Ralph Hovnanian, on Sept. 30, 1980).

"Warning Against the Hoxsey (herbal) Cancer Treatment .... Cancer can be cured only through surgery or radiation." - FDA poster, c. 1955-6AD, sent to 46,000 US Post Offices for display.

"Such letters ... from the FDA, are, ... filled with objectively demonstratable lies, practiced deceptions and deviousness, red herrings, directed mis-information, mis-directed information, etc.... Once ... FDA-NCI-AMA-ACS ... concedes that Laetrile anti-tumor efficacy was indeed even once observed ... a permanent crack in bureaucratic armor has taken place." - Dr. Dean Burk, co-founder, NCI, Head, Cyto-Chemistry Section; (open letter, July 3, 1973; in CCS, Cancer Control Journal, v.1,n.3,p.7, Sept. 1973).

"I was about the most negative person in the country about interferon." - Dr. Rauscher, (in Time, March 31, 1980).

"I would certainly not turn off Laetrile if it had an iota of activity that we could pinpoint. Unfortunately, there's no evidence at all." - Dr. Frank Rauscher, Director, NCI; Vice Pres., ACS; (on CBS-TV, 60 Minutes, March 31, 1974).

"... there is no basis for the use of Laetrile in man based on data derived from experiments in animals." - Dr. Jesse Steinfeld, Surgeon General, USPHS, 1974, (last 2 above, in W. Westover, See the Patients Die or Let the Patients Live, p.26-7).

"The data provided by the McNaughton Foundation certainly indicates some activity (of Laetrile) in animal tumor systems." - Dr. Carl Baker, Director, NCI, 1970-2.

(Laetrile) "may be useful in sickle cell anemia.... (Laetrile) used in animals with tumors show: a decrease in lung metastases; slower tumor growth; & pain relief." - Lloyd Old, MD, V. Pres., Sloan-Kettering Inst. for Cancer Res., (at FDA, July 2, 1974, obtained under Freedom of Information Act). (Last 2 above, in Ralph Moss, Cancer Syndrome, p.115 & 138.)

"In ... cancer, we simply do not yet have an adequate enough understanding of the problem to build the control procedure the public wants. The science base is lacking. .... Future NCI research efforts are going to be more narrowly defined." - Dr. Arthur Upton, Director, NCI, (in Family Health, Oct. 1977, p.6).

(Why is there frequent criticism that the cancer research system is unreceptive to unorthodoxy?)

"Because it's true. Not cancer research, all research systems. It's a very important issue.... The entire system ... tends to exclude people on the fringe who have ideas that are radical departures, and we ought to pay a lot more attention to them.... I try." - Dr. Vincent DeVita, Jr., Director, NCI; (N.Eng.J.Med., v.303, n.17, p.1014).

"The NCI will not investigate suggested treatments which are in the realm of the supernatural, or which are outmoded or generally recognized as having no value."

"If a new drug does not appear superior to those already available, it is not tested. Similarly, the NCI does not investigate methods of treatment that lack a reasonable scientific base." - "Policy of the NCI Regarding Investigation or Evaluation of Proposed Cancer Treatments", (Bulletin n.559, 1957 & 1961 rev., 0-708-948; in Suzanne Caum, Cancer Cures Crucified, p.576-581).

"Non-acceptable type of therapy, including Laetrile, Krebiozen, etc." - NCI, 1976 SEER Code Manual, p.68, (for gathering data for statistics on effectivity of cancer therapies); (Surveillance, Epidemiology & End Results; Biometry Branch; DCCP; NCI).

"BECAUSE of the vast areas of IGNORANCE that still exist in our understanding of the cancer problem,... areas of BASIC RESEARCH are ESSENTIAL.... This ... must be SUPPORTED at an adequate level" (by Congress, taxes). - Report of the President's Cancer Panel, 1975, p.4, ("Submitted to the President of the US for Transmittal to the Congress"). (Capitals by Editor)

(For) "selection of what research to recommend,...(here is) a set of values....,
'weighting' factors....:(assign) PRIORITY (of) LOW (where) CRITICAL KNOWLEDGE IS LACKING, & its availability can not be predicted.... (Further,) High Priority - High Impact Project Areas...., where ADDITIONAL KNOWLEDGE was REQUIRED (because "VERY LITTLE EFFORT has been DONE in the area" or "Proposed effort is technically or SCIENTIFICALLY BEYOND the PRESENT STATE-OF-THE-ART"),... would either be STARTED LATER ... or ... at a LOW level of EFFORT." - NCI, An Analysis of Mid-Range Resources ..., March 1973, p.II-14 to 16, (USDHEW Pub. n.(NIH) 74-571).

Q.2.5 RESEARCH vs. DEVELOPMENT, at NCI:

"Obviously, a very fundamental point is at issue here — there must be clear definitions of scientific discoveries (research - Ed.) & of development (... 'based on them') & an assessment of the importance of each." - NIH; J. Comroe & R. Dripps, The Top Ten Clinical Advances..., p.22, DHEW Pub. No. (NIH)78-1521.

"The main criterion for an award (of a research contract from the NCI) is the capacity to demonstrate the relevance of the project to the program's target. But the only sure way to prove this relevance is to have, in fact, already proved it." - June Goodfield, FRSM, The Siege of Cancer, p.179.

"We are attempting to analyze by apparently logical & rigorous methods the likelihood of the crazy ideas being right before they have been put to adequate test. ...denying...radical new ideas...to be tested. ...(&)saying that ideas which have not been tested should not be published."

"...I would beg that all workers in the cancer field should think seriously even about some of the wilder concepts." - D. Horrobin, Editorial, "Innovative Approaches to Cancer", Medical Hypotheses, 5: 1-3, p.1-3, 1979.

Q.2.6 HEW, SECRETARIES (& ASSISTANT):

"I think we are creating in the US a cancer program bureaucracy that is going to be very, very difficult to come to grips with in the years ahead."

"The vast amounts of money this nation has spent for biomedical research ... had only modest effects on ... health ...."

"But fundamentally, the search for knowledge about ... the problems we recognize as specific diseases ... cannot be compartmentalized." - HEW Assistant Secretary for Health, Dr. Charles C. Edwards, to US Senate, Nov. 12, 1975, (in Daniel Greenberg, NEJM(New England Journal of Medicine), v.293,n.26,p.1379, Dec. 25,1975).

"... Because of my strong commitment in reducing the morbidity & mortality which result from smoking, the Department (HEW) is conducting a major review of its programs in this field in order to introduce administrative & legistlative proposals to combat this problem." - HEW Secretary, Joseph Califano,Jr.,(p.ii).

"Beginning in the 1920's, a number of reports appeared which suggested a relationship between lung cancer & tobacco smoking."(p.263).

- CDC, The Health Consequences of Smoking, A Reference Edition, 1976, HEW Pub. No. (CDC) 78-8357.

"Some hallowed medical traditions must be questioned & some ancient practices curtailed." - HEW Secretary, John W. Gardner, (in Forward to Milton Silverman & Philip R. Lee, Pills, Profits, & Politics).

Q.3.0 TOP BIO-MEDICS & OTHERS:
Q.3.1 PREVENTION:

"The aim of medicine is to prevent disease & prolong life; the ideal of medicine is to eliminate the need of a physician." - William J. Mayo,MD, (in H. G. Bieler,MD, Food Is Your Best Medicine, p.14).

"During the 1960's...HIP,...study showed no gain from mammography to women under 50, ('yet') all women over 35 were invited to participate in the (Breast Cancer Detection) Demonstration Project (of the ACS &) NCI...."

"In 1973, Alan S. Rabson of the (NCI) Division of Cancer Biology & Diagnosis (said) mammography was the real risk,(the test itself causing cancer). William Pomerance (Chief, Diagnostic Branch, same NCI Division, wrote:) '...At a meeting of some contractors, ...I made the statement...I would...change the initial age to 45.... They "fell on me"...& went so far as to decide (to)...start with age 30.... Their reaction is hysteria....' ....John Bailer III (of NCI) published...in Jan. 1976...that for women under 50, the risk...might equal the chance of (detecting)...."

"(When) the controversy became public.... ...An independent NCI committee (found:) Of 1,850 women diagnosed (by mammography) as having cancer, the review of the (pathological) tissue showed that 66 did not have cancer at all.... NCI 'reclassified' (18) cases. For the remaining 48 cases, there appears to be no evidence of cancer; 37 of the 48 women have undergone mastectomies. The National Women's Health Network... complain(ed).... Dr. Vincent DeVita (Director), NCI...responded (in) 1980, that 'NCI chose not to inform the women...' & that 'NCI does not acknowledge that "there were serious problems" in this program.'" - Susan Rennie, National Women's Health Network News, v.6, n.2, p.4, March 1981.

"...when I submitted that manuscript for clearance, I was called ... in to the office of my (NCI) director. He said,'Now, the high medical official of the AEC (Atomic Energy Commission) objects against that. They said there are quite other reasons why the uranium miners develop cancer; it's not the radioactivity. You shall omit that from your presentation.'"

"My ... studies on occupational cancer ...in... industries was forcefully & abruptly brought to a halt in 1952 by an order of the Surgeon General.... (This followed) a protest to the PHS by ...(an) industry.... alleg(ing) that my activities were detrimental to their interests.... I was forbidden (by PHS) to contact, thereafter, state health depts. & industrial concerns on all matters of occupational cancer. (I was) to discontinue all field work...." - Dr. Wilhelm C. Heuper, Chief, Environmental Cancer Section, NCI, (in Larry Agran, The Cancer Connection, p.27).

"There are now over 200 (experimental carcinogenesis bioassay) results still waiting to be reviewed & published, while no substantial supportive staff is provided (by NCI top management).... I cannot accept any longer a situation which in fact deprives the regulatory agencies, industry, labor, consumers, & the scientific community of data of urgent public health value." - NCI Assoc. Director for Carcinogenesis, Dr. Umberto Saffiotti, resignation letter, 1976, (in The Miami Herald, April 23, 1978, p.20-A,col.4)

"In a NCI study of 120 compounds that looked carcinogenic because of their chemical structure, ... less than 10% caused cancer in test animals.... Instead of despair, we need determination." - Environmental Defense Fund & Robert H. Boyle, Malignant Neglect, p.212.

"The problem with 'prevention' is that it does not produce revenues. No health plan reimburses a physician or a hospital for preventing a disease." - NCI Deputy Director, Division of Cancer Cause & Prevention; & of Diet, Nutrition, & Cancer Program; Dr. Gio Gori, (in George E. Berkley,PhD, Cancer: How to Prevent, & How to Help Your Doctor Fight It, p.196).

"The NCI...(has) concerns about exposure to specific agents.... However, there is currently no identifiable program that assesses, on a holistic basis, ...the (combined-Ed.) carcinogenic insult of air & water pollutants, diet contaminants, & other composite stresses." - United Nations, International Register of Potentially Toxic Chemicals Bulletin 1, June 1978, p.4, (in Samuel Epstein,MD, The Politics of Cancer, p.351).

"'...Search for the cause may be a hopeless pursuit because most disease states are the indirect outcome of a constellation of circumstances.'" - Dr. Rene Dubos, Rockefeller Inst., Mirage of Health.

(Almost)"'any study undertaken with any pair of nutrients has...show(n) a significant interaction in terms of some nutritional or biochemical criterion. ...since...enzyme... apo-enzymes...coenzyme (mediate).'" - R.A. Harte; & Bacon Chow, Johns Hopkins.(p.65).

"The evidence is truly overwhelming that disease is pluri-causal."(p.43).

"(Host Resistance & Susceptibility) X Environmental Challenge = (Health or Disease)". (p.48). - E.Cheraskin,MD,DMD,Prof. Emeritus & of Med., & Chmn., Dept. Oral Med., U. Alabama Med.; W.M.Ringsdorf,DMD; J.W.Clark,DDS; Diet & Disease, p.43-4, 48, 65.

"In 1906, ...Upton Sinclair's sensational novel, The Jungle (appeared).... Meat consumption in the US fell by 25% in the year following publication of The Jungle. (In) ...1967, President Johnson signed the Wholesome Meat Act into law. Upton Sinclair, in a wheelchair, was at his side. ...130,000 cattle carcasses were held back by federal inspectors in 1969 for removal of carcinomas & cancer eye."(p.2-4, 24).

"...On fatal poisoning.... in Dade County, Fla., ...in the under 5-year (old) group, pesticides were the leading cause of death."(p.219).

"...Environmentalists...rarely leave energy in reserve for monitoring enforcement. ...The constituencies mobilized by the original event tend to equate enactment of a program with solution of the problem.... FCC Commissioner Nicholas Johnson...(to) Senate Subcom.: '...Then the pressure starts - on those who have been handed the job of investigation & reform. Corporate interests that will adversely affected move to delay, to water down, to remove "dangerous" people, & then finally to participate in the final whitewash.'"(p.330-1). - Harrison Wellford; Cambridge U., England; Harvard U.; Marshall Scholar; Danforth Fel.; Woodrow Wilson Fel.; Center for Study of Responsive Law; Sowing the Wind, p.2-4, 24, 219, 330-1.

"...Man is the only animal...destroying his food value by cooking...."(p.20).

"...It would prove of the highest benefit were the inmates of our prisons, lunatic asylums, &...all charitable institutions (hospitals-Ed.), confined to a fruit... & vegetable diet, which experience has so amply demonstrated to be ... conducive to the health of both body & mind."(p.67). - Robert Bell,MD,FRFPS; Pres.,Med. Assoc. for Reduction & Prevention of Cancer; Physician in Charge of Cancer Res., Battersea Hosp.; Hon. Mem.,Amer. Soc. Progressive Med.; The Prevention & Treatment of Cancer, Health Research, p.20, 67.

"The chief, if not the sole,cause of the monstrous increase in cancer has been vaccination." - Dr. Robert Bell; V. President, International Society for Cancer Research; British Cancer Hospital; (in Eleanor McBean, The Poisoned Needle, p.41, Health Research).

"Dr. David Grassetti ... said, 'The spread of cancer in mice ... is astounding after they are given a dose of Rifampin'...., a miracle anti-biotic.... In 1973, (a manufacturer of Rifampin) Dow Chemical, received almost $900,000 in contracts from ... the NCI. (The) research (results were) permitted to remain confidential." - Health Writers, Health Newsletter, v.3,n.1,p.3,Jan. 1974.

"'People who have had their appendixes removed are twice as likely to have colon cancer.'" - Dr. Birger Jansson, M. D. Anderson Hospital & Tumor Inst.(p.51).

"During 3 different strikes of MD's (in) the mid-1970's (in Israel, Columbia, & California), death rates fell between 18% & 50% ...."(p.69). - Peter Chowka, "The Failure of Specialty Medicine", Journal of the Nutritional Academy, v.2,n.3,p.51 & 69.

"Doctors ... make periodic surveys of their techniques. I don't know why. After they're done, nobody seems to pay much attention to them...."

"One of the first controlled community studies on tonsillectomy (in Rochester, NY, in 1922), showed it had no effect...; yet this past year (1970), 1/3 to 1/5 of all children hospitalized in that same area (Rochester) were admitted for tonsillectomies!" - Leonard Tushnet,MD, The Medicine Men, p.82, & 129.

"Ionizing radiation..(:) X-rays & radio-pharmaceuticals —...used in the diagnosis or treatment of disease — account for 90% of the man-made dosage."

"By...1906 some researchers suspected.... But the curious fact is that few physicians read research journals, & x-ray abuse persisted for decades." - EDF(Environmental Defense Fund: J. Highland, Marcia Fine, et.al.), R. Boyle, Malignant Neglect, p.154-6.

"... A total disregard ... occurs when treatments are continued in spite of the reports & the articles alerting physicians to the dangers (of some treatments)."

"In Japan there is a saying: 'Many people mistake Hiroshima for yesterday; it is really tomorrow.'" - Ronald Glasser, MD, The Greatest Battle, p.48, & 154.

"I have given orders to my Death Units to exterminate without mercy or pity men, women, & children belonging to the Polish speaking race.... After all, who remembers today the extermination of the Armenians." - A. Hitler, Aug. 22, 1939, (in James Nazer, The First Genocide of the 20th Century,... Armenian Massacres ..., back jacket).

Q.3.2 FDA, (SOIL to SOUL):

"... in Europe at the present time (1943, it is) a crime punishable by death to spread information in regard to nutrition in Norway, Belgium, Holland, and all other conquered countries." - D.T.Quigley, MD, FACS, in The National Malnutrition, p.58.

"A relation of stomach cancer with soil types & diet has also been suggested for some areas in Holland. (Source: W. Haenszel, Journal NCI, v.21, p.213, 1958)" - Cancer: A Worldwide Menace, Subcommittee on Reorganization ..., Committee on Government Operations, US Senate, July 17, 1959, p.14.

"It has been common ... to combine such unproven ingredients as bio-flavonoids, rutin ..., with such essential nutrients as Vitamin C ..., thus implying that they are all nutritionally valuable for supplementation of the daily diet. The courts have sustained FDA legal action to prevent such practices, and the new FDA regulations preclude this type of combination in the future.... Similarly, it has been common... to state or imply that the American diet is inadequate because of soil deficiencies, commercial processing methods, use of synthetic nutrients, and similar charges. FDA recognizes that these false statements have misled, scared, and confused the public, and is prohibiting any such general statements in the future.... The medical and nutritional professions have shown strong support of this policy, ..." - FDA (Ass't. Gen.) Council's letter to 5 US Legistlators, in: Vitamin, Mineral, Diet Supplements, part 1, p.151, Hearings, US Congress, Oct. 29-31, 1973.

"A citizenship of wholesale delegation & abdication to public & private power systems, such as prevails now, makes such periodic checks as elections little more than rituals." - Ralph Nader, (in Environmental Defense Fund & R. H. Boyle, Malignant Neglect, p.224).

"The (synthetic, processed -Ed.) food industry, its trade associations, and research foundations, is well financed and highly organized to pressure the FDA." - Ralph Nader.

"22 of 52 top (FDA) officials have worked for regulated industries, or organizations that cater to those industries.... During a hearing held in 1969 by the House Intergovernmental Relations Subcommittee, it was disclosed that of 49 high ranking FDA officials who had recently resigned or retired, 37 joined or served as consultants to regulated industries." -Michael Jacobson, Food for People, Not for Profit, p.374,377, (for last 2 paragraphs above).

"How many times have you heard...; 'You'd have to eat a carload of that to get cancer'? As if there was a known level below which any carcinogen ... not to cause cancer. As if all species reacted the same way to carcinogenic insult. As if there (was) was no such thing as co-carcinogenesis...."

"... a few of us have the capacity to harm a lot of us in the name of economics." - FDA Bureau of Veterinary Medicine Director, Lester Crawford, (in NFA, Natural Food & Farming, v.27,n.1,p.4, June 1980).

"The possibility for fraud is apparent when the consumer doesn't know if the storekeeper is honest, when the storekeeper can't tell if the distributor is honest, & when the distributor doesn't know if his suppliers are living up to their promises. ... Conventional foods at times have been substituted for organic foods...."

"Differences in the nutrient content of food from plants of the same species depend on their genetic nature, the climate, the nutrients available for growth, & the stage of maturity at which they are harvested. ...Wide variation in the Vitamin A content has been found in different varieties of carrots & in ... oranges grown in different parts of the country." - "The Confusing World of Health Foods", FDA Consumer, July 1978, HEW Pub. No. (FDA)79-2108.

Q.3.3 DOUBLE STANDARD IN RESEARCH:

"The investigation of plants as a source of new (cancer therapy) begins by collecting test samples.... ...largely at random (67,000 species to date)...."(p.2, 3).

"New (plants)...are simultaneously screened against the P388 ('in vivo...leukemia ...in(to)...mouse') & the KB ('in vitro, human cancer cells') (cancer therapy test systems) at a cost of $80.28 & $19.40, respectively."(p.7, 8).

"Both NPB (of NCI,) & USDA officials agree that the chemical makeup (against cancer) of a plant can vary with different geographical (soil - Ed.) areas. ...32 species contained anti-cancer active agents, 12 of which had shown no anti-cancer activity when obtained from other countries."(p.4). - USGAO, HRD-80-53, Review of the NCI's ... Plant Extracts , Feb. 28, 1980, report to US Senator Edward Kennedy.

"For some places you want harsh regulations backed by the full weight of the law - (we) have had IND's (request to test on humans an Investigational New Drug) for Laetrile, for example, & other hoax remedies.... Sometimes we say it is proper to hinder research."

(The FDA has) "what some people called the worst personnel in government.... Open drunkenness ... for months.... intimidation.... tittering in corners, throwing spitballs; I am describing physicians, (who) slouch down in a chair, not respond to questions, moan & groan with sleeping gestures, a kind of behavior I have not seen in any other institution as a grown man." - FDA, Bureau of Drugs Director, Dr. J. Richard Crout, (in Ralph Moss, Cancer Syndrome, p.270-273).

"... FDA was allegedly using one standard of safety, efficacy, and design of clinical tests for the little investigator ..., but a different (more lax) standard for government paid NCI investigators using the drugs of big drug companies." - Dr. Miles H. Robinson, inserted by US Senator Edward V. Long into Congressional Record, v.112, part 19, p.25187, Oct. 5, 1966, "Is the FDA Hamstringing Cancer Research?".

"The Establishment.... undismayed by the futility of funds dumped into the bottomless barrel of its 'proven' methods, it remains adamant in refusing to investigate 'unproven' methods...."

"Nobody in the science & medical departments (in the ACS) is capable of doing real science.... They don't know how to prevent cancer or cure patients; instead, they close the door on innovative ideas. ACS money goes to scientists who put on the best show to get grants, or who have friends on the grant-giving panels." - ACS Science Editor(25 yrs.), ACS Science Writers' Conference originator, Pat McGrady, Sr., (1st paragraph: in R. Moss, Cancer Syndrome, p.94; 2nd: in Peter Barry Chowka, NHF Public Scrutiny, Feb. 1981, p.19).

(It is) "a corrupt practice for the persons giving out ... & getting (the money) to be the same ... even when it is called 'peer review' or 'cancer research'.... (It is) not worth revamping & should simply be junked."

"It is almost impossible to get 'peer review' that will accept a study of iatrogenic (doctor caused) disease."

"For 30 years radiologists in this country have been engaged in massive malpractice, ... something that a doctor will not say about another doctor." - Irwin Bross, PhD, Director of Bio-Statistics, Roswell Park Memorial Institute for Cancer Research, & Prof. Johns Hopkins Med., author of 300 articles/letters, (1st paragraph: in Peter B. Chowka, East West Journal, March 1981, p.38; 2nd & 3rd: in Moss, Cancer Syn., p.60).

"I've heard of cancer politics, but I've never seen anything like this in my entire life. In fact, I wouldn't believe it, if I hadn't seen it with my own eyes."

"... everybody's afraid. Fear is overriding scientific inquiry & the ability to let an audience make up its mind."

"The whole set-up (NCI-ACS) is a farce & a fraud." - Joseph Gold, MD, Director, Syracuse Cancer Research Institute, (last 3 above, in: Cancer Syndrome, p.161; Chowka, East West Journal, March 1981, p.47; Spotlight, June 1, 1981, p.16).

"Promising preventions & cures to cancer are being hopelessly stifled, as long as cancer research funding is captive to certain members of the peer review system. Who are these 'peers'? Are they chosen fairly? Do they assure a fair evaluation of all promising, alternative, cancer approaches?" - Richard Ericson, JD, author of Cancer Treatment, Why So Many Failures?, What You Can Do About It.

"'The surgeons. They controlled medicine, & they regarded the X-ray as a threat to surgery. At that time surgery was the only approved method of treating cancer. They meant to keep it the only approved method by ignoring or rejecting any new methods or ideas. This is why I was called a 'quack' & nearly ejected from hospitals where I had practiced for years.' - Dr. Emil Grubbé,... discovered ... X-ray therapy (for cancer) ... in 1896....X-ray was not recognized as an agent for treating cancer by the American College of Surgeons until 1937.... Dr. Grubbé ... still was not recognized as late as 1951." - in Herbert Bailey, Vitamin E, Your Key to a Healthy Heart, p.23.

"... students were obliged ... to learn about an interminable number of drugs, many ... valueless,... useless, some ... harmful."

"... there is less intellectual freedom in the medical course than in almost any other form of professional education in this country." - Harvard Medical School Dean, Dr. David Edsall, (in G.E.Griffin, World Without Cancer, p.380).

"The condescending 'egg head' or 'ivory tower' attitude that something, as deceptively obvious & apparently simple to understand, as nutrition, is not important or worthy of attention or deserving of our research dollars...must be changed."

"It is clear to anyone who has even a basic knowledge of nutrition that the peer review group was not qualified sufficiently in nutrition to evaluate the proposal fairly." - Dr. Stanley J. Dudrick, Chairman, U. Texas Medical School; testimony to US Senate, Subcommittee on Nutrition, (in Ted Agres, "The Business of Cancer", Spring of Life, n.10, p.2).

"...Members of the US 'cancer cartel' have staked their reputations on their oft repeated claims that the non-toxic, nutritional therapy of cancer is ineffective.... The time will...come when (its) efficacy...will be officially acknowledged here in the US, as it already has been in many other countries." - Albert Schatz, PhD, FRSH; discoveror of streptomycin; Sloan Kettering Inst.; U. Penn. Med.; Washington U.; Temple U.; UNFAO; Phi Beta Kappa; Sigma Xi; hundreds of articles; much more; IACVF Board Chairman; (in A. Schatz, "The FDA & Truth Decay", IACVF, Cancer News Journal, v.11, n.4, p.11, 1976; & Schatz resume in v.10, n.6, p.2-5, 1975).

"Cancer research has no place for fixed concepts, for vested interests, for orthodoxy.... Scientific progress depends ... on the correction of errors, no matter how authoritative & traditional these errors may be ...(& on) the application of research findings." - Dr. Michael Shimkin, Assoc. Director of Field Studies, NCI; Prof. Oncology, U. of Cal., San Diego, (in Independent Citizens Research Foundation, Just Around the Corner, p.7).

Q.3.4 FAMOUS BIO-MEDICS:

"The history of medicine is replete with committees who criticized new discoveries, but did not experiment." - Andrew Ivy, co-author of 1,500 scientific articles; Director, ACS; et. al.; in Congressional Record, v.108, part 11, p.14288, July 20, 1962.

"(Dr. Andrew C.) Ivy cited the effectiveness of bread mold (e.g. penicillin) applied to wounds & infections, (was) known as far back as 500 AD." - (p.161, 1976 edition).

"...no scientific standards for testing cancer exist .... The competent & incompetent alike, the quack & the dedicated healer, the fraudulent & the genuine are damned equally...." - (p.86, 1976 ed.). - in Nat Morris, The Cancer Blackout, p.86, 161.

"Gregor Mendel, who had never received a teaching certificate because he couldn't pass in biology, began in 1856.... (His) work, which was virtually the birth of genetics, wasn't widely appreciated until the end of the century. ...Charles Darwin... dropped out of medical school because he couldn't stand science...." - C.R.Scriver,MD, "Inborn Errors of Metabolism: A New Frontier of Nutrition", Nutrition Today,Sep.1974,p.4.

Q.3.5 NOBEL LAUREATES:

"More than half of the great remedies known to medical history have come from empiricists...'irregulars'...of no or little scientific training. There is no reason to believe that conditions have essentially changed." -Alexis Carrel, Nobel Laureate (in Harry Hoxsey, You Don't Have to Die, p.8).

"Patients have been cured almost instantaneously of...lupus..., cancer, ...ulcers, tuberculosis.... In a few seconds, at most a few hours, the symptoms disappear & the anatomic lesions mend. The miracle is characterized by extreme acceleration of the normal process of healing." - Dr. Alexis Carrel, Nobel Laureate in Medicine, "Prayer", p.42, 43, (in Health Research, Is Cancer Curable?, p.10).

"It is not well known that in 1973 Tinbergan won a Nobel Prize in Medicine for demonstrating that changes in alignment of body structure can affect the health of the entire body. As a result, few practitioners consider body structure in their treatment plan." - Hulsey, DDS, MS; Steigerwald, DC(Chiropractic); "The Skeletal Dysfunction Syndrome", Price - Pottenger Nutrition Foundation Bulletin, v.6, n.3, p.22, 1981.

"The discovery of radium by the Curies was facilitated by observing a native witch doctor treating sick people by burying them up to their necks in radium-bearing mud." - Donald Law, A Guide to Alternative Medicine, p.5.

"Everyone should know that the 'war on cancer' is largely a fraud, and that the NCI and the ACS are derelict in their duties to the American people who support them."
-Linus Pauling, Nobel Laureate twice.

"The ACS tried to ruin my research foundation." - Albert Szent-Gyorki, Nobel Laureate, discoveror of Vitamins C & P.

"(The National Cancer Program is) a bunch of (obscenity)." &

"The American public is being sold a nasty bill of goods about cancer." - James Watson, Nobel Laureate, co-discoveror of DNA double helix. (All 3 above in P.B.Chowka, East-West J., Jan. 1978,p.23; & March 1981,p.36,47; & John Richardson,MD, Laetrile Case Histories,p.59). (1st quote by J. Watson also in: Phillip Nobile, "King Cancer", Esquire, v.6, p.103, June 1973.)

"The ACS has done the American public a really great disservice." - Dr. David Baltimore, Nobel Laureate in biomed., (in Ralph Moss, The Progressive, Feb. 1980, p.16).

"... cancer ... there is no disease whose prime cause is better known.... In the meantime, millions of men must die unnecessarily." - Otto Warburg, Nobel Laureate twice in Medicine, (in Nat Morris, Cancer Blackout, p.iv, 1977).

"Rous, ...in 1911...discovered a virus that caused cancer in chickens.... In 1966, ...Rous was awarded a Nobel Prize for the work he had done 55 years before...."(p.100).

"Howard Temin discovered that RNA viruses can translate their RNA into DNA.... After Temin's discoveries last year, the field suddenly exploded & too much work of a second-rate nature was done by people not well enough versed in virus lore."(p.102, 105).
- Lucy Eisenberg, "The Politics of Cancer", Harper's Magazine, Nov. 1971, p.100.

"'The historical phenomenon' of the 'long interval which' elapses 'between the making of a fundamental discovery & the general understanding of its importance & full realization of its benefits'.... Nowhere today is this delay more unhappily evident than in the field of cancer research. The accumulated data of **Rous**, **Shope**, **Coley**, **Bittner**, Strong, Andervont, Green, Greene, Williams, Taylor, **Furth**, Twombly, Cowdry, **Diller**, Bawden, Pirie, Stanley, Wycoff, Kunitz, & others indicate ... the path for ... something of practical benefit to the cancer patient ... other than surgery & radium."
- Frederick S. Hammett, Lankenau Hosp. Res. Inst., Science, v.103,n.2685,p.714,June14,1946.

Q.4.0 PRIVATE MEDICAL UNIONS & GROUPS:
Q.4.1 ACS, (UNPROVEN METHODS; WHOLISTICS):

The ACS "Committee on Unproven Methods of Cancer Management...("comprised of... representatives of the NCI, the FDA") ...is actively involved in strengthening & encouraging passage of state legistlation to control the use of worthless cancer remedies & tests." - ACS, "Fact Sheet on Laetrile",1977; & ACS,1978 Cancer Facts & Figures,p.23, (except that in parenthesis).

"In 1966 the ACS formulated a State Model Cancer Act which was instrumental in the enactment of anti-quackery laws now enforced in 9 states. ...In California, (it is a)... felony.... The use of unproven methods is also a criminal offense in Colorado, Illinois, Kentucky, Maryland, Nevada, North Dakota, Ohio, & Pennsylvania." - Jane Brody of New York Times, & Arthur Holleb,MD, of ACS, You Can Fight Cancer & Win, p.145, 150.

"The California cancer law places the burden of proof of efficacy & safety of a cancer agent on the proponent .... In Sept. 1974, the State of Cal. enacted new legislation which makes a conviction of a 'quackery' charge a felony ..., with jail terms of up to 5 years & fines as high as $10,000."

"The ACS is ... publishing articles of interest on unproven methods in Ca - A Cancer Journal for Clinicians, which is distributed to more than 360,000 physicians, medical students, dentists, & medical libraries throughout the nation." - ACS, Unproven Methods of Cancer Management - 1976, p.10, 11.

"When, in 1976-7, (the ACS) finally decided to remove the ban on 3 of **(over 66)methods** (from their Unproven Methods of Cancer Management) - listed for years - no apologies or explanations were offered. These treatments are ... Coley's toxin's, Staphage Lysate... by Dr. Lincoln, & Hyperthermia." - Richard Ericson,BS,JD, Cancer Treatment: Why So Many Failures?, p.165.

"On April 17, 1952 the Dickinson County, Iowa chapter of the ACS ran a full page ad in...'The Spirit Lake Beacon', asking the society to enter the new field of investigating cancer cure claims. They cited 4 such 'cures'. The chapter was expelled from the ACS. Its chair(woman), Mrs. Roy Tatman, felt compelled to declare: 'We were asked to help conquer cancer. We have tried to do just that. Has the society (ACS) another motive?'"
- Arlin J.Brown, March of Truth on Cancer, p.104.

"... we as doctors may begin to emphasize treatment of the patient as a whole as well as the disease .... to influence general body systems & through them modify the neoplasm which resides within the body. ... within one's mind is a power capable of exerting forces which can either enhance or inhibit the progress of this disease." - ACS President, Dr. Eugene P. Pendergras, 1959, (in International Association of Cancer Victims & Friends, Cancer News Journal, v.15,n.1,p.5, Spring 1980).

Q.4.2 **AMERICAN COLLEGE of SURGEONS:**

(You) "would be shocked ... at the amount of unneccessary surgery that is performed (for) Money.... And I can prove it." - Paul R. Hawley, MD, Director, American College of Surgeons, (in US News & World Reports, Feb. 20, 1953, in Is Cancer Curable?, Health Research, p.68).

"The (modern, orthodox) medical care system does some things very well - principally, emergency & acute care. Accident victims ... need ... mechanistic medicine - & fast." (with Alternative Therapy as an adjuvant (in combination) - Ed.) - R.J. Carlson, JD, (in Leslie J. Kaslof, Member, N.Y. Academy of Science; Founder, National Council on Wholistic ... ; Wholistic Dimensions in Healing, A Resource Guide, p.1.

"Investigators at Johns Hopkins reported...more than half of a group of automobile accident victims who had died from abdominal injuries 'should have had a reasonable chance of survival' if mistakes in diagnosis & treatment had not been made in the emergency rooms." - Spencer Klaw, (grad., Harvard U.; Assoc. Ed., Fortune; lecturer, Columbia U.), The Great American Medicine Show, p.42.

"The...Commission on Professional & Hospital Activities maintains a computer bank of information on...American hospitals, including comparative death rates for procedures, accidents, infections, errors.... ...with a vengeance the government would envy. ...the information is 'classified'.... ...this computer bank contains the potential for a 'Pentagon Papers' & 'Watergate' combined." - Robert Mendelsohn,MD; Chmn., Med. Licensing Comm., State of Ill.; Assoc. Prof. of Preventive Med. & Community Health, U. of Ill.; Pres., NHF; board director, Alternative Birth Crisis Coalition; med. dir., Project Head Start; Confessions of a Medical Heretic, p.136.

"The American College of Surgeons said that a little more than 10% of surgery was necessary." - Dr. Mendelsohn, NHF, Public Scrutiny, March 1981, p.18.

Q.4.3 **AMA, (ETHICS, FOOD, FLUORIDE):**

"It is derogatory to the dignity of the profession, to resort to public advertisement,... inviting ... individuals affected with particular diseases,... PUBLICALLY OFFERING ADVICE & MEDICINE TO THE POOR GRATIS or promising RADICAL CURES, or to PUBLISH cases ... in the daily prints,... to invite LAYMEN to be present in operations, ... to boast of CURES & remedies." - AMA, Code of Ethics, 1847 (first); (Capitals by Editor).

"...A class action effort by 150 Iowa chiropractors (is) seeking $300 million on charges of conspiracy by the AMA. Exhibits for evidence...include...a 1965 letter from ("an AMA organized") Quackery Committee, warning AMA members it was unethical to associate with 'the cult of the chiropractic'...."

"Last year the AMA adopted a new code of ethics allowing MD's to work with chiropractors." - Voice of Medical Freedom, March 1981, p.12.

"A physician should practice a method of healing founded on a scientific basis; & he should not voluntarily associate professionally with anyone who violates this principle." - AMA, Principles of Medical Ethics, 1977.

"A physician shall, in the provision of appropriate patient care, except in emergencies, be free to choose whom to serve, with whom to associate, & the environment in which to provide medical services." - AMA, Principles of Medical Ethics, 1980.

"The solicitation of votes for office...shall be considered a disqualification for election to any office in...this Association (, the AMA)." - AMA, (in G. Edward Griffin, World Without Cancer, p.388).

"The belief of some trustees & staff members (is) that the selection of (the new Chairman, Board of Trustees) was in part engineered from within federal prison (by the) former board chairman now serving an 18-month sentence for bank fraud."(p.51).

"...Control of the (AMA) is solidly in the hands of a layman of whom most AMA members have never heard of... , (a) former executive director of AMPAC - the American Medical Political Action Committee."(p.52).

"...Former AMA employees say that telephones at headquarters were tapped."(p.54). - "Turmoil at the AMA", Medical World News, May 10, 1974, p.51.

"... purely for pleasure.... In this perspective, there is no such thing as a junk food." - AMA Secretary, Council on Foods & Nutrition, Philip White, 1979.

(It is) "inappropriate at this time to adopt the proposed national Dietary Goals (of the Select Committee on Nutrition & Human Needs, US Senate, Feb. 1977).... There is a potential for harmful effects" (from it). - AMA Exec. V. Pres., James Sammons, to the Senate Committee. (Last 2 above, in CSPI, Nutrition Action, v.7, n.9, p.4 & 6, Sept. 1980.)

"About 30% of organic foods analyzed in 1972 by the NYS Dept. of Agriculture ... contain(ed) pesticide residues, as compared with 25% of regular foods." - T.H.Jukes, "The Organic Food Myth", Journal AMA, v.230,n.2,p.276, Oct. 14, 1974.

"...how frequently...(is) the patients' suffering made worse by...frank mismanagement, if not downright neglect, of the patients' nutritional health in our hospitals."

"...one of the largest pockets of unrecognized malnutrition in America...(is) in the ...hospitals."

"Entering a hospital & placing oneself in the hands of doctors engenders a feeling of security akin to that experienced by a fugitive when he reached the sanctuary of the cathedral doors in legendary times." - Charles E. Butterworth,Jr.,MD; Chairman, Council of Foods & Nutrition, AMA; Prof. of Med., & Dir. Nutrition Program, U. Alabama; "The Skeleton in the Hospital Closet", Nutrition Today, Mar. 1974, p.4.

"...malnutrition has for too long been identified with the 'classical' vitamin deficiency syndrome, by physicians...."(p.8).

"...malnutrition is often a complex medical & socio-economic problem.... (Yet, with) "simple adherence to basic diagnostic & therapeutic principles of nutrition.... -At times the results will seem nothing short of astonishing." - C.E.Butterworth; & George L. Blackburn,MD,PhD; Ass't. Prof. Surg., Harvard Med.; Dir., Nutrition...Boston City Hosp.; & New England Deaconess Hosp.; "Hospital Malnutrition", Nutrition Today, Mar. 1975, p.8, 18.

"Don't drink fluoridated water.... Fluoride is a corrosive poison which will produce harm on a long term basis." - AMA President, Dr. Charles Heyd (in Aid for Cancer Victims, ...Directory..., p.6).

Q.4.4 ADA, (FLUORIDE):

(In) "1916...that grand old pioneer of advancement in dentistry, G.V.Black... presented his epoch making studies on the role of fluorine in producing mottled enamel. ... The studies...by...the USPHS, led to a nationwide effort to eliminate...excessive ...fluorine in the drinking water (by) the USPHS...."

"...our knowledge of the subject certainly does not warrant the introduction of fluorine in community water supplies generally."

"Sodium fluoride is a highly toxic substance..., it may be definitely harmful."

"...the potentialities for harm far outweigh those for good." - Editorial Dept., J. Amer. Dental Assoc., L.P.Anthony,DDS,Editor, v.31, n.19, p.1360, Oct. 1, 1944.

Q.4.5 AMALGAMATIONS, (FOOD, FLUORIDE):

"Thus, under careful examination of original data, cross-examination under oath of scientific proponents, & critical followup assessments of effects, neither the efficacy nor the safety of fluoridation has been demonstrated. Nevertheless, it seems impossible to engage the scientific community or the public health authorities in any effort to examine the subject."

"The reexamination of subjects on which strong recommendations have been made challenges one's commitment & integrity. If, as scientists & public health advisors, we can't muster the courage to meet those challenges, perhaps we should all take up a more honest profession such as used car sales or TV repair where at least the results of our services are unequivocal." - Frederick I. Scott, Editor(ial), American Laboratory, v.12, n.9, p.12, Sep. 1980.

"Dr. Miller: 'The USDA made some examination.... (&)recommended to the farmers that fluorine not be added to the water...of (pregnant) sows because it did something to the pigs that were unborn.... Do you think it might be wise for the (US)PHS...to inquire what might happen to pregnant women & the unborn child...?'"

"Dr. Porterfield: 'No, sir; I think there is a difference. .... There is more money available for matters that have economic value than there is for health.'"
- Chemicals in Foods & Cosmetics, Hearings, Select Committee to Investigate the Use of Chemicals in Foods & Cosmetics, US House, 82nd Congress, 2nd Session, 1952, p.1702, (in A. Schatz, "The FDA & Truth Decay", Cancer News Journal, v.11, n.4, p.13, 1976).

"'It is certain that some day cancer & heart disease will be conquered. If they are controlled, the majority of people will live 10 to 20 years longer. It is no exaggeration to point out that elimination of these degenerative diseases, which at first glance might be a blessing, could easily constitute a major disaster.'" - AMA's official, A. I. Landis, (in the Pittsburgh Press, within Morris Bealle, American Capsule News, all in Arlin Brown, March of Truth on Cancer, p.105).

"...Dr. A. I. Lansing, the outgoing President of the Gerontological Society, who said on Nov. 8, 1958, that finding a cure for cancer & heart disease would be a major financial disaster which would bancrupt the social security system & the big insurance companies."
- J. I. Rodale, Prevention, 11/1961, (in Cancer Control Journal, v.3, n.1, p.14, 1975).

"Individual food faddism - the individual's food behavior or beliefs, stemming from food myths - has its origin '...in acute or chronic psychological aberration.'"
- ACS & NCI, National Conference on Nutrition & Cancer, (Proceedings of the), 1978, p.2122, "Editorial: ... Nutritional Fads", by William Darby, MD, PhD, Pres., Nutrition Foundation.

"In the feeding of hospital patients, more attention should be given to providing tasty & attractive meals, & less to the nutritive quality of the food."

"People say that all you get out of sugar is calories, no nutrients.... There is no perfect food, not even mother's milk."

"Have confidence in America's food industry. It deserves it." - Harvard U., School of Public Health, Nutrition Dept. head, Dr. Frederick Stare, (1st paragraph: Cancer News Journal, v.7, n.5, p.14, May 1972; 2nd, in: William Dufty, Sugar Blues, p.156; 3rd, in: The Dictocrats, p.195).

"Overcrowding 'decreases the number of well-trained men who can count on the profession for a livelihood ...Doctors(:)....the way to get them better is to produce fewer'. ...Medical education...should be reserved for those who could afford 'a liberal & disinterested educational experience'. ...Medical schools, with their admission requirements of 4 years of high school or its 'equivalent', attracted 'a mass of unprepared youth...drawn out of industrial occupations....' Neither 'the crude boy' nor 'the jaded clerk' were suitable.... (Abraham) Flexner proposed" (in his modern governing model: "Flexner Report" / Medical Education). - E. Richard Brown, Rockefeller Medicine Men, p.147-8.

Q.5.0 MASS MEDIA:
Q.5.1 PRESS:

"... attempts to make further reports were blocked by the requests of the Journal of the AMA, made to the (other) official journals, to refuse me the right to report my findings further."

"... so when the Cancer Quack conventions of the AMA annually proclaim that the sign of the quack is his refusal to report his work in official journals, they are putting on a gigantic fraud. It was so in my case." - in The Functional Carbonyl..., p.3, by William Frederick Koch, MD, PhD; Prof. Chemistry & Histology, U. Michigan Medical School; Prof. Physiol., Wayne St. U.; lauded in JAMA editorial for sparing para-thyroid from surgical removal; (nephew to Robert Koch, Nobel Laureate in Med); (praised by: Dr. J. Maisin, Pres., Internat'l Union Against Cancer; & Dr. W. Dow, Pres., Dow Chem.; & Dr. A. R. Mitchell, Chairman, Board of Trustees, AMA).

"'I see in him (Dr. Max Gerson) one of the most eminent medical geniuses in the history of medicine .... he was greatly impeded by adverse political conditions.'"

"'... try to tell the people of America about Dr. Gerson's merits &...results.... I wish you the best in your difficult task.'" - Dr. Albert Schweitzer"

"Dr. Gerson showed me letters of rejection from various medical magazines (for articles entitled): 'Cancer: A Deficiency Disease', ... 'Dietetic Treatment of Malignant Tumors'." - S. J. Haught, Has Dr. Max Gerson A True Cancer Cure?, p.21, 137, & title p.

"Ferdinand Sauerbruch, MD, (Nobel Laureate)...arranged a grand test for using Gerson's diet therapy (against cancer, etc.) on 450 'incurable' lupus (skin TB) patients. 446 recovered...."(p.7).

"Gerson was invited...on a...talk show by...host Long John Nebel.... ...Nebel was fired...the very next day & the radio network was threatened by the AMA."(p.18).

"Even when a rare Jew...escaped from a concentration camp & sneaked back to his people to warn them...they could not believe the escapee."(p.10).

"On 2 occasions Gerson became violently ill.... Lab tests showed...arsenic in his urine. Some of Gerson's best case histories mysteriously disappeared from his files. The manuscript & all of its copies for Gerson's almost completed book were stolen & never recovered. ...They spread the lie that Dr. Gerson had died of cancer."(p.19).

- Norman Fritz, space shuttle engineer, Healing, Journal of the Gerson Inst. & ... Therapy, v.1, n.1, p.7,10,18,19.

"When results of the (Laetrile) toxicity tests at Loyola (University, Chicago) were complete, (Dr. Harold Manner, Chairman Dept. Biol., author of 50 articles & 5 texts) asked NCI to publish the findings in Journal NCI. This the agency refused to do. Publication in other journals was also denied him." - in National Health Federation, Bulletin, Nov. 1977, p.2.

"When Dr. Manner reported on the total remission of breast cancer in lab animals (using 'Laetrile in conjunction with vitamins & enzymes')... , ACS President, Ben Byrd, criticized (him) for making his announcement in public, & said such announcements should be made only in a proper scientific forum."

"But, as all scientists know, there is a time lag of 12 to 18 months between the time a manuscript is submitted & the time it is published in a scientific journal."

"...Delay, says Dr. Manner, is a luxury which people with right-now cancers cannot afford." - Paul Harvey, "Cancer Remission with Laetrile", Los Angeles Times, (in The Laker, Oct. 10, 1977, p.2).

"The...experts of the FDA have declared Laetrile to be worthless...quackery & fraud.... These experts are the professional descendants of experts...confident that mental illness should be cured by drilling holes in the skull, the better to let the demons out. ...This is the Orwellian fashion in which the medical establishment throws its weight around...." - James Kilpatrick, Washington Star, (in Cancer News Journal, v.11, n.4, p.12, 1976).

(The) "NIH (including NCI) has permitted other nations to pull ahead of the US in vital fields of research. The critics blame stodgy old guard bureaucrats who pour govt. money into the same tired old research projects but won't take a chance on anything at all unconventional." - Jack Anderson, (in Gary Null, "Linus Pauling Could ... , But He Can't Get the Money...", Caveat Emptor, v.10,n.10,p.8, Oct. 1980).

"'Cancer Dialogue '80'...(was) sponsored by the Omega Inst., & co-sponsored by the Amer. College of Preventive Med., & the Amer. Holistic Med. Assoc. .... The New York Times reported on Oct. 13, 1980 that 9 of the 27 (speakers: NCI Directors, Drs. Arthur Upton & Frank Rauscher, Sr. V. President of ACS; Dr. Emil Frei III, Director, Sidney Farber Cancer Inst.; et. al.)... had withdrawn about 2 weeks before the opening ... from this discussion of traditional & 'alternative' approaches to cancer treatment.... Some of the speakers said that pressure had been put on them.... the Medical Tribune (Oct. 22, 1980, p.13, said:) 'Most of the 8 symposium dropouts received influence-wielding phone calls from (the) chairman of the ACS's committee on unproven methods of cancer management, or other ACS officials.'" - Linus Pauling, Nobel Laureate twice, (in The Linus Pauling Institute ... Newsletter, v.1,n.10,p.1,Winter 1980).

"...Terminally ill cancer patients, ...100...who took 10 grams of Vitamin C daily lived 4 times longer (from date of diagnosis as 'untreatable', than controls).... Dr. (Linus) Pauling submitted these findings in a scientific paper to JAMA (Journal AMA), & NEJM (New England Journal of Medicine), & both have refused to publish this illustrous, (twice) Nobel Laureate's work." - D. Ian Thiermann, Yale U. grad., (in IACVF, Cancer News Journal, v.14, n.1, p.9, Jan. 1979).

(There is) "suppression of this info. by the health food industry - based press.... My book, A Macrobiotic Explanation of Pathological Calcification ... contains more than 600 references directly dealing with (Vitamin) D - group toxicity. In spite of this massive documentation, magazines like Prevention, Let's Live, & Better Nutrition have repeatedly refused to publish any article dealing with (it)." - J. Y. Moon, "...Addition of...Vitamin D, to Milk increase(s)...Bone Cancer & Heavy Metal Poisoning?", IACVF, Cancer News Journal, v.13, n.1, p.6, April 1978.

"...Rodale Press (publisher of Prevention -Ed.).... In 1965, ...brought out a...book ...Health Finder.... On April 3, 1964, the FTC served the publisher with a show cause order in an administrative cease-&-desist proceeding.... Rodale...spent nearly 5 years fighting for a right guaranteed every American...."

(For) "instance(s) of a federal agency...censor(ing) publications.... a long list of books could be cited, including those of Gayelord Hauser, Dale Alexander, Lelord Kordel, Dr. Royal Lee, Dr. Herman Taller, ... Paul C. Bragg,.... Joseph Boardman,MD,.... H. Curtis Wood,Jr.,MD,...." - Omar Garrison, The Dictocrats, Our Unelected Rulers, p.246-262.

"...the National Enquirer. ('The nature of the material makes (it) a medical journal in the foregoing instance')",(of an isolated medical article in it. - Ed.).(p.9).

"...Copyrights(')...permission...to use material.... (:) I might well die from cancer myself, while waiting for releases necessary for an epistemological review...in ...accumulated knowledge.... For those who use copyright laws against the public interest, ...I feel sorrow...." - J. Gordon Roberts, developer of Vitamin D milk against rickets, Cancer: How & Why It May Be Wiped Out, p.9, 142.

"Cancer...; the plight of a group of maverick scientists ... working on their own .... Their work cannot be called controversial; it is being ignored.... That cancer is caused by a bacterium ... which, in its life cycle goes through several forms, including a virus like phase.... (like a) larva into a butterfly. Nearly all ... are doctors with bona fide degrees in science or medicine (Dr. Clara J. Fonti, Dr. W. M. Crofton,FRSM). (Yet each) must do his research privately & after that publish findings at his own expense.... In light of today's knowledge, science cannot be absolutely sure that they are absolutely wrong...." - Life, v.52,n.25,p.85, June 22, 1962.

"'The whole thing, as far as we are concerned, is a put-up deal to discredit Laetrile.'... says Robert Bradford of the Committee for Freedom of Choice in Cancer Therapy." - Time, May 11, 1981, p.55.

"Sometimes there is little regard for people's lives. ...A hospital tested a new NCI drug...on children. Their kidneys were lost within days. This was no big deal, because new drugs are routinely given out with literally no safeguards for people...." - FDA drug review section's Robert Young.

"We've been on a plateau for about 10 years. There've been virtually no breakthroughs" (in cancer therapy). - Dr. Gordon Zubrod, Dir., NCI Comprehensive Cancer Center for State of Florida, U. Miami Hosp. & Clinic.

"...It's been like swatting at flies with a sledgehammer. ...I suppose as far as end products are concerned it's been a bust, but then so is the over-all treatment of cancer." - Dr. Charles Moertel, Dir., NCI Comprehensive Cancer Center, Mayo Clinic.

"A 1-year study by the Washington Post has documented 620 cases in which experimental drugs have been implicated in the deaths of cancer patients. .... And they amount to merely a fraction of the thousands of people who in recent years have died or suffered terribly from cancer experiments...."

"...In the vast majority of drug experiments, it is not uncommon for none or 1 or 2 of 100's of patients to benefit from the drug."

"These human experiments have gone largely unchallenged & unquestioned by Congress, the medical profession, & the scientific community at large." - last 6 paragraphs above in Ted Gup & Jonathan Neumann, "Cancer Cures Often a Curse", Washington Post, (reprinted in Chicago Sun Times, Sunday, Oct 25, 1981, Section 2, p.1).

"The new medical-industrial complex is now a fact of American life ... with broad & potentially troubling implications ...." - Dr. Arnold Relman, Editor, New England Journal of Medicine.

"Corruption has permeated virtually every area of the Medicare-Medicaid health-care industry." - FBI Assistant Director, Francis Mullen,Jr., to Congress. - (last 2 above, in US News & World Reports, Aug. 17, 1981, p.50, & 53).

"Every person with a new theory is a quack until the value of the theory is demonstrated, but if all the quacks are arbitrarily suppressed how are their theories to be tested?" - Editorial from a Scribner's Magazine of 1891, (in IACVF, Cancer News Journal, Bicentennial Issue, p.20, 1976).

"'Many of our medical writers have a tendency to work with the establishment, to shoot for those $1000 prizes offered by the establishment organizations, in addition to the fee they get from the magazine. ...At the magazine, ...a query was sent to the ACS or ... NCI: 'What do you think about this idea?' And they would say:'...how can it be any good, because we've got the best right here.... So forget about it.'.' - Pat McGrady, Jr., President, American Society of Journalists & Authors; (who) wrote (an) article on ... Vitamin A & Enzyme therapy for cancer at the Janker Clinic in Bonn.... (His article) finally appeared in Esquire in April 1976, after 5 years of rejection by many other major magazines." - Gary Null & Robert Houston, "The Cancer Fraud", Penthouse, Sept 1979, p.78.

(A) "striking & disturbing" (pattern in magazines that accept cigarette advertising:) "I was unable to find a single article in seven years of publication, that would have given readers any clear notion of the nature & extent of the medical & social havoc being wreaked by the cigarette-smoking habit." - R.C. Smith, Columbia Journalism Review, 1978, (in "Conspiracy of Silence", ACSH,(American Council on Science & Health), News & Views.v.1,n.2,p.1,Feb. 1980).

"...The FDA is forcing pharm. mfg. firms to remove some 3,000 prescription drugs from the market because...none (were)...in compliance with the 1962 Kefauver-Harris legistlation, which required the makers of the drugs to show the FDA 'substantial evidence' of effectiveness for all the uses...suggested. ...The FDA...agreement (was) ending a...lawsuit.... ...brought by the National Council of Senior Citizens, & the American Public Health Association, a Ralph Nader organization...." - Spotlight, Nov. 24, 1980, p.10.

"Nearly 90% of the more than 10,000 publications about phenothiazines have been financially sponsored by the drug industry. Independent research studies conducted without drug company backing have failed to indicate overall usefulness of phenothiazines." - D. Springer, "Thorazine; Chemical for Social Control", Issues in Radical Therapy, v.4, n.2, p.13, Spring 1976.

"Henri Pradal, Guide des Medicaments les Plus Courants (Guide to Medicines Most Current),(Paris: Seuil, 1974), is a list of the 100 best selling (drugs with their) consequences. On publication day, 57 drug firms started separate legal actions to have the book withdrawn & sued for reimbursement for probate damages."

"To promote Valium, (its drug firm) spent $200 million in ten years & commissioned some 200 doctors a year to produce scientific articles about its properties.... A study conducted by the FDA (showed)...1/5 of (the MD's, 'on field research with new drugs',) investigated had invented (faked) the data they sent to the drug companies, & pocketed the fees (1973).... In 1973, the entire drug industry spent an average of $4,500 on each practicing physician for advertising & promotion...." - Ivan Illich, Medical Nemesis, p.60 & 66, (Aug. 1977 edition).

"'The dilemma of the (AMA) Board of Trustees (is that it) ... had no choice but to appease the pharmaceutical industry ... or forego income from advertising (in its journals).... The (AMA) Council on Drugs ... (made up of 'independent thinking scientists & practitioners ... was dissolved' & replaced) by the staff of the (AMA's) Dept. of Drugs ('obligated to do the bidding of their superiors, ... emasculated & worthless').... Thus the AMA has abrogated its responsibility of providing factual information on drugs to the physician in the public's behalf.'" - AMA Council on Drugs Chairman, Dr. John Adriani, Professor of Surgery, Tulane U. Med., to US Senator Gaylord Nelson's Subcommittee on Monopoly, (in Spencer Klaw, The Great American Medicine Show, p.125).

"'... the public should not be asked to accept risks resulting from purely internal govt. decisions if, without endangering national security, the information can be made public & the decisions reached after public discussion.'...." (This) "(panel's report was subsequently suppressed) ... despite the panel's explicit recommendation that it be released". - in Underground Nuclear Testing, USAEC Report n. TID 25180, Sept. 1969, p.51ff &52; & Underground Nuclear Weapons Testing, Committee on Foreign Relations, US Senate, Sept. 29, 1969, p.31ff; (both referred in Joel Primack & Frank Von Hippel, Advice & Dissent, Scientists in the Political Arena, p.107,& 115; F. Von Hippel, Chairman, Federation of American Scientists; founding member, Committee on Scientific Freedom & Responsibility, AAAS; Sr. Res. Physicists, Center for Energy & Environmental Studies, Princeton U.; J. Primack, Prof., U. Cal. Santa Cruz).

"The lowest standards of journalism, the greatest corruption, the most blatant pandering to advertisers goes on in the sections of the newspaper concerned with life's necessities...: food, ... , cars...." - Nicholas von Hoffman.

"Food pages...last year helped daily newspapers (to) $873 million in food ads." - last 2 quotes in Consumer Ed. Research Ctr., Caveat Emptor,v.11,n.9,p.16,Sep. 1981.

"... lack of communication & understanding between organic farmers & the agricultural research & Extension communities has hindered the transfer & application of research & educational information. The negative attitudes of many conventional farmers & of the agricultural establishment toward organic farming have sometimes limited the acceptance of this method of farming. Many ... strongly believe that organic farming is impractical or infeasible. To some extent, these views are the result of misperceptions & misunderstandings.... Agricultural policymakers are not fully aware of the environmental, conservation, & energy-related benefits of organic farming.... Little research & public information are available to help organic farmers...."

"...data showing adverse effects of high ingestion levels of pesticides on experimental animals are now extensive...." - USDA, Report & Recommendations on Organic Farming, July 1980, p.65 & 83.

"In Connecticut, recommended books on...nutrition are listed by the State Board of Health & issued to librarians. ...Silent Spring (was) placed on Conn.'s 'not recommended' list.... This...aroused...a protest by (US) Senator Abraham S. Ribicoff." - Beatrice Trum Hunter, Consumer Beware!, p.41.

Q.5.2 **TELEVISION:**

"CBS Reports, ..."The Silent Spring of Rachel Carson" caused almost as much anger as the book itself.... 3 of its 5 commercial sponsors withdrew their support." - PBS, WTTW, Chicago, Sep. 26, 1981, 9pm.

"We've heard...very little about the hazards, ...the failures, ...& yet the public ... was being asked to accept, ... to acquiesce..., & did not have the whole picture, so I set about to remedy the balance there." - Rachel Carson, in CBS Reports, "The Silent Spring ...", 1963.

"This is an era of specialists, each of whom sees his own problem & is unaware of or intolerant of the larger frame into which it fits....When the public protests, confronted with some obvious evidence of damaging results..., it is fed little tranquilizing pills of half truth." - Rachel Carson, Silent Spring, p.23; (8 awards: The Schweitzer Medal; Conservationist of the Year; 1963 Achievement (by A. Einstein College of Med.); etc., for book on pesticides.)

"...Last year when we discussed this book (S.Wolfe, Pills That Don't Work) on the (Phil Donahue Show).... 120,000 people ordered the book just from watching this (one hour total) program." - Sidney Wolfe,MD; Director, Health Research Group, & Public Citizen, (both Ralph Nader groups); on WGN -TV, Phil Donahue Show, Sept. 24, 1981.

"NBC in ... 1975 launched ... programs which portrayed doctors as being as afflicted with error & greed as the rest of us.... (The producer was) aided in preparing Medical Story by Dr. Sidney Wolfe of (Ralph) Nader's Health Research Group, a leading critic of unnecessary surgery; the producers of Marcus Welby, who would never dream of committing any medical sin, get their cues from the AMA." - David Hapgood, The Average Man Fights Back, p.50.

"In the first 5 years of his television 'practice', Marcus Welby, MD, received 250,000 letters from viewers seeking medical advice." - ACT solicitation letter.

"Each spring there is a media blitz in conjunction with ACS's fund-raising campaign. The vast majority of advertising space & time is contributed free of charge as a 'public service'." - "Overview Needed of Cancer Cabal", Spotlight, April 13, 1981, p.6.

"...The Annenberg School of Communications at the U. of Penn. ...study showed that ...the 'magic of (Orthodox -Ed.) medicine' (is advertized, since:) There are 5x as many ...health professionals on TV as...in real life. ...Daytime serials...may well be 'the largest source of medical advice in the US'. ....In the NEJM(,) a full report is to be released by the USPHS...." - Health Writers, Health Newsletter, v.11, n.10, p.5, Oct. 1981.

"'The industries that oppose (a bill for truth-in-packaging of food) represent 1/6th of the GNP.... Home economists (were) told to ... work against the bill or ... lose their jobs.... Editorial services in Washington ... send out editorials against truth-in-packaging; (editorials) used by hundreds of small newspapers across the nation; (to) papers that rely on canned editorials.... I was told advertisers had objected.... An educational television ...man... explained, '...the largest contributors to the foundations which feed money to (educational television) are the major industries.'.' - US Senator Philip A. Hart, (on the) virtual blackout on radio & television coverage for the entire 1963 truth-in-packaging hearings."

(We did)" '...discuss ... the facts of life covering advertising-media relationships .... We suggested to the publisher ...(that) their editorial department ... understand ... (that) their operations may affect the advertiser - their bread & butter. We invited them to consider publishing some favorable articles about the food industry.... (Television stations receive) about 65% of their advertising revenue from GMA (Grocery Manufacturers of America) members.'" - P. S. Willis, GMA head, in address to Television Bureau of Advertising, 1963. - (last 2 paragraphs above, in Beatrice T. Hunter, <u>Consumer Beware!</u>, p.25-6).

"...The (tv) cameras were not rolling when (US) Rep. John Dow gave an eloquent appeal against giving South Africa a larger sugar (import) quota (into the US). He lost ... on an unrecorded vote, with 'public' civil-righters.... voting against him."

"...The (tv) networks <u>refused</u> an offer by a group of anti-war (US) Senators to <u>buy</u> time to explain their position. 'I could buy time to sell soap...,' complained Senator Harold Hughes, 'but not to speak as a US Senator on issues of war & peace.'" - Mark J. Green, <u>Who Runs Congress?</u>, Ralph Nader Congress Project, p.68, 104.

"In support of ... my news release..., I wish to insert a petition to Congress, .. by the Massachusetts Womens Political Club:

"'...the FTC, the USPO, (&) the FDA, are being used ... to bring pressure on drugless doctors, small-business men, & private individuals who interfere in any way with the profits ... or who criticize the Federal bureaus who are protecting (special interests).'"

"'...control of press, radio, & television is made possible (1) by the voluminous advertising by (special) interests, (2) by a 'working agreement' whereby nothing pertaining to health ... is made public until it has been cleared through a representative of the local health dept. whose policy is dictated by the AMA.'"

"'The (US) Justice Dept. ...acts as prosecutor (against) doctors & businessmen whose only crime is telling the truth & exposing the illegal activities....'"

"'The FDA uses evidence furnished by a so called scientific dept. of a great university, a dept. largely supported by huge donations from the very concerns who are flouting the law....'" - inserted by US Congressman Usher L. Burdick, <u>Congressional Record, Appendix</u>, v.<u>103</u>,n.40,p.A-1853, March 7, 1957.

Q.6.0 <u>LAW vs. JUSTICE</u>:
Q.6.1 <u>FREEDOM of SPEECH & PRESS, (OFFENDED)</u>; <u>USPO</u>, <u>FTC</u>:

"'It is hereby ordered that the defendants ...are... prohibited from ... representing in any manner (e.g. speech) that by eating ... specific foods,... supplements..., the metabolism of any person ... is altered toward a ... state of better health or free of illness ...(, including prohibition of) publishing material in any form whatsoever (on this) directed at California...'" - Superior Court of California (in Riverside), Judge Rich, Injunction, n.123619, Aug. 2, 1978.

(Defendant)"Nord Davis (was accused) that he <u>INTENDED</u> to ... practice medicine without a license."

"Dr. (Carey) Reams was found guilty of practicing & conspiring to practice medicine without a license (&) ordered ... to Cal. Inst. for Men for a 90 day...." - in Arlin Brown Info. Center, <u>Cancer Victory Bulletin</u>, v.<u>4</u>,n.11,p.1, Nov. 1978.

"...Dr. Krebs...is facing the possibility of a jail sentence stemming from violation of a 1977 court order not to speak publicly about Laetrile." - Voice of Medical Freedom, April 1981, p.6.

"'5 hours after presenting a ... lecture on cancer before an audience of about 400 in L.A., the windshield was shot out of my car on the road back to S.F. The next night the glass window in the tailgate was shot out ('300 miles removed from the first shooting').... The late Arthur T. Harris,MD, was threatened by two men with assassination if he continued to use Laetrile.'" - Dr. Ernst T. Krebs, Jr.

"... the science of cancer therapy is not nearly as complicated as the politics of cancer therapy." - G. Edward Griffin, World Without Cancer, p.19, 460.

"Dr. (Howard H.) Beard (Sc.D., Ph.D., Yale; Prof. Biochem./Med., at 3 med. schools; Biochemist at 3 institutes; author of 150 articles & 3 books) 'was ... charged with... mail fraud ... rendering fake & medically worthless cancer reports.... Postal investigators satisfied themselves the reports were willfully falsified....' On Oct. 30, 1967, Dr. Beard was sentenced in US Federal Court, Ft. Worth, TX, 'to ... mail fraud.... He alleged he could detect the presence of cancer in urine in 95% of all tests made.'" - FDA Papers... 1967-8, (in ACS, Unproven Methods of Cancer Management, c. 1971, p.36).

"...the complaint that Health Research, Dr. R.G.Wilborn,DC ... are...conducting an unlawful enterprise through the mails ... The Undersigned, ... Assistant Solicitor, Fraud Division, Post Office Dept. ... alleges that (Health Research is) obtaining ... money through the mails for various books & pamphlets entitled: Commonsense About Cancer; The Grape Cure; ... ; Is Cancer Curable?; ... ; Tumors; & Back to Eden; by ... fraudulent pretenses...." - Post Office Dept., Office of the Chief Hearing Examiner, May 14, 1955, (in Eleanor McBean, The Poisoned Needle, Health Research, p.94).

"'...Johanna Brandt in her book, The Grape Cure,.... The FTC objected to this book...(because) it represented: ...that most diseases originate in the intestine & are caused by poisons due to uneliminated waste;... that salt, inorganic drugs, & 'patent medicines' cause cancer.... The (FTC) ordered that such misrepresentations be discontinued.... The USPO Dept. ... issued a Fraud Order ... against the distributor for use of the mails to advertize & circularize ... 'health books' advancing fraudulent claims for dietary cures of...high blood pressure (low salt / fat?-Ed.), faulty eyesight (Vitamin A?-Ed.), & grey hair.'" - Journal AMA;v.116,p.2525, 1941; & v.139,p.93, 1949; (in ACS, Unproven Methods ..., p.84).

"...the US Postal Service...issued an order to stop my...mail. ...I have had to report to the local...Postal Service...&open my mail in front of a local postal inspector. If any person...orders the herbal Cancer preventative formula...the letter...is confiscated..., stamped 'Fraudulent', & returned to the sender. The FDA recommended to the US Postal Service...that this...formula was not beneficially effective towards the treatment of Cancer. (The FDA) did not even know what the ingredients of the formula were."

"('Active chemicals'&) alkaloids are only (or much more - Ed.) harmful when extracted from the crude herb or botanical(;) becom(ing) imbalanced, causing contra-indications (&)'side effects'. ...Jurisdiction of the FDA is restricted only to those new drugs manufactured after 1938." - F. Joseph Montagna, Alternative Medical Assoc., "Editorial", p.2.

"In 1971, the (US) Postal Service attempted to ban (Arlin Brown's) book, March of Truth on Cancer, from the mail." - Arlin Brown, (in Spotlight, May 18, 1981, p.18).

"... The Cancer Biopathy ...was... forced out of print by an injunction that caused Reich's books to be witheld or destroyed by an agency of the US govt." - C.M.Raphael,MD, in Forward to The Cancer Biopathy by Willhelm Reich,MD,U.Vienna, associate of Sigmund Freud.

"'Also seized as labeling ... was a variety of literature ... containing ... therapeutic claims, charged to be false.... The Scientologists claimed religious persecution,... (L. Ron) Hubbard focused on the book seizures, which he referred to as 'book burning''" - FDA Report ..., 1963, (in ACS Unproven Methods ..., p.113).

"On Jan. 15, 1970, Dr. (William Donald) Kelley (DDS; post-grad., Wash. U., & U. Alabama, & U. West Va.) was ordered by (17th) District (Court of Texas) Judge W. E. Jordan not to practice medicine without a license & to cease distribution of (his) booklet titled One Answer to Cancer." - (in ACS, Unproven Methods ..., p.129).

"'(Robert) Nara (DDS) received a hearing.... (by) hearing examiner Wayne Lusk of the state Dept. of Licensing & Regulation. He ruled that the specialty advertising charges against Nara "failed to establish a violation". The dentistry board voted 6-2 to suspend Nara anyway, & also voted not to use Lusk as a hearing examiner anymore.'" - Jim Fitzgerald, Detroit Free Press.

"...Dental colleges.... ...manipulate or influence both the ADA & the many... governance agencies.... A suppressed doctorial thesis explored this twilight zone of interlocking bureaucracies. ....the university involved made absolutely sure (the thesis) would never be published." - Robert O. Nara,DDS, & S.A.Mariner, Money by the Mouthful, p.89, 136, (for last 2 paragraphs above).

"'All of the high protein diets, of which (XYZ's) is a typical example, set you up for heart disease & stroke & cause death', (Dr. Nathan) Pritikin said (to 'a television interviewer'). (XYZ) replied with a ('$5 million ') law suit, charging Pritikin with slander...."

"...The recent non-fiction best-seller list...included five diet books in the top 15...." - Jane Hall, "Holy Cholesterol! Watch Those Diet Doctors Roast Each Other", TV Guide, Nov. 14, 1981, p.49.

"... This ... is published for informational & educational purposes only, no matter how controversial; the right to so publish has been upheld by the US Supreme Court. ... (similarly,) to distribute.... References: Thomas vs. Collins, 323 US 516; Thornhill vs. Alabama, 310 US 88; Martin vs. City of Struthers, 319 US 141; Lamont vs. Postmaster General, 381 US 301; Lovell vs. City of Griffin, 313 US 444." - Myron Sylton, AFCV, International Directory of Alternative Cancer Tests & Therapies, p.6.

Q.6.2 FREEDOM of CHOICE in HEALTH CARE, (DEFENDED):

"That the percentage of efficient & beneficial treatments by respondent (Hoxsey-herbs) is reasonably comparable to the efficiency & success of surgery & radium, without the physical suffering & dire consequences"(of the last 2). - Judge William H. Atwell, US District Court for Northern Texas, Dallas, Dec. 20, 1950, Decision.

"I am of the firm opinion & belief that Hoxsey has cured these people of cancer (with herbs). Hoxsey has been done a great injustice &... articles & utterances by defendent Morris Fishbein (AMA chief & Managing Editor) were false, slanderous, & libelous." - Judge W. L. Thornton, Decision, Hoxsey v. Fishbein, (in Harry Hoxsey, You Don't Have to Die, p.239-243,&255 for last 2 paragraphs above).

(FDA's ban on Laetrile is)"arbitrary, capricious, an abuse of discretion, & as a matter of law, unsupportable." - (Dec. 1977).

(What) "disturbs me mostly ... is the willfull, deliberate denial (by the FDA, of) our own citizens, a fair chance to use Laetrile, when all the record (shows) it is not toxic ... is safe & ... is effective."

"... to say,... that Laetrile should not be continued to be used by those who are suffering from terminal cancer, I would have to hang my head in shame." (Aug. 5, 1980).

(The FDA is) "to refrain & desist from interfering with terminal cancer patients, in their use of Laetrile acquired through the 'Affidavit System'." - (May 1, 1981) - Judge Luther Bohanon, US District Court, Oklahoma City; Rutherford v. US.

"New methods of health care have been discouraged, restricted, & in some instances, eliminated (by the AMA)."

"...the AMA has prevented the dissemination of truthful, objective information that could provide substantial benefits to the public."

"Competition...potentially poses a threat to the income of physicians in private practice. The costs to the public in terms of less expensive or even, perhaps, more improved forms of medical service are great."

"... a conspiracy between the AMA & its constituent & component medical societies.... The record evidence contains a more than sufficient quantity of independently admissable evidence to establish the existence of the conspiracy."

"The means (of) restraints ... include ...the "Principles of Medical Ethics",... & communication with medical societies & individual physicians to promote compliance with these...."

(AMA's)"Judicial Council issues interpretations (on 'Ethics', &) is empowered to institute disciplinary proceedings ... against physicians ... & has appelate jurisdiction ...."

"... when a physician disregards 'local custom',... he has acted unethically."

"In 1976, (AMA's) AMPAC reported campaign fund transfers of more than $1 million, making it the second largest political action committee in the US." -FTC, Docket n.9064, (Initial Decision, p.37, 283-4; & Choice,v.6,n.3,p.24),Finding, Upheld by 2nd US Court of Appeals.

"The regulations imposed (by the Board of Medical Examiners) must be reasonably related to the public health & welfare, & must not amount to an arbitrary or unreasonable interference with the right to practice one's profession..., protected by the due process clause."

(There is no) "harmfulness as a reasonable basis for the Board's ... restricting use of this treatment."

(The Dr. had not) "defrauded his patients into believing that (the) treatment was a cure for their condition." - Florida Supreme Court, in State Board of Medical Examiners v. Robert J. Rodgers,MD, n.56,096 , (in NHF, Public Scrutiny, Dec. 1980, p.12).

"... Dr. McQueen-Williams, Mr. Sarkisian, ... filed suit in the US District Court ... for $5 million against the ACS for allegedly libelous statements ... in Ca - A Cancer Journal for Clinicians...."

"... the FDA seized (their herbs).... Court action was based on charges that the product was shipped ... as a drug without prior showing of safety...."

"Dr. McQueen-Williams said no (NDA) new drug application had been filed since they do not believe the law covers botanical compounds." - ACS, Unproven Methods..., p.124.

"21 USC 312 (f), the definition of 'food':'... articles used for food or drink for man....' ...Program Circular No. 7318.01A from the FDA Program Compliance Manual... & Section 125.2 (b) (5) of the FDA vitamin regulation(:) Both say that...'Non-Essential Food Ingredients' or 'NEFIs' can be sold as long as they are not represented as being nutritionally or therapeutically essential...(nor) combined with any essential nutrients. ... With 21 USC 321 (g) (1) (B)...a food only becomes a drug when...intended for... diagnosis, cure...of disease. ...This intent...avoided, the NEFI cannot be a 'drug'. ...Not represented as a vitamin...(nor) 'food for special dietary use'...(&) no false labeling, it cannot be 'misbranded' under 21 USC 343 (a)....(&) (j). To counter that (NEFIs are) 'food additives'...argument,...21 USC 321 (f)...show(s)...that a food is a food by definition & not an additive." - John J. Matonis,JD, (in IACVF, Cancer News Journal, v.10, n.6, p.21, 1976).

(The FDA) "is seeking, under the guise of (other) charges, to prohibit the sale of a food in the market-place simply because it is not in sympathy with its use." - Judge's finding, in US v. Dextra..., (in O.Garrison, The Dictocrats, Our Unelected Rulers, p.38).

"Amygdalin (Laetrile) is listed in the US Pharmacopea of 1870...so the Grandfather Clause in the Food & Drug (& Cosmetics) Act prevents FDA from claiming jurisdiction. The US Court of Appeals, 4th District, #71-1243, May 23, 1972, upheld this...."

"Amygdalin...is listed in (FDA's) GRAS(Generally Recognized As Safe) list...."

"...First Amendment to our Constitution.... God gave us food (per Bible, &)...our religious freedom entitles us to partake...."

"Perhaps (some) are in favor of these (cancer) deaths to take the load off Social Security." - Walter Ermer, IHC(International Health Council), letter of testimony, (inserted by US Senator Edward M. Kennedy, into Banning of the Drug Laetrile from Interstate Commerce by FDA, Hearing, Subcommittee on Health & Scientific Research, Committee on Human Resources, US Senate, June 12, 1977, p.378-383).

"Nothing in this chapter shall ... discriminate against any particular school of medicine or surgery, ... podiatry, or any other treatment, ... prayer, ... practice of religion." - California Medical Practice Act, Sect. 2146, (in L. Worthington, "Unorthodox Healing & the Law", Let's Live, Feb. 1975, p.53).

"Every human being of adult years & sound mind has a right to determine what shall be done with his own body." - US Supreme Court Justice B.N.Cardoza, decision, (in Cancer News Journal, v.11, n.4, p.10, 1976).

"It may be conceded that the legistlature has no constitutional right to compel any person to submit to vaccination." - Judge Woodward, New York State Appelate Court, 1903, Viemeister case, (84 N.Y. Suppl. 712), (in Hannah Allen, Don't Get Stuck!, p.89).

"I would like to maximize the level of human choice in the medical field.... The choice of a treatment in many ways is like the free exercise of religion."

"Everyone's heard about the military-industrial complex, but they know very little about the medical-industrial complex ...(in) a medical arms race...." - Jerry Brown, Governor of California, (1st paragraph in: National Health Federation, Public Scrutiny, June 1980, p.15; 2nd, in: Ida Honorof, A Report to the Consumer, v.7, n.143, p.2, Feb. 1977).

"In 21 states, statutes .... protect...physicians from liability for defamatory remarks that may be made about colleagues in connection with review committee functions designed to improve the quality of patient care & medical services." - AMA, Peer Review Manual, v.1, ch.6, "Legal Considerations...", p.3.

Q.6.3 MEDICAL INQUISITION; CANCER:

"In ... 1954, a permanent injunction was issued by the Federal District Court... enjoining Dr. Willhelm Reich, his wife, ... from distributing 'orgone energy' devices, on complaint of the USFDA, ... for treatment of cancer.... The decree was won by default, since Dr. Reich contended that the court had no jurisdiction (in) ... 'Basic Natural Law', & he failed to appear or answer the complaint.... The decree (was)... for destruction ...of...all the misleading labeling which included 10 (different) books by Dr. Reich.... His followers ... charg(ed) interference with freedom of the press.... Dr. Reich was sentenced to 2 years, & Dr. (Michael) Silvert to 1 year ... in jail. After appeals were carried to the Supreme Court & denied.... Dr. Reich died in prison; Dr. Silvert died shortly after he was released. (Their) Foundation was ... fined $10,000." - ACS, Unproven Methods of Cancer Management, p.176.

"'Following the Koch trial, a number of physical attacks were made upon me.... I was robbed & beaten in my office & on the street.... Similar attentions were paid other physicians who agreed with Dr. Koch.' - Anonymous MD."

"... 1 death from poisoning, & 1 from being run down by an automobile, both victims being physicians of distinction & prominent in the advocacy of the Koch treatment. Mail has often been opened, & cartons of certain chemicals often arrive empty...."

"('Dr. Koch himself was the target of at least 13 unsuccessful attempts on his life' - Riley H. Crabb.)" - M. Layne, The Koch Remedy for Cancer..., p.18, Borderland Sciences Research Foundation.

"...They forced (Chauncey Smith) to leave Loma Linda (U.).... So he went east... (&) resumed his research (on germs causing cancer). (Then) mysteriously, he had died...."

"It was in 1936 that I...copyrighted...Cancer, Its Cause & Control.... ...They forced me to serve a whole year in jail, ...where I was so fed & treated that I had to cure myself of cancer.... But when I had everything ready to put out a third edition... they notified in no uncertain terms 'Unless you stop...we will snatch you...& do a lobotomy on you....'" - Emerson Hartman, IACVF, Cancer News Journal, v.12, n.1, p.11, 1977.

"Dr. Helen Calvin ... spearheaded ... Indiana to approve Laetrile, & then she used the Laetrile & metabolic program ... until the FDA arbitrarily & illegally held up her Laetrile shipments.... Patients started dying.... When 4 of them had died, Dr. Calvin ended her own life." - Arlin Brown, Cancer Victory Bulletin, v.4, n.10, p.1, Oct. 1978.

"...an investigator for the State Medical Board appeared ... with warrants for (our) arrest...(for) practicing medicine without a license. (Our) Dr. ... protested that he was the only man in the clinic who treated patients, & produced his license.... But...it had been cancelled the day before.... I pleaded with them not to arrest my wife who (did paperwork, &) told (them) that we had a 6 month old infant at home who had to be nursed regularly.... (My wife was) locked up with ... degenerate females.... ... They ganged up on her, slapped her, knocked her down & kicked her." - Harry Hoxsey, You Don't Have to Die, p.183.

(Maurice Kowan, MD) "served 3 months in jail, paid a fine of $3,000, & was forbidden to see a cancer patient...for 3 years. Before sentencing, it had been suggested to Dr. Kowan...to sign a statement that...Laetrile...had proved of no benefit.... ...He refused any 'deals'...." - Betty Lee Morales, "The National Health Federation, Do We Need It?"

"The jury had never been allowed to see any evidence that Laetrile actually worked. ...Dr. Kowan...was...age 70...." - G.E. Griffin, Cancer Control Journal, v.5, n.3, p.120, 1977.

"...In treating approx. 100 cancer cases, most...terminal, (Dr. Kowan) was able to achieve dramatic relief from pain in virtually every single case. ...Several patients... told...that the fees Dr. Kowan charged were ridiculously low.... Dr. Kowan was sentenced (including) 30 days in the workhouse...." - David Martin, Staff member, US Senate Internal Security Committee, (in IACVF, Cancer News Journal, v.6, n.1, p.21, Jan. 1971).

"... The cancer statutes (are) discriminatory against the cancer patient.... No other disease is so restricted by politics.... It is also discriminatory against the Negro because Laetrile helps sickle cell anemia.... It is discriminatory against the poor because the poor can't afford to go to Mexico or Germany (for therapies outlawed in the US)...."(p.4).

"... In July 1974. About 15 agents (of Cal. Food & Drug)...arrested me on the charge of selling Laetrile & other substances in the diagnosis, cure, & alleviation of cancer. In Citrus Municipal Court, West Covina, on Feb. 3, 1975, Judge Sam Cianchetti declared this statute unconstitutional. On Oct. 1974, I received a phone call from ... police at 1 (am 'Saturday morning') & he told me that my office was broken into. I went down to my office...& 2 agents...arrest(ed) me on a felony charge - conspiracy.... ... The law...states that before you are even arrested, they must give you a hearing (Cal. Health Code 1707.4).... (Another) judge denied this motion for a...hearing & he gave no reason."(p.1-2). - Dr. James Privetera; Roswell Park Memorial Inst.; Scripps Clinic; "The Nutrition Battle".

"A doctor who wishes to prescribe ... Laetrile or any other vitamin or nutrient to his patient -... cancer victim, may do so as long as his intention is to treat the patient's general health & not the cancerous growth per se. ...The doctor (is) to articulate (this) to his patient...." - Ben Hamrick, Judge of the Superior Court, County of San Diego, Decision...., People v. ...James R. Privitera..., No. CR-32978; 1-2-75. - (Last 3 paragraphs above in Cancer Control Journal, v.3, n.3, p.1-6, 1975.)

"... testifying for Dr. Privetera .... To these 19 cancer victims, the enforcement of (California) Health & Safety Code Sect. 1707.1, the denial to them of medical treatment, albeit unorthodox, albeit unapproved by a state agency, must surely take on a Kafka-esque, a nightmare quality. No demonstrated public danger, no compelling interest of the state, warrants an Orwellian intrusion into the most private of zones of privacy." - California Supreme Court Chief Justice, Rose Bird, dissenting opinion, (in Spotlight, June 25, 1979, p.10).

"In 1964 (we) conduct(ed) an intensive investigation of Laetrile ... conclud(ing) that there was no justification for making (it) illegal.... Yet, 16 years after... , doctors are still being jailed for (it). Dr. James Privitera, ...was recently released from 55 days ... much of it doing hard labor ... on a road gang.... If he were solely interested in making money, as he points out, there is a great deal more to be made from traditional cancer treatments, than by the use of Laetrile." - Santa Ana, The Register, April 13, 1980, (in National Health Federation, Public Scrutiny, Oct. 1980, p.12).

"Not that there are not real quacks in the field of cancer.... But...no legitimate MD ... with a thriving practice & after years of study & faithful service would give all that up to become a quack & subject himself & his family to the Hell...." - John Richardson,MD, Laetrile Case Histories, p.101.

"Does it make sense that a (Laetrile) smuggler who is supposed, (by the Medical Establishment - Ed.), to be making millions of dollars off of what he is smuggling, would spend five years of his life trying to legalize it?" - Frank Salaman, grad., Northwestern U.(p.170).

"Federal, state, & local police raided Dr. (John) Richardson's Clinic, ... beat up a(n)... aide, manhandled a nurse, & dragged (the) business manager off in handcuffs."(p.11).

"20 Federal agents in 13 undercover cars ... arrested & ... jailed ... Robert W. Bradford (President, Committee for Freedom of Choice in Cancer Therapy)... on leave from Stanford University ...& 2 Mexicans ... on charges of conspiracy to smuggle (laetrile)."(p.9).

"The Food, Drug, & Cosmetics Act, ... defines any article 'intended for use in the diagnosis, ... treatment, or prevention of disease' as a 'drug'.... Water...to an individual dying of thirst could ... be called a 'drug'."(p.115). - Michael Culbert, Freedom From Cancer, p.9, 11, 115, 170.

(In) "1970, the Pennsylvania Health Dept., swooped down on a meeting ... after the movie Laetrile, ... was shown. The film was confiscated & the association president ... arrested."(p.28). - Michael Culbert, Vitamin B-17, Forbidden Weapon Against Cancer,p.28.

"Important Elements of FDA Policy: Encourage local medical licensing authorities to investigate & take appropriate action to deal with the use of Laetrile by physicians in their medical practice." - FDA, Division of Federal-State Relations Director, 1974.

(This MD) "utilized (Vitamin B-15 & 17) as therapeutic agents in the treatment of cancer. (These) are not recognized vitamins in human nutrition. Laetrile ... is unsafe for self medication...."

"The management of cancer patients with ... vitamins ... to the exclusion of ... conventional modalities is an extreme departure from the standard practice of medicine."

(MD)"Certificate... of John A. Richardson ... is revoked." - California Board of Medical Quality Assurance, 1975.

- (last 4 paragraphs above in John Richardson, Laetrile Case Histories, p.78 & 85).

"...Dr. Thomas J. Roberts.... one of the leading wholistic physicians in the metro. Wash.,D.C. .... had his hospital privileges suspended because he doesn't believe in the Establishment 'cut - burn - poison' (Surgery - Radiation - Chemotherapy) cancer 'treatments'." - Carol M. Dunn & William Carmichael, Spotlight, Oct. 22, 1979, p.18.

"The board of directors...decided (to end) Chelation Therapy in the very hospital that I owned! ....I donated (my) 109-bed...hospital &...50-bed nursing home to the church."

"...The State Medical Board of Examiners of Louisianna.... ...ruled that a doctor practicing Chelation Therapy or using...natural minerals & vitamins was 'incompetent', ...'defrauding the public'."

"The US Patent Office (, for my) chelating agents....granted a patent."

"...In a period of 30 days, 3 lawsuits were filed against me for malpractice for a million $'s each.... ...I lost my malpractice insurance."

"I have declared bancruptcy. My home & furniture have been auctioned off."

- H. Ray Evers,MD,Vanderbilt U.; BS,Biochem. & Biol.,Auburn U.; Knight, Order of Malta; (in G. Edward Griffin, & Mike Culbert (Ed.), Voice of Medical Freedom, Americans for Medical Freedom, v.1, n.12, p.14, Dec. 1981.

"Our present state law has a 100% conviction record before the board (of medical examiners). There's not a D.A. in the country that would not love that record...."

- Dan & Beverly Dotson, MD's, (by Ann Cinquina, in Americans for Medical Freedom, Voice..., Health World News, Feb. 1981, p.6).

Q.6.4 MEDICAL INQUISITION; CARDIOVASCULAR:

"Several 100 (ex-)patients...of the Shute Clinic...treated successfully with Vitamin E therapy for cardiovascular conditions, formed...'The Cardiac Society'. ... The AMA.... enlisted.... the US Post Office. Letters addressed to the Society were returned to the sender marked 'Fraudulent'." - Herbert Bailey, Vitamin E ..., p.127.

(Dr. Nathan) Pritikin...maintains that patients with atherosclerosis, heart disease, ...can be 'returned to normal function' by...diet...low in fat, cholesterol, protein, & high in complex carbohydrates...."

"Loma Linda...reported...that of the first 111 patients...with blood cholesterol between 260 & 279..., the average patient left...with...190.... Of 218 patients (on) anti-hypertension drugs, 186 left...with normal blood pressure...."

(Pritikin's diet is) "bizarre...fad". - AMA public relations official, F. Chapel.

"Until he (Pritikin) shows us more than anecdotal evidence, there is nothing to evaluate his work on." - AHA(American Heart Association)'s Mary Winston.

"We've seen atherosclerosis turned on & off in monkeys (by nutrition, etc.). The problem is you've got to be a monkey to get proper treatment for heart disease in this country." - Dr. William Castelli, Director, Framingham Project. - last 5 paragraphs in CSPI, Nutrition Action, v.7,n.4,p.3, April 1980.

"Blood from coronary thrombosis patients....(:) on about 60...patients.... hemoglobin was in all cases up (high).... For 3 years...examining blood of...several hundred people a day.... testing out various diets.... I came to the conclusion that (a vegetable - fruit diet &) 1/3 natural fruit juice, 2/3 water...are the most suitable liquid foods to drop hemoglobin number as quickly as possible to the normal level.... ...The Medical Society of NY accepted...my article & published it in NY Medicine for May 20, 1949.... On May 21, 1949, I was fired from my position at the hospital. My daughter, who also worked there, was fired, too." - Ernest Klein,MD, "A New Theory of Diet & Coronary Thrombosis", Prevention; J. I. Rodale, Ed.; Ruth Adams, Ass't Ed.; Dec. 1954, p.42.

(Coronary artery bypass surgery:) "5-40% of patients...experience a heart attack during or soon after surgery...(;) typical rate...15-25%. ...20-30% of vein grafts become occluded (blocked) within 1 year of surgery.... ...Grafts increase the likelihood that new total occlusions will develop in the arteries at points both before & after the graft (parallel bypass) insertion site. ...6 months after surgery....(;)New total occlusions developed in only 16% of arteries not bypassed, in 29% of arteries with a patent (open bypass) graft, & in 62% of arteries with an occluded graft."(p.225-6). (continued)

"The US has a ratio ("of thoracic surgeons to population")...many times greater than any other nation."(p.239).

"Questionable medical practice is not just the result of mistake, occasional incompetence, & faulty regulation, but is the outcome of vested interests."(p.242).

- Marcia Millman, The Unkindest Cut, p.225, 226, 239, 242.

Q.6.5 MEDICAL INQUISITION; INFANTS:

"...Many physicians who agree with...safe alternatives will not participate in them for fear.... ...Doing so would be tantamount to...professional suicide.(p.411).

"...Nearly 25% of all childbearing women in this country (US) are now having Caesarian sections!"(p.1). - David Stewart,PhD, Exec. Dir., NAPSAC, The Five Standards for Safe Childbearing, p.1, 411.

"...Nial Ettinghausen,DP,..Calif., has attended over 7,000 home births over the past 40 years. His Ceasarian rate is 1.1% & his perinatal mortality rate for the past 5 years (2,508 births) is 4.2 per 1,000 - a rate less than ¼ the national average. Dr. Ettinghausen lost his license to practice in Jan. of 1981...."

"Hai Abdul,MD, ...(is) offering natural childbirth.... Since 1978, the California (BMQA) Board of Medical Quality Assurance has sent investigators to his clinic.... On Christmas Eve, 1980, the investigator visited Dr. Abdul & his wife, who were in the midst of wrapping Christmas gifts, to inform them that the BMQA planned to level charges...'in two months'. ...Dr. Abdul lost his hospital privileges.... ...Said Dr. Abdul...'It is an attack against every family who wants to choose the place & manner of their births.'...."

"It has been estimated that of the physicians' in support of home birth & other safe alternatives, at least 90% are in trouble today. Either their licenses have been suspended or in threat ... , their hospital privileges are in jeopardy, their insurance coverage has been cancelled, or all...."

"Do medical licensing boards, insurance companies, & hospital boards judge all physicians by the same standards, or are there two sets - one strict, the other lenient - depending on whether a doctor supports alternatives or not?" - NAPSAC(InterNational Assoc. of Parents & Professionals for Safe Alternatives in Childbirth), NAPSAC News, v.6, n.1, p.1, Spring 1981.

"I concluded that mongolism was a genetic defect (related to cancer - Ed.) resulting in metabolic accumulations. I treated it as such by removing the accumulations."

"Even the NIH (has) written (my) medicines are safe."

"Why...was my office robbed & vandalized while I met with the FDA in Washington... a thief who only stole & destroyed patients' records...? Why was my telephone tapped...? Why were mail checks put on parents of my patients, friends, & relatives?"

"...The Japanese National Inst. of Mental Health came to Detroit to extend to me their gratitude for the 'U' Series (used).... in 60 universities & national hospitals .... (where) 3,000 children had been treated.... 1/3 ...improved both mentally & physically; an additional third improved physically only."

(My patient)"so impressed the (Michigan) legistlatures...that both Houses passed... (a) Resolution...signed by the Governor, to treat institutionlized mongoloids with (my) 'U' Series (of **'vitamins, minerals, enzymes, &...prescription drugs...in...small dosages'). The Michigan Dept. of Health turned down this Resolution....**"(p.105).

(US) "Senator George McGovern wrote...he had seen improvements in...his constituent, my patient...."(p.111).

"...South African doctors...were told by the US State Dept. that our FDA would no longer allow them to treat...."(p.123)

"...the National Assoc. for Retarded Children, the National Inst. of Mental Health (of NIH), & the March of Dimes had declined to investigate (my treatment)."(p.177).

- **Henry Turkel,MD, (Update) New Hope for the Mentally Retarded, p.105, 111, 123, 177, & un-numbered.**

"The Health...Dept. of the State of New Mexico 'took my children away.... One of the charges leveled against me was that I had been raising my children on a vegetarian diet. I try to show my children respect for animals.... I was outraged when I found out they fed my children meat.'" - Vegetarian Times, (in Health Writers, Health Newsletter, v.6, n.7, p.9, 1978).

Q.6.6 JUDICIARY; INTOXICANTS; COSTS:

"'In my legal practice, I have seen certain Federal judges controlled or influenced by large corporations....(,) by large law firms...on more than one occasion (, &)...by special interests.... (Some) ought to be thrown right off the bench because they are breaking every code of conduct....'" - US Senator Orrin Hatch.

"Dr. James D. Rogers, a general surgeon ... after being the victim of a frivolous malpractice suit, ...countersued a former patient & the attorneys involved for making 'reckless, slanderous, ... charges' against him.... He acted as his own attorney (,) when he couldn't find a lawyer who would help him...." - last 2 paragraphs above in HALT (Help Abolish Legal Tyrrany), Americans for Legal Reform, v.1, n.2, p.1&6, Winter 1980.

"I usually accept bribes from both sides so that tainted money can never influence my decision." - Sir Francis Bacon, Lord Chancellor of England, (in Charles Ashman, The Finest Judges Money Can Buy, p.3).

"Victimless crimes...account for half of all arrests.... ...The National Council on Crime & Delinquency declares, '(This) so preoccupies the criminal justice system that it prevents it from dealing effectively with real crime.'" - Anne Strick, Injustice For All, (How Our Adversary System of Law Victimizes Us & Subverts Justice), p.206.

"Employing...nutrition & vitamin therapy...one of the nation's largest alcoholism treatment programs reports a 71% success rate. This contrasts with...(a) national... rate (of) 25%, as reported by NIAAA."(p.66).

"...All patients reported a loss of craving for drugs while taking large doses of Vitamin C, during detoxification. Of the first 30 carefully monitored heroin addicts, 30 successfully withdrew from their addiction with no more than minor discomfort. None of the 30 were reported to have relapsed.... Similar results have been reported by other doctors...Archie Kalokerinos...." - Irwin Stone, Journal of Orthomolecular Psychiatry, v.6, n.4, p.300, 1977. (p.68, 73).

"...The cost of maintaining the criminal justice system range from 30 to 50 billion $'s per year. Add...the monetary damage caused by criminals & estimates approach 200 billion $'s per year."(p.vi). - Alexander Schauss, Diet, Crime & Delinquency, p.vi, 66, 68, 73, (for last 3 paragraphs above).

"...Similar to the 19th century Opium Wars against China...."(p.iii). (There is) "$50 billion in retail drug (marijuana, cocaine, heroin , etc.) sales alone in the US, & $200 billion world wide."(p.1). "... The price series for heroin at retail level in major American cities show virtual total uniformity."(p.64). "...A huge chunk of international banking (etc.) have been created solely to manage dirty money.... enjoy(ing) the sovereign protection of (many) govts. ...gold & diamonds...."(p.68-9). - US Labor Party team, Dope, Inc., p.iii, 1, 64, 68-9.

"Alcohol...can cause cancer.... ...traffic fatalities.... The (total US death) toll due to alcohol...(is) between 50,000 & 200,000 people a year."

"The Institute of Medicine, (NAS) National Academy of Science has calculated the price to society - including medical bills, time lost from work, property damage, (etc.- was) $60 billion in 1975 (Alcoholism, Alcohol Abuse, & Related Problems, 1980). Adjusting only for inflation, the 1981 figure will pass the $100 billion mark.... (Plus), Americans buy $45 billion worth of alcoholic beverages each year." - Michael Jacobson, CSPI(Center for Science in the Public Interest), Nutrition Action, Oct. 1981, p.6.

"Total national costs from cancer, both direct & indirect,.... Projections for 1978 are in the region of $30 billion.... These figures underestimate the true cost...."
- Samuel Epstein,MD, The Politics of Cancer, p.7.
(Total direct medical costs in the US in 1980 were over $ 220 billion. - Ed.; see Chicago Tribune, Oct. 10, 1980, p.10; ...or $250 billion, - WMAQ-TV, Chicago, Nov. 2, 1981, 6pm News.)

"Next to oil, coffee is the largest internationally traded commodity." - Earthwork Books, Earthwork.

"Pesticides Used in Foreign Countries on Food Exported to US: (abridged)

Commodity:	Number of Pesticides: Allowed:	Having no US tolerance:	Not detectable with FDA tests:
Bananas	45	25	37
Coffee	94	76	64
Tomatoes	53	21	28 "

- USGAO, CED-79-43, Better Regulation of Pesticide Exports & Pesticide Residues In Imported Food Is Essential, June 22, 1979, p.11.

"Tobacco pesticides had no tolerances & no instructions for waiting periods between use & harvest. .... In 1964...organic phosphates...parathion, have replaced the chlorinated hydrocarbons aldrin, chlordane, dieldren, & heptachlor...; however, residue of all...including arsenic...would remain.... Can it be, then, that the...cancer-producing quality of cigarettes is related to the pesticides used? ...I received no reply. ...embarrassed silence." - Laura Tallian, The Pesticide Jungle, p.32.

"How are our nutrition studies received by the Medical Establishment? We have papers turned down by Orthodox journals. We have me getting bounced from a committee in Washington because I was too controversial; this is a committee that would dispense LSD for experimental use in the US. We have me getting bounced off an editorial board while Co-editor of International Review of Neurobiology.... So, there are some prices to pay for being an innovator, but there (is) a lot of good fun to be had, & it's well worth it...." - Carl C. Pfeiffer,PhD,MD; head, Brain Bio Center, Princeton, NJ; author, Mental & Elemental Nutrients, & Zinc & Other Micro-Nutrients; in Lecture at NOHA(Nutrition for Optimal Health Association), Sept. 30, 1981.

Q.7.0 RELATED FIELDS:

Q.7.1 OLIGARCHY of MULTI-NATIONAL CORPORATIONS, (INSURANCE, DRUGS, OIL):

"While millions of dollars were being projected for research on radiation & other cancer 'cures', there was an almost complete blackout on research that might have pointed to needed alterations in our environment, our industrial organization, & our food." - Carol Lopate, in Health Policy Advisory Center, Health PAC Bulletin.

"...The asbestos industry...has for decades successfully suppressed & manipulated information on the carcinogenecity & other hazards of asbestos. Involved in this conspiracy network were senior industry executives, their medical staff, attorneys, insurance companies, trade associations, scientific consultants, & commercial labs."
- Samuel S. Epsteins,MD; Harvard Med.; Prof. Environ. ..., Case Western Med.; Pres., Rachel Carson Trust; The Politics of Cancer, p.310.

"...In the preceding chapters...are hypothesis linking scattered observations. ... Relevant research on the system as a whole has not been done...."(p.239).
"It is remarkable that with the continuing concern with the health care 'crisis', so few studies of the consequences of alternative modes of delivering care have been done. Such a paucity of studies is no accident; such studies would challenge structural interests of both professional monopoly (MD's) & corporate rationalization in maintaining health institutions as they now exist or in directing their 'orderly' expansion."(p.247).
- Robert R. Alford; Prof., UC Santa Cruz; Health Care Politics, p.239, 247.

"... to retain the insurance companies' role (in profits from national health insurance), was based on recognition of that industry's power to kill any legistlation it considers unacceptable. The bill's sponsors (US Legistlators Kennedy, Griffith, & Mills) thus had to choose between appeasing the the insurance industry, and obtaining no national health insurance at all." - New York Times, Editorial, April 7, 1974, p.E16, (in Vicente Navarro, Medicine Under Capitalism, p.151).

"The NCI is unable to run an honest, fair, unbiased, scientific test of an anticancer compound they pronounced ineffective prior to commencing testing."

"If insurance really wanted to cut costs, they would promote reimbursement for a wide range of simpler, more effective, cheaper procedures"(with fewer side-effects).

- Robert S. Mendelsohn, MD; GPD(Guest, Phil Donahue Show); Chairman, Medical Licensing Committee, State of Illinois; Assoc. Prof., School of Medicine, U. of Ill.; (in: NHF, Public Scrutiny, June 1981, p.7; & his Confessions of a Medical Heretic, p.216).

"Unless Laetrile is specifically excluded by contract terms & conditions, the use & administring of Laetrile, in compliance with Public Act 80-1096, shall be payable."

- State of Illinois, Dept. of Insurance (in IACVF, Cancer News Journal, v.14, n.3, p.13, April 1979). (Note: Chicago is headquarters for AMA, ADA(Amer. Dental Assoc.), another ACS(Amer. College of Surgeons), AHA(Amer. Hospital Assoc.), Blue Cross & Shield, others. - Ed.)

"A minimum of 30,000 Japanese (were) paralyzed & blinded, many permanently, after taking Quineform, ... manufactured & marketed by ...., under various trade names, ... still being sold throughout the world.... In 1964, British...ban(ned) (it even) for the treatment of dogs & cats. In 1965, ... circulated an alert across the European continent.... In 1970, Japan's Health & Welfare Ministry...banned (it)...while they assured their Pharmaceutical Assoc. that 'withdrawal...was not mandatory'.... The 7th revised Japanese Pharmacopoeia...(insert) reads 'This drug is non-absorbable, side-effects rarely seen.'.... In 1969, ...'s ...confidential memo...enumerated 56 reports on (its) side-effects.... In 1973, ...released a report which stated the drug was harmless...." - Ida Honorof, "The 'SMON' Tragedy...", The Provoker, v.18, Nov. 1978, p.25.

"Dr. (Henry K.) Wachtel ... after escaping the Hitler regime resumed work in NYC, aided by ... Columbia U. He served (9 years) as professor of physiology, & director of the Cancer Research Council at Fordham U. But when he began to test his pituitary substance, he was removed from both posts, (&) no other funds could be secured. Dr. Wachtel (is) outspoken in identifying ... an international drug cartel .... of controlling every phase of cancer research & therapy, including the allocation of grants from private foundations & government.... to maintain its monopoly, strangl(ing) every independent approach to cancer." - Nat Morris, The Cancer Blackout Amended, p.154.

"The info. that follows is taken primarily...from govt. hearings & reports published by various Senate & House committees." (8 listed).(p.245).

"By...WWII, I. G. Farben had become...part of the most gigantic & powerful cartel of all history.... interlocking agreements.... over 2,000 of them.... In the US, the cartel had established important agreements with" (very many major drug, oil, & chemical companies).(p.248-251).

"In 1938, I. G. sent a letter to (a major drug firm), one of its American subsidiaries, (that)...all advertising contracts must contain '...a legal clause whereby the contract is immediately cancelled if overnight the attitude of the paper toward Germany should be changed."(p.281).

"During the Nurenburg trials...Oswald Pohl, an SS Lieutenant General..., is shown here explaining how Farben operated such concentration camps as Auschwitz & Buchenwald." (Photo by)"US Army".(Picture section of book.)

- G. Edward Griffin, World Without Cancer, p.245, 248-51, 281, & picture section.

"On the very day that the NCI announced Laetrile's alleged worthlessness... , West Virginia became the 24th state to allow the use of Laetrile .... In signing the Laetrile bill into law, Gov. Jay Rockefeller said the study 'made no difference at all'."
- National Health Federation, Public Scrutiny, July 1981, p.5.

(John D.) "Rockefeller (Sr., was) concern(ed)... his money was being used to support the regular profession at the expense of the homeopaths. ...he scolded his staff in 1916: 'I desire that homeopathists should have a fair, courteous, & liberal treatment extended to them from all medical institutions to which we contribute.' In 1919 ... Rockefeller (Sr.) again warned his son & staff: 'Homeopathic teaching should not be excluded ... it should be provided for, the same as Allopathic". - in E. Richard Brown, Rockefeller Medicine Men, p.109.

"... a surgeon told John D. (Rockefeller) that everyone should have an appendectomy before the age of 16 as a preventative. The oil wizard saw the point at once. 'Why, you've got a better thing than Standard Oil!', he exclaimed." - in Nat Morris, The Cancer Blackout, p.199, (1977 ed.).

"Bankers regard research as most dangerous & a thing that makes banking hazardous due to the rapid changes it brings about in industry." - Charles Kettering, of Memorial Sloan Kettering Cancer Center, & V. Pres. of General Motors, (in Moss, Cancer Syn., p.276).

"'We have tremendous investment in facilities for (internal combustion) engines, transmissions, & axles, & I can't see throwing them away just because the electric car doesn't emit fumes.'" - Henry Ford II, (in Look, May 28, 1964).

"...In 1899 an electric vehicle captured the world land speed record (at) 66mph ...." - Peter Barry Chowka, East West J.,v.11,n.5,p.42,May 1981,(for last 2 parag.).

"Fundamental scientific breakthroughs seldom happen in giant company labs. They take place in bedrooms, garages, & makeshift labs.: for example, Moulton's bicycle, Carlson's Xerox, DeForest's vacuum tube, Wankel's rotary engine, Von Neumann's computer, etc. The dial telephone was invented by an undertaker, & the ball point pen by a sculptor. A French monk invented the principle of hermetically sealed refrigeration. Two concert pianists invented Kodachrome in their kitchens."

"It is possible ... to produce a vehicle for $150, a radio receiver for 9¢, & a $9 one-channel TV set.... need(ed) in underdeveloped countries...." - Richard Barnet & Ronald Müller, Global Reach, The Power of the Multinational Corporations, p.350 & 361).

"...President Truman's chief of staff, Admiral W.D.Leahy, told his boss about the atom bomb: 'This is the biggest fool thing we have ever done. The bomb will never go off, & I speak as an expert in explosives.'"(p.33).

"...The press as a whole refused to believe the Wright brothers for nearly 5 years (after their first flight). ...Editors discarded invitations to witness numerous flights ...."(p.32).

"...Dr. Thomas H. Moray.... used a simple antenna, (etc., per Nicola Tesla)...to generate...large amounts of...electricity.... During the 1930's he demonstrated (this)... even under the water.... (It) weighed about 55 lbs. & was capable of obtaining...50,000 watts of power on a steady basis. (It) utilized a transistor more than 20 years before anyone (else;of) germanium. The (REA)Rural Electrification Adm. ...was ordered (by Pres. FDR) to work with Dr. Moray on his invention, which took 20 years & $200,000 of his own money to develop. An REA engineer...smashed the Moray device with an axe. .... Dr. Moray was shot in a gun battle that took place in his lab.... In 1973, Lt. Col. Thomas Bearden, a nuclear engineer with the Army Missile Command, wrote of the Moray experiment which he had witnessed: 'It was...a legitimate, widely recognized demonstration that got electricity out of thin air.'"(p.41-43). - Tom Valentine, Editor, Newsreal, "Suppressed Inventions" issue, n.2, June 1977, p.32,33,41-43.

"Mr.H.H.Timken, the motor axle magnate, employed (Dr. Royal R.) Rife.... With his 150,000x microscope ... Rife showed that ...: (1) (Germs) gave off (one) wave-length of... uv light, at all times (alive).... (4) ... test animals (were) given lethal doses of pathogenic germs, ... : their lives (saved) by subjecting their bodies for a few minutes to the proper single wavelength of (electromagnetism). (5) ... by altering the environment & food supply, friendly germs ... can be converted into pathogenic germs...."

"Local MD's who ... tried to apply (this) to their clinical work, soon found their relations with the local medical society cancelled. Rife was called a quack."

(AMA chief Morris) "Fishbein ... is editor-in-chief of Index Medicus, the American source index for everything medical, & assoc. ed. for International Medical Index ... a position to determine what the doctor ... will not find out." - Royal Lee, DDS, (in Lee Foundation for Nutritional Research, Reprint n. 47; attachment to Journal of the Franklin Institute, v.237,n.2,p.103,Feb. 1944).

"Dr. Rudolph Diesel('s).... invention immediately threatened the whole steam engine industry, &...he permanently disappeared from the ship on which he was travelling to Europe."

"...William Bolon('s) Rialto, Cal., (auto)...steam engine....weighed less than 50 lbs. & eliminated the usual transmission & drive train.... Detroit...(asked) the inventor ...to sign forms releasing...his claims to the design before they would even look at it. After a Sun-Telegraph article...his factory was fire-bombed to the tune of $600,000."(p.13).

(Eric Cottel's) "ultra-sonic fuel system... 'vibrate'(s) existing fuels to much smaller particles.... (winning) congratulations from...("June 17, 1974, Newsweek, etc"). Later...silence. Cottel...explained that Detroit was so myopic that they would probably turn down even the wheel if it were a newly offered invention."

"In his Suppressed Inventions, Mike Brown.... tells of...Gulley (who) could supposedly get 115 mpg out of his big 8 cylinder Buick, using his (fuel) vaporizing"(carburetor). (p.4). - John Freeman, Suppressed & Incredible Inventions, p.4, 13;(available from Fry's, & Health Research).

"... the invention of Charles N. Pogue, of Winnipeg, Manitoba, Canada: 'Tests made with passenger ... cars equipped with this new carbureter will operate 200 mpg' - Mass Transportation, Dec.1936,p.406. We have personally interviewed several older citizens ... who remember the Pogue tests ... some were eye witnesses.... The last (Pogue) patent was filed Jan. 7, 1936, n.2,026,798."

(Another efficient fuel vaporizer is in:) "Argosy, Aug. 1977, p.23. (An) ERDA official ... gave a guarded evaluation ...but... did not think this was a hoax. Claims: ... a 4-cylinder engine will average 260-360 mpg."

(This most quickly causes a decrease in: air pollution, (respiratory) disease, inflation, unemployment, balance-of-trade deficits, foreign entanglements, war. - Ed.)

"'...ACS, established...by...(those) in the petroleum & drug businesses, ... were interested in looking for a solution to the cancer threat that involved the use of synthetic drugs...(that) have a coal tar base, ... derivatives of petroleum (as are pesticides - Ed.)'-Dr. John Richardson, testimony, US Circuit Court (in San Diego, Cal., Jan. 18, 1977)." - last 3 quoted paragraphs in J.E.Jackson, Gasolene Crisis Answers, p.9-12,& 142, by National Car Drivers Assoc.,POBox 1111,Tacoma,WA.

"I call this an organized conspiracy funded by the chemical industry & the ACS(American Cancer Society)...to take the public focus off of air pollution." - NJ State Senator John M. Skevin, Chmn., Cancer Incidence Comm., (in Betty G. Morales & John G. Clark, Eden Ranch - Organic Consumer Report, v.59, n.13, March 27, 1979.

"In a 24 hour day, the adult man uses...(approx.) 8 pounds of oxygen...."
- A. Schatz, discoveror of streptomycin, (in Cancer News Journal,v.12,n.2,p.6, June 1977.

Q.7.2 EPA

"... we accumulated roughly 1,000 studies on how carbon monoxide affects human(s) &...animals. One study can contradict another; studies ... have flaws...; or a single study may (be) highly significant ...,but... no other experiments have duplicated (it). .... If we wait for scientific proof before taking firm ... action, we will very likely ... have waited too long. ... We cannot delay writing sensible, balanced rules ...." – USEPA Administrator, Douglas M. Costle, remarks to National Coalition on Disease Prevention & Environmental Health, (in Natural Food Associates, Natural Food & Farming, v.27,n.4,p.5, Oct. 1980).

"'If it's a political decision, we want to make the most of it.'" – USEPA Deputy Administrator, B. Blum.(p.6).

"...Regional Administrators (of USEPA), appointed by the President.... jealously guard information about pollution violations, because information is power."(p.8).

"...Public health officials from HEW were squeezed out ... during the formation of EPA, snapping potentially productive ties between health care activists & environmental protectors.... An urban environment coalition...would push EPA into issues like safe drinking water."(p.9).

"One (EPA) official implied that if EDF (Environmental Defense Fund) & NRDC (Natural Resources Defense Council) were to close down tomorrow, EPA's already sluggish regulatory programs would come to a complete standstill."(p.12). – Gail Robinson & Deborah Baldwin, Environmental Action, June 1980, p.5-12.

Q.7.3 AGRI-BUSINESS, (PESTICIDES); USDA:

"An investigation was initiated by the FDA, EPA, NCI, & the Inspector General of HEW, & evidence revealed that IBT (Industrial Bio-Test Labs., Inc.) deliberately falsified data submitted on potential carcinogens, & 4 of the major pesticide manufacturers were aware...but...silent. ... 1,781 (tests) required auditing. ...94% of tests ...for cancer caus(ation) were invalid. (Pesticides are made from, & owned by OIL.-Ed.) .... The Wall Street Journal reported that EPA is asking 235 chemical companies to 'reexamine 4,363 IBT tests that were crucial in obtaining federal clearance to market 483 different pesticides.'(Feb. 21, 1978). ....The average (%) invalid,(of 1,781) tests...studied was 75%." – Ida Honorof, Report to the Consumer, v.11,n.252,Aug. 1981.

"Food imperialism, through the marketplace, by the rich over the poor, is one of the most crucial problems confronting man." – USDA Deputy Administrator, Lyle P. Schertz, (in R. L. Ledogar, Hungry for Profits, p.92).

"The living elements of food are either removed...or are preserved with chemicals.... ...easily transported long distances, stored without refrigeration... ...A few central (monopoly) manufacturers can saturate supermarket shelves across the country...because... (there is) no chance the food will spoil. ...Companies buy ingredients when they are cheap, produce & stockpile vast quantities of the processed results, then withhold the product from the market for months, hoping to manipulate prices upward & reap a windfall." – Bette Lamont, "Our Food, Our Minds", Issues In Radical Therapy, v.4, n.2, p.3, Spring 1976.

"... we are on a collision course with disaster. Our poor farming practices are laying the groundwork for a severe disaster in American agriculture.... By destroying farmland & water resources ... the erosion of American farmland today is probably at a record high ... this simply cannot go on ...." – Secretary of Agriculture, Bob Bergland, (in Herald of Health, v.84,n.10,p.2, Oct. 1979).

"North Dakota, Montana, Oklahoma, Arkansas, & Tennessee blindly passed the 'chemical trust protection law', & collaborating state officials are ... refusing to allow any natural soil building materials whatsoever sold in those states." – L.B.Taylor,Lieut.Colonel USAF,Ret., (in Herald of Health,v.83,n.8,p.1,Oct. 1979).

"...A lack of some of the minerals in the plant can also cause a lack of...vitamins .... Vit. B-1...contains sulpher & chlorine; Vit. B-12...contains cobalt & phosphorous. & where there is a lack of boron...in the soil, the plant may be deficient in Vit. C. A deficiency of zinc (lowers) Vit. B-2 in the plant...."

"Same vegetable...same variety.... Two tomatoes can be almost identical in color... size...taste...but...Dr. (Firman E.) Bear (; head, Agri. Dept., Rutgers U.; Editor in Chief, Soil Science;...finds:) One tomato will contain ...1938 times more iron (than the other tomato)!... One head (of lettuce) has...169 times the manganese (as the other head). ....The Vit. C content ...can vary (in) Muscadine grapes (by) 1800%! .... The Vit. A content...may differ (in) corn by...800%." - T.M.Rudolph,PhD, Miraculous Minerals, p.15-17.

"Using spinach, we had 2 rows of bugs, then (rows of) no bugs, 2 rows of bugs, then (rows of) no bugs. Not because we sprayed (pesticides), but because we got a different condition (natural fertilizer) in the soil under, (the rows of no pests)." - Dr. William A. Albrecht, U. Missouri, to US Congressman James J. Delaney, Hearings, Chemicals in Food Products, (in Robert L. Preston, Healthology...,p.37).

"Although evidence continues to accumulate that at least 25% of all marketed pesticides are potentially carcinogenic, the EPA has not made use of its Congressional mandate to protect the public." - US Congressman John Moss's report, Subcommittee on Oversight & Investigation, (in NFA, Natural Food & Farming, v.25,n.9,p.1, Feb. 1979).

"Despite a tenfold increase in the use of pesticides between 1947 & 1974 (in the US), crop losses due to pests have ... remained at an estimated 33%. Losses due to insects alone have nearly doubled, ...from 7% in the 1942-51 period, to about 13% in 1974."(p.60).

"During the drought years 1970-74, the total value of agricultural exports from Sahel (Africa) was 3 times that of all cereal imported....(p.89). The governments have pressured farmers & skewed every conceivable program to favor export production...(over) food crops (for native nutrition)....(p.90) (Exports) earn foreign exchange ... used to enable govt. bureaucrats, & better-off urban workers, to live an imported life style. (p.91). ...In its need to extract wealth from the colony, ... colonialism promoted the increasing concentration of landholding by the few, & the increasing landlessness of the many....(p.115). In Bangladesh ... a landlord (will) sabotage irrigation, (etc.) ... because he does not wish his tenants to prosper & become less dependent.(p.21)." - Frances Moore Lappé & Joseph Collins, Food First: Beyond the Myth of Scarcity, p.21, 60, 89-91, 115.

"Pesticides (banned) for use in the US because of hazards... are exported routinely .... The EPA ... has (not) informed other governments of pesticide (bans)."

"The FDA does not analyze imported food for many (pesticide) residues. It allows food to be marketed before testing ...." - USGAO, CED-79-43, Better Regulation of Pesticide Exports & ... Residues In Imported Food Is Essential, June 22, 1979,cover page.

"...I took a pen name for sending the leaflets (protesting pesticides).... Discovery...had...result (that):.... Planes had come, & had dropped their pesticides upon (my) apiaries...."

"Hugh McDonald, an organic farmer.... ...stated on television in LA that he did not use insecticide because of the relationship of cancer.... Within days, banks demanded payment of his loans, & packing house officials...(took) control of his grove prior to picking. ...They placed guards upon his ranch & threatened to spray all his trees."(p.45).

(Insects controlled by) "...native enemies.... ...parasitic fungi.... ...microbial insecticide.... Resistant plants.... A wasp...controlled cotton bollworm on the entire ...valley. Since other beneficial insects controlled other pests of cotton, no farmer needed to spray."(p.47, 53, 56, 61). - Laura Tallian, The Pesticide Jungle.

"Kenneth Little, San Diego Co. Agri. Commissioner: '(In) some of the Japanese beetle traps (used to assess need of pest control)...people are placing (on purpose)... Japanese beetles....'"

"Floyd Morrow, Councilman: 'And how did they know it was a Japanese beetle (they were putting in the trap)....'"

"K. Little: '...they are pretty expert at it.'"

"F. Morrow: 'You mean they ... to sell a lot of insecticide?'"

"K. Little: "I think it's (like)...a false fire alarm.'"

– Laura Tallian, People's Lobby, Politics & Pesticides, p.71.

"'4 distinct groups of bacteria survive pasteurization. ...the strep. of pasteurized milk are the most frequent cause of rheumatic fever – – the most deadly disease of childhood.'" – USDA.

"...Cartels...(drove) independent (milk) distributors out of business. .... The small (milk) producer couldn't afford the excessive cost of pasteurization machinery, ... manufactured by the (cartel)." – last 2 quotes above in American Capsule News, Jan. 19, & Feb. 9, 1957, (in Raymond Bernard, PhD, The Revolt Against Chemicals, Health Research, p.73, 85).

(A) "chairman of the NAS (National Academy of Science; Cereals Subcom.)...is director of (R&D of a major food co.).... The chairman of NAS's Food & Nutrition Board ...appeared at FDA...on vitamins on behalf of (major food & drug co.'s). ....(US) Senator William Proxmire charged in a Senate speech that NAS's Food & Nutrition Board 'is both the creature of the food industry & heavily financed by'(it)."(p.100).

"In...The Great American Grain Robbery..., Martha Hamilton reports that practically all of the government purchases are of processed food.... ...60% of the small companies had not been informed by...a request for bids from USDA.... ...A 29¢ can of tomatoes returned 3¢ to the farmer.(p.223). Supermarket chicken prices were running 80 to 90¢/lb. ...but chicken farmers were getting just 2¢/lb."(p.227). – Jim Hightower, Dir., Agribusiness Accountability Project; Legistlative Ass't to US Senator Ralph Yarborough, Eat Your Heart Out, p.100, 223, 227.

"Many of the (state & local) advisory groups, similar to those of the (US) Dept. of Agriculture (e.g. ARPAC, NASULGC – Ed.), are established along commodity & industry lines.... The rural non-farmer, the small farmer, the leaders of rural communities, & the consumer are not usually represented on experiment station advisory committees."
– USDA's Roland Robinson, Agriculture Economist, (in Jim Hightower, "Hard Tomatoes, Hard Times: the Failure of the Land Grant College Complex", in Richard Merrill, Ed., Radical Agriculture, p.99).

Q.8.0 PEOPLE:

Q.8.1 UNDERMINED MINORITIES:

(Circa 1970, in) "the scientific advisory groups of the NIH, ... fewer than 3% of the some 2,000 committee members shaping research projects have been women .... Less than a third of NIH advisory committees deciding on research & training funding have had any women as voting members ...." – Gena Corea, The Hidden Malpractice; How American Medicine Mistreats Women, p.48.

"The Federal Advisory Committee Act (5 U.S.C. App. I) requires advisory council membership 'to be fairly balanced in terms of the points of views represented.'"
– USGAO, HRD-81-18, Research Planning & Evaluation at the NIH & Aspects of Advisory Council Operations, p.15, Dec. 30, 1980, report to US Senator Edward Kennedy.

"In the long run, however, consumerists & patients' rights advocates are doomed to sterility & cooptation unless they decide to take on biomedicine itself." – Health Law Project, Library Bulletin, v.4, n.1, p.7, Jan. 1979.

"Threat of malpractice suits...inhibit(s) the clinician in...experiment(ing) with... unorthodox(y); but research scientists...failed to test (unorthodoxy since it has) not been written up in any of the major journals."

"...Healing & regeneration...are best facilitated by a spirit of cooperation with the homeostatic mechanisms of the body (the vigorous (mechanisms) perceived as symptom patterns), rather than militaristic attitudes ('fighting' disease, 'destroying the invader', etc.)... aggression & arrogant intervention (of male 'heroics' - Ed.)...." - Alan E. Lewis; & Phil; Lipson, CCRP (Comprehensive Cancer Research Project), "An Intro. ...", p.2, & comments.

"I must confess, I am very disturbed & concerned over the type of treatment a cancer sufferer receives here in the US, for I know that all possible treatments for cancer have not been given a fair evaluation. To me, such is a sin against God & humanity. (So) I believe God should take the treatment of cancer from those presently so empowered, & give it to those who will give a fair evaluation, clinically, to all cancer therapies ... of value ..., regardless of the status of the discoveror or proponent, (or) the location & type of organization responsible for the treatment." - Richard Ericson,BS,JD, patent attorney; author, Cancer Treatment, Why So Many Failures?; GE-PS Cancer Memorial; in letter of Aug. 26, 1981, p.3.

"Nutrition need not be left solely to the nutritionist.... To be an 'expert' in ALL the areas of food ..., one would need to be degreed in at least these fields: (23 listed) ...It doesn't make a big difference whether someone has a degree in one out of (dozens of) related fields, or in zero of (dozens).... ...There are times when being a specialist might be more of a hindrance than a help." - Stan Perrin, Pres., CAN(Center for Appropriate Nutrition), The Food Chain, v.1, n.2, p.2, March 1981.

"The American press is not free. It's dominated by the same rich, elite aristocrats that control everything else.... How long will press reporters stand by & take it before they find the Martin Luther King who will lead them...?"

"I called up (a very famous nutritionist).... I mentioned...things...like kelp. And, I didn't get no reaction. So I checked him out...: he's on the board of directors of ... Chem. Co., that makes so many of the food additives."

"We'd use salt & overcook everything to take the taint away (from leftovers during slavery- Ed.), & then put the taste back in with more spices. Soul food is the worst food on the market." - Dick Gregory, "Up From Soul Food; ... from Night Club to Juice Bar", East West Journal, v.11, n.7, p.30, July 1981.

"The inner city poor...suffer...diseases...from...bad air, polluted water, excessive noise, & continual stress. Hypertension, heart disease, chronic bronchitis, emphesymia, sight & hearing impairment, cancer, & congenital anamolies ... are half again (i.e. 50% higher than) the levels found in the suburban population. ... Incidence of behavioral, neurological, & mental disorders ... is roughly double that of the suburbs." - USEPA, 1978 Report, Better Health & Regulatory Reform, Feb. 19, 1979, p.17.

"If exposure to mutagenic (carcinogenic) substances plays a role in athero-genesis (causing athero-sclerosis), ... Workers being followed for occupational cancer should be followed as well for CHD (Coronary Heart Disease) mortality." - Report, NHLBI, Working Group on Heart Disease Epidemiology, p.44, June 1979, NIH Pub. No. 79-1667.

"'Today 1 out of 10 men in America is sterile.' This...was found...by Diane Swanbrow...for...New West. ...Sterility...is also an indicator of birth defects & genetically derived cancer. ...12% functional sterility...in parts of of Michigan, to 23% in Houston.... compared to a 1938 study showing only 0.5% functional sterility in America. .... (A 20-fold increase in 40 years. - Ed.) ...Caused by pesticides...chemicals... radiation...pollution...emotional stress." - Health Writers, Health Newsletter, v.11, n.6, p.1, June 1981.

"...Several thousand food additives. In 1970 each of us consumed approx. 5 lbs. of these chemicals.(p.4). (& more chemicals in air & water! - Ed.).

"According to the National Foundation / March of Dimes, every year 250,000 American babies are born with such (gross anatomical) defects...."(p.30). - Michael Jacobson, AB, U.Chicago; PhD, Microb., MIT; Eater's Digest, p.4, 30.

"Nitrosamines ... given to rats near the end of pregnancy, induced kidney, lower brain, & spinal cord cancers in the offspring. (These are very common sites of human infant cancers. - Ed.) (It) did not affect the pregnant animals...." - Beatrice Trum Hunter, Mirage of Safety, p.168.

"Immunizations are mandated child abuse. ...Cancer? .... Have you ever asked what is in the needle?" - Jo Sesny; Assoc. Board Member, NOHA(Nutrition for Optimal Health Assoc.); in WGN-TV Rebuttal, Chicago, Oct. 1, 1981.

(For) "Deaths of children under 15 years attributed to scarlet fever, diptheria, whooping cough, & measles.... 90% of the improvement in death rate had already occurred prior to the introduction of immunization & the use of antibiotics."(p.151-2).

"Where is the counterveilling force to the immense power of multinational drug companies? ...The ill are too old, too young, too poor, too inarticulate, too disabled or debilitated..., too transient.... They do not parade..., present no briefs. They have no organization & exert no pressure."(p.175-6).

"...Research...counter to the profit-maximization role of any particular industry. ...might be cut off at the grant level."(p.162). - Alan Klass,BA,MD; FRCS, Edinburgh; FRCS, Canada; Dept. Anat. & Surg., U. Manitoba; Chmn., Med. Advis. Brd., Cancer Inst., & Pres., Col. of Physicians & Surg., Manitoba; There's Gold In Them Thar Pills, p.151-2, 162, 175-6.

"I see little hope for a nation which values the health of its livestock more than that of its people. .... Farmers are not criticized for routinely giving their (live)-stock (nutritional) supplements.... ...superior to any sold for humans....(p.340). .... Millions of families could plant home gardens if they truly wanted health.(p.343). ... Refined foods are...practically unknown in Russia.(p.347). .... The life expectancy of a 40-year-old American is near the lowest in the world."(p.337). - Adelle Davis,MS, Bio-chem., USC Med., Let's Get Well, p.337, 340, 343, 347.

"A key to the entire problem lies dominantly in the area of public education.(p.210). .... People who would not think of feeding a dog (junk)...eat such foods with abandon.(p. 211). .... There has never been a successful continuous feeding of a synthetic diet to several successive generations of animals."(p.224).

"...Whole personalities can be changed by good nutrition.... ...17 delinquent girls .... When their diet was changed to...more nutritious & diversified...quickly became less aggressive & quarrelsome."(p.43). - Roger J. Williams,PhD; discoveror, Vit. B-5; pioneer, Folic Acid; Pres., Amer. Chem. Soc.; Member, NRC(National Research Council); Prof. Emeritus, U. Texas; Nutrition Against Disease, p.43, 210-1, 224.

"Artificial vitamins...are not balanced by...associated factors...& lead...to compensatory deficiency of other vitamins (, minerals, enzymes, co-factors, etc.-Ed.)"(p.11).

"Crystalline vitamins are made...by the treatment of...natural source material with ...chemical solvents: Ether..., Benzene..., Toluene.... ...then...precipitant(:)barium ..., lead..., aluminum...."(p.10).

"Synthetic vitamins...(are) made from cheap materials."(p.12). - Raymond Bernard, PhD, "Natural vs. Synthetic Vitamins", Health Research, p.10-12.

"Chlorophyll reduced the toxicity of several carcinogens. .... Chlorophyll is widely distributed in plants.... The clinical use of chlorophyll for treatment of infectious (disease) has been known for many years." - Dr. Chiu-Nan Lai, U. Texas System Cancer Center, M.D.Anderson Hosp. & Tumor Institute; (in Dr. Gio B. Gori, Ed., (NCI Deputy Director,) Nutrition & Cancer, v.1, n.3, p.19, Spring 1979.

"...Two women...each...got rid of a tapeworm 200 feet long, 2" wide, that measured 3" around the head.... on bentonite (clay; psyllium seeds), herbal laxative, & liquid diet, (no food from animals), with...enemas.... Her daughter...passed a 40' tapeworm.... Bentonite seems to make (worms) turn loose their hold." - Eloise Allison, Unveiled Mysteries of Natural Healing, p.179.

Q.8.2 **PATIENT, PRACTITIONER, RESEARCHER:**

"The degree to which patients desire to control their own fate is continually underestimated by physicians. For most people, diet is the easiest health measure to manipulate." - Jan van Eys,MD,PhD, in ACS, Nutrition & Cancer, 1978, p.16.

"...the words of Tolstoy's Cossack, ... about West European doctors, 'All they can do is cut. Well, they're fools. But up in the mountains you get real doctors. They know about herbs.'"(p.107).

"He picked up a ... book ... 'Abrikosov & Styukov, Pathological Anatomy.... It's written here ... "It happens rarely but there cases of self induced healing."'."(of cancer).

"'...the relationship between the potassium & sodium salts ... depends on a man's attitude of mind!'"(p.133-4).

"'...he noticed ... there was no cancer among the peasants who came to him. ...the peasants, ... instead of tea, brewed ... chaga .... not really a birch (tree) fungus, it is a birch cancer....'"....

"'If the mushroom's that good, why don't the doctors ... put it in their standing orders?'"

"'It's a long business.... Some people don't believe in it, some don't like learning new things..., some try to stop it to promote their own remedies....'"(p.141-3).
- Alexander Solzhenitsyn, Cancer Ward, p.107, 133-4, 141-3.

"In spite of the severe shortage of nurses, somewhere between 500,000 & 600,000 qualified nurses are currently inactive because of low pay & the lack of intellectual stimulation." - E.K.Faltermayer, "Better Care at Less Cost Without Miracles", Fortune, Jan. 1970, p.89.

"...the NCI ... Annual Planning Project Requirements (says that) by July 1, 1975, it is estimated that 670,000 people in the US will be working on cancer." - June Goodfield, FRSM, The Siege of Cancer, p.179.

"... Biological Transmutation is a phenomenon completely different from the atomic fissions or fusions of physics; ... it reveals a property of matter not yet seen prior."

"... Exaggerated specialization ... condemns the modern scientist, isolating him from other disciplines. For many, science today is just another job...."

"I have found great support among known personalities, but they are a minority. They ... cannot vanquish the obstacles & inertia created by the too many." - Prof. Louis Kervran, Biological Transmutations, p.xiii, 20, 156.

"...Modern biomedical science clings to the Inquisition.... Censorship by the reviewers for a journal...is anonymous.... ...Most biomedical scientists cannot keep up with the volume of even specialized articles. ...In times of limited funding.... A lottery could equally well...distinguish the 'worthy' from the 'unworthy' grant proposals. .... The anonymity of the closed peer review (is a) dire threat(;)... signing reviews will dispell this threat. .... No true censor can tolerate public exposure." - T.J. Sernka,PhD, "Biomedical Free Speech", Physiol. Chem. & Physics, v.10, p.89, 1978.

"We are aware of many cases in industry, government laboratories, & even universities where scientists have been retaliated against when their professional standards interfered with the interests of their employers or funders. This retaliation has taken many forms, ranging from loss of employment & industry-wide blacklisting to transfers & withholding of salary increases & promotions. We are convinced that the visible problem is only the tip of the iceberg." - American Chemical Society (another ACS) President Alan C. Nixon, (in AAAS, Science, v.182, n.4116, p.1002, Dec.7, 1973).

Q.9.0 **AUDITS & ANALYSES, OFFICIAL:**
Q.9.1 **HEW, NIH, (LAGS in RESEARCH):**

"...Lag...occurred between an initial discovery & its effective clinical application. We analyzed the length of 111 such lags: 8% amounted to 0.1 to 1 year; another 18% were 1 to 10 years; 17% (lagged) 11-20 years;... 39% (lagged) 21-50 years; only 18% required more than 50 years for application."(p.3)

"...NIH...should contract for interdisciplinary research on ('research') problems such as lags...."(p.61, 4).

"Some causes of long lags: (1)The initial discovery was lost.... ...buried in an earlier civilization. ...language not widely read. ...little known journal. ...title did not accurately describe the contents.... ...ignored in...a comprehensive review article. ...huge accumulation of scientific literature.... published only as a patent. (2)The author delayed in the publication.... (3)The scientist did not fully appreciate ...his own discovery. (4)The scientist...unwilling to speculate...or...editor...deleted his speculation. (5)The initial report...was premature. (6)...(Only) appreciated by scientist working in other fields. (7)Many intermediate advances were needed.... (8)...Concept...was opposed by leading authorities.... (9)...Reluctance of university clinicians to try new ideas. (10)Editorial policies of journals.... (11)...FDA...or commissions on human investigation...block...research. (12)The initial failure... inhibited continuing efforts. (13)...No perceived clinical need for it. (14)... Corporate decisions...delayed widespread use.... (15)...Personal(ity) attributes.... (16)An insufficient number of...scientists...in research....specialties.... (17)Lags in utilization...by practicing physicians & in acceptance...by patients...."(p.62-76).

"Scientists now share their ideas freely (verbally), ...but few put untested ideas in print for others, (widespread). Such sharing of ideas might...greatly increase the productivity of researchers who now do 'me-too' research for lack of original ideas. ...Of a random sampling of 50 articles in which authors did speculate, only 4 proved later to be wrong."(p.81). - NIH; Julius Comroe,Jr.,MD, & Robert Dripps,MD, The Top Ten Clinical Advances in Cardiovascular - Pulmonary Medicine & Surgery 1945-1975, Jan. 31, 1977, p.3, 4, 61-76, 81, DHEW Pub. No. (NIH)78-1521.

"Every effort should be made...to ensure that ('peer review by Study Sections') form of decision making provides support for truly innovative ideas. Such proposals may appear controversial & involve risks but may be highly significant for the progress of science."

"... medical schools almost ignore the field of nutrition."

"Nutrition is today a neglected field...."-(Interdisciplinary Cluster on Nutrition).

"... all the items of high technology ... have always turned out to be much less complex than the methods used in the preceding period of transitional technology. And in each instance, the measures for preventing or curing disease have also tended to become much less costly, at the same time that they become decisively effective."-(Overview Cluster: **Chairman:** Lewis Thomas,MD,V.Pres.,Mem.Sloan Kettering Med.Ctr.; Members: R.W. Berliner,MD,Dean,Yale Med.; S.S.Kety,MD,Prof.,Harvard Med.; Arthur Kornberg,MD, Prof.Biochem.,Stanford; N.E.Miller,MD,Rockefeller U.; W.Rosenblith,MD,Provost,MIT; C.Wharton,PhD,President,Mich. St. U.; & others, of fame).
- Report of the President's Biomedical Research Panel, DHEW Pub. No. (OS)76-500, & Appendix A, -501, (in Nutrition Today; v.11,n.1,p.26,Jan. 1976; & v.12,n.3,p.15,May 1977).

"Sound procurement procedures were often bypassed in favor of expediency.... ... Little initiative was evident on the program side to monitor contractors' technical progress & adjust errant performance.... ...Weak controls over patent arrangements could also allow contractors to retain greater rights than warranted." - HEW Inspector General, Thomas D. Morris, NCI Contracting Operations, May 1, 1978, letter to HEW Secretary.

"...Contract extension...was awarded, totalling $64.5 million for bioassays (in) the Carcinogenesis Testing Program.... ...An NCI official stated that 'An arbitrary distinction has been made between resource & research contracts to avoid scrutiny by chartered HHS technical review committees....(p.31) ...The Deputy Ass't Sec'y for Health Oper'ns...stated '...We are placed in a position of not having sufficient & critically important time to consider alternative courses of action.'"(p.46-7)

"During FY 1979, NCI submitted...late...in the last 2 weeks of the FY...19 contracts amounting to $80 million. Late submissions limited the (NIH) Board's (of Awards) ability to perform an adequate review."(p.78).

"...NCI awarded 3 contracts...for the 'Clinical Neutron Therapy Program'.... ... exceeding $40 million.... ...Any chance of resolving the (NIH) Board (of Awards) comments prior to the award was precluded.... The Board had serious reservations...."(p.79).

– HEW, OIG(Office of the Inspector General) Audit Agency, Report on Follow Up Review Contracting Operations, NCI, Draft copy only, not finalized, (mailed to Author officially by HEW/HHS), tentative pages 31, 46-7, 78-9.

Q.9.2 GAO:

"Several nutrition experts ... believe that nutritional activities in general ... are not adequately supported at the (NIH Clinical) Center."(p.15)

"Harvard School of Public Health officials reported in the Oct. 1973 ... Journal, American Dietetic Assoc., ... that half of the Nation's medical schools' catalogs did not mention nutrition in any course description, & only 4% ... showed an independent course in nutrition as a requirement for all medical students."(p.17). – USGAO, Human Resources Division, HRD-79-46, Use of Nutritional Supplementation During Cancer Treatment at the NIH, p.15, 17, Report to US Senator George McGovern, Jan. 22, 1979.

"...A grants peer review study team appointed by the Director of NIH.... sent letters to 30,000 people ("whose names were on the mailing list for the NIH Guide for Grants & Contracts").... Of the 1,493 people responding...167 commented on...innovative research. About 89% believed that the (peer review) system was biased against innovative research proposals...."

"...The team recommended in Dec. 1976 that the (NIH) Director consider...limited support for certain speculative, high risk, innovative research proposals. As of Dec. 1980, the Director had not implemented this recommendation...."(Enclosure I,p.4,5).

"...Nutrition grant applications were approved & funded at rates lower than the average rates.... ...(Of) a total of 8,374 research project grant applications.... over 74% were approved as eligible for funding, & 35% were funded. ...Included (were) 699 nutrition grant applications.... ...The Nutrition Study Section — reviewed only nutrition....(&) recommended approval of 57% of the 191 applications it reviewed, & 26% of the applications were funded."(Enclosure I,p.8,9). – USGAO, HRD-81-95, Nutrition Research Peer Review at the NIH, June 1, 1981, Enclosure I, p.4, 5, 8, 9; requested by US Senator George Mcgovern, Report to US Congressman Frederick W. Richmond.

"If a staff fellow('s) research interests are not congruent with those of his Institute, his appointment can be terminated."(Appendix I, p.46, "Comments of the DHEW...")

"...NIH cannot terminate a research grant due to poor research progress."

"...If a cure for a disease were found or other research breakthroughs occurred, NIH could not end grant support of (obsolete – Ed.) projects having similar objectives...." (p.9). – USGAO, HRD-76-58, Better Controls Needed Over Biomedical Research Supported By The NIH, July 22, 1976, p.9, 46.

"...The National Cancer Advisory Board, & the President's Cancer Panel.... ...are appointed.... ...Reviewers (of nominees) attempt to insure equitable distribution of members in regard to geographic origin, sex, race, & discipline ("e.g. clinician vs. researcher, disease area of expertise")."(Enclosure II,p.1,2).

"...NCI — does not view evaluations as a process distinct from program operation;... there is no specific evaluation staff at NCI."(Enclosure I,p.5). – USGAO, HRD-79-74, April 25, 1979, Report to US Senator Edward M. Kennedy; Enclosure I,p.5; Enc. II,p.1,2.

"...4 of the 5 advisory groups that can influence the (NCI) carcino-genesis programs have given little attention to cancer prevention & carcinogenesis research."

"Since the first meeting of the President's Cancer Panel in 1972, there has been minimal discussion of cancer prevention & carcinogenesis research at its meetings."(p.3).

"21 of the 47 organizations represented by advisory group members had a total of 49 active contracts from the carcinogenesis programs. ....Members of the Panel & the (NCAB, National Cancer Advisory) Board being appointed by the President. ...a conflict of interest investigation is not required before making these appointments ; nor appointments to) other NCI advisory groups...."(p.5-6). - USGAO, HRD-78-143, (Advisory Groups to the NCI's Carcinogenesis Program), July 26, 1978, p.3, 5, 6; Report to US Congressman Henry A. Waxman.

"In 1976, NCI directed Tracor - Jitco to...produce draft reports on all completed bio-assays (of carcino-genesis, done) before...1976 — (a total of) 207 bioassays."(p.5).

"Further, there are more bioassays, which qualified for inclusion in the backlog, than were reported to the Congress by NCI. We (at GAO) identified 223 unreported bio-assays, but we are not certain these are all that exist. Thus, NCI has not disclosed to the Congress the full extent of the bio-assay backlog."(p.9).

"...Included in these 223 bio-assays were saccharin, cyclamates, hair sprays, & dandruff control shampoo."

"We also found that the Carcinogenesis Research Program performed 37 small-scale bioassays...between 1970 & 1972, which were not included in the reported backlog. ...As of...1979, ...papers on the remaining 16 (of 37) are in preparation."(Enclosure I, p.21-22).

"...Regulatory agencies are reluctant to act on data until it is finalized. ... (into) technical reports...published...."(p.6).

"We believe the single most important factor that contributed to the backlog was the lack of commitment by NCI to preparing bioassay reports until 1976."(Enclosure I,p.23). - USGAO, HRD-79-51, March 30, 1979; p.5, 6, 9; Enclosure I, p.21-3; Report to US Congressman Henry A. Waxman.

"'...NCI will be advertising the results of the Eppley tests which otherwise (will) remain buried in the scientific literature without the public acclaim.'" - Manager of Bio-assay Segment, Carcinogen Testing Program, NCI. (p.29).

"...There was unauthorized use of Federal funds & equipment by Eppley (Cancer Research Institute)...."

"...The justification for non-competitive procurement (by NCI) was not based totally on facts."(p.i).

"...Animals ("mice, rats, & hamsters") were bred.... The veterinarian at Eppley... provided records showing that...53,015 (animals) were killed before any research use was made of them. ...The total cost of breeding & caring for them was charged to the (NCI) contract."(p.39). - USGAO, HRD-78-44, Need to Improve Administration of a Carcinogen Testing & Carcino-genesis Research Contract, Feb. 10, 1978, p.i, 29, 39; Report to US Congressman David R. Obey.

"NCI did not effectively manage 4 of the 5 contracts we examined.... 3 of the (5) contracts (were) not fully achieving their intended goals."(p.14).

(NCI) "project officers fail to notify the (NCI) contracting officers of contractors' poor performance."(p.16). - USGAO, HRD-80-57, The Objective of the Cancer Control Program, & the NCI's Administration of Program Contracts, June 13, 1980, p.14, & 16, Report to US Congressman David R. Obey.

"...Of the 12 institutions NCI has scheduled for review (as future Comprehensive Cancer Centers), 6 are in cities that do not qualify for centers based strictly on population, & 3 are in cities that already have centers. (Yet) 3...(other) cities which the (evaluating) contractor found needed centers the most ... are not among the 12 institutions the NCI has selected for review ...." - USGAO, Manpower & Welfare Division, MWD-76-98, Comprehensive Cancer Centers... , Mar. 17, 1976, p.10.

"GAO is also recommending that the FDA have all ... food additives tested for their cancer causing potential ... (even) when ... ('unintentionally added') to the food in amounts less than 1 or 2 (ppm) parts per million. (HEW) disagrees, saying the risk of cancer is remote, & the costs for testing would be substantial."(p.ii).

"7 Federal agencies have principal authority for (carcinogens): NCI, NIEHS, NIOSH, FDA, EPA, OSHA, CPSC."(p.2).

"PHS ... publishes ... animal carcinogenecity experiments.... About 1,000 of the 6,000 (chemicals it published) have been reported in the literature to cause cancer in animals."(p.15). - USGAO, MWD-76-59, Federal Efforts to Protect the Public from Cancer Causing Chemicals Are Not Very Effective , June 16, 1976, p.ii, 2, 16.

"Although coal tar hair dyes are subject to FDA labeling requirements, the agency has not used this authority to require a cancer warning on labels of (these) dyes containing known ... carcinogens.... ...absorbed through the skin...."(p.i, ii).

"Coal tar hair dyes are exempt from...provisions of the FD&C Act, & therefore, coal tar color additives banned...may continue to be used in...hair dyes."(p.6). (This) "exemption does not apply to...vegetable dyes."(p.17).

"...before the Subcommittee on Health, Senate Committee on Labor & Public Welfare, ... FDA testified that: 'coal tar hair dyes should not receive priviliged treatment....'"(p.19). - USGAO, HRD-78-22, Cancer & Coal Tar Hair Dyes: An Unregulated Hazard to Consumers, Dec. 6, 1977, p.i, ii, 6, 17, 19, Report to US Congressman John E. Moss.

Q.9.3 SELF ANALYSIS:

"Many research ... activities have been subject to a phenomenon called problem displacement, i.e. the substitution in organizational concern, of trivia for significant problems, since the latter appear to be unsolvable. Furthermore, in some organizations, goal displacement is evident: turning away from original goals & substituting means for ends." - NCI, Planning Biomedical Research Programs, Feb. 1974, p.6-1, by Dr. Ralph Ingersoll.

"The war on cancer is really two wars ...; the other has cancer researchers fighting each other."(p.31).

"'Much of what is done in the treatment of cancer, by surgery, irradiation, & chemotherapy, represents halfway technology ....'" -Dr. Lewis Thomas, President, Memorial Sloan-Kettering Cancer Center.(p.32).

"'... A defect of the (National) Cancer Plan (NCP)...: too little acknowledgement is made of the genuine possibility that any or all of today's leads ... could turn out to be the wrong leads.'" - Institute of Medicine - National Academy of Science, committee to review the NCP.(p.37).
-Medical World News, July 12, 1974, p.31.

"The members of the American Association for Cancer Research (AACR) were polled.... 97% ... felt that additional basic knowledge was absolutely essential or probably essential for ... the goals of the (NCP) National Cancer Program...."

"Fewer than 1 in 100 favored exclusively intramural review, the method used with great frequency in the past for the review of contracts."

"...the AACR...consist(s) of multidisciplinary specialists in...the cancer problem ....(with) 1865 active members in...1974." - Cancer Research, v.35, p.1109, May 1975.

"The composition of any committee (to review grants or contracts) is at the discretion of NCI management.... Under the...Federal Advisory Committee Act (PL 92-463), ...Jan.5,1973, all advisory committees with any non-Federal participants are required to be chartered & approved by the (OMB) Office of Management & Budget." - NCP, Operational Plan, FY 1976-80, Aug. 1974, DHEW Pub. No. (NIH)75-777, page VII-11.

"...The DCT (Division of Cancer Treatment, NCI) program is a highly structured one, ... A detailed linear array convergence technique has been developed, &...every project within the NCI must fit into this picture puzzle." - Carl Fretts, Chief, Research Contracts Branch, Office of the Director, NCI, in "Contracts", Cancer Chemotherapy Reports, part 3, v.4, n.3, p.73, May 1973.

(NCI) "Division of Cancer Treatment, (&) Division of Cancer Control & Rehabilitation, (have no) NCI Programs & Awards (for) Nutrition." - Guide to NIH Programs & Awards, March 1, 1976, p.24, DHEW Pub. No. (NIH)76-33.(Compare to date below, next.)

"July 23, 1974 - The National Cancer Act Amendment of 1974, PL 93-352, was signed. (It) encourages the NCP to explore the role of nutrition in the treatment, rehabilitation, & causation of cancer."(p.1).

"Institutions Receiving More Than $1,000,000 ('Total') From the NCI in FY 1975: Litton Bionetics, $26,271,000;..Tracor Jitco, $8,475,000;..Pfizer,Inc., $2,526,000;..TRW Systems, $1,308,000;..Merck & Co., $1,296,000;..Upjohn Co., $1,248,000."(p.35).

"NCI Regular Grant Award - 1975 - Competing, New (Grants): Awarded Amount, $30,605,000"(which is only 4% of the total NCP budget - Ed.).(p.47).

- NCI, NCI Fact Book, Rev. Dec. 1975, p.1, 35, 47, DHEW Pub. No. (NIH)76-512.

"...From a review of the recent NCI contract programs, ...over 50% of the contract funds were awarded to commercial industrial firms." - NCP, An Analysis of Mid-Range Resource Requirements ..., March 1973, p.II-52, DHEW Pub. No. (NIH)74-571.

"NCI Frederick Cancer Research Center ('Litton Bionetics, Inc.'). Title: (Litton performs the) Operation & Maintenance of the Frederick Cancer Research Center...."(p.128).

"Subcontract with Dow Chemical Co. Objective: To evaluate the potential carcinogenecity & chronic toxicity of 5 selected environmental chemicals used in commerce & industry.... Major Findings: The overall survival was good in (animal) studies, the only exception being that of the positive control groups."(p.170-171).

"Subcontract with Industrial Bio-Test Labs.... To investigate the carcinogenecity of selected compounds."(p.175).

- NCI, Report of the Carcinogenesis Program, FY 1976, p.128, 170-1, 175, DHEW Pub. No. (NIH)77-991.

"Chemical Carcinogenesis: n.40254; ... General Electric Co. ('Contract' to:) Evaluate chemicals ... for carcinogenic activity.... Supported by USHEW (NCI)." - NCI, Current Research on Cancer Etiology & Epidemiology: Non-Viral..., DHEW Pub.No.(NIH)76-936.

Q.10.0 RESEARCH of RESEARCH:
Q.10.1 STATISTICS, (SURVIVAL, DELAYED TREATMENT):

"The ACS, ... FDA, & all major cancer centers & cancer researchers, totally reject Laetrile ... in the treatment of cancer. Legalization of an unproven remedy can defraud the public, endanger the lives of countless persons, & open the door to a wave of worthless preparations."

"In 1980, about 785,000 people will be diagnosed as having cancer.... This year (1980), about 405,000 will die of the disease." (USA only.)

- ACS, Cancer Facts & Figures, 1978, p.23, & 1980, p.3.

"On Feb. 17, 1964 ... US District Court, at Pittsburgh, 'Judge Rosenberg ruled that Mucorhicin, as a hope-giving treatment, could cause "irreperable injury to the public" by inducing patients to delay competent medical treatment until they are beyond help.' - FDA Report ..." - ACS, Unproven Methods ..., p.162.

"The use of Laetrile in early cancer cases to the exclusion of conventional treatment might well be dangerous since ... - surgery or radiation - would thereby be delayed ... until ... metastases had occurred & the cancer, therefore, might no longer be curable." - California Dept. of Public Health's Dr. R. Weilerstein, (in G. Edward Griffin, World Without Cancer, p.171).

"It is not possible to make a certain evaluation ... that cancer may be arrested if 'caught early'." - Hardin B. Jones, "Demographic Consideration of the Cancer Problem", Transactions, New York Academy of Sciences, series 2, v.18, n.3, p.322, Jan. 1956.

"...No studies have established the much talked about relationship between early detection & favorable survival after treatment (by surgery, radiation, etc.).... Neither the timing nor the extent of treatment of true malignancies has appreciably altered the average course of the disease." (e.g.: Cancer treated early shows a better 5-year survival rate, by merely observing the earlier, optimistic, part of an unswerving(?) cancer course. - Ed.) - Hardin B. Jones, (Prof. Donner Lab. of Med. Physics, U. Cal., Berkely & Davis; aids by AEC, USPHS, Guggenheim Found.; Speaker at ACS 11th Annual Science Writers Conference); in Cancer Control Society, Cancer Control Journal, v.5, n.3-6, p.148, 1977/1979; & p.147:

"My studies (show) untreated cancer victims actually live up to 4 times longer than treated individuals." - Dr. H.B.Jones, (in Spotlight, May 18, 1981, p.18).

"The detection of occult (hidden) metastases from radio-nuclide & (x-ray) imaging studies (has)... apparent futility.... Post-mortem examination showed an unsuspected high incidence of metastatic disease despite an extensive pre-operative investigation."

"(In) metastases (cancer spread: to) bone (from) melanoma, (to) liver (from) breast or testes, (& to) lung (from) fundus-uterus, incidence (is under-diagnosed) at 1% (or) less (on) detection by (x-ray) or radio-isotope, (but actually is) 30% (to) 80% (with) autopsy." - ACS, Metastases & Disseminated Cancer, p.40.

"Percentage of patients...(with) no tumor directed therapy within 4 months of diagnosis, (i.e.) No Rx; White, Male ; (by) Cancer Site, (& year diagnosed):
1940-49: Colon: 40%. Stomach: 65%. Lung: 63% Esophagus: 66%
1965-69: Pancreas: 73%. Stomach: 37%. Lung: 25% Esophagus: 23%"
(Partial data of "hopeless" cases beyond Orthodox Therapy. - Ed.) - ACS, Cancer Statistics, 1975 — 25-Year Cancer Survey, p.2.

"Percent of patients, (with no) treatment initiated within 4 months (2 months for leukemia) of diagnosis; White, Male & Female; Primary Cancer Site; Year Diagnosed:
1950-54: Liver: 91%. Gallbladder & Ducts: 63%. Chronic Leukemia: 53%
1970-73: Liver: 57%. Gallbladder & Ducts: 43%. Chronic Leukemia: 43% Pancreas: 63%."

"Percent of patients (surviving), e.g. Relative Survival Rates, (at) '1-year' or '5-year(s)' after diagnosis; Distant (spread of cancer); Year diagnosed; White:

Female:	Breast:		Corpus Uteri:		Cervix Uteri:	
Survival:	1-year	5-year	1-year	5-year	1-year	5-year
1950-54:	64%	21%	35%	19%	42%	15%
1960-64:	40%	7%	26%	13%	28%	7%

(Partial data on negative progress with Orthodox Therapy.-Ed.)

Male & Female:	Colon:		Bladder:		Pancreas:	Kidney:	Esophagus:	Pharynx:
Survival:	1-year	5-year	1-year	5-year	1-year	1-year	1-year	1-year
1950-54:	36%	9%	33%	6%	12%	24%	10%	47%
1960-64:	27%	5%	11%	3%	4%	20%	6%	35% "

- NCI, Cancer Patient Survival, Report Number 5, 1976, DHEW Pub.No.(NIH) 77-992, (for data above, & the reference just before & after this).

"Cancer Survival Data ... (1960-73), Median Survival Time (Years & Months):

Primary Site:	Corpus Uteri:	Bladder:	Melanoma:	Connective Tissue:	Penis:
Median Survival:	Years,Months	Yr.,Mo.	Yr.,Mo.	Yr.,Mo.	Yr.,Mo.
White:	12,3	4,0	9,1	2,7	5,1
Black:	1,8	1,1	1,9	4,6	8,5 "

- partial data from Dr. John Richardson, "Health Statistics for the US", The Richardson Clinic Reports, v.1, n.5, p.9, (from NCI, Cancer Patient Survival, Report Number 5, 1976).

"... Over the last 25 years.... The overall cancer incidence for blacks went up 8%, while for whites it dropped 3%. Cancer mortality for blacks increased 25%, while for whites it rose only 5% .... Most of the differences...were attributed to environmental & social factors...."

"For children, cancer is responsible for more deaths in the 3- to 14-year-old group than any other disease."

"Cancer is the leading cause of death among women aged 30 - 54."

- ACS, Cancer Facts & Figures, 1980, p.5, 6.

"US 1958, Ratio of Cancer Deaths to all Deaths: Women, age 40 - 50; 1 in 3 (deaths is due to cancer)." - ACS, Slides on Cancer Statistics, p.6.

"Complete Expectation of Life in Years (Remaining), for Each Sex at Selected Ages, Massachusetts, 1789-1929: (Partial data to show negative progress.-Ed.)

1789: Expectation of life in years, at...age...60: Male: 14.8 years; Female: 16.1 yrs.

1929: Expectation of life in years, at...age...60: Male: 14.0 years; Female: 15.4 yrs."

- E. Sydenstricker, Health & Environment, p.164.

"In 1972 the (WHO) World Health Organization issued its statistical report...for 34 countries...the life expectancy for persons who had already reached 65. ...23 of the 34 nations reporting showed a drop in the life expectancy of their 65-year-olds from the previously recorded 1958 figures. (Except) Japan, all the highly industrialized nations were in this group of 23." - Ivan Popov,MD, Stay Young, p.22.

"...United Nations...Population & Vital Statistics (said that:) 88 nations of the world have a lower death rate, (fewer deaths/1,000 people), than we (in US) have!"

"'Although in America today life expectancy at birth is near the best of any civilized country in the world...at the age of 40, life expectancy is near the bottom....'"

- New York State Medical Journal, Sept. 15, 1955.

- last 2 quotations above by Dr. P.M. Lovell, in Blanche A. Leonard (Editor), Check That Chick! Evidence on Meat Consumption as a Cause of Cancer & Other Diseases, p.62.

"...The incidence of cancer in children under 14 has almost doubled in little more than a decade, & that of leukemia has increased almost sixfold in the 50-year period ending in 1951." - Emanuel Cheraskin,MD,DMD, Professor Emeritus & of Med., & Chairman, Dept. of Oral Med., U. Alabama Med.; W.M. Ringsdorf,DMD,Dept. Oral Med., U. Alabama; J.W. Clark,DDS; Diet and Disease, p.208.

"The large range (in patient survival rates) presented (herein) at each stage (of a cancer) is due to patient selection & associated medical disease." - ACS, Clinical Oncology for Medical Students & Physicians, A Multidisciplinary Approach, 1974, p.273.

"'Beginning in 1940, ... questionable grades of (low) malignancy were classed as cancer. ...the proportion of 'cancer' cures ... increased rapidly....'"

"'If persons in the untreated ... group die at any time in the study interval, they are reported.... In the treated group, however, deaths which occur before completion of the treatment are rejected from the data, since these patients do not then meet the criteria ... of the term 'treated'. The longer it takes for completion of the treatment, ...the worse the error....'"

"'...The likelihood of treatment (of any one patient) increases with the length of time since origin of the disease. ...Those cases in which the neoplastic process progresses slowly ... are more likely to be transferred to the "treated" category than to remain in the "untreated"....'" - Hardin B. Jones, PhD, ACS 11th...,New Orleans,Mar.7,1969.

"... One of the side-effects of (surgery, anasthesia,) X-ray ..., & chemo-therapy, is the suppression ... of the patient's immunological defenses.... A simple cold often leads to death from pneumonia - & ('pneumonia') is what appears on the death certificate, not cancer." - G. Edward Griffin, "The Hoax of the Proven Cancer Cure; A Second Look at Orthodox Therapy", Cancer Control Journal, v.5, n.3-6, p.126, 1977/1979.

"'In the only 2 categories of cancer where good results from chemotherapy are generally acknowledged...(i.e.) in acute lymphocytic leukemia in children & in choriocarcinoma, the validity of (chemotherapy is)...challenged. ...In leukemia the real benefit (is from)...concomitant use of corticosteroids & antibiotics; & in choriocarcinoma, the (differential) diagnosis between this & benign precursor, hydatid mole, is unreliable.'" - Miles H. Robinson,MD, "who has taught & done research in physiology & pharmacology at the U. of Penn. & Vanderbilt medical schools"; - in Congressional Record, v.112, part 19, p.25194, Oct. 5, 1966.

"Hodgekin's disease.... ...is considered by many to be neoplastic in origin, but neither an infectious origin nor an immune response...has been excluded." - Dorland's Illustrated Medical Dictionary, 25th Edition, p.457.

"... Recognizing the capacity of tuberculosis to masquerade as other conditions (e.g. cancer, lung metastases) is stressed, especially since there is (less) ... suspicion with the decreasing prevalence of a disease." - M.Sievers,MD, Chief of Med., USPHS Indian Hosp., "The Second 'Great Imitator' - Tuberculosis", Journal AMA, v.176, n.9, p.810, June 3, 1961.

"...What we call 'spontaneous'...may result from external factors which are as yet unknown to us. ..Spontaneous remissions...may be more common than is generally realized, but...may be unrecognized as such because the patient is receiving some form of therapy." - Solomon Garb,MD,FACP; Co- Chairman, CCCC(Citizen's Committee for the Conquest of Cancer); Sci. Dir., Amer. Med. Ctr. at Denver; Prof. Pharm., U. Missouri Med.; Cure For Cancer, A National Goal, p.38-9.

"...More end result studies, (comparing) the treatments that cancer patients receive (, are needed).... The...NCI...End Results in Cancer, Report No. 4 (& 'No.5') contains valuable statistical data. However, it does not divulge (relative effectivity & safety of various Orthodox & Un-orthodox) treatments that were used (or not)." - Richard Ericson,BS,JD, Cancer Treatment, GE-PS Cancer Memorial, p.50.

"... Every alternative cancer therapy would be judged in comparison to the so-called 'treatment of choice', not only in ... survival, but in ... costs of treatment, freedom from pain, necessity of hospitalization, (etc.).... Statistics...should be available from the Cancer Establishment; (but) they have no reliable statistics, (or) records (are)...unobtainable & every effort to obtain them would be evaded.... Once reliable figures are obtained, the bitter controversies over therapies can be resolved once & for all." - Nat Morris (Maurice Natenberg), International Assoc. of Cancer Victims & Friends (IACVF), Cancer News Journal, v.14, n.1, p.4, Dec.-Jan. 1979.

Q.10.2 PROOF:

"Most shocking, from the point of view of scientific ethics, is...that...every one of their (SRI - Southern Research Institute) errors was in the direction of lowering the efficacy of the (Laetrile) treatment (of animals). ...There is essentially zero probability that such a systematic misrepresentation is inadvertant. There is no doubt to give anyone the benefit of!" - Dr. Bernard Kenton, City of Hope National Medical Center, (in G.E.Buddy Diamond, "Who Profits from Cancer Research?...", Harvard Political Review, Spring 1977).

"One simply cannot conclude from a large body of negative evidence, that positive evidence, however occasional, does not exist or is of no importance...." - Dr. Dean Burk, NCI co-founder; (in David Rorvick, Time med. reporter, "...Laetrile...Watergate ..."); (last 2 quotes above in Tom Valentine (Ed.), "The Great Cancer Ripoff", Newsreal, n.4, p.26 & 57, Aug. 1977).

"Even a schoolboy, fishing in a lake...& drawing out a fish on the first cast, but none on the 2nd cast, would (not) conclude that there were no fish in the lake." - Dr. Dean Burk, Head, Cyto-chemistry Division, NCI, (in Cancer Control Journal, v.1, n.3, p.8, Sept. 1973).

"... Extremely few of the published policy statements on breast cancer screening are supported by discussions that address even a majority of the issues, & it is difficult to find examples of good reasoning. Medical problems are very complicated, yet the profession does not appear to have developed the tools to manage this complexity. .... The randomized controlled trial...has its own shortcomings. ...It is tempting to assume that a study done in one place, at one time, to a given population, using one technique, is applicable to other(s)....", David Eddy,MD, U.Va.; PhD, Engineering-Econ., Stanford U.; Chief of Bio-Engineering Research Branch, US Army Med. R&D Com.; in The Stanford Engineer, v.3, n.1, p.22, 26, Spring 1980.

"The relevant matter in examining any form of treatment is not the reputation of its proponent, the persuasiveness of his theory, the eminence of its lay supporters, the testimony of patients (e.g.placebo - Ed.), or the existence of public controversy, but simply - does the treatment work?" - David Karnofsky, chemotherapist, Mem. Sloan Kettering Cancer Ctr., (in Ralph Moss, The Cancer Syndrome, p.86).

"The best estimates are that the medical system ... affects about 10% of the usual indices for measuring health." - AMA President, Dr. Richard Palmer.

"Only 10% - 20% of all procedures currently used in medical practice have been shown to be efficacious by controlled trial." - Office of Technology Assessment, US Congress, Assessing Efficacy & Safety of Medical Technology, 1978.

(Reply on what constitutes scientific proof:) "The question is much too difficult for me." - Albert Einstein, (quoted by Dr. O.Carl Simonton; Chief, Radiation Therapy, USAF Med. Ctr., Travis AFB; author, Getting Well Again).

Q.10.3 EXPERIMENTAL TECHNIQUE CRITIQUE:

"...There is one essential difference between the initial investigator's approach & that of those attempting to reproduce his work (:) the idea was his to begin with (&) he was very enthusiastic — a quality...lacking in...subsequent investigators. (He,"with interest, excitement") explain(ed) to the patients & their families the basic mechanisms & the expected results.... The subsequent experiments by other(s) showed approximately ½ as good results as his initial work had shown. After these less favorable reports were published,(still later) investigators were even more skeptical,(further) decreas(ing the) response of the patients treated." - Carl O. Simonton, MD, radiation oncologist, "The Role of the Mind in Cancer Therapy", Acad. of Para-psychology & Med., (in CCS, Cancer Control Journal, v.3, n.5, p.14 & 18, Sep. 1975, (for last 2 paragraphs above)).

"(In) some double-blind studies involving students in boarding schools.... ...the older boys exchanged their tablets with one another. ...mischievous.... (In) a double-blind...study with 190 employees of the NIH.... although a placebo indistinguishable from the Vitamin C capsule was available to them, the investigators used one containing only...sugar... , easily identified as lacking the acid taste of ascorbic acid."
- Linus Pauling, Nobel Laureate twice, Vitamin C, the Common Cold, & the Flu, p.176-8.

"Constraints in the Generation of Data:(A)...Initial Design: 1. ...Too few animals. 2. ...Premature animal deaths.... 3. Doses too low... 4. ...Premature sacrifice of animals for other 'studies'.... 5. Premature termination of the test.... (B)...Husbandry: 1. Poor housing, diet, & care resulting in infections, sickness, & premature death. 2. Failure to...treat...as originally intended. 3. Failure to inspect cages regularly.... 4. Inadequate autopsies. 5. Failure to examine appropriate tissues & organs for histological (tissue) study. 6. Poor record keeping. 7. Alteration, falsification,...destruction of records." - Samuel Epstein,MD; Chief, Lab. of Environ. Toxic. & Carc., Children's Cancer Res. Found'n; The Politics of Cancer, p.300.

"'It has been found that...changes in age, sex, hormonal status, diet & nutritional status, genetic factors, individual variation in the metabolic handling of chemicals, or the combined effect of different chemicals, all can alter the response of an individual to a chemical carcinogen; differences in response as high as 100-fold or 1,000-fold can be obtained by changing only one factor at a time.'" - NCI Assoc. Director for Carcinogenesis, Dr. Umberto Saffiotti.

"Since 1% of 50 experimental rats, is half a rat, such cancer would be totally overlooked...-& yet.... 1% of our (US) population is 2 million persons!"

"...Species sensitivity...individual susceptibility...."

"There are all kinds of ways to juggle scientific results(:)...species...('...extraordinarily resistant to (certain) tumors'), the stage at which you give the chemical ('...conception, ...days of pregnancy...'), the time you look for damage...."(p.46-50).

"...Lifetime feeding studies. ...Multi-generational studies.... ...Watch...for birth defects, ...fertility, infant mortality, viability of offspring (including tissue micro-exam - Ed.), life spans.... ...The chick - embryo study in which chemicals...are injected into the egg sac or yolk of fertilized eggs. ...is relatively inexpensive, gives a large sampling ('1,000's of eggs...'), &...it can quickly - within 21 days, the hatching period for chickens - sound the alarm about potential causes of birth defects. (It revealed)...thalidomide...birth defects...."(p.42-43).

"...(Humans) were 60x more sensitive to thalidomide than mice, 100x...than rats, 200x...than dogs, & 700x more sensitive than hamsters."(p.46). - Dr. Jacqueline Verrett, FDA, first to alert on cyclamates, top FDA chick-embryo tester; & Jean Carper, Eating May Be Hazardous to Your Health, p.42-43, 46-50.

"'...The convenience of these (animal) tumors as research tools tends to obscure the need for cancer research in man.'" - Charles Heidelberger, a chairman, McCardle Labs, U.Wisconsin; J. Holland, Roswell Park Mem. Inst.; Cancer Research, v.20, p.975, 1960.

"'Thus a screening system or evaluation program (in animals) limited to measurement of local tumor growth may miss compounds which produce therapeutic effects without extensive inhibition of tumor growth.'" - A. Goldin; J. Venditti; N. Mantell; all, of NCI; Cancer Research, v.21, p.1346-8, 1961.

"'It seems most unlikely from results obtained during the last decade, that any single drug evaluation system...can be expected to predict the potential of all classes of drugs against all of the many classes of human cancer.'" - F. Schabel, et. al., SRI (Southern Research Inst.), Cancer Research, v.21, part 2, p.235, 1961.

"'It would be really too much to ask that any one, or a few, types of cancers in animals would have the same responses as the hundred-odd different types of cancer in man.'" - Michael B. Shimkin, MD; Assoc. Editor, Cancer Research; author, NCI's Science & Cancer; USPHS Pub. # 1162, Rev. 1969, p.136.

- last 4 paragraphs above, in The McNaughton Foundation, "The Evaluation of Cancer Drugs", (in NHF Bull., April 1971; referred in CCS, Cancer Control J., v.3, n.4, p.10, July 1975).

"...NCI...tested on CDF mice using P388 lymphocytic leukemia.... The % increase in survival over controls, T/C.... must be greater than 135% for further testing." - Richard Ericson, BS, JD, Cancer Treatment ..., p.96.

Q.10.4 BIOMEDICAL INFORMATION EXPLOSION:

"The literature has become too vast to be comprehended.... It is...difficult to grasp even for the workers in closely neighboring fields. ...There is much more reliance on word of mouth for the transmission of scientific data.... gossip."

"Some of the shrewdest insight into natural processes have been greeted at the outset by the exclamation 'But that's ridiculous'."

"The (most) solid...piece of scientific truth I know of, ...is that we are profoundly ignorant about nature. Indeed, I regard this as the major discovery of the past 100 years of biology." - Memorial Sloan Kettering Cancer Center President, Dr. Lewis Thomas, "Hubris in Science?", AAAS (American Association for the Advancement of Science), Science, v.200, p.1459, June 30, 1978.

"...The (biomedical) literature has been growing at a rapid but essentially unchanging pace for more than a century, doubling in size every 25 years.... In 1969... (some) 20,000 active journals...(were) estimated to contain ... 2,000,000 new articles (yearly)...within the biomedical sciences broadly outlined." - S. Jablonski, "The Biomedical Information Explosion", Bull. Med. Libr. Ass., v.59, n.1, p.94, Jan. 1971.

"...The role of the (biomedical) journal is changing. Publication speed in a journal is not of vital importance to members within an 'invisible college', but is important to those conducting research in fields outside of their 'invisible college' contacts. Distinction will have to be made between the archival function & the rapid dissemination function...."(p.251).

"...Delayed recognition that a finding has a clinical significance may be a greater factor...."(p.253). - Gail Yokote, & R.A. Utterback,MD, "Time Lapses in Information Dissemination: Research Lab. to Physician's Office", Bull. Med. Libr. Assoc., v.62, n.3, p.251, July 1974.

"... A random examination of 18 recent reports in the English literature on therapy & survival in lung cancer showed that 8 different systems of histo-patho-logical nomenclature were used. Evidently, valuable data is being wasted due to poor comparability." - L.H. Sobin, "The (WHO) World Health Organization's Programme for the Histo-pathological Definition & Classification of Tumors", Meth. Inform. Med.,v.10,n.2,p.120, 1971.

"... $\frac{1}{4}$ to $\frac{1}{2}$ of medical & paramedical terminology consists of synonyms, some ... obsolete ....The micro-organism Candida albicans has...more than 170 different names. ...Terms...have multiple, sometimes opposite, definitions. 'Nyctalopia' means night blindness in English, but in French it means day blindness. Some assign the designation 'petit mal' to 3% of all forms of epilepsy; others classify 80% of all seizures (thusly)." - Jean Kennedy, & C.E. Kossmann,MD, "Nomenclature in Medicine", Bull. Med. Lib. Assoc., v.61, n.2, p.238, April 1973.

"Let's do now what we can do with existing data. It takes years for the medical profession to pick up things that are well reported in the literature. It can take 5 to 10 years. Our task is to cut that down." - NCI Director, ACS V. Pres., Frank Rauscher, PhD, (in Washington Post, May 26, 1972, in ICRF, Newsletter, v.2, n.2, p.1, Summer 1972).

(Continued on p.131 & 169.)

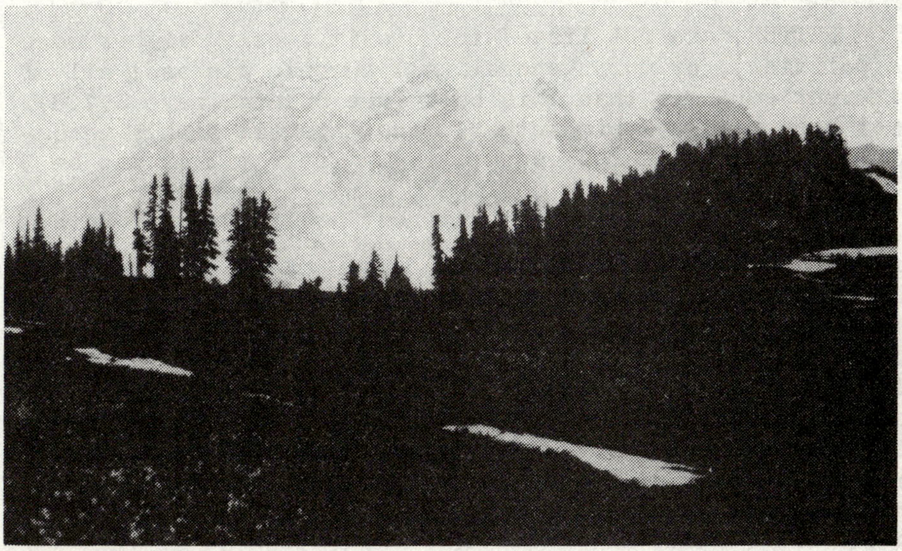

Mt. Rainier National Park. Breathtaking scenery, clean air, ions, sun. (Photo by R.H.)

READINGS RECOMMENDED, BOOKS:

The Author's motivation here is not to be partial, but to save newcomers any despair from pitfalls in this field, by guiding them:(a) towards rapid familiarity with this field's many facets, & (b) away from specialized books more readily valued by those with specialized needs (e.g. patients committed to a single therapy) or vaster perspective (e.g. cancer scholar).

As a quick learning library on cancer politics, the following books are highly recommended. They survey very interesting highlights, & are generously richer in their contents, than quotes & data from them inserted herein. (They are listed in alphabetical order by author. Their total cost is less than ½ the cost of a day in a hospital. They can be bought from "Public Interest Health Groups" listed later herein. A photocopy of this book list might be used as part of an order form.)

SURVEYS of Alternative Therapies of Cancer & Their Politics:
- ACS, Unproven Methods of Cancer Management, (1971), (free of charge from local ACS).
- George E. Berkley, Cancer, How to Prevent It, & How to Help Your Doctor Fight It, (Prentice Hall, NJ; 1978).
- Arlin J. Brown, March of Truth on Cancer, (Arlin Brown Info. Ctr., P.O.Box 251, Fort Belvoir, VA 22060; 1976).
- Suzanne Caum, Cancer Cures Crucified, (1968).
- Richard Ericson, Cancer Treatment; Why So Many Failures? What You Can Do About It!, (GE-PS Cancer Memorial, 519 Austin Ave., Park Ridge, IL 60068; 1980).
- G.Edward Griffin, World Without Cancer, (American Media, P.O.Box 4646, Westlake Village, CA 91359; 1974).
- Health Research, Is Cancer Curable?, (P.O.Box 70, Mokelumne Hill, CA 95245; 1962).
- Nat Morris, The Cancer Blackout Amended, (1976).
- Ralph W. Moss, The Cancer Syndrome, (Grove Press; 1980).

SINGLE Alternative Therapy of Cancer & Its Politics:
- Michael Culbert, Freedom From Cancer, ('76 Press, P.O.Box 2686, Seal Beach, CA 90740; 1974); & Vitamin B-17, Forbidden Weapon Against Cancer.
- John Richardson, Laetrile Case Histories, (725 So. Center St., Reno, NV 89501; 1977).
- Harry Hoxsey, You Don't Have to Die, (Bio Medical Center, 611 General Ferreira, P.O. Box 727, Tijuana, B.C., Mexico; 1956).

MISC.:
- Julius H.Comroe,Jr., & Robert D.Dripps, The Top Ten Clinical Advances in Cardiovascular - Pulmonary Medicine & Surgery 1945-1975, (USDHEW No. (NIH)78-1521; 1977; free from NIH).
- Samuel Epstein, The Politics of Cancer, (1978-9; prevention).
- Max Gerson, A Cancer Therapy, Results of 50 Cases, (Gerson Inst., P.O.Box 430, Bonita, CA 92002; 1958; no politics).

OTHER BOOKS, EQUALLY GREAT OR BETTER, are not listed for brevity, being either more specific (one therapy; little/no politics), or more general (all chronic disease; all of medicine), or otherwise of a different emphasis than this book (see "Scope" save S.1.8). Or, more likely, they have not yet been read by this Author. They are all highly recommended (respectively for patients & health scholars, especially). Their titles can be gleaned from all the references in "Cancer Quotations Collage", many references interspersed in "Table / Matrix", book lists from "Public Interest Health Groups", etc.

Some of the literature cited herein, are available FREE from these groups publishing them:
- ACS (local unit, then state division, then 777 Third Ave., NY, NY 10017).
- USGAO (DHISF, Box 6015, Gaithersburg, MD 20760).
- US Senate (Wash., DC 20510). US Congress (Wash., DC 20515).
- NCI / NIH (Public Inquiries Section / Division, NCI / NIH, Bethesda, MD 20014).
- HEW(now HHS): FDA; CDC; etc. USEPA. USDA.

This is a laudable use of donor & taxpayer moneys. Yet, another note to a similar address list cautions that the: "ACS...AMA...FDA...NCI...are generally hostile to unorthodox treatments." - R. Moss, Cancer Syndrome, p.304. This same free government literature costs if ordered from: USGPO (Wash., DC 20402).

(Continued on p.235.)

PUBLIC INTEREST HEALTH GROUPS; JOURNALS & ADDRESSES:

(Continued on p.236.)

● CANCER / ACTIVIST / FREEDOM OF CHOICE / ALTERNATIVE THERAPY

International Association of Cancer Victims and Friends (IACVF)
(Cancer News Journal)
7740 Manchester Ave., Suite 110
Playa Del Rey, CA 90293
(Tel. 213-822-5032,-5132)

Committee for Freedom of Choice in Cancer Therapy (CFCCT) (Choice)
146 Main St., Suite 408
Los Altos, CA 94022
(Tel. 415-948-9475)

Arlin J. Brown Information Center
(Cancer Victory Bulletin)
P.O.Box 251, Ft. Belvoir, VA 22060
(Tel. 703-451-8638)

Americans for Medical Freedom
(Voice)
790 Hampshire Rd., Suite H
Westlake Village, CA 91361
(Tel. 213-889-1231)

Richardson Ctr.(Newsletter defunct)
1000 Ryland, Reno, NV 89502
(Tel. 702-348-7744)

National Health Action Committee
(Bulletin)
6439 Taggart Rd.
Delaware, OH 43015
(Tel. 614-548-6202,-4067)

Report to the Consumer
P.O.Box 5449
Sherman Oaks, CA 91403

East-West Foundation (Journal)
17 Station St.
Brookline, MA 02146
(Tel. 617-232-1000)

GE-PS Cancer Memorial
519 Austin Ave.
Park Ridge, IL 60068
(Tel. 312-823-5425)

International Health Council
(defunct)

Comprehensive Cancer Research Project (CCRP)
(defunct)

International Health Institute / Nutritional Academy
(Journal of Health Science)
1238 Hayes, Eugene, OR 97402
(Tel. 503-687-1248)

Foundation for Alternative Cancer Therapies (FACT)
(Cancer Forum)
P.O.Box HH, Old Chelsea Station
New York, NY 10011
(Tel. 212-741-2790)

Independent Citizens Research Foundation (ICRF) (Newsletter)
P.O.Box 97, Ardsley, NY 10502
(Tel. 914-948-3399)

National Health Federation (NHF)
(Bulletin; & Public Scrutiny)
P.O.Box 688, 212 W.Foothill Blvd.
Monrovia, CA 91016
(Tel. 213-357-2181)

Cancer Control Society (Journal)
2043 No. Berendo St.
Los Angeles, CA 90027
(Tel. 213-663-7801)

Eden Ranch
(Organic Consumer Report)
P.O.Box 370, Topanga, CA 90290
(Tel. 213-455-1336)

American Natural Hygiene Society
(ANHS) (Health Science)
698 Brooklawn Ave.
Bridgeport, CT 06604
(Tel. 203-366-6229)

Omega Institute
P.O.Box 396, New Lebanon, NY 12125
(Tel. 518-794-8850)

American Academy of Healthology
P.O.Box 786, Ventura, CA 93001
(Tel. 805-648-7147)

Linus Pauling Institute of Science & Medicine
440 Page Mill Rd.
Palo Alto, CA 94306
(Tel.415-327-4064)

National Foundation for Cancer Research
7315 Wisconsin Ave., Suite 851-W
Bethesda, MD 20014
(Tel. 301-654-1250)

Aid for Cancer Victims, Inc.(ACVI)
People Against Cancer (PAC)
RFD 1, Box 415, Mashpee, MA 02649
(Tel.: 617-477-9862)

Alternative Medical Association
7915 S.E. Stark St.
Portland, OR 97215
(Tel. 503-254-7555)

Cancer Information Crusade
7335 Monticello Way
Ravenna, OH 44266
(Tel.: 216-296-4419)

PUBLIC INTEREST HEALTH GROUPS; JOURNALS & ADDRESSES; (continued):

Syracuse Cancer Research Institute
600 E. Genesee St.
Syracuse, NY 13202
(Tel. 315-472-6616)

Spring of Life
World Medical Health Foundation, Inc.
2 East 37th St., NY, NY 10016
(Tel. 212-684-2291)

International Foundation for Preventive Medicine (IFPM)
6932-B Little River Turnpike
Annandale, VA 22003
(Tel. 703-256-8845)

● NUTRITION

Lee Foundation for Nutritional Therapy
2023 W. Wisconsin Ave.
Milwaukee, WI 53201
(Tel. 414-933-2100)

Center for Science in the Public Interest (CSPI)
Nutrition Action
1755 "S" St.,NW
Washington, DC 20009
(Tel. 202-332-9110)

Price / Pottenger Nutrition Foundation (PPNF)
P.O.Box 2614
La Mesa, CA 92041
(Tel. 714-582-4168)

North American Vegetarian Society (NAVS)
(Vegetarian Voice)
P.O.Box 72
Dolgeville, NY 13329
(Tel. 518-568-7970)

Center for Appropriate Nutrition (CAN)
P.O.Box 10696
Chicago, IL 60610
(Tel. 312- 764-5470)

Nutrition for Optimal Health Association (NOHA)
P.O.Box 380
Winnetka, IL 60093
(Tel. 312-251-3700)

Feingold Foundation for Child Development
1050 North Point St.
San Francisco, CA 94109
(Tel. 516-543-4658)

Nutrition Resources, Inc.
392 Franklin St.
Cambridge, MA 02139
(Tel. 617-864-5237)

● SOIL to HEALTH

Natural Food Assoc. (NFA)
(Natural Food & Farming)
P.O.Box 210 (Linden Hwy.)
Atlanta, Texas 75551
(Tel. 214-796-3612)

Rodale Press (Prevention)
Soil & Health Found. (News)
33 E. Minor St.
Emmaus, PA 18049
(Tel. 215-967-5171)

Earthwork
3410 19th St.
San Francisco, CA 94110
(Tel. 415-626-1266)

Herald of Health
(defunct; merged with Natural Food Assoc.)

The Provoker Press
Lakeshore Rd.
St. Catherine's
Ontario, L2R 7C9
CANADA
(Tel. 416-934-2534)

Bio Dynamic(s) Assoc'n
Box 253
(Richmond Townhouse Rd.)
Wyoming, RI 02898
(Tel. 401-539-2320)

● WORLD HUNGER

Food First / IFDP (Inst. for Food & Dev. Policy)
1885 Mission St.
San Francisco, CA 94103
(Tel.: 415-864-8555)

Earthwork (see Soil to Health)

Oxfam-America
115 Broadway
Boston, MA 02116
(Tel. 617-482-1211)

Meals for Millions/Freedom from Hunger Found.
1800 Olympic Blvd.
P.O.Drawer # 680
Santa Monica, CA 90406
(Tel. 213-829-5337)

● NUTRITION, Retail

Vegetarian Times
41 E. 42nd St., Suite 921
New York, NY 10017
(Tel. 212-490-3999)

Vegetarian Voice
North American Vegetarian Society (NAVS)
P.O.Box 72
Dolgeville, NY 13329
(Tel. 518-568-7970)

Bestways
400 Hot Springs Rd., Suite 12
P.O.Box 2028
Carson City, NV 89701
(Tel. 702-883-7311)

Let's Live
444 N. Larchmont Blvd.
Los Angeles, CA 90004
(Tel. 213-469-3901)

Diet Times
Human Research Lab., Inc.
519 Madison Ave.
NY, NY 10022
(Tel. 212-751-8145)

New Health
1680 South Main St.
Springville, UT 84663
(Tel. 801-489-9486)

PUBLIC INTEREST HEALTH GROUPS; JOURNALS & ADDRESSES; (continued):

● HEALTH / ACTIVIST / CONSUMERISM

Caveat Emptor
Consumer Ed. Research Grp.
(defunct)

Health PAC (Policy Advisory Center)(Bulletin)
17 Murray St., NY, NY 10007
(Tel. 212-267-8890)

(Library Bulletin)
Health Law Project
(defunct)

Health Research Grp.(HRG)
(Public Citizen)
2000 "P" St., NW
Wash., DC 20036
(Tel. 202-872-0320)

Medical Self Care
P.O.Box 715
Inverness, CA 94937
(Tel. 415-669-7360)

Total Health
Trio Publications Co.
1800 N. Highland Ave.
Los Angeles, CA 90028
(Tel. 213-464-4626)

Health Writers Newsletter
306 N. Brooks St.
Madison, WI 53715
(Tel. 608-255-2255)

Consumers' Health Group(CHG)
(defunct)

● PSYCHIATRY

(Biosocial, J.Behav.Ecology)
(Diet, Crime, & Delinquency)
915½ Pacific Ave., Suite 206
Tacoma, WA 98402
(Tel. 206-565-0911)

Citizens Commission on Human Rights (CCHR)
(defunct address)

Cooperation Corp., IRT
(Issues in Radical Therapy)
P.O.Box 5039
Berkeley, CA 94705

Himalayan Internat'l Inst. of Yoga Science & Philo.
RD 1, Box 88 (Res.Bull.)
Honesdale, PA 18431
(Tel. 717-253-5551)

(See list in: H.Otto & J.Knight (Ed.), Dimensions in Wholistic Healing,(1979); Leslie J.Kaslof (Ed.), Wholistic Dimensions in Healing,(1978).)

● DENTAL

Holistic Dental Assoc.(HDA)
P.O.Box 1427
Carlsbad, CA 92008
(Tel. 714-729-6345)

Oramedics International
200 E.Montezuma Ave.
Houghton, MI 49931
(Tel.906-482-1419)

● WOMEN / BIRTH

National Women's Health Network
224 7th St., SE
Wash., DC 20003
(Tel. 202-543-9222)

NAPSAC (National Assoc. of Parents & Professionals for Safe Alternatives in Childbirth)
P.O.Box 267
Marble Hill, MO 63764
(Tel. 314-238-2010)

SPUN (Society for Protection of Unborn Through Nutrition)
(defunct)

HOPE (Home Opportunity for the Pregnancy Experience)
P.O.Box 78, Wauconda IL 60084
(Tel. 312-438-5271) (See list)

La Leche League, Internat'l
9616 Minneapolis Ave.
Franklin Park, IL 60131
(Tel. 312-455-7730)

(See list in: Gena Corea, The Hidden Malpractice, p.301, New York: Harcourt Brace Jov., 1977; & by NAPSAC.)

● MULTI-DISCIPLINARY SCIENCE

Health Research
Box 70
8349 or 70 Lafayette St.
Mokelumne Hill, CA 95245
(Tel. 209-286-1324)

National Exchange; & Newsreal
(defunct)

Progressive
408 W. Gorham St.
Madison, WI 53703
(Tel. 608-257-4626)

Mother Jones
Found. for National Progress
625 Third St.
San Francisco, CA 94107
(Tel. 415-495-6326)

New Age Communications Inc.
32 Station St.
Brookline Vill., MA 02146
(Tel. 617-734-3155)

Groundswell
(defunct)

Natural Life, Box 444, Oakville
Ontario, CANADA L6J 5A8

Science for the People
897 Main St.
Cambridge, MA 02139
(Tel. 617-547-0370)

Borderland Science Research Found.(J.Borderl. Res.)
P.O.Box 548 or 549
Vista, CA 92083

PUBLIC INTEREST HEALTH GROUPS; JOURNALS & ADDRESSES; (continued):

MULTI-DISCIPLINARY SCIENCE (Cont'd)

Mother Earth News
P.O.Box 70
Hendersonville, NC 28739
(Tel. 704-693-0211)

Applewood Journal
(defunct)

The Community of Eden Voice
(defunct)

Heartland Journal
7000 N.Glenwood
Chicago, IL 60626
(Tel. 312-465-8005)

● ENVIRONMENT/POLLUTION

Environmental Defense Fund
444 Park Ave. So.
NY, NY 10016
(Tel. 212-686-4191)

Environmental Action
1346 Connecticut Ave., NW
Wash., DC 20036
(Tel. 202-833-1845)

Natural Resources Defense Council (NRDC)
122 E. 42nd St.
NY, NY 10017
(Tel. 212-949-0049)

(See list in: Environ. Action, v.12, n.9, p.14, Mar. 1981; & Samuel Epstein, The Politics of Cancer, App. V.)

● ENVIRONMENT / ECOLOGY

Cousteau Society, Calypso Log
777 Third Ave., NY,NY 10017
or 8430 Santa Monica Blvd.
LA, CA 90069
(Tel. 213-656-4422)

Greenpeace
240 Fort Mason
San Francisco, CA 94123
(Tel. 415-474-6767)

Center for Environ'l Educ.: Whale/Seal Rescue Funds
624 9th St., NW
Wash., DC 20001
(Tel.: 202-737-3600)

● ENVIRONMENT / ENERGY

NCDA (National Car Drivers' Assoc.)
P.O.Box 1111, Dept. F
Tacoma, WA 98401
(Tel. 206-474-2318)

Fry's
22511 Markham
Perris, CA 92370

Solar Lobby (Sun Times)
1001 Conn. Ave., NW, 5th floor
Wash., DC 20036
(Tel. 202-466-6350)

(See: list in Fred Wilcox (Ed.), Grass Roots, p.17, 22, 57, Crossing Press, Trumansburg, NY 14886 (Copyr. 1980); & Multi-Disciplinary (National Exchange, Health Research) above; & Political (Spotlight) below.)

● POLITICAL / ECONOMIC / LEGAL

HALT (Help Abolish Legal Tyrrany / Americans for Legal Reform) (Suite 319)
201 Mass. Ave., NE
Wash., DC 20002
(Tel. 202-546-4258)

National Taxpayers' Union (NTU) Dollars & Sense
325 Penn. Ave., SE
Wash., DC 20003
(Tel. 202-546-2040, -2085)

Liberty Lobby (Spotlight)
300 Independence Ave., SE
Wash., DC 20003
(Tel. 202-544-1794)

New Solidarity Internat'l Press Service
304 W. 58th St.
NY, NY 10019
(Tel. 212-247-8820)
(credible on world hunger)

Citizens Party
2000 P St., NW, Suite 200
Wash., DC 20036
(Tel.: 202-659-8878)

Planetary Citizens
POBox 426
Menlo Park, CA 94026

Amnesty International, USA
304 W. 58th St.
NY, NY 10019
(Tel. 212-582-4440)

● PEACE

Physicians for Social Responsibility, Inc.
P. O. Box 295
2464 Mass. Ave.
Cambridge, MA 02238
(Tel. 617-661-9095)

Mid-Peninsula Conversion Project/Plowshare Press
867 W. Dana, Suite 203
Mountain View, CA 94041
(Tel. 415-968-8798)

(Many others; see F. Wilcox, Grass Roots, (above), p.26.)

● DEMOCRACY

People's Lobby
3456 W. Olympic Blvd.
Los Angeles, CA 90019
(Tel. 213-731-8321)

Foundation for Rational Economics & Education, (Ron Paul's Freedom Report)
POBox 1776
Lake Jackson, TX 77566

(See lists on many topics in: V. Kulvinskas, Survival Into The 21st Century, p.288, C.1975, Omangod Press, Wethersfield, CT; C. Lerza & M. Jacobson (Ed.) Food for People, Not for Profit, p.451; New Age Directory, O Mango Press, P. O. Box 64, Woodstock Valley, CT 06282.)

PUBLIC INTEREST HEALTH GROUPS;
JOURNALS & ADDRESSES; (continued);

APPENDIX:

● CANCER...

Healing, J. Gerson Institute
PO Box 430, Bonita CA 92002
(Tel. 714-267-1150)

Metabolic Research Foundation
518 Zenith Dr., Glenview, IL 60025
(Tel. 312-299-7180)

J. Natural Health & Parapsychology
Canadian Society of Geobiology/Biomagnetism
(defunct)

Foundation for Health
337 East Ave.
Watertown, NY 13601
(Tel. 315-782-6664)

● NUTRITION

The Shute Institute
10 Grand Ave., London, Ontario
CANADA N6C 1K9
(Tel. 519-432-1884)

Fruitarian Network
POBox 4333, Wash., DC 20012
&,
7202 Trescott
Tacoma Park, MD 20912
(Tel.: 301-270-3444)

The Sproutletter
POBox 10985
Eugene, OR 97440

(Continued on p.236.)

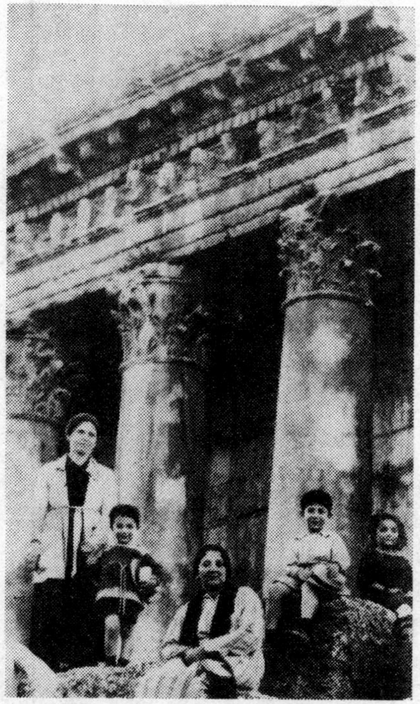

Family of author's grandfather, MD, survivors of 1915AD genocide of 1.5 million Christian Armenians; in front of ancient columns in Fertile Crescent.
"(The) Viet Nam...war involved...a deep incompatibility of culture...& from that lie others flowed...endlessly."
-Time, April 15, 1985, p.25.

NOTE: Please send Stamped Self-Addressed Envelope to groups in lists adjacent.

DIRECTORIES & DISTRIBUTION;
DOCTORS & ADDRESSES:

Lists of cancer therapists /MD's are provided by the following:

GROUPS (see addresses just above):
- Cancer Control Society.
- International Assoc. of Cancer Victims & Friends.
- Aid for Cancer Victims, Inc.
- (last 3 groups above have similar lists)
- Americans for Medical Freedom.
- Metabolic Research Foundation.
- American Natural Hygiene Society.
- International Found'n Preventive Med.
- American Holistic Medical Assoc./Inst.
- Omega Institute.

BOOKS:
- R. Ericson, Cancer Treatment..., GE-PS Cancer Memorial.
- A. Brown, March of Truth on Cancer, Arlin Brown Info. Center
- Bettie Towner, Cancer Holiday.
- Nutrition Minded Physicians, Alacer, Box 6448, Buena Pk., CA 90622.
- V. Kulvinskas, Survival into 21st Cent.
- D. Law, A Guide to Alternative Medicine.
- Ann Hill, A Visual Encyclopedia of Unconventional Medicine.
- Robert & Raye Yaller, The Health Spas.
- John Heinerman, The Treatment of Cancer with Herbs.
- Dick Richards, The Topic of Cancer, (Pergamon, 1982).
- Ruth Yale Long, No More Cancer, (similar to CCS list).
- Arthur & Stuart Frank, MD's, The People's Handbook of Medical Care.

BLANK TABLE / MATRIX for FUTURE ENTRIES: Author/Editor:

TREATMENT (Mode, Theory)	BENEFITED, % of total, or #	TREATED, total #	MEASURE of BENEFIT	DISEASE SEVERITY	RESEARCHER, Credentials	REFERENCE, Publication

ADDENDUM A to CANCER QUOTATIONS COLLAGE

TABLE of CONTENTS for ADDENDUM A to CANCER QUOTATIONS: (Continued from p.65-123, & onto p.168-234.)

ADDENDUM A to CANCER QUOTATIONS COLLAGE:

A.Q.1 HISTORY, CIVICS:

"'If too much salt is used in food, the pulse hardens.'" - Ch'i Po, 2600 BC, (in Lloyd Rosenvold, MD, Drop Your Blood Pressure, p.14).

"'It is changes that are chiefly responsible for diseases, especially the greatest changes, the violent alterations both in the seasons & in other things. (:)... regimen & temperature, &...one period of life to another.'" - Hippocrates.

"The doctors of Chaucer's day (1343-1400 AD, England).... ...had...a more practical, workaday code(:).... 'Do not disparage your fellow physicians. If you do not know them personally, say you have heard nothing but good of them. Avoid the company or fellowship of layman. .... Do not look lecherously on the patient's wife, daughters, or maid-servants, or kiss them, or fondle their....'" - E.S. Turner, Call The Doctor; A Social History of Medical Men, (1959), p.15-17.

"Men of learning began to set experience aside...to form theories...& to substitute these in the place of experiments."

"As theories increased, simple medicines...were forgotten, at least in the politer nations. ...Medical books, were immensely multiplied, ...(towards) an abtruse science, quite out of reach of ordinary men."

"Physicians now began to be...more than human. And profit attended employ.... (for) keeping the bulk of mankind at a distance.... They filled their writings with abundance of technical terms, utterly unintelligible to plain men.... Those who understood only how to restore the sick to health, they branded with the name of Empirics. They introduced...compound medicines consisting of so many ingredients, that it was scarce possible for common people to know which it was that wrought the cure; ...; of chemicals, such as they neither had skill, nor fortune, nor time to prepare; yea, & of dangerous ones, such as they could not use...but by the advice of a physician."
- John Wesley, Founder of the Methodist Church; MA, Oxford; (1703-1791); Primitive Remedies, preface.

"Medicine is a social science & politics is medicine on a large scale.... The very words 'Public Health' show those who are of the opinion that medicine has nothing to do with politics the magnitude of their error." - Rudolf Virchow, (1821-1902), founder of cellular pathology, (in P.B. Chowka, "Good News!...", J. Nutritional Acad., v.2, n.1, p.66, 1979).

"It is because cancer is so grim that some humor should - indeed, must - be included. Besides, a bit of humor helps to remind both scientists & physicians that they are, after all, fallible human beings - not gods."(p.X).

"In 1889 Dr. Roswell Park made this proposal to the NYS Legistlature: If they would give him $10,000, within two years he would find the cure for cancer."(p.169).
 - Ira Pilgrim, The Topic of Cancer, (c.1974, TY Crowell Co., NY), p.X, 169.

"In early 1978 I sent a serious article on the approaching trends of unorthodox cancer treatment to a major British doctor's publication, ... , to which I had frequently contributed before. It was declined, as was the editor's privilege. This decision I accepted without comment.... But when I published a similar article for a more general readership in a non-medical publication, the Deputy Editor of ... published a most offensive attack on me & my views. .... This year another major medical publication, Doctor, was pleased to accept & print my views. A huge correspondence from doctors seeking further information ensued."(p.4,5).

"The violent disagreements & vehement proclamations of different 'experts' at cancer symposia are now well-known, as each defends his own pet programme."(p.10).

"In most European countries amygdalin (laetrile) has never been illegal. ... Bitter almond, ...peach (are some) sources of amygdalin..... Celsus in ancient Rome used almond to treat 'putrid flesh'. Largus, another Roman, used it for bladder tumours. Galen...used almonds for 'scirrhus of the liver'. .... Avicenna also used (almond) oil for tumours of uterus, spleen, stomach & liver."

"...The psychosomatic element.... ...in cancer causation & treatment.(:) Gendon in 1701, Burrows in 1783, Nunn in 1822, Walshe in 1846, the famous Sir James Paget, describer of Paget's disease, in 1879, Snow in 1893, & Elida Evans in 1922, are the names of just a few (Drs.)."(p.50). - Dr. Dick Richards, Kent Private Clinic, England, The Topic of Cancer: When the Killing Has to Stop, (c.1982, Pergamon Press Ltd.), p.4, 5, 10, 50, 51.

"As early as 1759, Sir Richard Guy suspected that cancer of the breast was particularly predominant among women showing hysteric & nervous signs of distress, especially melancholy." - Hans Selye, CC, MD, PhD, DSc; Pres., Internat'l Inst. of Stress; et.al., Cancer, Stress, & Death, p.13, (of Sloan Kettering Inst. Cancer Series; R.A.Good, S.B.Day, eds.).

"'Glyptolythic humanity (of dinosaur era?) left.... ...clues to the anti-cancer molecule...taken from the blood of pregnant women at certain times. Acupuncture ....'" - Dr. Javier Cabrera Darquea, surgeon & cardiologist, & archeologist of Ica, Peru, (in Anne-Sophie Mileweska, "An Earlier Humanity?", Planetary Citizens, UN, (Norman Cousins, Honorary Chairman), Planet Earth, Spring 1982, p.8).

A.Q.2 TOP OFFICIALS, RECENT, & RESEARCH:

"Americans should have freedom of choice in the selection of physicians, hospitals, & health delivery systems." - Jimmy Carter, Pres. of US, (in Journal of the Nutritional Academy, v.2, n.1, p.34, 1979).

"Thousands of common household items are available to consumers, which contain potentially harmful substances. Hundreds of new uses for such products as food additives, food colorings, & pesticides are found each year, adding new potential hazards." - Lyndon Johnson, Pres. of US, (1964 message to Congress; in Booth Mooney, exec. ass't to Sen. Johnson, The Hidden Assassins, p.4).

"Our knowledge about health hazards in food is like the tip of an iceberg. .... Those of us who use the products (food) also have to defend ourselves. All of us need information & the determination to force consideration of health & safety among those who seem to be unwilling to take such considerations upon themselves, whether in producing, processing, or consuming publics." - Walter Mondale, Vice Pres. of US, US Senator, (in Ruth Winter, Poisons In Your Food, Intro.).

"The point is that we are not offering the best that the knowledge, wealth, power, & vision of this nation will allow—...to good health care.... ...I believe deeply that the people have been given less say in the area of health care than in almost any other area of American life. In no other area do they have so little choice or control. In no other area is the provider of services given such total freedom & authority."(p.XXI).

"...The hospitals & physicians take no responsibility for making sure the ambulances are properly equipped or the attendants properly trained. Nor...that the service is fast.... (A) metropolitan...County (had) the ambulance service operated there by funeral homes." (Conflict of interest? - Ed.) (p.76).

- US Senator Edward M. Kennedy, In Critical Condition: The Crisis in America's Health Care, p.XXI, 76.

"I spent a part of...1923 with...Dr. W.W.Keen. ....In the...Civil War ... he was a surgeon...& had seen many men die from the suppuration of wounds after he had operated. ...He would hold the sutures in his teeth, & sharpen his knife on the sole of his boot, after he had raised up his boot from the muddy ground. That was the accepted practice at that time."

"...He went to Scotland & studied under Lister. .... ("Lister was persecuted by the (BMA) British Medical Assoc. He was threatened with having his license revoked.") Yet in Lister's hospital virtually no one died as a result of operations because Lister had developed a carbolic acid wash & disinfectant. Dr. Keen came back from Scotland.... He was referred to as a crazy Listerite. .... He was denied an opportunity to practice in every hospital in Phila. ...."

"Finally there was one openminded surgeon in the great Penn. General Hosp. He said, 'Let us give this young fellow a chance'. So they let him operate."

"...No one died from infection under Keen. .... He (Keen) began to chronicle the results in statistical articles. He was threatened with expulsion from the Penn. Medical Soc. .... This was in the 1890's. .... Finally he was accepted as the greatest surgeon in the US. The old man told me — & he started to cry....'I nearly went under. I was nearly shut off.'."

- US Senator Paul Douglas, Congressional Record, v.109, part 18, p.23618, Dec. 6, 1963.

"In 1946 Dr. Gerson became the first physician to demonstrate recovered cancer patients before a US (Legistlative) committee. This Senate committee was holding hearings on a bill to find means of curing & preventing cancer. Unfortunately the lobby supporting surgery, radiation, & chemotherapies caused the defeat by 4 votes of the Senate bill which could have supported extensive research into the Gerson therapy."

- Max Gerson, MD, A Cancer Therapy: Results of 50 Cases, (2nd ed.), back cover, (statement probably not by Dr. Gerson). (Bill by US Senators Claude Pepper & Matthew M.Neely.)

"(...The Congress had exhibited) unequaled liberality in protecting our domestic animals against every sort of disease & pest." - US Senator Matthew Neely, 1928.

"'Federal aid was extended...to the studies on the health of farm animals, while almost no funds were available for direct work on the diseases of man.... This was ...prior to 1885...partly because human welfare brought no direct financial return. Hogs did.'" - Richard Shyrock, American Medical Research, (1947), p.44, (in Stephen Strickland, Politics, Science, & Dread Disease, (Harvard U.Press, 1972), p.5).

"'Human cancer research...by the NIH....(:)results...of prevention or cure have been very limited. As a contrast, the research on cancer involving animals & poultry conducted by the (USDA) through its (SEA) Science & Education Adm. with comparatively miniscule funding has yielded some positive results.... A successful vaccine has been developed that prevents (Marek's Disease) type of cancer in poultry." - US Senator John Melcher, Animal Cancer Research Act, Hearing, Subcom. on Agricultural Research, Comm. on Agri., Nutrition, & Forestry, US Senate, Dec. 10, 1979, (in Robert E. Netterberg, DDS, & Robert T.Taylor, MA, The Cancer Conspiracy, p.176).

"'The provisions of this Act shall not be so construed nor shall they be so administered as to discriminate against any system or method of treating human ailments.'" - Illinois Medical Practice Act, 1923, Section 20. (p.8).

"'Medicine based exclusively on the empirical use of pills & potions is becoming obsolete. ...Physical agents, produce striking biological responses (&) psychic reactions more potent than the effects of many of the drugs.... ...This extensive field of medical practice includes the employment of...light, heat, cold, water, electricity, massage, manipulation, exercise, & mechanical devices - in the diagnosis & treatment of disease.'" - Ray Lyman Wilbur, MD; President, AMA; Pres., Amer. Acad. of Medicine; Pres., Assoc. of Amer. Medical Colleges; Secretary of the Interior (under US President H. Hoover); Prof., & Dean of Medical School, President (1915-42), & Chancellor, Stanford U.; "Report of the Baruch Committee on Physical Medicine". (p.12).

- last 2 paragraphs in James Bishop, LLB, & A.M.Parker; Joint Council of Natural Healing Professions; Natural Medicine vs. Drug & Surgical Medicine, or, The Battle for National Health & Survival, p.8, 12.

"'The fundamental proposition originally announced by Dr. Albert Abrams must be regarded as established to a very high degree of probability.'" - Lord Thomas Horder, Chairman, committee to investigate radionics.

"Radionics...emerged from...Dr. Albert Abrams...MD.... ...Heidelberg U.Med. ... gold & silver medals.... ...Prof. Pathology & Director...Dept. Medicine, Stanford U."

- Ann Hill (ed.), A Visual Encyclopedia of Unconventional Medicine, p.167.

"'"Rigged research" — (is) the study that was set up & written to support a claim, rather than to seek for scientific proof. .... Only enough work is done to point in the proper direction & to get the report published in a medical journal; only enough to raise a doubt, or to put the Government to the task of proof by a preponderance of evidence.'" - FDA Commissioner George Larrick, (in J. H. Young, The Medical Messiahs; A Social History of Health Quackery in Twentieth-Century America, (Princeton U.Press, 1967), p.404).

"Food additives are far safer in actual use than the basic natural foods themselves." - Dr. Frederick Stare, Dept. Nutrition, School of Public Health, Harvard U.

"It is wholly unscientific to state that a well-fed body is more able to resist disease than a less well-fed body." - FDA's nutrition dept. head, Dr. Elmer M. Nelson.

"The manufacturer is entitled to reach his own conclusions, based on his scientific evidence that a subject is, in fact, generally recognized as safe (GRAS). & he is not required to come to us then & get the material (e.g. additive) added to the (GRAS) list." - FDA (Deputy /) Commissioner Winton Rankin.

- (in Gene Marine & Judith Van Allen, Food Pollution: The Violation of Our Inner Ecology, p.21, 60, 79; for last 3 paragraphs above).

A.Q.3 TOP BIO-MEDICS & OTHERS:

"The incidence of gastric (stomach) cancer has been related to diets low in fresh vegetables, fruits, & vitamins (Ernst L. Wynder, Pres., Amer. Health Found'n; et. al.). (There are) apparent relationships between the zinc - copper ratio of garden soils & the householders death from cancer of the stomach." - Ackerman & del Regato, Cancer: Diagnosis, Treatment, & Prognosis, (1970 ed.), p.429.

"'Up until 1972 there was a taboo that said if you fed a cancer patient, you would accelerate the growth of the tumor. We've found that to be untrue.'" - Dr. Stanley Dudrick, chairman, U. of Texas Medical School, (in Dr. Richard Passwater, Cancer & Its Nutritional Therapies, p.66).

"...Next to tobacco & alcohol, meat is the greatest single cause of mortality in the US." - John Scharffenberg, MD, MPH, Assoc. Prof. Applied Nutrition, Loma Linda U., Problems With Meat, p.101.

"'As any trauma in a cancer area tends to dislocate & disseminate tumor cells.... No doubt many curable cases of external cancer have been made incurable by biopsy.'"
- D.T.Quigley, MD, FACS, (author, The National Malnutrition). (p.40).

"...J.Ellis Barker's book, Cancer, Surgeon, & Researcher, ...shows the cancer mortality rate of (:) Physicians & Surgeons - 70, as compared to Coal Miners - 61, ... Agricultural Labourers - 54, Clergymen & Priests - 45."(p.29). (i.e. MD's have less survival, if cancer).
- John Tobe, Provoker Press, Cancer: How To Prevent & Gain Remission From Cancer, p.29. 40.

"The health establishment is a blood brotherhood known by the company it keeps, & these moguls need no oath or ritual as they work hand in glove with & for each other — if medicine benefits in the process, all to the good."

"...They are wise to the ways of wall street — &...getting their fair share of the loot.(:)...from who will be the head of the NIH, to which honorary degree will go to whom, which congressman gets the campaign funds from AMPAC ("the political arm of the AMA"), & whether Medicare fees can be hiked a bit for the suffering specialist. ...(or) to nominate their favorite for a Nobel Laureate...."

"Cancer has pizzazz, box office, & glamour, & in actual dollars & prestige, even heart & mental can't hold a candle to it. It's a health dodge with a future & everybody who's anybody is jumping in...."(p.169).

"But cancer can also be fun with its luncheons, theatre parties, & fund-raising luaus. ....What will they all do if a cure comes out of it? Considering how easily the March of Dimes conglomerate shifted gears after the polio vaccine, it should pose no problem."
- Edgar Berman, MD, (teacher, Johns Hopkins Med.; Pres., MEDICO; surgeon with Dr. Albert Schweitzer; author, 24 research articles; Moscow Internat'l Fellow.Award; 1st plastic transplant on human; 1st successful heart transplant on animal (dog); med. consultant to V.Pres. Hubert H. Humphrey, State Dept., & White House; med. school fellowships at 9 countries), The Solid Gold Stethoscope, p.167-170).

"...Vitamins in combination with their natural concomitants. The latter are not to be dismissed as 'excess baggage', but must be thought of as the result of millions of years of evolution of optimal combinations."(p.51).

"Over the years, cancer research has become the domaine of specialists in various fields. ...This specialized work...(has) had the peculiar result of becoming an obstacle to the study of the whole."(p.V).

"...Adaptation to an unsuitable environment is possible, but such adaptation necessitates hundreds of generations...."(p.122). - Alexander Berglas, Member, Cancer Research Found'n, Institute Pasteur, Cancer: Nature, Cause & Cure, p.V, 51, 122.

"...The truly fraudulent claims must be discarded. But novel methods of therapy should not be rejected just because they are novel, or because they run counter to some generally accepted belief ("which may just be bias"), or because we do not understand the mechanism of the proposed treatment, or because it has come from an unconventional source." - Linus Pauling, PhD, Nobel Laureate twice (Chemistry, & Peace); & Ewan Cameron, MB, ChB, FRCS (twice), Cancer & Vitamin C, p.86.

"'Explore higher plants for biologically active structures that up to now have eluded the imagination of the synthetic chemist.'" - N.Farnsworth, "Problems...".

"'For every disease that afflicts mankind, there is a treatment or a cure occurring naturally on this earth.'" - Dr. Norman Farnsworth, Prof., College of Pharmacy, U.Illinois, (in L.Aikman, Nature's Healing Arts, p.186, (in John Heinerman, Science of Herbal Medicine, p.xxviii)).

"That's the trouble with the conventional doctors. They always say, 'How does it work?' but often there isn't any neat little answer.... Something simply works.... We don't really know how it does. We say we do. We know one or two things we can see & measure...."

"There are plenty of quacks in this field. Fewer than you'd expect, though still plenty" (in Alternative Medicine). - John Bradshaw,MD, Doctors on Trial, p.273, 277.

A.Q.4 PRIVATE MEDICAL UNIONS & GROUPS:

"'The profession to which we belong, once venerated...— has become corrupt & degenerate to the forfeiture of its social position....'" - Dr. Nathaniel Chapman, first President, AMA, 1848. (p.77).

"'Any system of medicine that offers complete coverage & relieves the recipient of making any direct contribution for his own medical care will lower his sense of responsibility for his own health.... Such a system is inherently wasteful. .... It offers endless opportunities for 'chiseling' on the part of both dispenser & receiver & tends to the corruption of both.'" - AMA House of Delegates, June 1952. (p.98).

"'...In lay magazines...the favorable articles on new drugs, methods of treatment, & modern miracle surgery have in some instances been sufficiently exaggerated ....'" - AMA Law Dept. Director, C. Joseph Stetler. (p.239).

- Richard Carter, The Doctor Business, p.77, 98, 239, (for last 3 paragraphs above).

"It is not a question for the medical profession to say whether or not (medical insurance) laws shall be put in force. That is a question for economic groups & forces outside the profession." - AMA, Committee on Social Insurance, 1919.(p.105).

"The doctor is essentially a small business man. He is selling his services, & is as much in business as anyone else selling a commodity." - AMA, Bureau of Medical Economics, Dr. F.G.Dickinson.(p.33).

- (in Roul Tunney, (Yale U. grad.& Prof.; Look mag. promo.head); The American Health Scandal, p.33, 105; for last 2 paragraphs above).

"'Some of our members are giving lectures in osteopathic & optometric schools & addresses before their societies. Some members are associated by a common waiting room with them. ...(or) partnership in practice. All of these voluntarily associated practices are unethical....'" - AMA Judicial Council. (p.243).

"'There can never be a majority party & a minority party in any science. There cannot be two distinct sciences of medicine, or two different, yet equally valid, systems of medical practice.'" - AMA, Proceedings of the House of Delegates, 1961, p.174. (p.251).

- Elton Rayack, Professional Power & American Medicine: The Economics of the AMA, p.243, 251, (for last 2 paragraphs above).

"'The individual who violates the rules in a zealous search for an answer to the problem may overstep the bounds & thereby suffer loss of his relationships to the organized medical profession.'" - Journal AMA editorial under chief Morris Fishbein.

"Today, expulsion is again mustered into service in a war of ideology. ....Modern society makes its heresies out of political economy.... Ethics has always been a flexible, developing notion in medicine, with a strong flavor of economics from the start." - Oliver Garceau, Dept. of Govt., Harvard U., The Political Life of the American Medical Association, (1941), p.106.

"I shall never cease to be astonished at the number of people who would not invest a penny in any enterprise without full assurance of its safety, yet who will hop on the operating table & permit anyone to cut into their bellies." - Paul R. Hawley, MD, Director, American College of Surgeons, (in Herbert Denenberg, Commissioner, Pennsylvania Insurance Dept.; Member, Inst. of Medicine, NAS (National Academy of Sciences); The Shopper's Guidebook to Life ..., Health ..., Auto ..., Homeowner's, Insurance, ..., p.103).

"'The dentist has the obligation of not referring disparagingly, orally or in writing, to the services of another dentist, to a member of the public.'"

- ADA Code n.8. (p.290).

"...Life insurance.... companies are constantly making it more complicated because it is more profitable that way for agents & companies."(p.180).

- Consumer News Inc., Help: The Useful Almanac, 1976-77, p.180, 290, (for last 2 paragraphs).

A.Q.5 MASS MEDIA:

"'I invite your attention to the latest piratical development commonly known as the "radio trust". It would seem that human cupidity could not reach so far, or human insolence become so gross as to attempt...to withhold from the public use the instrumentalities of communication through the air; & yet that is exactly what a group of great capitalists are attempting through the organization of a huge monopoly.'"

- US Senator James A. Reed, (first term: 1911-), this speech cut off air. (p.238).

"The American consumer has about one billion dollars invested in radio sets, ... ten times greater than the inflated capital of commercial broadcasting companies. Yet the consumer...has delegated — by default — to the broadcasting companies & the program sponsors a power that he should have retained: that of regulating the traffic through his own receiving set. ...an unending stream of...false statements on the supposed merits of a long list of advertised foods, dentifrices, medicines, cosmetics, ..."(p.3-4).

"Radio frequencies are recognized as public property by the Congress of the US." (p.248). - Peter Morell, Poisons, Potions, & Profits, c.1937, p.3, 4, 238, 248, (for last 3 paragraphs above).

"(For) a company introducing a new, patented drug product... The goal is obvious: to associate the (company) brand name with the product so that the physician will continue to prescribe it by that name long after the patent has expired. ...Part of this strategy (is)...to select public or generic names that are far more complex than their respective brand names, & far more difficult to remember, spell, or pronounce. .... Since 1964 (naming is by) the US Adopted Names Council...." - Milton Silverman & Philip R.Lee, HEW Task Force on Prescription Drugs Chairman & Staff Director, Pills, Profits, & Politics, p.36.

"Most patent medicines depend for their success upon utterly false curative claims. ...Many people automatically believe anything (anything) they see in print — doubtless a holdover from early childhood, when the textbook was regarded as the acme of truthfulness...."

"...A prize of $50,000 was offered for a successful treatment for cancer. ... Before the prize offer had expired almost 4,000 cures had been submitted. .... Not one was judged worthy of being tested in a cancer lab.",(by ACS's precursor, ASCC).

- August A.Thomen, MD, Doctors Don't Believe It — Why Should You?, c.1941, p.258-261.

"Advertising space in (the top nutritional supplement magazine) is not cheap. As of...1979, the general advertising rate was $12,355 for a black-&-white page, $21,715 for a color page, & $28,225 for the back cover. ...Several 1979 issues of the magazine have carried each month at least 100 pages of ads ("including inserts"), nearly all of which were devoted to food supplements, health food nostrums, ..."(p.223).

"(An) incident (was) reported in JAMA (Journal, AMA).... After more than 20 physicians failed to find the cause, the woman finally made the diagnosis herself. An investigation of the medical literature convinced her that she was suffering from lead poisoning. Subsequent testing revealed that she was right."(p.233).

- Consumers Union, Health Quackery, p. 223, 233.

"'Just go on as you used to go on & I will not take any action to seize your goods or...take any case into court....'" - Secretary of Agriculture, James Wilson.(p.202).

"Advertising is well known to be the mainstay of sales of fraudulent & dangerous drugs & adulterated & substitute foods."(p.181).

- Arthur Kallet & F.J. Schlink, Consumers' Research, 100,000,000 Guinea Pigs, c.1933, p.181, 202, (for last 2 paragraphs above).

"'...Your company...will send drugs to all the underdeveloped countries of the world, & since they do not have any standards, we will fool them all we can & make a great big profit & never tell the doctors that there is a risk.... ...You will meet the standards of the country in which you are advertising, not the...proper standard.... I would think that you would not sleep at night.... I do not think this country will stand for it.'" - US Senator Gaylord Nelson.(p.77-78).

"100,000,000 Guinea Pigs sparked a rising wave of consumer indignation. But...it takes a major catastrophe to carry legal & enforcement action over the hump of lethargy & inaction. .... Today, nearly 40 years later, the situation is worse, not better." - John Fuller, (Emmy Award producer of The Great American Dream Machine, 1970-1), 200,000,000 Guinea Pigs, c.1972, p.9, 10, 77, 78, (for last 2 paragraphs above).

"'...The governments in the first world countries (should) stop their own companies from exporting drugs that are already banned or withdrawn or severely restricted in their own countries....'" - CAP (Consumers' Assoc. of Penang, (Malaysia)).

"'...The company...(:) ...they omit 'contra-indications', they omit 'side-effects' indications, they enlarge the spectrum of 'indications'...in order to make of each drug ...a best selling....'" - a famous health activist writer.

"The pharmacist says its the doctor's responsibility, the doctor says its the government's or its the manufacturer's responsibility, the government says its the manufacturer's responsibility, now the manufacturer is saying its the government's (or local distributor's) responsibility. Everybody is passing the buck to somebody else."

"The International Organization of Consumers Unions has recently helped establish a global health information network."

- Robert Richter, Producer, "Pesticides & Pills: For Export Only", Non Fiction Television, WNET, Ch. 13, NY, (on WTTW, Ch. 11, Chicago; 9pm, Oct. 7, 1981; for last 4 paragraphs above).

"'The association between cigarette smoking & wrinkling was striking in both sexes.... Smokers in the 40-49 year age group were as likely to be prominently wrinkled as non-smokers who were 20 years older.... Encourage young women (against) smoking.... (It is) ironic much of the successful cigarette ads use youth & sexiness.'" - Dr. H. Daniell.

"Dr. Herlich found that 75% of the (balding) men between 21 & 22 years of age were heavy smokers." - Don C. Matchan, We Mind If You Smoke, p.41-42, (for last 2 paragraphs).

"...Modern children.... ...grow fast & large.... ...The natural needs & aspirations of the body & soul still torment young people.... Desire for earthly goods, for power, for sexual satisfaction are constantly stimulated by the mass-communications media. But social mores still dictate...." - Dr. René J. Dubos, Prof., Rockefeller Inst.; (Mary) Lasker Award; Prof., Harvard Med.; "Beyond Traditional Medicine", (in Marion K. Sanders, Ed., The Crisis in American Medicine, p.139, 141).

"'Health experts working on a union backed screening program to detect bladder cancer in a Georgia chemical plant were stunned when the local (ACS) cancer society chapter not only didn't support the program, but tried to discourage participation in it.'" - Jack Anderson, "Big Charitable Funds Bully Their Smaller 'Competitors'".

"A recent EPA action(:)... That agency (EPA) is not only not publishing booklets, but they are destroying 86 of the 104 publications they have on hand. Most are objectionable to the chemical industry because they emphasize the dangers of pesticides & chemicals...." - Caveat Emptor, v.12, n.2, p.19,20, Feb. 1982, (for last 2 paragraphs above).

"On Dec. 1, 1977...NBC Nightly News presented to the nation...that the possibility for a universal cancer preventive vaccine does exist.... NBC News spent several months checking out the data before airing the presentation. What was the result...? Three years of silence (to date) from the cancer establishment."(p.XVI).

"...The AP & the UPI did not report upon the NBC News telecast, so nothing further appeared in the newspapers across the nation."(p.118).

"...20 research institutions receive 50% of all the NCI funding for cancer research annually!"(p.113).

- Dr. Robert Netterberg & Robert Taylor, The Cancer Conspiracy, p.XVI, 113, 118, (for last 3 paragraphs above).

Preston: "Medicine is...an exceedingly lucrative business.... It's a closed shop (union - Ed.).... ...Licensure(:).... In credentialling physicians... the medical profession....is protecting itself, not the public. ...Why don't we revoke the licenses of all the incompetent physicians...who are alcoholics, ...drug abusers...? ...The medical profession controls state licensure boards. ...."

Donahue: "...Oncology is 'grab bag' out there! You have no idea what kind of attention you're going to get! ... ...A program I (did had)...young people who have...cancer...(&) how they used their own attitude to change themselves. .... It's one of the most important shows I've ever done."

- Dr. Thomas Preston, cardiologist, (author, The Clay Pedestal), on Phil Donahue Show, WGN-TV, Ch.9, Chicago, Dec. 17, 1981.

"'...Physicians who are members of medical societies flock to the defense of their fellow member charged with malpractice, & the plaintiff is relegated...to the occasional lone wolf or heroic soul who, ...has the courage to run the risk of ostracism by his fellow practitioners & the cancellation of public liability insurance policy....'" - Justice Jesse Carter, Cal. Supreme Court, 1951. (p.241).

"...The AMA Public Relations Dept.'s activities...for 1957....(:)conventions... conferences & symposia.... Weekly releases.... Liaison was maintained with the National Assoc. of Science Writers.... assisted in the preparation of copy for newspapers & magazines, & some of the publications actually submitted the manuscripts to the AMA for review.... (&) close contact with the television industry, (on:) March of Medicine, Medical Horizons, Dr. Christian, Dr. Hudson's Secret Journal, Frontier Doctor, (& 9 other shows listed). .... There was Medical Education Week, with...repeated screening of AMA slides & film clips on 133 tv stations."(p.223).

- Richard Carter, The Doctor Business, p.223, 241, (for last 2 paragraphs above).

A.Q.6 LAW vs. JUSTICE:

"'No right is held more sacred or is more carefully guarded by the common law, than the right of every individual to the possession & control of his own person.'"

- Justice Cooley, US Supreme Court.

"'No laws are binding upon the human subject which assault the body or violate the the conscience.'" - Blackstone. (back cover).

"'Predatory medicine on the loose, the greed of a national charity racket, & thousands of little white coffins....'" - Morris Beale, Super Drug Story. (p.59).

"'...A clumsy public relations effort of the (US Presidential) Administration (was) designed to aid the re-election of the incumbent. .... The press has also been condemned as the hand-maiden of the medical establishment in selling (the swine flu vaccine) program to the public. .... Few dissenters to the program were quoted... & spokesmen for the government viewpoint had a virtual monopoly of the air waves & news columns.'" - David Rubin, "Swine Flu, the Media as a Mirror of Confusion...", Journalism Review, July 1977. (p.85-86).

- Ida Honorof & Eleanor McBean, Vaccination, the Silent Killer, p.59, 85-6, back cover, (for last 4 paragraphs above).

"...Loss of medical society membership....(:) Ethical condemnation can result in professional embarrassment & disgrace, loss of referrals & other patronage, deprivation of malpractice insurance, the withholding of claims reimbursement by health insurance carriers, possible loss of hospital staff privileges, & denial of speaker & exhibitor status at professional society meetings. ...."

"The most notorious application of AMA contract practice restrictions resulted in the criminal conviction of AMA...for violating the Sherman Act by attempting to restrain the development of...(an HMO) through use of boycotts.... AMA vs. US. This conviction did not deter AMA & its affiliates from continuing to implement the same underlying contract practice restrictions against similar proposed arrangements..."

"In fact, petitioners' (AMA's) long history of illegal behavior strongly supports the need for a remedy to reverse the effects of the restraints of trade they have imposed. And although petitioners (AMA) are now quick to admit that their past conduct was unlawful, they have not been so quick to mitigate the effects of their past violations."

- US Dept. of Justice, brief filed in US Supreme Court, (in Caveat Emptor, v.12, n.1, p.4, Jan. 1982).

"...The patient, being unlearned in medical science, has an abject dependence upon & trust in his physician.... thus raising.... a resultant requirement, for divulgence by the physician to his patient of all information relevant to a meaningful decisional process.... (including) the available choices with respect to proposed therapy & of the dangers...in each." - Supreme Court of California, Cobbs vs. Grant, unanimous decision, (in Frank Wood, Attorney, "Doctors' Dilemma: Who Are the Real Quacks?", Cancer Control Journal, v.1, n.4, p.5, Nov. 1973).

"'I shudder to think what a Martian astronaut...would think of our courts & what goes on, or does not go on, in them. As to the judges, what would he think of certain of them, in theory elected by the public but in fact hand-picked by political leaders for purely political purposes irrelevant to merit?'" - Francis Plimpton, President, NYC Bar Assoc., (in Richard Ney, The Wall Street Gang, p.314).

"...The IACVF (Internat'l Assoc. of Cancer Victims & Friends)...tells of a (recent) raid against one of their public meetings by the Nassau County (NY) D. A., during which several people were arrested, handcuffed, & dragged away.... Their homes were searched...."(n.217, Mar. 1975).

"In Georgia, after the Civil War, a vendor of 'unwholesome bread, or pernicious liquor' drew a $1,000 fine, 39 strokes with the lash, or a term on the chain gang of up to a year." - Inst. of Nutritional Research, Nutritional Therapy.

"...The AMA, National Health Council, FDA, (APA) American Pharmaceutical Assoc., FTC, ACS, Arthritis Found'n, Council of Better Business Bureaus (BBB), & the USPO. (were together) Operating under the name 'Coordinating Conference on Health Info.' (CCHI). ...Minutes of these meetings (were) ("obtained through the Freedom of Information Act"). ...The prime mover of the gathering was (the) head of the AMA's Department of Investigation... (who) also was overseeing...AMA's Committee on Quackery...."(p.11-12).

"...The FDA...against chiropractic.... not only intended to 'take the products off the market, but it would initiate criminal actions involving advertising agencies ...promoters, & also the people doing the research'."(p.13).

(In contrast) "...although the Federation of State Medical Boards estimates that 16,000 doctors are unfit to practice medicine, an average of only 66 licenses a year are revoked, nationwide."(p.19-20). - Mark Shaeffer, American Citizens for Honesty in Government, "The Great Conspiracy to Stamp Out Quackery", Freedom, Oct. 1978, (condensed in NHF Bull., v.25, n.5, p.11, 12, 13, 19, 20, May 1979).

"...Except for very superficial complaints ("about fees, poor communication..."), peer review ("dentists judging other dentists")...allows...the (patient's) complaint ....(to) be...stalled past the statute of limitations in a civil suit.... (Peer review) deliberations are secret; even in a civil suit, with a subpoena, the patient can't get (deliberation records)." - Faye Willard, AADV (Amer. Assoc. of Dental Victims, 3320 E. 7th St., Long Beach, CA 90804), "Dialogue With A Doubting Thomas".

"...Galen...was...forced to flee from Rome to escape the frenzy of the mob. .... Vesalius was denounced as an imposter & heretic.... William Harvey was disgraced as a physician.... William Roentgen...was called a quack & then condemned...."

"In...1535, when...Jacques Cartier found his ships...in...the St. Lawrence River, scurvy began.... & then a friendly Indian showed them (that)....Tree bark & needles from the white pine —both rich in...Vitamin C — were stirred into a drink (for)... swift recovery. Upon returning to Europe, Cartier reported this incident to the medical authorities. But they were amused by such 'witch-doctor cures of ignorant savages' & did nothing to follow it up. ...."

"...It took over 200 years & cost hundreds of thousands of lives before the medical experts began to accept.... Finally, in 1747, John Lind...discovered that oranges & lemons produced relief from scurvy.... & yet it took 48 <u>more</u> years before his recommendation was put into effect. ...'Limeys' soon became the rulers of the 'Seven Seas'. ...."

"(In) 1914...Dr. Joseph Goldberger had proven that (pellagra) was related to diet, & later showed that it could be prevented simply by eating liver or yeast. But it wasn't until the 1940's...that the 'modern' medical world fully accepted pellagra as a vitamin B deficiency." - G. Edward Griffin, (Publisher & Editor, <u>Voice of Medical Freedom</u>; Chairman, Americans for Medical Freedom), <u>World Without Cancer</u>, p.47-50.

"Marzari in Italy in the 1850's, & earlier Lumin in a Basel lab., pointed out that pellagra was a disease which resulted from some sort of dietary deficiency. .... In 1887 Takaki eliminated beri beri from the Japanese Navy by reducing the amount of milled rice...." - John Richardson, MD; Diplomate, National Board of Medical Examiners; (author, <u>Laetrile Case Histories</u>); "...Vitamins...Through the Miasma of Political Manipulation", <u>Richardson Newsletter</u>, v.<u>1</u>, n.9, p.3, 1979.

"'In the mind of the Court this fact, considering the enormous proportions to which the ("so-called") alum baking powder industry has grown in this country, & the length of time such baking powders have been in use, stands as a stone wall against the deductions of the most eminent scientists who presented their theories on the part of the prosecution.'" - <u>State of Missouri vs. Whitney Layton</u>. (p.347).

"'(In) 1828.... Dr. ...held that ...alum was poisonous.'"(p.39-40).

- Ernest E. Smith,MD,PhD; Pres., NY Acad. of Science; Fellow, NY Acad. Medicine; <u>Aluminum Compounds in Food</u>, c.1928, p.39, 40, 347.

"Susceptibility to chemical additives & contaminants of air, food, water & biological drugs & chemically derived drugs has been demonstrated to be the leading factor in the causation of chronic illness in approximately one-third of the writer's chronically ill patients. It appears to be a contributing factor which cannot be ignored for best results in the management of another third."(p.11).

"The fuel-oil-burning space heater & kitchen range are <u>major causes</u> of indoor air pollution & respiratory symptoms...."(p.39).

- Theron Randolph, MD & chief of Allergy Clinic, U. Michigan Medical School; fellowship, Harvard U. & Mass. General Hosp.; Staff Member: Northwestern U. Medical School; Swedish Covenant Hosp.; Lutheran General Hosp.; Henrotin Hosp.; <u>Human Ecology & Susceptibility to the Chemical Environment</u>, c.1962, p.11, 39. (Continued)

"(In) 1949, Randolph.... ...(did) testify in the FDA's bread hearings.... (He) requested that food ingredients, especially corn & cane & beet sugar, be listed on the labels of processed food products. .... Shortly after Randolph returned to Chicago, he was no longer allowed to mention his medical school affiliation in his articles; he was soon deprived of his position at ___ & his hospital privileges at ___-affiliated hospitals. A major food manufacturer suddenly cancelled his research grant, which had previously been approved for extension."(p.5).
- Theron Randolph, MD; & Ralph Moss, PhD, Ass't Director, Public Affairs, Memorial Sloan-Kettering Cancer Center; An Alternative Approach to Allergies, p.5.

"I went to the administrators of Loyola U. (Chicago).... They indicated that they...would support my research out of university funds (non-govt.). This did not mean that...I could indicate publically that our position was Loyola U.'s position."
- Dr. Harold Manner, The Death of Cancer, p.4.

"Dr. Alexis Carrel, ...(winner of the Nobel Prize in 1912 for his success in suturing blood vessels & the transplanting of organs)....(:) After his book was published in 1935, titled Man the Unknown, he was slowly eased out of the Rockefeller Institute of Research, & he went to France.... When he arrived, he was arrested on a false charge & put in prison.... Two months later (he) died." - Prof. Hilton Hotema, Health Research sheet.

"...The influence of the factory upon the physiological & mental state of the workers has been completely neglected."

"The modern city consists of...dark, narrow streets full of gasoline fumes, coal dust, & toxic gases, torn by the noise...."

"Enormous amounts of money are spent for publicity. As a result, large quantities of alimentary & pharmaceutical products, at the least useless, & often harmful, have become a necessity for civilized men."
- Alexis Carrel, MD, ScD, LLD; Nobel Laureate; Prof. Emeritus, Rockefeller U.; Man the Unknown, p.24-25.

"...Li Chung-yun, of tropical China...died in 1933 at the great age of 256. He buried 23 wives,,,,"

(In) "1923, Sadhu Swami, of Karimganji, India, was...over 330 years old. He remembered events that occurred over a period of more than 3 centuries."

"...Numa De Cugna of Bengal, India...died in 1566AD at the age of 370. ...Cugna grew four new sets of teeth & his hair turned from black to grey 4 times."(p.32).

Per "London, Thomas Carn died in 1795 at the age of 207."

"Dando, the Illyrian, lived over 500 years."(p.62).
- Prof. Hilton Hotema, Live Longer Now, p.32, 62.

A.Q.7 RELATED FIELDS:

"Pension fund stock already amounts to 37% of all stock held by all categories of institutional investors.... Institutional votes decide a wide range of social, economic, environmental & ethical issues which are considered at stockholder meetings." (Conflict of interest? - Ed.)

"Voting power of the large institutional investors is especially concentrated in 56...corporations, including two major broadcasting networks."

"More than half of these 600-plus key positions as a 'top-5' identified stock-voter are held by only 21 institutions.... & who controls the major voting rights in the dominant banks? Other large banks. ....Stockholdings below 5% can... constitute control. ...often augmented by two other powerful levers of control, interlocking directorates & debtholdings." - Voting Rights In Major Corporations, Subcommittee on Reports, Accounting & Management, of the Committee on Governmental Affairs, US Senate, Jan. 1978, p.1, 2, 3.

"...The (giant cereal) company had published in 1942 (that:) The rats who got nothing but water & vitamins lived for about 8 weeks.... But the (company's) own laboratory study showed that rats given vitamins, water, & all the Puffed Wheat they wanted died in 2 weeks. ...Putting the grain under 1,500 psi (pounds per square inch) of pressure...may produce...a poison.... ...The President of the company (said:) 'I know people should throw it (Puffed Cereals) on brides & grooms at weddings, but if they insist on sticking it in their mouths, can I help it? Besides, we made $9 million on the stuff last year (early 1970's).'" - Paul Stitt, Fighting the Food Giants, p.62-64.

"Nearly half of the world's rain forests have been destroyed.... (Ed. - This partially causes, intercontinentally sometimes, that:) Every year we are losing some 6 million hectares (1 hectare = 2.47 acres) of arable land, going out of agriculture to...desertification. ...29 million acres of agricultural lands were converted to non-agricultural uses (e.g. urban sprawl - Ed.) in the US in the past 10 years. ... Coastal land & breeding grounds for over two thirds of the world's fisheries are being degraded or destroyed...Over 1,000 animal & some 25,000 plant species are today threatened with extinction. - From the United Nations Environmental Programme (UNEP)."(p.9).

"...A leading shampoo manufacturer in Japan...had admitted the possibility of hair loss & scalp damage with the use of shampoo. ...Synthetic detergents are a factor contributing to birth defects. ...Prof. M.Mikami of Mie U., in 1973, (showed that) pregnant mice...applied with synthetic detergent...developed embryos with deformed spines ("in 70% ...", &) harelips & damage of internal organs."(p.5).
- CAP (Consumers' Assoc. of Penang (Malaysia)), Utusan Konsumer, Bil. 71, p.5, 9, June 1980.

"Of 82 food dyes permitted in 22 countries, only one is permitted in all."(p.86).
"...In 1965, the French Ministry of Health banned the use of all antibiotics, hormones, & other drugs in the feed of animals intended for human consumption."(p.158).
"Hungary prohibited the use of all persistent pesticides."(p.182).
- Beatrice Trum Hunter, (author of: Great Nutrition Robbery; & Mirage of Safety; & How Safe Is Food In Your Kitchen?; & Gardening Without Poisons; & Natural Foods Cookbook; & Food Additives & Your Health; & Fermented Foods ...; & The Sugar Trap ...; etc.); MS, Columbia U.; grad. work, Harvard U.; (columnist, "The Book Hunter": Herald of Health; & NFA, Natural Food & Farming); (Member: Advisory Board, PPNF; & Board of Directors, HEAL); Consumer Beware!, p.86, 158, 182.

A.Q.8 PEOPLE:

(In) Leicester....Clean streets, clean markets & dairies, efficient garbage removal, sanitary housing & a pure water supply, took the place of vaccination scars, with the notable result that...in the much vaccinated & revaccinated British Army & Navy, the death rate (from smallpox) was 3 times as high (as Leicester's)."(p.78).
"...The population of England & Wales is more than 4 times that of the Philippines, (&) the number of vaccinations per 100 persons in the (Philippines) Islands was over 26 times that in England. Yet the total of smallpox fatalities in England & Wales for...1911-1920 was only...14 for each year, as against a yearly average of 7,533 fatalities in the Philippines."(p.94).
- Anne Riley Hale, The Medical Voodoo, (c.1935), p.78, 94.

"...If the ...immunization studies done by Shope, Andervont, Bittner..., Glover, Gregory, & L'Esperance had been taken more seriously, cancer treatment would now be far advanced."(p.89).
"Someone of the (ACS) or affiliates who was high up in the hierarchy called the dean at Columbia U. & had Eleanor (Alexander Jackson)'s work terminated there."(p.104).
"On...1971, Louis F. Saylor, MD, Dir. of Public Health of...Cal., as Plaintiff tried to obtain an injunction against the (IACVF) Internat'l Assoc. of Cancer Victims & Friends, & their officers, editor, & publisher, as well as the (NHF) National Health Federation."(p.223).

(Continued)

"...My father (an MD) became very ill.... ...A prayer (was) offered...to heal the sick.... (The) chief of...surgeons, said...'We have opened your father...(&) his stomach also. There is absolutely nothing the matter with him. Yet only yesterday a large mass was present in his stomach both by exam. & by x-ray.'"(p.91).

– Virginia Livingston,MD, NYU; BS, Vassar; Assoc. Prof. Biol., Rutgers U.; Assoc. Prof., U. San Diego; Cancer: A New Breakthrough, p.89, 91, 104, 223, (for last 4 paragraphs above).

"...The coronary care unit.... ...The psychological impact of this scene. The patient is continuously aware (of) his heart.... ...(This) can in itself create tremendous panic & anxiety. ....He is denied access to support from those whom he especially needs.... The touching...between human beings? It is often the small, 'insignificant' actions which determine whether a patient lives or dies."

"...Most people...perceive their life & their experience dualistically & hence negatively." – Dolph Ornstein, MD, Pres., San Francisco Medical Research Found'n, Medicine Today, Healing Tomorrow, p.82, 153, 154.

"The effective way to oppose Laetrile('s & some other alternatives') suppression is to enlist & band together those interests which would economically benefit most by (cure) of cancer. ...includ(ing): life (&) medical insurance companies, tobacco co.s, ...all manufacturers of carcinogenic substances, beef & poultry growers, ..."(p.5).

"The individuals comprising the industrial-medical-government triumvirate against Laetrile (& some other alternatives) are...choosing between...a comfortable... status-quo & severe economic sacrifice to promote the general welfare."(p.4).

– Stewart Jones, PhD, MS; MD, Stanford U. Medical School; Nutrition Rudiments in Cancer, p.4,5.

"The National Wildlife Federation now counts 2.5 million members nationwide; the National Audubon Society, 325,000; the Sierra Club, 200,000; Greenpeace, 250,000; Natural Resources Defense Council, 45,000; Environmental Defense Fund, 52,000; National Wilderness Society, 100,000. Friends of the Earth has 25,000 members in the US & 175,000 worldwide...."

"The World Directory of Environmental Organizations lists more than 200 national & multi-state environmental groups.... California has 45 separate groups working on local water issues alone."

"A Louis Harris survey in (1981) showed....(:) Only 12%...favored making the Clean Air Act less strict..., & only 4% favored weakening the Clean Water Act(s). Only 5%...would not mind living within 5 miles of a toxic waste dump."

"...Environmentalists have made progress...in joining forces with labor."

– Anne Jackson, & Angus Wright, "Nature's Banner: Environmentalists have just begun to fight", the Progressive, (founded in 1909 by Robert M. LaFollette, Sr.), v.45,n.10,p.26, Oct. 1981.

"The coalition...to achieve the Health Era has not yet formed. ...Candidates... include...the women's health movement, ...victims of...medicine. ...neighborhood organizations.... ...unions.... (&) older Americans...."

"The Health Era demands a loosening of the power structure that presently allocates to the medical sector control of so much money, so many people, & so many tools. This power attracts & misdirects millions." – John McKnight, Prof., Northwestern U.; Assoc. Director, Center for Urban Affairs, NU; Evanston, Ill.; "Health in the Post-Medical Era", Health & Medicine, v.1, n.1, p.2, Winter 1982.

"The practice of laying birthing mothers flat on their backs was initiated to satisfy...Louis XIV ! (who) got his kicks by peering from behind a curtain while his mistresses...gave birth. ...His vision was obscured when the women were seated on birthing stools. ...The law of gravity had been repealed. ...Intra-abdominal pressure...during labor.(:)...the greatest pressure was exerted in the sitting position. ...Squatting alters the pelvic shape (&) makes it advantageous for delivery." – Robert Mendelsohn, MD, Evanston, Ill., MALe Practice: How Doctors Manipulate Women, p.152-153.

"...In miso...a byproduct of the...yeasts...remove(s) from the body...pollutants & radioactive poisons. .... Sea vegetables actually inhibit the absorption of radioactive strontium & cadmium." - Keith Block,MD, & Penney Block,MA, Evanston, Ill., "Macrobiotics...", (in E.Esko, (Ed.), East - West Foundation, The Cancer Prevention Diet, p.46-47).

"Samuel Gompers, the 'Father of the AFL'.... In 1902...co-authored a pamphlet... entitled 'Some Reasons for Chinese Exclusion: Meat vs. Rice, American Manhood Against Asiatic Coolieism - Which Shall Survive?'" - Council on Interracial Books for Children, Stereotypes, Distortions & Omissions in US History Textbooks, p.38.

"Publisher's Warning: ...In North America, some well intentioned laypeople & some medical charlatans have adapted the image, but not the substance, of acupuncture. ....In China...personnel...have been trained intensively.... While...herbal treatments...may...be...harmless...they require...knowledge.... The treatments...may well prove to be as effective, & less costly, than...methods employed by Western physicians."(p.xi).

"...On the prevention & treatment of cerebral hemorrhage (type of "stroke").... ...needle the...points...for...acupuncture."(p.391).

"Parasites...."(p.331-350). - A Barefoot Doctor's Manual, (1977 reprint of DHEW Pub. #(NIH) 75-695), p.xi, 331-350, 391.

"Though it is hard to believe, it is conservatively estimated that 25 to 50 million Americans carry trichina larvae in their muscles & internal organs. .... If the (trichinosis) worms affect the heart, respiratory system, or the nerves, severe symptoms or even death may result."

"Amebic dysentry is endemic throughout the world, affecting 17.6% of the population. In the US, it affects 13.6%. .... No one...really knows the extent of the parasites & the diseases they cause."

- Ruth Winter, Poisons In Your Food, p.139-140.

"People with type-A blood manufactured mucous & catarrh when digesting dairy...& animal products.... Type-O (blood) people...were not able to derive their protein needs from a vegetarian diet." - Dr. James D'Adamo, One Man's Food ..., p.35.

"...Keep in mind the comparative effects of different altitudes, latitudes, temperatures & races, &...note the similarity of the reactions of these (14) primitive groups when (dietary) contact is made with our modern civilization(:) ... Susceptibility to dental caries (tooth decay)....data reveal an average increase in susceptibility of 35 fold (3,500%)." - Weston A. Price,MS,DDS,FACD; Member Research Comm., ADA (American Dental Assoc.); Member, Amer. Assoc. of Physical Anthropologists; Hon. Fellow, Internat'l Coll. of Dentistry; Hon. Member, Am. Acad. Appl. Nutrition; Nutrition & Physical Degeneration, (Intro. by E.A.Hooton, Prof. Anthropology, Harvard U.), p.5.

"...Pets are found suffering from all the ailments known to the human...."(p.142).

"...Humans were the only creatures in the world that ate their food cooked. You'd never find a gorilla frying up some bananas for dinner or a lion charcoal-broiling a zebra steak. Cats don't often run to the oven with a mouse or bird they've captured, & a dog wouldn't naturally prepare its rabbit dinner in a stew."(p.144).

- Dick Gregory, comedian, & Alvenia Fulton, Dick Gregory's Natural Diet for Folks Who Eat, p.142, 144.

"...I had to depend on Braille for my reading & a guide for my walking...I am now wearing no glasses, reading, & all without strain...by taking lessons in seeing... optometrists hate the method..."(back cover).

"Every guild & trade has its own...private patriotism, which makes it resent all rebellion from within & all competition or criticism from without. ...Vested interests. The manufacture of optical glass...."(p.10). - Aldous Huxley, (author of 45 books: Brave New World), The Art of Seeing, (c.1942, 1975), p.10, & back cover.

"...The various clubs, of persons afflicted with cancer in the US, learned that medication was available for cancer but that it was kept a secret. .... (because)... Hyaluronidase Enzyme (&) Vitamin A...Carotene may be obtained readily without a prescription...."(p.1,3).

"...Pesticides mfgd. by...Oil Co. are...why such a high percentage of farmers are sick with cancer. The Medical people...blame the sun for their cancer. Is the sun any different today than it was in the past?"(p.18). - Anon., Cancer: American Holocaust, p.1,3,& 18.

A.Q.9 AUDITS & ANALYSES, OFFICIAL, &

A.Q.10 RESEARCH of RESEARCH:

"'We don't have any pesticides showing up in the food chain anymore.'" - NCI Director, & ACS Vice Pres., Dr. Frank Rauscher.

"'... Around 1972 or '73, we stopped including in our calculations all skin cancers except melanoma, the only one that's fatal, & also in situ cervical cancers, because many experts don't consider these to be cancers at all. Since together they account for a large number of cases, that could be why the incidence has gone down.'" - ACS Vice Pres. of Public Info., I. Rimer.

"'I never even heard from the ACS — in 5 years no one from there has even called me.'" - Benno Schmidt, Chairman, President's Cancer Panel (including ACS Pres., Dr. Lee Clark, for 5 years); member, NCAB (National Cancer Advisory Board, chaired by Dr. J.Rhoads, an ACS officer; & including many ACS officials); in Hearings, US House.

"When 253 of the professionals on the NCI staff were asked in a 1974 survey to indicate problems adversely affecting their job performance at the Institute (NCI), half cited 'widespread lack of confidence in the scientific acumen of the decision-making hierarchy' & a third complained of the 'shortage of qualified & technical personnel'." - Ruth Rosenbaum, "Why America Is Losing The War On Cancer", New Times, (reprinted in Journal of the Nutritional Academy, v.1, n.1, p.13, Summer 1978; for last 4 paragraphs above).

"In the year following the 1979 NIH Consensus Conference which deemed the radical mastectomy obsolete, 11,000 women received this treatment." - Maryann Napoli, (Editor, Health Facts), "Breast Cancer: A Critical Look at Early Detection", National Women's Health Network Newsletter, v.7, n.3, p.4, May 1982.

"Analysis of survival curves of women with breast cancer suggests that two or more populations exist, with about 40% suffering fatal outcome unaffected by treatment. The remaining 60% exhibit a relative mortality only modestly different from that of women of similar ages without evidence of disease. Increasing detection of an entity that is histologically defined as malignant but biologically relatively benign (exists)." - Maurice S.Fox, PhD; Biology Dept., MIT; Journal AMA, v.241, n.5, p.489, Feb. 2, 1979.

"6 of the 10 leading causes of death in the US have been linked to poor nutrition. .... Various nonfatal conditions have also.... (e.g.) dental decay."

"The AMA & the Nutrition Foundation sponsored a 1962 conference...after an AMA survey found that 'Medical education & medical practice have not kept abreast of the tremendous advances in nutrition knowledge'. .... The situation has not changed, according to an August 1978 Senate Committee Report...." (p.2).

"(A) review (of) the 1978 National Board Exam for...nutrition questions.(shows) 3 to 4 % of the questions were on clinical nutrition...." (p.7).

"...Social, ethnic, economic, & cultural factors...affect food selection."(p.9).

"...We suggest that interested groups outside of the Federal govt. initiate action...." (p.14).

- USGAO, CED-80-39, Greater Federal Efforts Are Needed to Improve Nutrition Education in US Medical Schools, Jan. 2, 1980, Enclosure I, p.2, 7, 9, 14.

(Continued on p.169.)

SECOND EDITION ADDITIONS

to

MEDICAL DARK AGES CIRCA 1984

or

CANCER ALTERNATIVE THERAPIES' CURE RATES

by Ralph R. Hovnanian,
Programmed Genetically as Homo Sapien;
De-institutionalized in Planet Earth, a Halfway House

NOTE: The headings, sequence, & numbering of sections in Additional Editions closely match those in the First Edition. Most (99%) of the 1st Edition has not been revised from the original, but added on to as follows:

COPYRIGHT:

DISCLAIMER: (Continued from p.2)

This Author/Editor/Publisher/Distributor/Charity takes no legal responsibility whatsoever for the contents herein.

"(Some) rely for (their) livelihood on continuing placid relations with organized medicine. All are entitled to pick their own quarrels on their own terms & in their own time & do not need me to fling down the gauntlet for them. That is why the only persons quoted by name in this book are those whose remarks were made in public or in print or in the line of official duty."

"...My acid was directed at ideas rather than at the ladies & gentlemen whose function it is to protect those ideas."

"Like all other writers of books about current history, I merely picked up where hundreds & hundreds of other journalists had been obliged by time or employer to leave off." – Richard Carter, The Doctor Business, p.273-274.

FUNDING & FURTHERING; DONATIONS:

To aid in donating this book to those who are most likely to use it well, the entity, "Medical Dark Ages" was formed, & has received tax-deductible charity status from the IRS, (see "Funding...", p.3). Please make any donation checks payable to: "Ralph Hovnanian, Pres., Medical Dark Ages"; & address it to same, at: 2128 Prospect Ave., Evanston, IL 60201. This charity welcomes any who want to share in this adventure, & will provide most effective & efficient use of their donations. Yet, please do not feel obligated to contribute, if that would preempt your generosity to other equally pressing concerns, with no conflicts of interest, especially some of the organizations listed in "Public Interest Health Groups...".

TABLE of CONTENTS, GENERAL, for SECOND EDITION:

PREAMBLE: (Continued from p.4.)

"An Athenian citizen does not neglect his state because he takes care of his own household; even those of us who are engaged in business have a very fair idea of politics. We do not regard a man who takes no interest in public affairs as harmless. We do not say that such a man 'minds his own business'. Rather we say he has no business here at all." - Pericles, (495-429 BC), (in Donald K. Ross, A Public Citizen's Action Manual, (Ralph Nader group), p.iv).

"Anyone can become angry - that is easy; but to be angry with the right person, & to the right degree, & at the right time, & for the right purpose, & in the right way - that is not within everybody's power & is not easy." - Aristotle, (384-322 BC), (in Walter A. Heiby, Live Your Life, p.65).

"There is nothing more difficult to carry out, nor more doubtful of success, nor more dangerous to handle, than to initiate a new order of things. For the reformer has enemies in all those who profit by the old order, & only lukewarm defenders in all those who would profit by the new order, this lukewarmness arising partly from fear of their adversaries, who have the laws in their favor; & partly from the incredulity of mankind, who do not truly believe in anything new until they have had experience of it." - Machiavelli, (1469-1527 AD), The Prince, ch. 6.

"...A democracy always collapses over loose fiscal policy.... The average age of the world's greatest civilizations has been 200 years. These nations have progressed through this sequence: from bondage to spiritual faith; (next) to great courage; ...to liberty; ...to abundance; ...to selfishness; ...to complacency; ... to apathy; ...to dependence; ...back again into bondage." - Alexander Tyler, Cycle of Democracy, 1770 AD, (in US Congressman Ron Paul, Freedom Report, v.7,n.3,p.3.

"...Substantially all ideas are second-hand, consciously & un-consciously drawn from a million outside sources.... ...It takes a thousand men to invent a telegraph, or a steam engine, or a phonograph, or a photograph, or a telephone, or any other important thing - & the last man gets the credit & we forget the others. ....I stole his dedication, without knowing it, & used it to dedicate my (prose)." - Mark Twain, (in Ira Pilgrim, The Topic of Cancer, c.1974, (TY Crowell Co., NY), p.225).

"First a new theory is attacked as absurd. Then it is admitted to be true but insignificant. Finally it is seen to be so important that its adversaries claim that they themselves discovered it." - William James, (1842-1910), (in Michael Culbert, Save Your Life, p.284).

"...The press has become the greatest power within the Western countries; more powerful than the legistlative, the executive, & the judiciary." - Alexander Solzhenitsyn, (author, Cancer Ward), (in The Stanford Magazine, Summer 1982, p.21).

"Unfortunately, many have been so busy making a living, that they have failed to take the time necessary to protect & preserve the system that makes their individual efforts, their businesses & their security possible." ....

"Still, we get the kind of government we deserve. It's absurd to expect officials in Washington to behave like statesmen, when we demand that they act like demagogues to get elected & re-elected. The main problem is thet the leaders of our communities, successful businessmen & women, haven't led. .... It doesn't mean contributing $1,000 to each candidate in a national race in hopes of having an 'open door' no matter which one wins." - US Congressman Larry McDonald, MD, Emory U., (in Robert White, Ed., The Duck Book Digest, March, 1983, p.36).

ABBREVIATIONS for TABLE / MATRIX (mainly), of 2nd Edition: (Continued from p.11-12.)

AACR: American Association for Cancer Research
AB: Arts Bachelor
ABM: Anti-Ballistic Missiles
ADA: (American Dietetic Association, is not so abbreviated herein; see ADA (Dental) of 1st Ed.)
AEC: Atomic Energy Commission
AHA: American Hospital Assoc. (Amer. Heart Assoc. not so abbreviated herein; see "ACS", p.11)
AMA: (does not stand for Amer. Manufacturers Assoc., nor Amer. Management Assoc., herein; see "AMA",p.11.)
AML: Acute Myelo-genous Leukemia
AMPAC: Amer. Medical Political Action Committee
ANHS: American Natural Hygiene Society
ASCC: Amer. Society for the Control of Cancer; (now ACS)
Adm.: Administrat(or/ion)
Anat.: Anatomy
blk.: black
CCS: Cancer Control Society
CPSC: Consumer Product Safety Commission
cu.: cubic
DMSO: Di-Methyl Sulph-Oxide
DoT: Dept. of Transportation, US
D. Phil.: Doctor of Philosophy
DSc: Doctor of Science, ScD
Dip.: Diploma
EDTA: Ethylene Di-Amine Tetra-Acetic Acid
Ed.: Education
Exec.: Executive
FASEB: Federation of American Societies for Experimental Biology
Fel.: Fellow
GH3: Gerovital H3, Procaine
Gazz.: Gazzette (Italian)
HMD: Homoeopathic Medicine Diploma, DHM
ICAN: International College of Applied Nutrition
ICRF: (Ivy Cancer Research Foundation, is not so abbreviated herein; see ICRF of 1st Ed.)
Ital.: Italian
Jap.: Japanese
kg.: kilo-gram
LSU: Louisianna State University
Ltr. Letter
MPH: Master of Public Health
MSKCC: Memorial Sloan-Kettering Cancer Center
NAPSAC: National Assoc. of Parents & Professionals for Safe Alternatives in Childbirth
NCAB: National Cancer Advisory Board
NHTSA: National Highway Traffic & Safety Administration
NIEHS: National Institute of Environmental Health Sciences
NIOSH: National Institute for Occupational Safety & Health
NYAS: New York Academy of Science
OSHA: Occupational Safety & Health Administration
PAC: Political Action Committee
Pres.: President
RN: Registered Nurse
ScD: Science Doctor, DSc
SKI: Sloan-Kettering Institute
Soc.: Society
Subcom.: Subcommi(ssion/ttee)
Suppl.: Supplement
Tech.: Technical
USAF: US Air Force
USDoD: US Dept. of Defense
V. Pres.: Vice President
yr.: year

TABLE of CONTENTS for TABLE / MATRIX, APPENDIX C, of 2nd Edition:
(Continued from p.15-17.)

C.9.6.5 Vitamin C; (Stone)
C.9.6.6 " ; (DeCosse)
C.9.6.7 " ; (McCormick)
C.9.6.8 " ; (Knight)
C.9.7.6 Vitamin A, Vegetables
C.9.7.8 " , inject
C.9.7.9 " , Carotene
C.9.7.11 "
C.9.7.13 " , Retinoids
C.9.7.14 " , acid, external
C.9.8 Super-Nutrition; (Cheraskin)
C.9.10.1 Vitamin B-6, Pyridoxine
C.9.10.2 Celiacs get Lymphoma
C.9.10.7.1 Selenium
C.9.10.7.2 " ; (Schrauzer)
C.9.10.7.3 " ; (Shamberger)
C.9.11 Potassium Magnesium Orotate; & Bromelain; (Nieper)
C.9.14 Sprouts; (Wigmore)
C.9.15 Vitamin B-2, Ribo-flavin
C.9.18.1 Anti-Oxidants; (Passwater)
C.9.18.2 " ; (Shamberger)
C.9.20 Zinc; (MIT)
C.9.22.1 Germanium; (Asai)
C.9.22.2 " &... ; (Jurasunas)
C.9.23 Rubidium & Cesium; (Brewer)
C.9.23.3 " ; (Sartori & ")
C.9.23.4 " ; (Nieper & ")
C.9.23.5 " ; (Tufts & ")
C.9.24.1 Indium; (Schroeder)
C.9.24.2 " ; (Bonadio)
C.9.25 Butyric acid
C.9.26 Vitamin B-15, Pangamic acid
C.9.27 Lipo-tropes: Choline, Folic acid, Cyanocobolamine; &, Methionine; (MIT)
C.9.28 Inositol

C.10.0 LAETRILE, VITAMIN B-17
C.10.1 " , historical
C.10.2.1-2 " ; (Contreras)
C.10.4.1 " ; (Bouziane)
C.10.4.2 " ; (Morrone)
C.10.4.3 "
C.10.4.4-6.1 Laetrile; (Harris)
C.10.6.2 " ; (Restifo)
C.10.6.3-4 " ; (H.H.Beard)
C.10.11 Benz-aldehyde
C.10.14 Chelation, EDTA
C.10.20.7.1 Apricot Kernels

C.11.0 NUTRITION, ENZYMES
C.11.2 Tropical Fruits; &, Sweat
C.11.5 Individualized; (Kelley)
C.11.7 Raw Food; (Bircher)
C.11.9 Protease Inhibitors; (NYU)

C.12.0 NUTRITION, ANTI-BIOTIC, ANTI-VIRAL
C.12.1 CULTURES
C.12.1.1.1 Lacto-bacillus; (Bogdonov)
C.12.1.2 Lactic Acid; (Keating)
C.12.1.2.1 " " ; (Argonne)
C.12.1.2.2 " " ; (Stock, SKI)
C.12.1.5.2 Brewer's Yeast; (Sugiura)
C.12.1.5.5 Glucan; (DiLuzio)
C.12.2 PLANTS
C.12.2.1 Mushroom

C.14.0 NUTRITION, HERBS
C.14.4 Herbs, Scope, Statistics
C.14.4.1 " " " (Hartwell)
C.14.4.2 " " " (Duke)
C.14.4.3 " " " (NCI)
C.14.5 Essiac; (Caisse & Brusch)
C.14.21 Herb, Chinese
C.14.22 " , Indian
C.14.23 Fruit, " , Nasally

C.16.0 ANIMAL (CELLULAR) EXTRACTS INJECTED
C.16.2 Immuno-Therapy; (Issels)
C.16.10.1 Urea; (Danopoulis)
C.16.10.2 " ; (Aiken)
C.16.11 Insulin

C.17.0 IMMUNOLOGY, Injections, FEVER
C.17.1 Immuno-Augment. Therapy (Burton)
C.17.11 Pleomorph Vaccine; (White)
C.17.16 Mixed Bacterial Toxins; (Coley)
C.17.22 De-Shielding Ca. Cell Surface; (Alivizatos)
C.17.23 Immuno-Stimulant
C.17.24 Allergens, Bacteria & By-products, Minimized; (Gardner; Mattoon)
C.17.25 Cimetidine, toxic; (Martin)

C.18.0 CHEMICALS
C.18.2.3 Kerosene; (Ganner)
C.18.4 Hydrazine Sulfate

C.23 ACID-ALKALINE (pH) BALANCE
C.23.1 Acids: Hydro-chloric, Benzoic, & Salicylic; (Guy)

C.24 SLEEP & REST

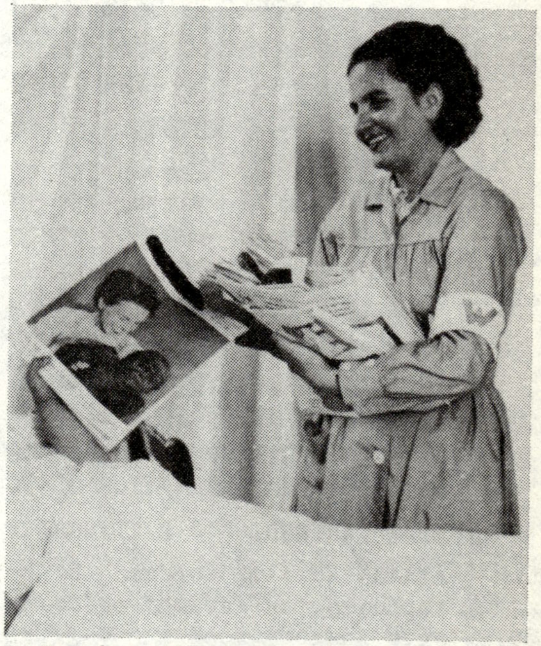

Author's mother as volunteer in Women's Auxilliary of hospital.

TABLE / MATRIX, APPENDIX C: (Continued from p.18-64.)

TREATMENT (Mode, Theory)	BENEFITED, % of total, or #	TREATED, total #	MEASURE of BENEFIT	DISEASE SEVERITY	RESEARCHER, Credentials	REFERENCE, Publication
APPENDIX C	APPENDIX C		APPENDIX C		APPENDIX C	APPENDIX C
C.1.0 CONTROLS for COMPARISON C.1.2.2 Chemo-THERAPY CAUSES recurrence of CANCER, & worsens survival.	32% 60% 37% 61%	patients, treated control treated control	after 3½-5½ years: free of ca. " : survival	cancer	Switzerland	Judith Glassman, The Cancer Survivors, p. 50-51.
C.1.2.3 Chemo- & Radio-THERAPY of Hodgkins disease, CAUSES Secondary CANCER (not metastases) of leukemia (AML).	90% 99.996%	patients: treated control	free of secondary ca., AML, at 10 years	Hodgkins disease	Stanford U. Med.	
C.1.3 NO THERAPY vs. ORTHODOX THERAPY C.1.3.2.1 Surgery, not affect ALS (Average Life Span), (since detect/treat). Surgery: / No Surgery:	same#, both	patients: treated control	ALS: unchanged	cancer, stomach	K. Bauer	Leon Chaitow, An End to Cancer?, p.117.
C.1.3.2.2 Radical Surgery, of adjacent organs, too, shortens ALS survival by 40-50%.	worse, 40-50% same	patients: treated control	ALS: 40-50% worse on radical surg.			
C.1.4 ORTHODOX THERAPY SURVIVAL RATES C.1.4.1 All Cancers.	17.9%	patients: 10,000	survival, 5 years	ca.: skin, for 2/3 of cases	" & W. Fischer	" , p.113; ref. to: The Cancer Problem, 1949.
C.2.0 SPIRITUAL, MENTAL, etc. C.2.1.1 FRIENDS & ACQUAINTANCES, a close & broad SOCIAL life, prevents early death by factor of 2.3 for men, & 2.8 for women.	averaged	populace: 7,000 in Alameda Cty., Cal.: men: women:	reduced incidence by factor of: 2.3 2.8	early death	Lisa Berkman, Yale Med.	Health & Longevity Report, v.1, n.6, p.1, Feb. 1983.
C.2.1.2 PETS, bring withdrawn people out of shells. Pets: / No Pets:	94% 56%	patients: treated control	survival, 1 yr. after hospital	heart disease	Dr. Aaron Katcher	Vegetarian Times, n.54; ref. in: NHF, Public Scrutiny, v.28, n.4, p.4, April 1982.
C.2.4 Imagery, Encounter Groups, Meditation. ALS (Average Life Span) of treateds' is 2x controls: Path from Limbic brain, to Hypothalamus, to Pituitary, to Adrenal, to Thymus (...Immunity).	averaged 10% 51%	patients, treated: 240	ALS twice controls dramatic remission as active as ever	cancer, incurable	O.C. Simonton, MD, & Stephanie Simonton, (authors, Getting Well Again), trained 5,000 therapists, & few MD's; (see 2.4).	Judith Glassman, The Cancer Survivors, p.278. (Barbara Waters, Say No to Cancer.)
C.2.8.2 Stress, releases adrenal hormones that weaken immunity (white blood cells (T-lymphocytes)).	93% 0-20%	mice, stressed: high low	free of ca., at age: 14 months 8-18 months	cancer prone genetically (breast cancer)	Dr. Vernon Riley	"Mouse Mammary Tumours:... Incidence...Stress", Science, v.189, p.465, 1975; ref. in: Jeffrey Bland, Your Health Under Siege, p.140.

CONTINUED from p.64 of 1st Edition.

TREATMENT (Mode, Theory)	BENEFITED, % of total, or #	TREATED, total #	MEASURE of BENEFIT	DISEASE SEVERITY	RESEARCHER, Credentials	REFERENCE, Publication
C.2.13.1 Mental, Spiritual, Life-style, Low Stress; De-toxify, Metabolic: fresh, organic, whole, fruits & vegetables, sprouts, & sun-dried; Laetrile; Enzymes.	75% 50% whole	patients, self	completely reverse condition	cancer: advanced terminal melanoma & metastases	Robert W. Stickle	A Rational Concept of Cancer, p.18. Cancer - One Man's Fight to Control Malignancy.
C.2.13.2 PSYCHO-SOMA; HYPO-CHONDRIA, Placebo, Stress, Autogenics (Bio-feedback, Relaxing, Release of bad emotions, Breath), Exercise: Physical inactivity is greatest stressor. Stretch, Aerobics. Holistics: Do All.	72% aver-aged	patients, treated :1	improve 50-100% 21% pain disabled, at 6 months free of ca., 6 years	invalids, 6+ years arthritis, 82% pain disabled ca., 3 mos. "to live"	C. Norman Shealy, MD, PhD; Pres., Amer. Holistic Med. Assoc.; Dir., Pain & Rehab. Ctr.	Address, IAPM (Internat'l Acad. Prev. Med.), Oct. 1978; ref. in: ICRF, ...: Self-Help for Patients, p.21.
C.2.13.3 PARA-PSYCHOLOGY, Mental Healing.	3 in #	patients, treated	amazing results	cancer	(Para-psychology Assoc. of Riverside (PAR), Cal.)	H. Denning, PAR, letter to Ed., Dec. 14, 1981.
C.2.14 BELIEF BY PHYSICIAN in Therapy, & by PATIENT in Physician. Therapy, when first introduced: Same Therapy, after a newer therapy supercedes it:	 70-90% 30-40%	patients, treated	effectivity	angina pectoris (chest pain)	Dr. Herbert Benson, Harvard Med.; author, The Relaxation Response.	"Angina Pectoris & the Placebo Effect", NEJM, v.300, p.1424, 1979; ref. in: Judith Glassman, The Cancer Survivors, p.299.
C.2.15 GOALS: Survival thru 3 month period: Before Birthday: After Birthday: (also ASTRO-LOGY, see TIME 20.)	92% 50%	newspaper obituary: 747 tot.	survival	total mix	Dr. Phillip Kunz, Prof. Sociol., Brigham Young U.	" , p.345; ref. to: "Relat. ...Suicide & Month of Birth", Psychological Rep., v.42, p.794, 1978.
C.3.0 EXERCISE C.3.1 Exercise, enhances psyche, circulation, metabolism. Bio-feedback of natural sensations.	aver-aged	mice	ca. incidence prevented by 50%	carcino-genic chemicals	Calacino & Balke	Herbert Devries, Physiol. of Exercise, p.277.
C.3.6 Exercise & limited Caloric Intake.	84% 12%	mice, ca. prone: treated control	free of ca.	genetic predis-position to ca.		O. Carl Simonton, Getting Well Again, p.209; ref. in: Cameron Stauth, The New Approach to Ca., p.245-7.
C.4.0 HEAT C.4.9 Heat, (108°F, 1hr./day), by Diathermy Current, onto body surfaces & cavities accessible.	some all	patients, treated " " early	cachexia & tumor gone alive	tumors	Albert Geyser, MD	"Non-Surgical Treatment of Ca.", NY Med. J., v.107, p.203, 1918; ref. in:
C.4.10 Heat (with needles), & Radiation.	92% 50% 12 in #	patients, treated: 47	tumor: shrank 50% all gone free of ca., 2 years	cancer cancer, terminal	Dr. Michael Manning, U. Arizona	Judith Glassman, The Ca. Survivors, p.218-9; ref. to: "Clinical Hyperthermia...", Cancer, v.49, p.205, 1982. (**Cancer Research, v.39, n.6, part 2, p.2231-2340, June 1979.**)

TREATMENT (Mode, Theory)	BENEFITED, % of total, or #	TREATED, total #	MEASURE of BENEFIT	DISEASE SEVERITY	RESEARCHER, Credentials	REFERENCE, Publication
C.4.11 Heat, whole body perfusion Hyperthermia, (body temp.: 41.5°C for 4 hours; 43°C for 15 minute spikes).	14%	patients, treated: 200	complete regression	ca., 92% of cases no better with Orthodox Therapy	Leon Parks, MD, Dept. Surg., U. Mississippi Med.	Judith Glassman, The Cancer Survivors, p.20. (Ned Hornback, MD, Chair., Dept. Rad., Indiana U. Med., Hyperthermia & Ca.: Clinical Trial..., (CRC Press).)
	30% average	139 control	survival (ALS) months: 11 / 1-2			
C.6.0 AIR C.6.1 HIGH Altitude; (less air & water pollution; more: sun rays, negative ions, ratio of oxygen to air). Few Waterveins. High Altitude, Few Waterveins:	99.94%	pop., German towns: 2,000 in Gratenau	free of ca., annually; (ca. incidence prevented by 96%, for high alt.)	cancer incidence per year, averaged	Freiherr von Pohl (See: 5.4; 5.5.1; A.5.4.1; A.5.5.1.1; A.6.1.1; A.6.3.3; A.6.4.1; B.5.1; B.6.1)	Earthradiations: the Cause of Many Diseases & Cancer; ref. in: Ludwig Siedersberger, J. Natural Health & Para-psychology Sept. 1982, p.27.
Many Waterveins, Clay Soil	98.50%	3,000 in Vilsbilburg				
C.6.5.1 Hydrogen Peroxide, (1% in drinking water). Toxic, (lose body weight). (Note: Rosenow found neurotropic strep. bug caused mental ills.) Exp. #F-6:	67% / 7%	mice: Swiss: treated: 21 / control: 15	survival, after 15 days	Ehrlich tumor, 5-6 million cells, injected subcutaneous	(Father Richard Willhelm, Chief Chaplain, VA Hosp., Dayton.) (Dr. Ed Carl Rosenow; Mayo Clinic; Longview Hosp., Cinci.; author, 450 articles).	"Cumulative...Results of ...Experiments, Mar. 25, ...1982", at Metabolic Res. Found'n, (Dr. Harold Manner, Dir.), Mtg., Sept. 25, 1982, Chicago.
Exp. #B-2, G-7, & RH-8:	70-80% / 20%	Boontucky: treated: 45 / control: 30				
C.6.5.2 Hydrogen Peroxide/Ozone. Anti-septic: destroys most viruses, bacteria, & parasites. Ozone gas over open lesions prevents amputations. (i.v.)	100% / some	patients, treated: dozens	recovered ", 5-10 yrs.	cancer, advanced	Joachim Varro, MD. (Internat'l Oxidation Inst.; " Ozone Assoc.)	Norman Fritz, "Progress Report", Gerson Inst., Aug. 1983. (Robert Bradford & Michael Culbert, International Protocols in Ca. Mgmt., IIMP, p.17-24)
	100%	3	tumor shrink (1 by 95%)	melanoma	Charlotte Gerson (see 9.2) Norman Fritz; many MD's.	
	85%	patients	success	herpes	Heinz Konrad, MD.	
C.6.5.3 Hydrogen Peroxide, oxygenates, selectively destroys cancer cells.	averaged	treated	success	skin cancer	Dr. F.B. Exner.	"Immuno-...", Med. Trib., Nov. 18, 1972; ref. in: N. Pritikin, & Pat McGrady, Jr., The Pritikin Program..., p.385.
C.7.0 WATER C.7.1 DRINKING C.7.1.3 Chlorination causes high serum cholesterol & atherosclerosis. No chlorine (in drink water) lowers a high serum cholesterol (caused from low Calcium) by 33%.	prevents 33%	pigeons, 12 tot.: drink water chlorine: low: 6 / high: 6	cholesterol (mg/100cc): 135 / 200	serum cholesterol, atherosclerosis	Richard Bull, Head, Toxicology & Microbiol. Div., USEPA. (Lecture, Amer. Soc. Pharmacalogy & Experim. Therapeutics.)	J. Kaloff, "Calcium, Chlorine, & Heart Disease Linked", Science News, (Glenn T. Seaborg, Pres.), v.124, n.7, p.103, Aug. 13, 1983
C.8.0 FASTING C.8.1 Fasting		patients	much statistics			Hayward Carrington, Therapeutic Fasting.
C.8.2 NATURAL HEALING, NATUROPATHY. (Less side-effects.) (See 6.7).	40%	patients, treated: 100	no return of ca. in 5 years	cancer	Rees Evans, Cardigan, South Wales.	Picture Post, Sept. 1950, ref. in: Health Research, Is Cancer Curable?, p.14.

TREATMENT (Mode, Theory)	BENEFITED, % of total, or #	TREATED, total #	MEASURE of BENEFIT	DISEASE SEVERITY	RESEARCHER, Credentials	REFERENCE, Publication
C.8.3 Naturo-pathy (therapies in nature, humans adapt to by genetics, over 1,000's of generations); & hot springs, colonic, Aztec herbs, chelation, HBO, GH-3, vit. C, DMSO, Laetrile.	5 in #	patients, treated	recovery	cancer, metastases, terminal	Edward Carl, ND, HMD; Pres., Natural Health Assoc., Mexico; International College of Naturopathic Physicians.	Patients' testimonials. (Alan Immerman, "The Scientific Basis of the Hygienic Diet", ANHS, Health Science, v.5, n.4, p.2, July 1982.)
C.9.0 NUTRITION, GENERAL C.9.1.1 Diet change: Hormone & Diet change: (Trace dose only, of hormone.)	80% almost all	patients, treated: 20,000	excellent recovery	degenerative disease	Dr. M.E. Page, DDS, & Page Found'n, 200 Drs. (MD, DO, DDS...). Amer. Soc. Anthropo-metric Med. ...	Howard Beard, PhD, A New Approach to the Conquest of Cancer ..., p.7 & 113.
C.9.2.1 Gerson Therapy (see 9.2) cured Albert Schweitzer's family of many "incurable' diseases; his daughter had 1,000 skin ulcers of an unknown cause & disease.		Albert Schweitzer family: Dr.	off of insulin, back to work, to age 90	diabetes, cannot work, at age 75	Dr. Max Gerson; (see 9.2) invited to show cured ca. patients in US Senate; bill lost by 4 votes. (13 authors acclaim Gerson Therapy to control skin TB.)	J. Gerson Inst.: Healing, v.2, n.1, p.10 & 20, 1982.
		wife	lived 25 more years	lung TB, hopeless		
		daughter	healed	skin ulcers		
C.9.2.2 Gerson Therapy is effective against many chronic degenerative diseases.	averaged	patients, treated: 124/127	marked improvement	skin TB (tuberculosis)	Jacobson & Brill, Russia. Gowalowski, Czech.	" , p.33; ref. to: Dr. Erich Urbach, Skin Dis., Nutr., & Metab., 1946.
C.9.3.6 Coffee, orally, causes ca. of colon (& bladder & pancreas). Thiamine, which aids bowel movement, is depleted by coffee. Pesticides, banned for use in US, exported to 3rd world, & imported back in coffee.	deaths /100,000:	populace: Cal., 7th Day Advent.:	incidence prevented 29%	cancer of large bowel	Roland Phillips, & David Snowdon, Schools of Health & Med., Loma Linda U.	"Assoc. of Meat & Coffee Use with Ca. of Large Bowel...", ACS, Work. Conf. Nutrition in Ca. Caus. & Prev., AACR, Ca. Res. v.43, n.5 Suppl., p.2403s, Chart #4, May 1983.
	22 31	no coffee drink coffee	mortality per 100,000 people			
C.9.3.8 Bowel movements, frequent, prevented 80% of abnormal cells in breast fluid (linked to breast ca.) of women with (high risk of, or frank) breast ca., (see 2.2.1).	averaged	patients, women: 1,481	incidence of abnormal cells in breast fluid: 5% 23%	breast ca. /?; & bowel movements/day: 2.00 0.21	Dr. Eileen King, UCSF Med.	"Constipation...Linked to Ca.", Eden Ranch, Organic Consumer Report, v.62, n.26, June 29, 1982.
C.9.4.2 Diet Taylored to Urine-Saliva Test.	100%	patients, treated: 25	recovered	leukemia	Carey Reams; (see 9.4.2).	A. J. Brown, Ca. Victory Bull., v.3, n.1, Jan. 1977.
C.9.4.3 Tests on cultured cells from ca. patient, predicts to 97% accuracy, a (drug) therapy's lack of effect on that patient. Saves time; risk/benefit trade.	97%	patients, tested: 200	accuracy of prediction of anti-ca. drug's effectivity	in vitro, ca. cells from ca. patient	Dr. Sydney Salmon, U. Ariz. Health Sci. Ctr.	"Customized Drug Treatment", Reader's Digest, July 1980, p.24; ref. in: J. Heinerman, Treatment of Ca. with Herbs, p.129-130.
						(Barbara Waters, Say No to Cancer.)

TREATMENT (Mode, Theory)	BENEFITED, % of total, or #	TREATED, total #	MEASURE of BENEFIT	DISEASE SEVERITY	RESEARCHER, Credentials	REFERENCE, Publication
C.9.5.4 Vegetarian, low-protein diet.	aver-aged	patients, children, treated	do better than controls	leukemia, acute	Stanislaw Garwicz, U. Hosp., Lund, Sweden; &, another MD, & hosp.	Lancet, 1976, v.2, p.1413; &, Brit. Med. J., 1966, i, p.979; ref. in: Wayne Martin, We Can Do Without Heart Attacks, p.197.
C.9.5.9 Fruits & Vegetables, fresh, organic, whole:	60% 1200 in #	patients: treated	cure	cancer, many beyond help	L. Duncan Bulkley, MD, Founder, & Sr., Phys., NY Skin Ca. Hosp.; Founder, Am. Assoc. Study/Cure Ca; Member, AACR (ACS's origin)	Health Research, Is Cancer Curable?, p.12, 32. (Bulkley, Ca. & Its Non-Surgical Treatment.)
Surgery:	8%	control	survival			
C.9.5.10 Pritikin Diet, high in: fresh fruits & veg., grains, legumes; low in: fat, animal products, salt. Reverses artery closure. Aids athletic stamina.	32 in #	patients, treated	proven reversal	artery closure	Nathan Pritikin, Dir., Pritikin Longevity Ctr., Santa Monica, Cal.; & many MD's	medical literatute; ref. in: Pritikin Ctr., Lifeline. N. Pritikin, Guest Editor, Preventive Med., v.11, p. 733, 1982.
		athletes	1st, 2nd, 4th place wins	aerobics: triathalon		
C.9.5.10.1 Pritikin Diet & Exercise (see3.). (No: tobacco, alcohol, or caffeine.)	aver-aged	patients: treated: 29 64	tri-glycerides (mg/dl): post: 147 126±7 follow up at 5 yrs.: 140	pre: 174 179±16	R. James Barnard, PhD, Physiol., UCLA.	Barnard, ..., "Effect of... Nutrition & Exercise... on Coronary...", Med. Sci. Sports Exer., v.14, p.179; ref. in: Lan Barnes, (AB Princeton), Anabolism, v. 2, n.2, p.7, Feb. 1983.
C.9.5.11 Vegan diet (no animal food), some yoghurt; Stretch, Relax; Breath; Meditate, Visualize; Psycho-social Group Support; Rural Environs (clean air & water; & sun). Treateds can work more, with less chest pain, than controls.	aver-aged	patients, treated: 23 (control: 23)	exercise duration: +44% total work: +55% plasma cholesterol: -20% angina (pain): -91%	ischemic heart disease	Dean Ornish, MD; &, 7 MD's; & 2 PhD's; & 1 MPH; & 2 RN's; & 1 DPhil.; at: Baylor Med.; U. Texas Public Health; U. Conn. Med.; etc.; now: Harvard Med.; & Mass. Gen'l Hosp.	"Effects of Stress Management Training & Dietary Changes in Treating Ischemic Heart Disease", JAMA, v.249, n.1, p.54, Jan. 7, 1983.
C.9.6.5 Vitamin C (Oxygen-ates, see A.6.8).	1 in #	patient, male	complete remission	leukemia	Irwin Stone, PhD, 26 US Patents; (see A.9.6.5)	Medical Times, 1955; ref. in: Ruth Yale Long, PhD, No More Cancer, p.12.
C.9.6.6 Vitamin C; & no Surgery:	aver-aged	patients, treated	reduction in # of polyps after 2 yrs.: 67%	cancer precursor lesion: familial poly-posis	Jerome DeCosse, MD, Dept. Surg., MSKCC (Sloan Kettering); Med. College of Wisc.	"Effect of Ascorbic Acid on Rectal Polyps...", Surg., v.78, p.608, 1975; ref. in: W. R. Bruce, ..., "... Dietary Intervention...Colon Ca.", ACS, Proc. National Conf. on Ca. Prev. & Detect.-1980, Cancer, Supp., v.47, n.5, p.1121, Mar.1, 1981; ref. to: "Risk...", Am. Surg., v.182, p.511, 1975.
No vitamin C; only Surgery:		control: 154	78%			

TREATMENT (Mode, Theory)	BENEFITED, % of total, or #	TREATED, total #	MEASURE of BENEFIT	DISEASE SEVERITY	RESEARCHER, Credentials	REFERENCE, Publication
C.9.6.7 Vitamin C, (100mg/kg of body weight)		patients, treated: children	inhibited, some regressed	leukemia	W. J. McCormick, MD. (Fred Klenner, MD, Duke MS; FCCP; AAFP; Honor, Int'l Acad. Appl. Nutr.; Fellow AAAS; Royal Soc. Health; ICAN; over 28 articles)	D.B.Cater, J. Path. Bact., v. 63, p.599, 1951; ref. in: Klenner, The Key to Good Health: Vitamin C, p.64-7; (ref. to: A.L.Waldo, Cancer, v.8, p.187, Jan. 1955).
C.9.6.8.1 Vitamin C	usually	14	cured in 1 week	polio	Granville Knight, MD; Columbia Med.; Pres., Price-Pottenger Nutr. Found'n; Hon. Fel., ICAN; Dir.& Speaker, Assoc. Amer. Phys. & Surg.; Pres., Pure Water Assoc. Amer.; Chief Ed., J. Applied Nutr.; Dir., Inst. Nutr. Res.; Dipl., Am. Brd. Clin. Immun. & Allergy; Dir., Int'l Acad. Metabology; Fellow: NYAS, &, Soc. Clin. Ecology, &, Am. Col. Allergists, &, Int'l Assoc. Allergists.	"
C.9.6.8.2 Vitamin C		8		4 paralyzed	Dr. Edward Greer, Ill.	"
C.9.7.6 Vitamin A; daily intake of green & yellow vegetables.	50%	populace of: Japan	ca. incidence prevented: 50%	lung cancer	Dr. T. Hirayama, Japan	Nutrition & Cancer, v.1, n.3, p.67, 1979;
Blood levels of retinoids not low.	83%		83%		J. D. Kark	J. Chronic Diseases; " & ", both ref. in: Dick Richards, The Topic of Cancer, c.1982, p.89.
C.9.7.8 Vitamin A (300,000iu/day, intra-muscular), & Vit. C (1g/day, iv), 21 days; &, oral, 6 months. No side effects.	averaged	patients, treated: 218	tumor growth stop or regress	cancer	Germany	H.Reinhold, "Vitamins A & C in the Treatment of Ca.", Nutrition Abstract Reviews, v.31, p.601, 1961;
C.9.7.9 Vitamin A, Carotene, oral, (1,000iu/day).	averaged	mice, treated: small #	positive results	tumor tissue implanted	Clifford Kuh, doctoral student, Yale Med.	"A Study of Vitamin A in ...Ca.", Yale J. Biol. & Med., v.5, p.123, 1932; ref. in:
C.9.7.11 Vitamin A	averaged	patients, treated: 346	tumor slowed very much	tumor cells inoculated	Germany, 1936	Judith Glassman, The Cancer Survivors, p.83.
C.9.7.13 Retinoids (Synthetic Analogues of Vitamin A), in soaked sponge on cervix.	33%	patients, women, treated: 18	remission, after 4 days	pre-cancer of cervix	Dr. Frank Meyskens, Jr., U. Arizona	Wall St. J., Nov. 15, 1982; ref. in: Maureen Salaman, MSc., Nutrition: the Cancer Answer, p.xv.
C.9.7.14 Vitamin A acid applied topically (to skin).	1 in #	patients, treated: 2	complete regression	melanoma		Lancet, v.2, n.8188, p.224, 1980; ref. in: Total Health; ref. in: NHF, Health Freedom News, v.3, n.1, p.24, Jan. 1984.
	1 in #		partial response			
C.9.8.1 Vitamin C, & Zinc, & Magnesium. Prevented anemia from Vit.C loss from adrenal hypertrophy from cachexia. Killed tumor.	90% 75% 91% 82%	patients, treat., tot: 200 stomach: 23 lung: 28	pain relief, in days: 10 2 days	ca., most biopsied, advanced; (autopsied)	B.A.Meyer, MB, ChB; G.G.Exner, FDS, RCS, DMD, LRCP, MRCS; Great Britain.	"A Treatment for Inoperable Ca. & an Adjunct to All Treat. ...", Medical Press, Dec. 30, 1953AD, p.651.

TREATMENT (Mode, Theory)	BENEFITED, % of total, or #	TREATED, total #	MEASURE of BENEFIT	DISEASE SEVERITY	RESEARCHER, Credentials	REFERENCE, Publication
C.9.8.2 Super-Nutrition, (see 9.7.3 & 6.3.2), kills cancer cells. (Only 1 week of:)		patients:	killed ca. cells per patient:	cancer	Emanuel Cheraskin, MD, DMD; Prof. Emeritus & of Med., & Chair., Div. Oral Surg. & Med., U. Alabama; author, 16 books, 800 articles.	AP (Associated Press), on: Mtg., Amer. Col. Surg., Oct. 14, 1975; ref. in: Richard Passwater, Cancer & Its Nutritional Therapies, p.60.
Super-Nutrition & Radiation:	100%	treated	90%			
Only Radiation:	56%	control	70%			
C.9.10.1 Vitamin B-6, Pyridoxine.	averaged	patients, treated	help	cancer	Dr. Balfour Mount, McGill U., Royal Victoria Hosp.	George Berkley, PhD, Cancer: How to ..., p.53.
C.9.10.2 Celiac Disease (allergy to gluten in grains) increases susceptibility to malignant lymphoma by 100-fold. Villi in intestines cannot absorb nutrients, or make blood; (see 17.3).	averaged	patients	causes 10,000% more incidence of malignant lymphoma	celiac disease		Wayne Martin, letter to Ed., June 17, 1983. (Hilda C. Hills, Good Food, Gluten Free. K. Morishita, MD, The Hidden Truth of Cancer.)
C.9.10.7.1 Selenium.		sheep:	free of ca.; incidence prevented	adenocarcinoma	Dr. Wedderburn, veterinarian.	Ruth Yale Long, PhD, No More Cancer, p.13.
Selenium added to drink water:	100%	treated				
No Selenium in soil:	98%	control				
C.9.10.7.2 Selenium, added to drinking water.		mice, female:	free of ca.; incidence prevented	breast cancer, spontaneous	Dr. Gerhard Schrauzer, Prof., U. Cal., San Diego; Pres., Internat'l Assoc. Bio-inorganic Sci.	Annals Clin. Lab. Sci., v.4, n.6, p.441, 1974; ref. in: Rich. Passwater, Ca. & Its Nutritional Therapies, p.140.
	90%	treated				
	18%	control				
C.9.10.7.3 Selenium, (painted on skin, near site of carcinogen applied topically too).		mice:		ca. from chemicals:	Dr. Raymond Shamberger, Cleveland Clinic; (see C.9.18.2).	Biochem. J., v.111, p.375, 1969; JNCI, v.44, p.931, 1970; Experientia, v.22, p.116, 1966; Nature, v.213, p.617, 1967; all ref. in: Dr. Richard Passwater, Cancer & Its Nutritional Therapies, p.144-5.
	83%	treated		": DMBA		
	57%	control				
" & different timing of applications.	55%	treated				
	11%	control				
	32%	treated		": MCA		
	13%	control				
Selenium, (fortified in diet).	60%	treated: 35	after 20 weeks	": DMBA & croton oil		
	28%	control: 36				
	55%	treated: 36		": benzopyrene		
	14%	control: 36				
C.9.11 Potassium Magnesium Orotate; & Bromelain (enzyme, see 11.2).		patients, treated: over 140	survival, years:	coronary heart disease	Hans Nieper, (see 2.3).	Ampex Bio-Res. Inst., "Heart Disease Treated with Orotates & Bromelain".
	98+%		2			
	98+%		4			
Nitrates & Anti-coagulants:	79%	control:	2		Cleveland Clinic	
	64%		4			
With / without Anti-coagulants:	81%	1,550	2		Erkelens, Rotterdam, Holland	
	68%		4			

TREATMENT (Mode, Theory)	BENEFITED, % of total, or #	TREATED, total #	MEASURE of BENEFIT	DISEASE SEVERITY	RESEARCHER, Credentials	REFERENCE, Publication
C.9.14 Sprouts (wheat), Grasses, Weeds; fresh, organic, whole. (See B.9.19). (Seeds' proteins converted to vitamins, when sprouting; e.g. Vitamin B-2 in oats increases 20x. Chlorophyll absorbs solar energy.)	100%	patients, treated: 48	cured or improved greatly	cardio-vascular disease, incurable, in hospital 1 month already	Ann Wigmore, DD, ND, PsD, PhD, MsD, DBM, DHM; Recognition Award, Nobel Prize Found'n, Finland; Dip., Anglo-Amer. Inst. Drugless Therapy. Dr. Datey, Bombay, India	Hippocrates Health Inst. letter. (Why Suffer? ... Wheatgrass, God's Manna!); (Garden Indoors); (Viktoras Kulvinskas: Nutritional Eval'n of Sprouts & Grasses; &, Survival Into the 21st Century).
C.9.15.1 RIBOFLAVIN & CASEIN.		rats	free of liver ca.; incidence prevented	low protein diet & chemical (DMAAB) carcinogen	SKI (Sloan Kettering Inst.)	Howard H. Beard, A New Approach to the Conquest of Cancer ..., p.118.
Riboflavin & Casein:	97%					
Riboflavin only:	14%					
Synergism, (see 10.19.2) — Only Casein:	14%					
Neither:	14%					
C.9.15.2 Ribo-flavin, is extremely deficient, per urine test, in 80% of 1,000 cancer patients. (See A.6.8). (Vitamin Antagonists (e.g. Anti-Folates) used as Orthodox ca. therapy.)	80%	patients, adults: 1,000	virtually no urinary riboflavin	cancer	(Otto Warburg, Nobel Laureate twice in Med.)	Mark Renneker, UCSF, & Steven Leib, MD, UCLA, Understanding Cancer, p.394. ("...Riboflavin: Warburg ...", Anabolism, v.2, n.6, p.4, June 1983.)
C.9.18.1 Anti-Oxidants: Vitamins A, C, & E; Selenium. Synergism; aid each other.	85-95%	mice: treated control	free of ca.; incidence prevented	chemical carcinogen	Dr. Richard Passwater, PhD.	Amer. Lab., June 1973; ref. in: R. Passwater, Cancer & Its Nutritional Therapies, p.129.
C.9.18.2 Anti-Oxidants: Vit. E:	63%			" : DMBA	Dr. Raymond Shamberger, Cleveland Clinic (see 9.10.7.3)	", p.130; ref. to: JNCI, v.48, n.5, p.1491, 1972.
Vit. C:	32%					
C.9.20 ZINC. Activates Vit. A, for thymus to create T-lymphocytes, to fight cancer.		rats:		"	Drs. Paul Newberne (see C.9.23), &, Y.Y. Fong, Profs., MIT.	", p.187; ref. to: Science, News, v.113, n.6, p.88, Feb. 11, 1978.
	71%	treated				
	21%	control				
C.9.22.1 GERMANIUM. In Ginseng, Garlic, Mushroom. Fights heavy metal poisoning. Attracts oxygen to ca. cells. Useless in inorganic matrix, a mineral is useful in an organic matrix made by bacteria in water. Acts as in semi-conductor, bio-transmitting electric signals between brain & nerves.	100% 0%	mice: treated control	survival	injected with ca. cells	Dr. Kazuhiko Asai, discoveror of Asai diode in electronics; Coal Res. Inst., Japan.	Kurt Donsbach, PhD, ND, DC, DSc; &, Morton Walker, DPM, Metabolic Ca. Therapies, p.48.
	some	patients	marked improvement	cancer mix	Dr. Serge Jurasunas, PhD, Biol., London College Appl. Sci.; ND; DSc; Gold Medal Dag Hammarskjold... Med. Res.; Knight, Malta; Knight, Royal Order Justice; Commander, St. Gereon; Member: AAAS, &, NYAS; & 2 MD's; Portugal.	(Naboru Muramoto, Healing Ourselves, p.120. Eden Ranch, Organic Consumer Report, v.59, n.25, June 19, 1979, &, v.63, n.23, June 14, 1983.)
C.9.22.2 Germanium, & herbal/bio-catalyst/vitamin/mineral, & enzyme, & glutathione, & yeast, & plant hormone, & Gerson Diet.	85%	patients, treated: 5,000	very good results	cancer:		Mike Culbert, (Ed.), Comm. Freedom of Choice..., The Choice, v.9, n.2, p.14, Fall 1983.
	80%	male: 84	response	prostate		

TREATMENT (Mode, Theory)	BENEFITED, % of total, or #	TREATED, total #	MEASURE of BENEFIT	DISEASE SEVERITY	RESEARCHER, Credentials	REFERENCE, Publication
C.9.23.1 RUBIDIUM Carbonate, (.06mg./g.body weight/day). Treateds had 1/10th the tumor mass of controls'.	averaged	mice, C57blk/6J strain, treated:8 control:8	tumor weight (g.): .275 / 2.90	mammary adeno-carcinoma transplant	A.Keith Brewer, PhD, U. Wisc.; National Res. Fel., Cal.Tech.; Chief, Mass. Spec.& Isotope Sect., NBS (National Bureau of Standards); Chief, Sci. Sect., Naval Operations; Distinguished Civilian Award, US Navy; Member, Sigma Xi; Wisc. St. Legistl. Award; (see B.9.16); & 3 Drs. Biol., Amer.U.	A.K.Brewer: "The Effects of Rubidium on Mammary Tumor Growth in...Mice", Cyto-bios, v.24, p.99, 1979. " (& Richard Passwater, Amer.Lab.: (Nov. 1973); April, June, &Nov., 1974; Jan. & Oct., 1975.) " (et.al.: Ca.Res., v.1, p.775, 1941; &, Nature, v.149, p.357, 1942; &, v.213, p.718, 1967.)
C.9.23.2 High Rubidium & CESIUM food (from volcanic soil), & living, of Hopi Indians.	some	patients, treated	complete regression	cancer		" "...Mechanism...Carcinogenesis: Comments on Therapy", JIAPM (J. Internat'l Acad. of Prev. Med.), v.5, n.2, p.29 & 49.
C.9.23.3 Cesium Chloride (3-6g./day, oral); (side effects: diarrhea, nausea); & Potassium Chloride (2mg./day), & Zinc, & Selenium. (See C.9.23.7)	95%	patients, treated: 30 total	tumor gone	ca.: advanced to mostly terminal:	" & Hellfried Sartori, MD, MPH, MS, U.Graz Med., Austria; Pres. Life Sciences Universal (3 teaching hosp., 1200 Med.Ctrs. in world); in Who is Who in Bio-Behav. Sci.; US Navy Surg.	" & M.Tufts, High pH Therapy for Cancer, (draft copy): Ch. IV, "Clinical Tests on Humans". (H. Sartori, "Patient ... Eu-metabolic Ca. Therapy".)
	100%		ca. pains & effects gone in 36 hours			
	100%	3	complete regression	pancreas		
		2		liver		
		3		bronchogenic ca.		
	8 in #		back to work	" & incapacitated		
C.9.23.4 Cesium Chloride, Zinc Orotate, Vitamins A & C.		patients: many	pain gone in 36 hours	ca., 50% terminal	" & Hans Nieper (see: 2.3; 9.11; 10.10).	" ", "Tests on Mice & Humans", p.9.
C.9.23.5 Cesium Chloride, (Intraperitoneal (abdominal) inject.)	97%	mice, treated	curative	cancer	" & Marilyn Tufts, Prof. Biol., U. Wisc.	" " ", p.8;
C.9.23.6 Cesium & LITHIUM. (Do psych. patients have low ca. incidence due to Lithium or Insulin Therapy?-Ed.; see C.16.11.)	averaged	mice	drastically shrink tumor mass	tumor	" & Dr. F. Messiha, Med. School, Lubbock, Texas.	ref. to: Messiha, "Effects of Lithium & Cesium Salts...", Neuro-behavioral Tech., I, 27, 1979.
C.9.23.7 (C.9.23.3 continued). Cesium Chloride (6-9g./day, 3x/day (over 20g./day depletes body's Potassium, toxic); Vits. A, C, &K; Zinc; Potassium; Magnesium; Selenium; Laetrile; whole grain& veget. diet; EDTA; & DMSO.		patients, treated:	survival, 1-3 years	cancer, metastases, terminal (except 3)	H.E.Sartori, med. license, 7 states; Cert., Am.Brd. Family Practice; FAA Aviation Med. Exam.; Mem.: Am. Soc. Clin. Pharm. &Therap.; AMA; So.Med.Assoc.; National Acad.Res.Biochem.	"Cesium Therapy in Cancer Patients", Pharmacology, Biochem.& Behav., v.21, Suppl. 1, p.11, (&p.7), 1984. (Food for Mankind (in press)). (Cancer 1984).
	50%	tot.: 50				
	50%	pancreas: 4				
	33%	liver: 3				
	60%	lung: 5				
	100%	5	no tumors	autopsied		

TREATMENT (Mode, Theory)	BENEFITED, % of total, or #	TREATED, total #	MEASURE of BENEFIT	DISEASE SEVERITY	RESEARCHER, Credentials	REFERENCE, Publication
C.9.23 (Note: RUBIDIUM & CESIUM pass thru ca. cell membrane even faster than Potassium, raising pH of ca. cell, & neutralizing toxic acid enzymes. Carcinogens, on ca. cell surface, dis-orient & stop Phosphorus-Oxygen double bond radical from energizing the transport of lighter cations, Calcium & Magnesium, into ca. cell. So, pH control is lost inside ca. cell. Calcium carries Oxygen into cells, & metabolic byproducts out, but it cannot enter ca. cell. Calcium level in ca. cell is 1% of normal; (Hydrogen vibration is changed, as seen by NMR (Nucleo-Magnetic Resonance)). Heavier cations, Potassium, Rubidium, & Cesium can enter ca. cell. Potassium carries water & Glucose into ca. cells (having no Calcium & hence no Oxygen); so for energy, Glucose ferments, forming Lactic acid(-osis), rather than Oxydizing. Rubidium (cont.) & Cesium, preferentially enter ca. cells but not normal adult cells, & do not carry Glucose, so they raise pH but not Lactic acid. (Low pH therapy does not neutralize toxic acids; see 6.4.)						
C.9.24.1 INDIUM, (5ppm in drink water); optimal dose may be higher, due to poor absorption by animals, of Indium in this form. For humans, Sulfate form, orally, is better metabolized.	88.9% 86.2% 85.4%	mice: treated:87 control:100 :80	free of ca. (19-23% of incidence prevented, of cancer)	limited environmental metal exposure	Dr. Henry Schroeder, Dept. Physiol., Dartmouth Med.; 100's of articles, 7 books; (see 9.10.5). M. Mitchener, Brattleboro Mem. Hosp., Vt.	"...Indium in Mice: Effects on...Life Span", J. Nutrition, v.101, n.10, p.1431, Oct. 1971. National Heart Inst. grant.
C.9.24.2 Indium. Acts on pituitary, & creates insulin; normalizes thyroid & blood sugar	90%	patients, treated: 100	glands better in 7 days	cancer	George Bonadio, Found'n for Health	letter to Ed., Oct. 1984.
C.9.25 BUTYRIC ACID, (Sodium Butyrate). Fatty acid in milk & butter. (& used Staph Lysate).	1 in #	patients, treated: 1, self	all tumors gone, in 1 year	lymphocytic lymphoma	Cecil Pitard, MD, (diagnosed as Stage IV, hopeless, ca., by Mayo)	Michael Culbert, Save Your Life, p.149; (250 articles on Butyric a.&ca.)
C.9.26 PANGAMIC Acid, Vitamin B-15. (See: 9.3.3; 9.10.1; 10.6; A.6.8; B.9.15). Stimulates Oxygenation (see: 6; A.6; A.9.10.7; B.9.18).	88%	patients, treated: 203	practically healthy	atherosclerosis, obliterating, of legs, ready to amputate	Prof. Shpirt, Moscow Clinic n.60. (Biochem. Inst., Acad. of Sci.; & 30 assoc. U.'s; & Kazan Med. Inst., USSR. & 10 foreign nations.)	Culture & Life (Moscow), Aug. 1964; ref. in: Ernst Krebs, Jr., Physician's New Weapon (Vit. B-15), p. 35; (p.v-vi ref. to: Chem. Abstracts: v.62, p.8298b; v.63, p.2289g; v.66, p. 15737d; &, Jap. Heart J., v.2, n.2, p.147, 1961.
C.9.27 LIPO-TROPES (Choline; Folic acid; Cyano-cobal-amine (Vit. B-12); all B-vitamins; see: 10.1; 12.1.1.1; 12.1.2; A.6.8; B.9.15); &, METHIONINE (has Sulfur & Butyric acid; see: 13.4.2 & C.9.25). Deficiency lowers immuno-competence.	averaged	animals	incidence prevented	cancer	Paul Newberne (see C.9.20), Kathleen Nauss, & Joao de Camargo; Dept. Nutrition & Food Sci., MIT.	"Lipo-tropes, Immuno-... & Ca.", ACS, Work. Conf. on Nutrition in Ca. Caus'n & Prev'n, AACR, Cancer Res., v.43, n.5, Suppl., p.2426s, May 1983.
C.9.28 INOSITOL (B-vitamin), (injected).	averaged	patients, treated: 6	tumor size reduced, no blood in urine	bladder cancer		J. Urology, 1948; (& Science, 1943); ref. in: George Berkley, PhD, Cancer, How to ..., p.53.

TREATMENT (Mode, Theory)	BENEFITED, % of total, or #	TREATED, total #	MEASURE of BENEFIT	DISEASE SEVERITY	RESEARCHER, Credentials	REFERENCE, Publication
C.10.0 <u>NUTRITION</u>, <u>LAETRILE</u> C.10.1 Laetrile, Amygdalin		patients, treated	successful	2 fungus like tumors	Fedor Inosemsov, Prof. Surg., Imperial U., Moscow, Russia, 1845AD.	Arlin J. Brown, <u>Health Victory Bull</u>., v.<u>10</u>, n.4, April 1984.
				tumors	Chinese, 1,500BC.	
C.10.2.1 Laetrile. (3g/day (3 grams per day), i.v. (Intra-Venous route of administration) for 4 weeks, & longer. Phase II Studies; Retrospective.		patients, treated: 1,200	Objective Response:	cancer; advanced (for 87% of patients); no hope in Orthodox Therapy (for 73% of patients)	Ernesto Contreras, MD, (see 10.2); Jose E. Contreras, MD; Abel M. Prince, MD. (Over 600 MD's using Laetrile. - E.T. Krebs, Jr., in Bill Stover, <u>Don't Let Cancer Throw You</u>, p.62.)	<u>Kemdalin News</u>, ref. in: <u>Ca. Control J</u>., v.<u>6</u>, n.1-6, p.61, Jan.-June, 1978, (1982) (N. Tasca, "Clinical... Therap. ...Cyano-...Human Malignant...", <u>Gazz. Med. Ital</u>., v.<u>118</u>, p.153, April 1959; Manuel Navarro, "...Laetrile in Ca.", <u>J. Philippine Med. Assoc</u>., v.<u>33</u>, p. 620, Aug. 1957; both ref. in: Kittler, <u>Laetrile...</u>, p.281.)
	32.6%		Any, Total Remission:			
	3.6%		Complete			
	7.1%		Partial			
	21.9%		Stable			
			Subjective Response:			
	45.7%		Any, Total Remission:			
	8.3%		Complete			
	37.4%		Partial			
C.10.2.2 Laetrile, Vit., Min., Enzymes, & Non-toxic food. Phase III Studies; Prospective.		257 (average age: 56 years)	survival, 12 months after:	lung ca., in-operable, diagnosed, (for 54 Oat Cell, &, 151 extensive, ca. cases)	(Note: For cures of metastasized cancer patients by Pancreatic Enzymes: Maureen Salaman, <u>Nutrition, the Cancer Answer</u>, p.70-2, ref. to: <u>JAMA</u>, Dec.15, 1906, p.2003, &, Jan.19, 1907, p.225, &, Mar.23, 1907, p.1030; <u>Med. Rec</u>., Nov.24, 1906, p.812, &, Dec.8, 1906, p.918, &, May 8, 1909, p.804; <u>Brit. Med. J</u>., Aug. 31, 1907, p.525, &, Mar. 2, 1907; <u>General Practitioner</u>, Jan.11, 1908, p.22, &, Mar.21, 1908; etc.)	
	55%		diagnosis			
	34%		treatment			
			Objective Response:			
	49%		Any, Total Remission:			
	5%		Complete			(John Beard, DSc., <u>The Enzyme Treatment of Cancer</u>, 1911AD.)
	6%		Partial			
	37%		Stable			
C.10.4.1 Laetrile	most	patients, treated	ambulatory	cancer, terminal, some hopeless	N.R. Bouziane, MD, PhD; Prof. Path. & Biochem., U. Montreal; Dir., Res. Lab. & Chemo., Tumor Board, Hosp. Ste. Jeanne D'Arc, Montreal, Canada; Dean, Amer. Col. Bio-Analysts.	Glenn Kittler, <u>Laetrile: Nutritional Control for Cancer with Vitamin B-17</u>, p.76 & 82.
	some		resumed normal activity			
C.10.4.2	100%	patients, treated: 10	pain relief, appetite gain	cancer, not operable, metastases	John Morrone, MD, FICS; ASAS; Surgeon, Jersey City Med. Ctr.	", p.82 & 269, ref. to: Morrone, "Chemo. of In-operable Ca.: ... 10 cases Treated with Laetrile", <u>Experim. Med. & Surg</u>., n.4, 1962.
	80%		adeno-pathy decreased			

TREATMENT (Mode, Theory)	BENEFITED, % of total, or #	TREATED, total #	MEASURE of BENEFIT	DISEASE SEVERITY	RESEARCHER, Credentials	REFERENCE, Publication
C.10.4.3 Laetrile	12% 40% 48%	patients, treated: 3,000	cure steady state lost	cancer	Dr. Weedell, outpatient clinic, Salem, Oregon	Glenn Kittler, Laetrile ..., p.212.
C.10.4.4 Laetrile	29% 4% 67%	patients, treated: total:82	at 16 months of practice: comfortable clinically free of ca. temporary help only	cancer, all terminal (except 3 patients)	Arthur T. Harris, MD, U. Edinburgh (under John Beard); PhD, Med.; DSc., Biochem.; LittD.	" , p.42, (& 281, ref. to: E. T. Krebs, Jr. & Sr., & H. H. Beard, "The Unitarian or Trophoblast. ...Ca.", Medical Record, v.163, p.158, July 1950).
C.10.6.1 Laetrile, Vitamins, & Enzymes.	100%	patients: first 17 from 61 early cases	clinical recovery, for 6 years	cancer, biopsy & clinical symptoms		H. H. Beard, A New Approach to the Conquest of Cancer, Rheum. & Heart Diseases: p.192-3.
C.10.6.2 Laetrile	100%	patients, treated: 12 4 2 12	alive, responded well, over 1 year	cancer: leukemia lung Hodgkin's mix	J. A. Restifo, MD, PhD, Med. & Surg. Path.	", p.216.
C.10.6.3 Laetrile, Vitamins, & Enzymes.	72% 90%	patients, treated: 252	clinical recovery ", or improved	ca., clin. symptoms / biopsied, for 50% of patients	Howard H. Beard, Yale U. Porter Fellow, Physiol.; MA, Columbia U.; Dir., Biochem. Dept., LSU; Mtg. Chair, FASEB; Dir., John Beard Lab.; (see 10.6).	", p.197. (Frank Hourigan, The Shape of the Elephant, (draft)).
C.10.6.4 Laetrile, Vit. B-15, & Pancreatic Enzymes.	86% 62% 92% 51% 13%	patients, treated: 70 40 73 524 350	clinical recovery cure	cancer, Anthrone Test diagnosis (95-99.8% accurate)	Assoc. MD's. (100 Drs., 20 big hosp., Canada. 100 Drs., 6 other nations.)	Report n.: ref. in: H. H. Beard, PhD, ScD, The Anthrone Test & Your Cancer Problem Today, p.II-9. 1 2 3 ...5 ...4
C.10.11 Benz-aldehyde, (& Potassium, & vermifuge (anti-worm)), all in Figs. (Note: See Bible: Isaiah, Ch. 38, V.21.)	averaged	patients, treated	tumor weight 39% less	malignant tumor	Setsuo Takeuchi, Japan	"Benz-aldehyde as a Carcino-static Principle in Figs", Agri. & Biol. Chem., v.42, p.1449, July 1978; ref. in: John Heinerman, The Treatment of Cancer with Herbs, p.58.
C.10.14 Chelation (EDTA), (15x, over 8 years), prevented 90% of human cancer.. (See: C.18.)	averaged	patients, treated	incidence prevented by 90%	cancer	Walter Blumer, MD, Netstal, Switzerland	Hellfried Sartori, MD, "... Life Sci. Universal Eumetabolic Ca. Therapy", p.4.

TREATMENT (Mode, Theory)	BENEFITED, % of total, or #	TREATED, total #	MEASURE of BENEFIT	DISEASE SEVERITY	RESEARCHER, Credentials	REFERENCE, Publication
C.10.20.7.1 Apricot kernels in diet increased life span (from date of ca. detect./treat.) by 50%.	averaged	mice, treated	50% ILS (Increased Life Span)	leukemia	Dr. Vern Von Breeman, (see B.10.20.7.1)	Arlin J. Brown, Health Victory Bull., v.10, n.4, April 1984
C.11.0 NUTRITION, ENZYMES C.11.2 COCONUT Water (instead of i.v. feeding; has very easily used protein & minerals), Pineapple, Papaya, Sugar Cane, (& raw juices). Exercise, SWEAT, Breath.	1 in #	self	cure	ca., throat, hopeless, (anaplastic epidermoid carcinoma)	Wong Hon Sun, med. student	How I Overcame In-operable Cancer; ref. in: Ruth Yale Long, PhD, No More Cancer, p.27.
C.11.5.1 Individualized Metabolic Protocol; (see 9.4). (Patients selected from many (100's) more.)	100% of select group	patients, treated: 20 selected	remission, at 5 years, no symptoms left	ca., metastases, terminal	MD's using computer consultation by William Donald Kelley, DDS, (see 11.5).	Cameron Stauth, The New Approach to Cancer, p. 291-300.
C.11.5.2 Individualized Therapy based on test. Nutrition, Exercise. (See 9.4)	50%	patients, treated	success	cancer	Dr. Michael Cessna	NHF, Health Freedom News, v.2, n.4, p.32, April 1983.
C.11.7 Raw food, 99% of diet. Enzymes are not all destroyed in stomach: 50-80% reach colon, (esp. if stomach is neutral pH)	1 in #	patients, treated, female: 1	blooming health, at 25 months	leukemia, diagnosed hopeless	Dr. Ralph Bircher, (& Dr. Max Bircher-Benner, &, Dr. Zabel), Switzerland	Ebba Waerland, Cancer: Disease of Civilization, p.45-9.
C.11.9 Protease Inhibitors, survive inactivation by stomach digestion; & form complexes with (chymo-)trypsin; prevents ca. of intestines.		animals	incidence prevented	cancer, intestinal	Drs. J. Yavelow, &, W. Troll, Dept. Env. Med. &, T.H. Finlay, Dept. Ob. Gyn., NYU Med.; & Ann R. Kennedy, Harvard Public Health.	"...Soybean Protease Inhibitor(:) Anti-carcinogen", ACS, ...Nutr. in Ca. Caus. & Prev., AACR, Ca. Res., v.43, n.5 Suppl., p.2454s, May 1983.
C.12.0 NUTRITION, ANTI-BIOTIC, ANTI-VIRAL C.12.1 CULTURES C.12.1.1.1 Anabol, a lysozyme lysate/extract of Lacto-bacillus B. bacteria. Oral, at home.	45 in # (4 melanoma; 4 pancr.)	patients, treated	complete regression, follow up exam, same hospital	ca., biopsy, incurable, no Orthodox Therapy	Ivan Bogdonov, MD, Lab. Res. & Product. Biol. Active Substances, POB 272, Sofia, Bulgaria.	Observ. ...Anti-Ca. ... Lactobacillus B. ... on 100 Oncologic Patients, Digest, p.3, 18, 20.
Anabol, 10mg, 7 days after insult.	100%	mice, treat: 10	tot. regress	sarcoma	Dr. William Hardy, SKI	", p.13; ref. to: letter.
C.12.1.2 Lactic Acid. Injected i.v., inhibits an enzyme (LDH), from making Lactic out of Pyruvic acid, so frees Pyruvic into Krebs Cycle. Dilates blood vessels. For optimum enzyme action, adjust heat & pH; (see 4. & C.9.23).		patients; wife	tumor burst outward	dying of cancer	Dick Keating, Keating Found'n, veterinarian, Chicago.	D. Keating, A Cure for Cancer in Animals, p.1-3; &, letter to Dick Ericson, (GE-PS Ca. Mem.), Nov.19, 1980.
	averaged	animals, treated: 1,000's	tumor destroyed, massive	tumor transplant	Dr. Siedler, Head, Nutrition Dept., Agri. Col., U. Ill.	
	100%	some	necrosis			
		horse, female	alive $3\frac{1}{2}$ yrs. biopsy benign	malignant melanoma, biopsy		
C.12.1.2.1 Lactic Acid	100%	mice, nude, treated: 4	ca. killed (necrosed)	ca., cervix, (Bittrick)	Dr. Harold Jefferson, & 3 PhD's, Argonne Ca. Res., U. Chi.	

TREATMENT (Mode, Theory)	BENEFITED, % of total, or #	TREATED, total #	MEASURE of BENEFIT	DISEASE SEVERITY	RESEARCHER, Credentials	REFERENCE, Publication
C.12.1.2.2 Lactic Acid. (150cu. mm/kg/day.) Stop tumor totally.	100%	animals, treated:5	survival, halt tumor growth	Ehrlich carcinoma	Dr. Chester Stock, SKI (Sloan Kettering Inst.)	Keating; A Cure ..., ref. to: SKI report n.24,501.
C.12.1.5.2 Brewer's Yeast, as a % of diet, of 15%:	100%	rats, treated: many	free of ca.: thru lifetime	liver chemical carcinogen	Dr. K. Sugiura, PhD, Kyoto Imperial U., Japan; BS, Brooklyn Poly.; ass't chem., Harriman (Ca.) Res. Lab., 1911; (see 10.20.7.1).	J. Nutrition, June 10, 1951; ref. in: George Berkley, PhD, Cancer: How to ..., p.52.
6%:	70%					
3%:	30%					
0%:	0%	50	at 150 days			
C.12.1.5.5 Glucan; modifies viral, bacterial, fungal, & parasitic infections, in plants & animals (vertebrate & invert.), & fights ca.			inhibited (Note: see A.12.1.5)	cancer	Nicholas DiLuzio, PhD, U. Tenn. Med.; Prof. & Chair., Physiol. Dept., Tulane Med.; author, 500 articles.	"Immuno-pharmacology of Glucan ... Broad Spectrum...", TIPS (Elsevier Sci.), Aug. 1983, p.344.
C.12.2 PLANTS C.12.2.1 Mushroom (variety of: Polyporus umbellatus; Zhu-ling, #757. Mushroom & Chemotherapy:	aver-aged	patients, treated	ILS (Increased Life Span), months: 23	cancer	Dr. Chang, Inst. Chinese Materia Medica, PRC (People's Rep. China)	"Alternative Healing: Medicinal Mushrooms", Heartland J., n.17, p.21, Spring 1984.
Mushroom only:			12.5			
Only Chemotherapy:		control	9.8			
C.14.0 NUTRITION, HERBS C.14.4 (See: 14.1; 14.4; 14.10; A.14.4; B.14.4) C.14.4.1 Plants. (39 listed, most with location of Primary tumor treated.)		patients, treated		cancer	Dr. Jonathan Hartwell, NCI	"Plants Used Against Ca.: a Survey", Lloydia, v.30, p.379-436, 1967; v.31, p.71-170, 1968; v.32, p.79-107, & 153-205, & 247-296, 1969; & v.33, p.97-194, 1970; &, "Plant Remedies for Ca.", Ca. Chemo. Reports, v.7, p.19, May 1960; ref. in:
C.14.4.2 Herbs, Chinese, are 3/4 of Chinese medicine. Out of 796 herbal & animal remedies observed, 47% have scientific validity.		patients, treated	valid therapy	cancer	NAS; &, Dr. James Duke, Chief, Economic Botany Lab., USDA, (see 14.4).	John Heinerman, The Treatment of Cancer with Herbs, p.123-8. " , p.109.
C.14.4.3 Random Screening: Tests of 108,330 extracts (from 35,000 plant species), showed 4,149 extracts (from 2,935 species) were active against cancer.		rats, in-vivo	activity against cancer	cancer: tumor	NCI	" , p.132.
		cells, in-vitro		naso-pharynx (human, KB)		
C.14.5 Essiac. (Note: Proponents: King of England; Dr. Russell, Royal Marsden Ca. Hosp., Liverpool; Sir Fred Banting, co-discoveror, insulin, (wanted to test it); Evita Peron, V.P., Argentina, (wanted to use it); Mr. Funasaka, Pres., Toyoto, Canada.)	380 in #	patients	cured	cancer	Renée Caisse, (see 14.5). Dr. C. Brusch; med. award, Governor's Council, Mass.; Citation, Cambridge, Mass.; Mathew Dymond, MD, Health Minister, Ontario Province. U. Toronto Gen'l Hosp. 350 MD's, Canada	" , p.191-200. (Note: A Canadian Bill to allow Caisse to treat ca. was supported by 55,000 signatures.)

TREATMENT (Mode, Theory)	BENEFITED, % of total, or #	TREATED, total #	MEASURE of BENEFIT	DISEASE SEVERITY	RESEARCHER, Credentials	REFERENCE, Publication
C.14.21 Herb, Astragalus Membranaceus, aids immunity, via T-cells.	 67% 4 in #	patients, treated: 500 31 control	 survival, 1 year	cancer: mix liver, terminal	Sun Yan, Peking Cancer Inst., China; &, M.D. Anderson Hosp. & Tumor Inst., Houston	T.Chan, "Ancient Remedies: Clues to Ca. Cures", NHF, Health Freedom News, v.3, n.5, p.12, May 1984.
C.14.22 Herbs, Indian, (secret: White Rosin, Lavender, Linseed, Blood Root, Cranberry). External, topical, poultice. Black & Yellow salve. Pulls tumor; in external ca., patients survive.	100%	patients, treated 100 tot.	pulls out tumors: all some	ca., of: breast brain, pancreas, liver	Anonymous	CFCCT, The Choice, v.8, n.1, p.1, Win. 1982. (Robert Bradford, & Michael Culbert, International Protocols in Ca. Mgmt., IIMP, p.93.)
C.14.23 Fruit (Luffa Purgans), extract drawn into nostrils, INTRA-NASALLY: Brain Drain.	some	patients	cure	brain tumors	Indians, Columbia, So. Amer. (Dr. Asuaro; Anita Backhaus, Germany)	J. Natural Health & Parapsychology, Jan. 1984, p. 47.
C.16.0 ANIMAL (CELLULAR) EXTRACTS INJECTED						
C.16.2 Immuno-Therapy. Surg./Rad./Chemo., & Immunotherapy: Only Immunotherapy: " " " "	 18% 26% 24% 39 in #	patients, treated	survival: 5 years no sign of cancer for 15 years	ca., metastases, relapses, beyond Orthodox Therapy	Dr. Joseph Issels. (Independent audit by Dr. A.G. Audier.) (See 16.2).	Dr. A. G. Audier, Die Medizinische, n.40, 1960; ref. in: Dick Richards, MD, The Topic of Cancer, p.60.
C.16.10.1 Urea, topical. (See 12.1.2).	some 2 in # 1 in #	patients, treated 18, total	dramatic regression alive & well: 36 & 57 months 57 months	squamous cell carcinoma liver ca.: Primary as Metastases	Evangelo Danopoulis, Prof.; Hellenic Anti-Cancer Inst., Greece.	Lancet, Jan. 26, 1974, p.132, ref. in: Wayne Martin, "...Unused Ca. Therapies", IACVF, Ca. News J., v.16, n.3, p.27, Fall 1981.
ILS (Increased Life Span) of 5x. Liver less enlarged from ca.	averaged 100%		ILS: 500% shrink liver			Wayne Martin, "Treating Ca. Metastases", in press.
C.16.10.2 Urea	1 in #	woman: 1	doing well	" ", from: breast ca.	Nevin Aiken, MD	Wayne Martin, IACVF, Ca. News J., v.17, n.2, p.22, Sum. 1982.
C.16.11.1 INSULIN, lowers blood sugar level, leaving more Oxygen available; so, raises blood pH. Used in Psychotherapy. (See: C.9.23.6; C.23; 6; A.6; B.9.18; C.9.18; C.9.20; C.9.24; C.9.26.) (Note: Ernst T. Krebs, Jr., (see 10.1), & C.L. Bartlett, MD, "...Pregnancy ... Trophoblast...Pancreas", Medical Record, v.162, n.10, p.1-12, Oct., 1949.)	100% 100%	patients, treated: 1 1	biopsy: ca. gone ca. gone	ca., metastases, biopsied: adeno-carcinoma melanoma	S. Koroljow, MD. (Dr. C. P. Rhoads, Dir., SKI) (Dr. Philip Schein, Div. Med. Onc., V. Lombardi Ca. Res. Ctr., Georgetown U. Med.; NCI Grant)	"Two Cases of Malignant Tumors with Metastases... Treated Success...", Psychiatric Quarterly, v.36, p.261, April 1962. (Schein, ..., "...Insulin ...", Proc. ACS & NCI National Conf. Nutr. in Ca. 1978, Cancer, v.43, p.2070, 1979.)

TREATMENT (Mode, Theory)	BENEFITED, % of total, or #	TREATED, total #	MEASURE of BENEFIT	DISEASE SEVERITY	RESEARCHER, Credentials	REFERENCE, Publication
C.16.11.2 Insulin; missing in ca. cells; promotes Oxydation, (not Fermentation), of sugars in cells. (Injected)	25%	patients, treated: 16	complete remission	cancer	USSR. (Dr. Sam Beale, Mass. Many MD's in Italy, Spain, & So. America.)	Dr. Lynn Dalin, Cancer Causes & Natural Cures, p.167.
	87%		"/temporary remission			
C.16.11.3 Insulin. Diabetes causes a 3-fold increase in cancer incidence.		patients	cancer incidence 300% higher	diabetes		Wm. Cleare Filer, & IACVF, Holy Cancer, p.10.
C.17.0 IMMUNOLOGY, (Injections), C.17.1 Immuno-Augmentive Therapy (IAT). No toxic response.	FEVER	treat.: 1,800		cancer	Lawrence Burton, PhD, (see: 17.1; A.17.1; & D.17.1)	IAT, "Prelim. Report...", May 14, 1983.
	averaged	patients, treated: 14 tot.	good: weight, appetite, & function	proven malignant mesothelioma of:		
		6	survival, months: 34	pleura		
		7	22	peritoneum		
Un-treated:		controls	4.2	pleura		
General prognosis:			12	peritoneum		
C.17.11 Vaccine against Pleomorph bugs (Progenitor Cryptocides).		patients, treated: 100 tot.	cure	cancer, pathology proven:	Dr. John E. White, Surgeon, (author with: Dr. Thomas Glover, of: The Treatment of Ca. in Man: Results ... with a Specific Anti-Serum; (see 17.9)).	"Report of 100 Pathologically Proven Cases of Malignancy Treated by a Specific Anti-serum", 3rd. Internat'l Conf. on Micro-biol., 1953, (Rome); ref. in: V. Livingston, ..., The Microbiol. of Ca.; ref. in: R. Netterberg, ..., The Ca. Conspiracy, p.41-2, 48, 153.
(Note: "...29 bacteria of various kinds isolated from human & rat tumors. All appeared to be Pleo-Morphic" (i.e. many-phased: virus to bacteria & back, & forth) - Dr. Robert Netterberg, & Robert Taylor.	54%			mix		
	100%			colon; bone		
	10%			prostate		
	0%			tongue; liver		
C.17.16 Coley's Mixed Bacterial Toxins; injections. 4 months of Injections & Surgery:	85%	patients, treated: part of 126 tot.	well for 4-60 years; ALS: 4-13 years	osteogenic sarcoma:	William Bradley Coley. Helen Coley Nauts, Exec. Dir., (NY) Ca. Res. Inst.; (see 17.16; A.17.16).	Nauts, "Bacterial Products in the Treatment of Ca. ...", Internat'l Colloq. Bacteria & Ca., Mar. 16, 1982; ref. in: Bacteria & Ca., J. Jeljaszewicz, et. al., Eds., p.1-25.
Only Surgery:	10% to 15%	control	survival, ALS: 1 year	long bone		
Injections & No Amputation:	57%	treated, 128 tot.	remain well	ca. of extremities:		
" & " " :	96%			Giant Cell bone tumor		
" & " " :	80%			sarcoma, operable		
Only Amputation:	32%	control: 166				
C.17.22 De-Shielding ca. cells by removing its protein coat protection. Serum injected into patient. (See: 9.7.4; 10.6; 11.3; 17.)	55% to 60%	patients, treated: 100's	ca. arrest, except very advanced cases	cancer, terminal: 90% of cases	Dr. Heriton Alivizatos, Athens, Greece.	NHF, Health Freedom News, v.2, n.6, p.45, June 1983.

TREATMENT (Mode, Theory)	BENEFITED, % of total, or #	TREATED, total #	MEASURE of BENEFIT	DISEASE SEVERITY	RESEARCHER, Credentials	REFERENCE, Publication
C.17.23 Anti-gens of lung cancer, as immuno-stimulant against lung cancer.	78% 18%	patients; 52 tot. treated control	survival, for 7 years	lung ca.,& surgical therapy	Dr. Ariel Hollinshead, & Dr. Thomas Stewart, U. Ottawa Med., Canada	1973; ref. in: Judith Glassman, The Cancer Survivors, p.211.
C.17.24 Less: bacteria (endo-toxin), & bacterial by-products (exo-toxin) allergens (sterilized or not) in environs. Bugs (& by-products) are on old: dust, wool, feathers; & old food: sprout/ferment/sour, or, dry/cure/smoke - chocolate, cheese, malt (infant formula milk), liquor.	many	patients, treated: 19,000	dramatic benefits	allergy, disguised as many diseases	William Holmes Gardner, MD, RPh; Appl. Immun. Clin., NY Med.; EENT Hosp., Chicago; St. Luke's Hosp., Cleveland. Sue Gardner, RN. Stan Mattoon. 100's of MD's. Theodore Nelson, MD.	Stanley Mattoon, & Theodore Nelson, (MD, U. Kansas; post-grad., U. Vienna), Allergy Today, p.vi.
C.17.25 CIMETIDINE, (see 17.21; drug), enhances immunity by raising ratio of helper to suppressor T-lymphocytes. Toxic.	2 in #	patients, treated	became well	cancer, lung, hopeless	James Armitage, & Robert Sidnor, U. Nebraska Med.	Lancet, Apr.21, 1979, p.882; ref. in: Wayne Martin, IACVF, Ca. News J., v.17, n.1, p.3, Spr. 1982.
C.17.25.1 Cimetidine; & Warfarin (very toxic; like Coumarin, refined from moldy sweet clover).	3 in #	patients, treated	became well	melanoma, far advanced		Lancet, Aug.7, 1982; ref. in: Wayne Martin, "An Open Letter...", p.5.
C.18.0 CHEMICALS (See C.10.14) C.18.2.3 Kerosene, toxic unless specially processed. Spoonful dose. (Med. patent in France.)	3 in #	patients, treated	cured	cancer, metastases	Paula Ganner, (see 18.2.3). (Dr. Kossakowska, Warsaw, Poland.)	FACT, Cancer Forum, v.7, n.9, p.10, Spring 1984. (Patents, 5 nations, W. Europ)
C.18.4 Hydrazine Sulfate	44%	patients, treated: 41	aids glucose metabolism	cancer, advanced	Dr. Roman Chlebowski, Harbor-UCLA Med. Ctr.	CFCCT, Choice, v.10, n.2, p.20, 1984.
C.23 ACID-ALKALINE (pH) BALANCE (See: 6.4; 9.4.2; 12.1.2; 16.2; 17.10; C.9.23; C.12.1.2)						
Ca. cells killed above pH 8.5 & below pH 6.0. C.23.1. HYDRO-CHLORIC ACID (HCl), & BENZOIC & SALICYLIC ACIDS, (i.v.), raises white blood cell count.	many in #	patients, treated	dramatic recovery	cancer	Dr. Walter Guy, Fla. 100's of MD's. (Sir Hans Krebs, Nobel Laureate, used Benzoic a. against fungi ferment - Lancet, Nov.12, 1983.)	3 Years of HCl Therapy, Med. World, 1935; ref. in: IACVF, Ca. News J., v.15, n.4, p.28, Win. 1980-1. (Wayne Martin, "An Open Letter...", p.6.)
C.24 SLEEP & REST (See: Mental 2.; Light 5.; Gravity 19.; Time 20.; Noise 21.; (Feet) 22.)						
C.24.1 Sleep: too little or too much increases mortality. (Sleeping pills associated with 50% increase in mortality.)	55% 100% 38%	populace	survival relative to standard base of 100% for 7-8 hours sleep/night	nightly hours slept: under 4 7-8 over 10	Dr. Kripke; Dir., Sleep Disorders Clin., VA Hosp., La Jolla; UCSD (U.Cal. San Diego)	Archive of General Psychiatry, Jan. 1981; ref. in: Cal. Chiro. Assoc. J., n.17; ref. in: NHF, Public Scrutiny, v.28, n.4, p.4, April 1982.

CANCER QUOTATIONS COLLAGE

ADDENDUM B, 2nd Edition, Continued from p.65(-123), & 131(-146) of 1st. Ed.:

TABLE of CONTENTS for CANCER QUOTATIONS:

ADDENDUM B to CANCER QUOTATIONS COLLAGE:

B.Q.1.0 **HISTORY, CIVICS:**
B.Q.1.1 **REMEDIES' HISTORY:**

"Kill neither men, nor beasts, nor yet the food which goes into your mouth. .... And your bodies become what your foods are, even as your spirits, likewise, become what your thoughts are. .... For burned, frozen, & rotted foods will burn, freeze, & rot your body also. .... Cook not.... Be content with 2 or 3 sorts of food.... ...If you mix together all sorts of food in your body, then the peace of your body will cease, & endless war will rage in you. ....Never eat unto fulness."
– Jesus, The Essene Gospel of Peace, Book I, (Internat'l Biogenic Society; Szekely, 1978), p.48-52.

"'...In ancient times the people lived to be over a 100 years, & yet they remained active.... But nowadays people reach only half of that age & yet become decrepit & failing.... There was temperance in eating & drinking. Their hours of rising & retiring were regular & not disorderly & wild. ....Nowadays, people ...adopt recklessness as usual behavior.... They devote all their attention to the amusement(s)....'" – The Yellow Emperor's Classic on Internal Medicine, (c. 479 - 300 BC), (in G. Majno, The Healing Hand...in the Ancient World, p.241).
"'Their food was then (before the Flood) fitter for the prolongation of life. ...'" – Flavius Josephus, (c. 80-100 AD).
"...In ancient India, organ transplants involving bone, earlobe, nose, & other tissues, were pretty much 'a matter of routine' some 5,000 years ago." – John Heinerman, Understanding Herbal Medicine, (Studies in Medical Anthropology ...), p.7 & 8, (for last 3 paragraphs above).

"He who would eat much must eat little, for by eating less he will live longer, & so be able to eat more." – Luigi Cornaro, 1538 AD, (in Robert & Raye Yaller, The Health Spas, p.27).

"Only by understanding the wisdom of natural foods & their effects on the body, shall we attain the mastery of disease & pain, which shall enable us to relieve the burden of mankind." – William Harvey, (1578-1657 AD).

"Every one should be his own physician. We ought to assist, & not to force nature. Eat with moderation.... Nothing is good for the body but what we can digest. What medicine can procure digestion? Exercise. What will recruit strength? Sleep."
– Voltaire, (1694-1778 AD).
(last 2 quotes above from Ford Heritage, BSME, Composition & Facts About Foods, c.1968; 1971, Health Research; p.117, 119).

"The famous physician Dumoulin said when dying, 'I leave two great physicians behind me, simple food & pure water.'." – Voltaire, (from Helene S. Feingold, co-author, with Benjamin Feingold, MD, of The Feingold Cookbook for Hyperactive Children).

"The best doctors are Dr. Diet, Dr. Quiet, & Dr. Merryman." – Jonathan Swift, (1667-1745), (in Soaring Bear, Natural Dental Wellness, p.60).

"Those who neglect the cleanliness of their mouth are at least amateurs of life.... the teeth serve for the re-establishment of health...." – Pierre Fauchard, treatise, 2nd Ed., 1746 AD, p.183, (in Joseph E. Phillips, DDS, MS, Acquiring & Maintaining Oral Health, Through the Blotting Procedure & Total Mouth Hygiene, c.1972, p.8).

"The mischievous effects from lead have been known to scientists for at least 60 years. You will observe how long a useful truth may be known to exist before it is generally received & practiced on." - Benjamin Franklin, (1706-90), 1786, (in NHF, Health Freedom News, v.2,n.3,p.15,March 1983).

"You have just dined; & however scrupulously the slaughter-house is concealed in a graceful distance, there is complicity." - Ralph Waldo Emerson, (1803-1882), (in Alvenia Fulton, ND, PhD, Vegetarianism: Fact or Myth? Eating to Live, p.119).

(Save) "opium, which the Creator himself seems to prescribe, for ... pain to be soothed; ...(&) wine ... ; & I firmly believe that if the whole (remaining medicines of) materia medica, as now used, could be sunk to the bottom of the sea, it would be all the better for mankind - & all the worse for the fishes." - Oliver Wendell Holmes, Sr., MD, (1809-1894), (address to Mass. Medical Soc., 1860).

"It is not as if our homeopathic brothers are asleep: far from it, they are awake — many of them at any rate — to the importance of the scientific study of disease." - Sir William Osler, (1849-1919; "Father of Modern Medicine"), (in Dana Ullman, MPH, "Homeo-pathic Ed. Serv.").

"We labor under the fatal delusion that no disease can be cured without medicine. This has been responsible for more mischief to mankind than any other evil. .... Disease increases in proportion to the increase in the number of doctors in a place."
"Illness or disease is only Nature's warning that filth has accumulated in some portion or other of the body; & it would surely be the part of wisdom to allow Nature to remove this filth, instead of covering it up with the help of medicines." - Mahatma Gandhi, The Health Guide, c.1965, (in The Sproutletter, Jeff Breakey, Ed., n.15, p.7, Mar. 1983).

B.Q.2.0 TOP OFFICIALS, RECENT & RESEARCH:
B.Q.2.1 PRESIDENTS, US, RECENT:

"I think doctors care very deeply about their patients, but when they organize into the AMA, their responsibility is to the welfare of doctors, & quite often, these lobbying groups are the only ones that are heard in the state capitals & in the capital of our country." - Jimmy Carter, US President, (in "Carter Draws Sharp AMA Response", Amer. Med. News, May 19, 1978, p.1, (in John Heinerman, Understanding Herbal Medicine, p.xv)).

B.Q.2.2 FEDERAL LEGISTLATORS, US, RECENT:

"(My chemotherapy is) death in a bottle"" - Hubert H. Humphrey, Vice President, US, & US Senator, (in Judith Glassman, The Cancer Survivors, p.45).

"...The NIH have become bureaucratic, because of the great amount of money that has been poured into them, & have fallen under the control largely of the pundits of the AMA & are ruled by the prejudices of organized medicine. The prejudices of medicine go far.... ...The NIH have in part abused the trust & the money which have been given them." - US Senator Paul Douglas, "NCI Seeks to Delay or Avoid Clinical Tests of Krebiozen", speech in US Senate, July 20, 1962, (in Suzanne Caum, Cancer Cures Crucified, c.1968, p.517).

"...It seems that public officials are afraid that if they make any move, or say anything antagonistic to the wishes of the medical organization, they will be pounced upon & destroyed. ...Public officials seem to be afraid of their jobs & even of their lives." - US Senator Elmer Thomas, in Morris A. Bealle, The Drug Story, c.1949 & 1976, p.97.

"'It is our understanding that the NIH with FDA approval, clinically test at least 100 products a year on cancer patients. We feel Krebiozen deserves a similar test. Why should either side be afraid of the truth?'" - US Senators Paul Douglas, Clifford Case, Edward Long, Harrison Williams, John J.Williams, Hugh Scott, Joseph Clark, George Smathers, Jacob Javits, Steven Young, & Ralph Yarborough, (in Chicago's American, April 1, 1966 (in Citizens Comm. for Cancer Survivors on Krebiozen, Inc., Newsletter, May 12, 1966)).

"'I think every doctor should know the shocking state of affairs.... ...We discovered they (the FDA) failed to effectively regulate the large manufacturers & powerful interests while recklessly persecuting small manufacturers. .... (The FDA is) harassing (small) manufacturers & doctors....(&) betrays the public trust." - US Senator Edward V. Long, (in AMA News, May 8, 1967).

"'I could not move them. They would not even agree to a modification, of the ruling (banning the Rand vaccine), which would at least allow the 100 (cancer) patients at Richmond Heights (Ohio) to complete their injections. The Justice Dept. was prepared to go along, but the FDA Commissioner, Dr. James Goddard, was adamant, even belligerent. It's wrong of the Govt. to snatch away this hope when there is no evidence against its use offered in court. It's damnably wrong.'" - US Senator Stephen Young, (in Len Guttridge, "How the US Govt. is Blocking a Cancer Cure", Saga, May 1968).
- (last 2 paragraphs above in:) Howard H. Beard, ScD, PhD, Yale U., The Anthrone Test & Your Cancer Problem Today, p.6 & 13.

"Dr. Lawrence Burton.... ...in fighting cancer.(:) Many of his patients are now living normal lives after being told there was nothing more the conventional treatments could do for them, & that death was imminent. .... Why are Americans being forced to go off shore for treatment for cancer from an American doctor & for a program that was developed in America?" - US Congressman Larry P. McDonald, "Dear Colleague" letter, Sept. 24, 1980.

"Regulation of life-saving drugs by the FDA prompts people to go abroad for medication. Drug laws are such that prices of illicit drugs are higher than they would be otherwise, causing crime rates to soar & underworld mobs to flourish. Even vitamins are regulated by government." - US Congressman Ron Paul, Freedom Report, v.8,n.7,p.5,Aug. 1983.

"You can be sure that I will do all I can...that treatment is not denied to the millions suffering from this dreaded disease (cancer) because of our country's often restrictive policies." - US Congressman John Edward Porter, (letter, cc to Richard Ericson, Oct. 30, 1980).

"...At best the RDA's (Recommended Daily Allowances, of nutrients) are only a 'recommended' allowance at ante-diluvian levels designed to prevent terrible disease. At worst, they are based on conflicts of interest & self-serving views of certain parts of the food industry. .... The RDA standard is established by the Food & Nutrition Board of the (NRC) National Research Council, which is influenced, dominated, & financed in part by the food industry. It represents one of the most scandalous conflicts of interest in the Federal Government." - US Senator William Proxmire, (in Michael Culbert, Save Your Life, p.108).

"In 1962, the FDA tried to prohibit the sales of vitamins & minerals in all but very limited potencies & combinations, by first classifying, & then regulating them as prescription drugs. Congress blocked it at that time, unanimously adopting a resolution offered by Senators Bill Proxmire & Dick Schweiker...."

"However, FDA attempted to reverse this clear congressional intent in March, 1979, by proposing to regulate vitamins & minerals as 'Over-The-Counter' drugs...."

"As was noted in the Wall Street Journal, last March 21st, FDA approval of drug labelling, '...requires 7 to 10 years, & costs each applicant an average of $70 million.'" - US Senator Orrin Hatch, Chairman, Comm. on Labor & Human Resources, "Dear Colleague" letter, Oct. 20, 1981, (in NHF, Public Scrutiny, v.28, n.1, p.10, Jan. 1982).

"Indeed, after the testimony ... I was convinced that the NCI does not adequately protect patient safety. ....Every hearing we have held on this subject this year is evidence to the world that there is critical need for better management at NCI. ....When the NCI did learn of this drug's life-threatening effects in humans, the NCI did not promptly inform the FDA & all of its clinical investigators."

"Your assurances to me ... that the adverse reaction controversy was resolved have left a significant question of credibility. Each time we meet, you tell me you have solved the problems that we are now pointing to." - US Senator Paula Hawkins, Oversight of the National Cancer Institute, 1981, Hearings, Subcom. on Investigations & General Oversight, Com. on Labor & Human Resources, US Senate, Nov. 3 & 6, 1981, p.309, 310, & 406.

"...We in America have created a health care system that can be so callous to human suffering, so intent on high salaries & profits, & so unconcerned for the needs of our people. American families, regardless of income, are offered health care of uncertain quality at inflated prices. (It's) an industry which strongly protects the profits but only weakly protects the healing & rights of people." - US Senator Edward M. Kennedy, Chairman, Subcommittee on Health, (in Milton Friedman, "Holistic Health: Is Washington Listening?", National Journal of the Nutritional Academy, v.1,n.2,p.42, Fall 1978).

"The AMA puts the lives & well being of the American citizens below it's own special interest.... It deserves to be ignored, rejected, & forgotten. No amount of historical gymnastics can hide the public record of AMA opposition to virtually every major health reform in the past 50 years. ...The AMA has turned into a propaganda organ purveying 'medical politics' for deceiving the Congress, the people, & the doctors of America themselves." - US Senator Edward Kennedy, (in UPI, National Chronicle, 1971, (ref. by Kitty Schumacher)).

"The AMA...is concerned only about the wealthiest doctors in this country, & indifferent to delivering adequate health care to the people of this nation." - US Senator Howard Metzenbaum, (Akron Beacon Journal, Dec. 19, 1982, p.A-16).

"Medical authorities say that there is no question that this nation should be educated to consume more of the natural foods & discontinue the use of so many unworthy substitutes! Today it is being realized that the best medicine is food." - US Senator Royal S. Copeland, (in Alvenia Fulton, ND, PhD, Radiant Health Through Nutrition, p.19).

"Of all the dumb ways to save money, the dumbest is not to feed kids." - US Senator Mark Andrews, Hearings, Appropriations Committee, US Senate, (in Health Writers, Health Newsletter, v.13, n.3, p.8, March 1983).

"...You can extend your life tremendously by eating the right things. By eating right you can combat almost everything: disease, fatigue, over-work." ....

"Holland gets by on a total of 4 food additives; we have over 1,400."

"... Other countries are way ahead of ours in nutrition." - US Congressman Fred Richmond, Chairperson, Subcommittee on Domestic Marketing, Consumer Relations, & Nutrition, (in Journal of the Nutritional Academy, v.2,n.2,p.41).

"I am a former state health director.... It is disturbing to me when the men in the (PHS) Public Health Service, who, as late as 1950, were not ready to endorse the universal use of fluorine, have now (1952), almost to a man, come out for the endorsement."

"It is difficult for me to understand how high officials in the PHS could change their mind, over a 3-month period,& completely reverse the field. Where once they advocated the go-slow sign on the use of fluorides, they now apparently have gone overboard, & put out large amounts of propaganda favoring the fluoridation of water. I am certain that the dental profession merely echoes & endorses the opinions of the PHS."

"...I cannot find any public evidence ... that the AMA, the Dental (ADA), or several other health agencies, now recommending the fluoridation of water, had done any original ("experimental") work of their own. These groups were simply endorsing each other's opinions."

"You will note that all of the experts grounded in the science of biochemistry have advocated the go-slow sign on the use of fluorides in drinking water. I believe that the dental profession & other public-minded individuals, like myself, have been misled by the PHS, because all of the facts have not been made available upon this subject." ....

"I sometimes wonder if (a major aluminum co.) might not have a deep interest in getting rid of the waste products from the manufacture of aluminum, because these products contain a large amount of fluoride. In this connection it is interesting to know that (a bureaucrat), who now heads up the Federal Security Adm'n (precursor of the USPHS), & the firm of attorneys he was with ... represents (that aluminum co.)." - US Congressman Dr. A. L. Miller, Chairman, Special Committee on Chemicals in Foods, "Fluoridation of Water - Extension of Remarks", Congressional Record, March 25, 1952, p.A1899, (in John Yiamouyiannis, PhD, Fluoride: the Aging Factor, c.1983, p.140-2, 196).

"The practice of adding chemicals to water supplies...violates the fundamental principle that people should not be forced to ingest medicines or chemicals against their will, except...." - US Congressman John Seiberling, (in Spotlight, April 8, 1985, p.8).

"I came to Washington from a place where you can drink fresh water & the air smells good. I think my family is going to be a lot more unhealthy here than in Wisconsin because of the rotten air & the lousy water from the Potomac. My biggest frustration as a human is in not being able to control the environment I live in except by opting out & leaving. I frankly don't give a damn how much it costs. I think it is insane. It doesn't make any logical sense or moral sense or economic sense." - US Congressman David Obey, (in Newsday, Jan. 10, 1977, (in Nutrition & Cancer Research, Hearings, Subcom. on Nutrition, (George McGovern, Chairman), June 12 & 13, 1978, p.104)).

"This is a blatant attempt (by OSHA supervisors) to rid the government of a competent scientist who happened not to agree with an industry whose profits are at stake. (Govt. scientists) may be forced by political hatchetmen to abandon widely held views, in favor of the line currently advocated by industry." - US Congressman Albert Gore, Jr., in subcommittee, July 16, 1981, (in NRDC (Natural Resources Defense Council), The Amicus Journal, v.4, n.2, p.22-31, Fall 1982).

"...Prevent postal investigators from aggressively interfering with, or closing, a commercial enterprise merely because it has been deemed not to adhere to the prevailing body of scientific opinion — whatever they have determined that to be."

"After examining some of these recent cases which the Postal Service has pursued, I cannot find any overriding or compelling national interest which would warrant such vigorous prosecution of, for example, a health food advocate." - US Congressman Vin Weber, Congressional Record, v.128,n.82, June 24, 1982.

"Drinking driving is the most often committed violent crime in the nation &...our youth. This year another 26,000 people are projected to be killed by drinking drivers & about 750,000 seriously injured.... ...one of the nation's most serious health & safety problems.... ...Take immediate action to help stem the carnage occuring routinely.... The human suffering inflicted on the American public by drunk drivers can no longer be tolerated by a sane society." - US Congressmen James V. Hansen, Michael D. Barnes, & Glenn M. Anderson, ("Dear Colleague" letter, Oct. 6, 1981).

"If the administration is really serious about free-market energy policies, then I suggest we join together to root out the billions of dollars of subsidies we now give each year to petroleum, gas, coal, & nuclear industries. But if this administration will not or cannot do this, then they should at least stop trying to kill the emerging new technologies that are arising to compete with those older sources of energy." - US Congressman Berkley Bedell, (in Solar Lobby, Sun Times, Mar. 1983,p.4).

"I can't be bought, but I can be rented." - US Congressman J. Breaux, (in Common Cause, Common Cause, v.8, n.4, p.75, Aug. 1982).

B.Q.2.3 FDA COMMISSIONERS:

"The thing that bugs me is that the people think the FDA is protecting them. It isn't. What the FDA is doing & what the public thinks it's doing are as different as night & day."

"First, it is providing a means whereby key individuals on its payroll are able to obtain both power & wealth through granting special favors to certain politically influential groups that are subject to its regulation. This activity is similar to the 'protection racket' of organized crime; for a price, one can induce FDA administrators to provide 'protection' from the FDA itself."

"Secondly, as a result of this political favoritism, the FDA has become a primary factor in that formula whereby cartel-oriented companies in the food & drug industry are able to use the police powers of government to harass or destroy their free-market competitors."

"And thirdly, the FDA occasionally does some genuine public good with whatever energies it has left over after serving the vested political & commercial interest of its first two activities." - Dr. Herbert Ley, Commissioner of the FDA, (in Dore Deverell, How I Healed My Cancer Holistically,c.1978, p.49, (from G.E.Griffin, World Without Cancer, p.395, (from Autopsy on the AMA, Student Research Facility, Berkeley, 1970, p.42, (from San Francisco Chronicle, Jan. 2, 1970)))).

B.Q.2.4 NCI/NCAB/FDA/USPHS/NIOSH/OSHA/USDA/USDoD, OFFICIALS, RECENT:

"The basis of sound science is solid difference of opinion. When I was Director of NCI, I found myself rescuing people who incurred the displeasure of certain groups or their superiors. I did it 3 or 4 times. And I did it because they were good scientists." - Dr. Arthur Upton, Director, NCI. (Continued)

"...Research has been a special target of this administration. Health research is most damaging to an administration which doesn't want to do anything to upset things. A lot of scientific discussion is...dampened." - Dr. Anthony Robbins, Director, NIOSH (National Inst. of Occupational Safety & Health).
- last 2 paragraphs above in NRDC (Natural Resources Defense Council), The Amicus Journal, v.4,n.2,p.22-31, Fall 1982.

"...We are not aware of any scientific basis for introducing Laetrile into clinical trials & deplore the efforts of individuals & organizations, who by touting quick & easy solutions to a serious problem, would divert cancer patients from their only real prospects for help. There is obviously no ethical, scientific or legal foundation for any claims regarding laetrile or any other unproven therapy, unless it can survive the rigorous scientific examination...." - Dr. Kenneth Endicott, Director, NCI, (in G.M. Rosen, PhD, JD, "Laetrile: A Survey of Judicial & Administrative Activity", Annals of Internal Medicine, v.94,n.4,part 1,p.532,April 1981).

"I am not a proponent of unorthodox drugs, by any means, but I am a proponent of allowing individuals to search for relief when all else has failed. .... Laetrile itself, as you know, is toxic." - Henry C. Pitot, PhD; Chairman, NCAB (National Cancer Advisory Board); Director, McArdle Lab. for Cancer Research.

"Excuse me, but...I happen to know an individual...who had skin cancer, & (no) hope, &...took Laetrile, & 2 years later, is supposedly cured. ...The public is unaware of that." - US Senator Paula Hawkins, (p.25).

"Publication of an article...does not constitute effective transfer of information....It must be implemented.... (Perhaps) there are 1,500 cancer publications a month." - T.G. Sawyer, MD, Orlando Reg. Med. Ctr., (p.91).
- all in Oversight of the National Cancer Program, Hearing, Subcom. on Investigations & General Oversight, Com. on Labor & Human Resources, US Senate, May 21, 1981, (p.25, & 91).

"Toxicity of Laetrile in dosages currently employed for human cancer is assumed to be minimal." - NCI Clinical Protocol for Laetrile, (in Judith Glassman, The Cancer Survivors, & How They Did It, p.108).

"Despite intensive effort over many years, the FDA, the AMA, the ACS, the NCI, & independent researchers have been unable to find any scientific evidence that Laetrile has any effect on cancer." - FDA, (press release, P77-8, Feb. 17, 1977).

"The cyano group of vitamin B-12 (cyano-cobal-amin) is more labile & potentially more harmful than the cyano group found in Laetrile. Yet we know how safe & essential vitamin B-12 is." - Dr. R.A. Passwater, testimony, FDA Docket # 77N-0048.
- Dr. Richard Passwater, (author, many articles on cancer in Amer. Lab.), Cancer & Its Nutritional Therapies, p.167, 170.

"I have had some very interesting work with Dr. (Andrew C.) Ivy, & have had, what I think, unusually good results with Krebiozen. Due to the controversy which was stimulated by adverse quarters, it was the Army policy not to allow me to continue with this particular type of research project. I feel that Krebiozen, or perhaps a similar substance, is certainly on the threshold of finding the answer to some of our malignant (cancer) problems." - Wallace H. Graham, Major General, USAF; Physician to the President (of the US); letter to Lt. Col. Nick Stepanovich, April 9, 1952, (courtesy of Kitty Schumacher, Cancer Information Crusade).

"The NCI has a long history of correspondence with Mr. Ericson & with other Congressmen regarding Mr. Ericson's concerns. .... Lung cancer can be cured if treated before it spreads to other organs. .... Mr. Ericson recommends studies of the value of prayer as an adjunct to cancer treatment. .... The NCI would not support research attempts to draw up 'dependable principles' for prayer. .... Mr. Ericson is very interested in helping cancer patients find alternative methods of treatment that may be better than standard therapies. Comment: The NCI urges cancer patients to remain in the care of qualified physicians who utilize accepted & proven methods of treatment. .... I hope my comments have assured you that Mr. Ericson has not provided a suitable basis for a Congressional investigation." - Mary C. Knipmeyer, PhD, Legistlative Analyst / Congressional Liason, NCI, (letter to US Congressperson Henry J. Hyde, Nov. 18, 1982).

"Variety is not only the spice of life, it may be the staff of life." ....
"Unfortunately, in a terrible blow to natural-products chemistry in the US, the Board of Scientific Counsellors, Div. of Cancer Treatment, NCI, voted on Oct. 2, 1981, to abolish the NCI research contract program concerned with the development of anti-tumor agents from plants. On the other hand, the synthetic drug development program was left intact, though reduced. ...Pharmaceutical firms... have clearly signaled their relative disinterest in natural products. .... The search for natural drugs, the safest & economically &/or ecologically most desireable types, has been abandoned in the US." - James Duke, PhD; Chief, Germplasm Resources Lab., &, Economic Botany Lab., Agri. Res. Serv., USDA; "The Spices of Life", ("Unedited discussion draft, neither approved nor expected to be approved by NIH or the USDA.").

"I never have & never will approve a 'new drug' to an individual, but only to a large pharmaceutical firm with unlimited finances." - FDA, Bureau of Drugs Director, Dr. J. Richard Crout, (in <u>Spotlight</u>, Jan. 18, 1982, p.14).

"...Over a 1,000 medical studies have demonstrated DPH (di-phenyl-hyd-antoin) to be one of the most widely useful drugs.... Yet (its) only listed indication-of-use with the FDA is as an anti-convulsant."
"...For 8 years I...saw 3 secretaries of HEW, 2 assistant secretaries of HEW, 2 commissioners of the FDA, members of the staff of the FDA, a surgeon general,.... ...No official seemed to think he had the authority or responsibility to get it done."
"When an FDA listing is granted, it entitles a company to advertise & promote a drug for the purposes for which it has been approved. .... When patents expire, competition comes in & drives the price down. Thus, financial incentive to look for a new drug is far greater than it is to look for new uses of an old drug."
"...The (PDR) <u>Physicians' Desk Reference</u>...carries only those uses for a drug that are listed with the FDA." - Jack Dreyfus, open letter to President R. Reagan.
"'Once the new drug is in a local pharmacy, the physician may...vary the conditions of use from those approved in the package insert, without informing or obtaining the approval of the FDA.'" - FDA Commissioner Charles C. Edwards, <u>The Federal Register</u>, v.37, n.158, Aug.15, 1972.
- Jack Dreyfus; President, Dreyfus Fund; Partner, Dreyfus & Co.; head, Dreyfus Medical Foundation; <u>A Remarkable Medicine Has Been Overlooked</u>, c.1970 (1982), p.xxi-xxv, 110.

"In 1950, the NCI of the USPHS established a program for study of environmental chemical factors in cancer. Within a few years, a Dr. ... , then director of the Institute of Industrial Medicine at NYU, told me that he had been retained by a group of chemical industries to call upon the Surgeon General & object to studies conducted under this program. He stated that his objection had been successful, & that all field studies by the NCI in this program would be stopped. They were."

"A few years later, I showed this same gentleman data indicating a cancer hazard for men employed in another industry that had retained him as a consultant. He advised me to keep out of this problem, & shortly thereafter, notified me that my appointment as associate professor of industrial medicine at NYU would not be renewed. It was not renewed." - Dr. William E. Smith; chair, symposium on cancer prevention, Sixth International Cancer Congress; Hearings, Subcommittee on Health & Science, US House of Representatives, July, 1957, (in William Longgood, Pulitzer Prize winner in journalism, The Poisons in Your Food, c.1960, 1976, p.196-7).

"In 1981, the AFL-CIO &...the Teamsters, urged (Thorne) Auchter (Dir., OSHA (Occupational Safety & Health Administration)) to act immediately. ...3 authoritative govt. studies had projected 999 cancer deaths out of every 1,000 workers exposed to EDB (Ethylene Di-Bromide, a pesticide) at the existing OSHA limit. .... Instead Auchter embarked on a time-consuming rule-making process that ignored the urgency...." - Ida Honorof, Report to the Consumer, v.14, n.324, p.4, Aug. 1984.

"...A charge of conflict of interest against former OSHA (Occupational Safety & Health Adm.) Director Thorne Auchter (is) being examined by the FBI. ...Auchter resigned as head of OSHA to become President of (a co.). Earlier, he had dismissed a series of 12 OSHA violations against the same co. ...." - Health Policy Advisory Center, Health PAC Bulletin, v.15, n.3, p.21, May 1984.

B.Q.3.0 TOP BIO-MEDICS & OTHERS:
B.Q.3.1 PREVENTION / NUTRITION:

"In my practice as surgeon, I am impressed by the alarming increase of cancer cases lately brought to my notice; an increase, which in the light of the general hygenic & sanitary improvements of our time, can point to no other cause than an indulgence in certain foodstuffs detrimental to the normal life of the body." - Dr. Charles Mayo, Mayo Clinic / Found'n, (in Richard E. Welch, MD, New Hope for Cancer Victims, p.3).

"... The opinion has frequently been advanced by ancient & modern writers that there is a direct relationship between diet & cancer frequency, & particularly ... in regard to the excessive consumption of salt & meat. The per capita rise in the meat consumption of the principal civilized countries has often been referred to as a causative factor in the corresponding rise in the cancer death rate." - Dr. Frederick L. Hoffman, chief statistician, Prudential Life Ins. Co.; (author, Cancer & Diet); The Mortality From Cancer Throughout the World, c.1914, (in Maureen Salaman, Nutrition: the Cancer Answer, p.16).

"Some of the more severe (cancer cases) showed very markedly the benefit of dietetic...measures. ...shown by occasional cases of unquestioned cancer known to have entirely disappeared for many years, (as) sometimes reported, & also by my own experience during the last 30 or 40 years...." - L. Duncan Bulkley, MD; Founder: Am. Assoc. for the Study & Cure of Cancer, &, Senior Physician, NY Skin & Cancer Hosp.; Member, AACR (Amer. Assoc. for Cancer Research, now the ACS); Author, Cancer & Its Non-Surgical Treatment, (in Judith Glassman, The Cancer Survivors, p.60).

"Think back over the years of cancer research, of the millions spent, the time consumed, the pains expended...& where are we today? Isn't it time to take stock of our basic concept to see if there isn't something radically wrong to account for the years of utter & complete failure to date? .... We have come to regard these processed foods as the hallmark of civilization, when it is a fact that these very foods set the stage for every sort of ill, including cancer." - Dr. William Howard Hay, (in Cancer Journal, 1927 AD).

"In the past, money has been spent like water in so-called cancer research, all of which is utterly wasted...." - Dr. W.H.Hay, A New Era, 1935.

(To) "avoid cancer...eat whole wheat bread, raw fruits & vegetables & their juices.... Drain the body of its poisons, feed it properly...." - Sir William Arbuthnot Lane, "noted English surgeon", in lecture at Johns Hopkins Med., 1940's.

- Dr. Lynn Dallin, Cancer Causes & Natural Controls, p.14, 82, & 83, (for last 3 paragraphs above).

"Food is infinitely the most important problem of the present day &, if properly dealt with, must result in the disappearance of the vast bulk of disease, misery, & death." - Sir Arbuthnot Lane, MD, famous surgeon, England, (in Alvenia Fulton, ND, PhD, BTh, Radiant Health Through Nutrition, p.23).

"The relationship of nutrition to cancer has received much attention in the past ten years.... ...Diet & nutrition must be considered by all investigators in the cancer field, & not only by those who happen to be specifically interested in nutrition.... It is now well established that a diet restricted to approx. 2/3 of ...ad libitum (max. desired) effects a significant reduction in...tumors...;in the mouse (; &) the incidence of spontaneous breast tumors is significantly increased ...by a high-fat diet; (as are)...skin tumors...." (Aug. 4, 1944).

"At the present time, there is widespread interest in the relationship of nutrition to tumors.... ...A natural diet contains a more adequate quality, quantity, & balance of essential components than our present day synthetic diets."

- Albert Tannenbaum, MD, Dir., Dept. Cancer Research, Michael Reese Hospital, Chicago; conference, AAAS (Amer. Assoc. for the Advancement of Science), 1944, & 1945, (in Peter Barry Chowka, "The NCI & the 50 Year Cover-Up", East West Journal, v.8, n.1, p.22, Jan. 1978).

"To prevent cancer, it is therefore proposed, first, to keep the speed of the bloodstream so high that the venous blood still contains sufficient oxygen; second, to keep high the concentration of hemoglobin in the blood; third, to add always to the food...the active groups of the respiratory enzymes.... If at the same time, exo-genous carcinogens are excluded rigorously, then most cancers may be prevented today." (Preface to the First Ed.).

"...Dean Burk...of the NCI...shows.... ...fermentation increases with the malignancy...." (p.7).

"...A cancer...precursor...Plummer-Vinson syndrome. ...can be healed (with dietary) respiratory enzymes...: iron salts, riboflavin, nicotinamide, & pantothenic acid. ....With...nicotinamide, tuberculosis can be healed quite as well as with streptomycin, but without the side effects...." (p.14, 15).

- Otto Warburg, Nobel Laureate in Medicine twice; Dir., Max Planck Inst. of Cell Physiol.; honorary degrees, Harvard U., & Oxford U., & Heidelberg U. ; The Prime Cause & Prevention of Cancer, (English Edition by Dean Burk), p.7, 14, 15, & Preface to First Ed.

"...Personal activity is ... essential to produce any significant decrease in cancer incidence. We need to change our lifestyle to eliminate smoking, reduce exposure to sunlight, & avoid pollutants, but most of all, change our diets to include all known nutrients, & exclude (if at) all possible, processed, devitalized food that has been depleted of its protective nutrients." - Dr. John Higginson, Director, IARC (International Agency for Research on Cancer); Universities Associated for Research & Education in Pathology, Inc. (p.ix).

"Dietary deficiencies lead to malfunctions of the body that cause cancer." - Ernst L. Wynder, Pres., American Health Found'n. (p.1).
- (in Ruth Yale Long, PhD, & 2 Masters in Nutrition; JICAN (Journal, International College of Applied Nutrition) Award; (author: Crackdown on Cancer; & Nutrition & Cancer Update); No More Cancer, p.ix, 1, for last 2 paragraphs above).

"Nutrients, food additives, or contaminants, may act as carcino-gens, co-carcinogens, or both; nutrient deficiencies may lead to biochemical abnormalities which, in turn, promote neoplastic processes; & excess intake of certain nutrients may produce metabolic abnormalities that promote neoplasms." - Dr. Ernst Wynder, Pres., Amer. Health Found'n, & Dr. B.S.Reddy, "Diet & Cancer of Colon", Nutrition & Cancer, M.Winick, et.al.,Eds., (in Dr. Lynn Dalin, Cancer Causes & Natural Controls, p.76).

B.Q.3.3 DOUBLE STANDARD IN RESEARCH, MODERNS:

"...the self-satisfied dogmatism with which mankind at each period of its history cherishes the delusion of the finality of existing modes of knowledge."
- Alfred North Whitehead, (in Robert E. Netterberg, DDS, & Robert Taylor, Prof., The Cancer Conspiracy, c.1981, p.98.

"Now & then, in all ages & at all levels, exceptional individuals appear who rise above current concepts, who seem to be actuated by higher principles & greater humanity. Perhaps such individuals are outstanding in that they refuse to accept the commonly held basic assumptions." - Karl Menninger, MD,(Founder, Menninger Clinic / Foundation, & Winter VA Hosp. (world's largest psych. training program); author, The Human Mind), The Vital Balance; (in Robert W. Stickle, (author: Cancer - One Man's Fight to Control Malignancy), A Rational Concept of Cancer, p.6).

"In 1946, Oxford University in England was offered large funds to create a new Institute of Human Nutrition. The University refused the funds on the ground that the knowledge of human nutrition was essentially complete, & that the proposed Institute would soon run out of meaningful research projects." - René Dubos , Prof. Emeritus, Rockefeller Univ., "The Intellectual Basis of Nutritional Science & Practice", Critical Food Issues of the Eighties, (M. Chou & D.P.Harmon, Ed.), p.95.

"...These healers...my intellect has been unable to assimilate their theories .... But their facts are patent & startling; & anything that interferes with the multiplication of such facts, & with our freest opportunity of observing & studying them, will, I believe, be a public calamity." - William James, in Boston Transcript, 1894.

"...The inertia of the human mind, & its resistance to innovation are most clearly demonstrated...by professionals with a vested interest in tradition & in the monopoly of learning. Innovation is a two-fold threat to academic mediocrities; it endangers their oracular authority, & it evokes the deeper fear that their whole laboriously constructed intellectual edifice may collapse." - Arthur Koestler, The Sleepwalkers.
- Brian Inglis, The Case for Unorthodox Medicine, p.238-9, (for last 2 paragraphs above).

"...As Thomas Kuhn pointed out in The Structure of Scientific Revolutions, new scientific theories in any field are regarded with skepticism because scientists become attached to the old perspective earlier in their careers." ....

"Whatever the rationale, the suppression of unorthodox cancer theories & the sustained persecution of their proponents by govt. & colleagues runs counter to freedom of thought, much less freedom of choice." - Marilyn Ferguson, (author, The Aquarian Conspiracy; Editor, Brain / Mind Bulletin), "Are Promising Treatments Being Blacked Out?", Leading Edge Bulletin, M.Ferguson, Editor, v.1,n.6,p.3,Dec.1,1980.

"...Innovation is necessarily alternative.... The advance is early branded as heresy ("quackery, charlatanry, fraud, hoax") to be condemned & proscribed without serious testing by all respected, responsible members of the virtuous elite." ....

"In the past century over 100 methods have been offered by independent researchers as aiding in recovery from cancer. ...contrary to the nihilistic litany of cancer bureaucrats that there is 'no evidence'." - Robert Houston, "The War on Answers", Our Town, Sept. 3, 1978, (in CCS, Cancer Control Journal,v.6,n.1,p.116-9).

"A frequent criticism of holistic medical practices is that they have not been scientifically validated by research studies, published in peer-reviewed journals. Individuals making this criticism imply that they, the established conformists, are peers of those innovative, unorthodox, & truly creative individuals who are bringing about the next step in the evolution of medicine. The fact is that such innovators have no peers. They stand alone on the leading edge of science."
- Elmer M. Cranton, MD, Pres., AHMA (Amer. Holistic Medical Assoc.), (in HDA (Holistic Dental Assoc.), The Communicator, v.2,n.2,p.1,Nov. 1981).

"A theory appears to be a prerequisite for a diagnostic system to be accepted; further, it has to be a theory that is in agreement with currently accepted medical beliefs. This is unfortunate...."

"Karagulla, a neurologist, studied a clairvoyant individual who claimed to see directly the energy fields of the physical organs of the patient's body.... In several dozen observational tests, the clairvoyant was able to accurately diagnose...." - Arthur Hastings, PhD; Prof., Stanford Univ.; Research Assoc., Inst. of Noetic Sciences; Prof., Cal. Inst. of Transpersonal Psych.; Adj. Prof., JFK U., Orinda, Cal.; (co-author, Argumentation & Advocacy, Group Communication Through Computers,v.2, & Changing Images of Man); "Alternative Forms of Diagnosis", Health for the Whole Person, Arthur C. Hastings, PhD, James Fadiman, PhD, & James S. Gordon, MD, Editors, (Foreword by US Senator Ted Kennedy), c.1980,(1981, Bantam), p.462, 471.

"...Arigo saw as many as 300 patients a day.... ...Under pressure from the medical establishment & the Catholic Church, he was charged with practicing 'illegal medicine'. ....(Brazil's) Pres. J. Kubitschek granted Arigo a presidential pardon. ...."

"In the test,Arigo gave an immediate verbal diagnosis of each patient who stepped in front of him. Of 1,000 such patients, chosen at random, 545 had brought their official medical records with them. In 518 of these cases, Arigo's spontaneous diagnosis matched that of the patient's own doctor."
- Reader's Digest, Mysteries of the Unexplained, p.279, 281.

(The system is)"'fostering...a climate of conformity, not by the total suppression of dissent, but by the presentation of views which fall outside the consensus as curious heresies, or, even more effectively, by treating them as irrelevant eccentricities, which serious & reasonable people may dismiss as of no consequence.'" - R. Miliband, The State In Capitalist Society, c.1969, p. 268.

(Continued)

"...The system of influence & control...is highly skewed in favor of the corporate & financial value system. And this dominant influence is felt not only in universities, foundations, & institutions of higher learning, but also ...from the media to all other instruments of communication." - Vicente Navarro,(Prof. of Health & Social Policy, Johns Hopkins U.; Editor-in-Chief. International Journal of Health Services; author, Social Security & Medicine in the USSR: a Marxist Critique); Medicine Under Capitalism, c.1976,(1977), p.153, (for last 2 paragraphs above).

"'It's not what you know, but who knows what. .... At the heart of the matter is society's tendency to insist on credentials before listening seriously to a claim of new discoveries or ideas. .... Only rarely...does the public acknowledge that an unknown & unanointed person may have noteworthy capacities.'" - Fred Hechinger, of &in New York Times, June 2, 1981, review & comment.

"'Everything that has happened in publishing during the last 2 decades has conspired to focus greater & greater emphasis on the few big moneymakers ... (&) to exclude...those venturesome books....'" - C. Lehmann-Haupt, of NY Times.

"'...That genius is a rare exception(:) It's not true. Talent & genius have been wasted on an enormous scale throughout our history; this is all I know for sure.'" - Eric Hoffer, (author. The True Believer, &, Thinking & Working on the Waterfront, ...).

"...Sigmund Freud, ...John Stuart Mill, Charles Darwin, Albert Einstein, ... achieved intellectual preeminence without benefit of a faculty position."

"...Self publishing (was done by:)...Walt Whitman, Gertrude Stein, Mary Baker Eddy, James Joyce...." - Ronald Gross, The Independent Scholar's Handbook, p.xv, 36, 101, 140-1, 145.

"We live in a society that penalizes highly creative individuals for their non-conformist autonomy. This makes the teaching of problem solving in design both discouraging & difficult. A...student (has) massive blocks against new ways of thinking, engendered by some 16 years of mis-education...."

"Only a handful of American corporations & design offices are seriously engaged in facing up to challenges such as global minimal shelter needs, off road vehicles for roadless terrain.... The list is endless...."

"Discrimination against the poor by designers & their employers is reflected in the pricing...."

"...The school bus. ...give(s) insufficient protection to children & driver."

"Where are well designed, low cost inserts that would convert any station wagon to an ambulance....?" - Prof. Victor Papanek,(Dean, School of Design, Cal. Inst. of Arts; UNESCO Internat'l Design Expert; Prof.: Purdue U., & SUNY; student of: Frank Lloyd Wright, & MIT; co-author, Nomadic Furniture), Design for the Real World, (Intro. by R. Buckminster Fuller), c.1971, p.142, 146, 147, 163, 189.

"'Some colleagues...accused me of 'arrogance' for thinking that I could contribute to a field of research in which I had no experience. ....Funding agencies are discouraged from 'risk-taking'.... ...'Compartmentalization'(:)... The peer review system tends to give truly innovative ideas — especially those that cross disciplinary boundaries — mixed reviews because the peers do not understand it. ....Recommendations:...award...a contract or grant monitor for having recognized an innovative project in its early stages & having supported it.'" - Richard A. Muller; recipient of Alan T. Waterman Award; testimony, US House, Subcommittee on Science, Research, & Technology, Sept. 11, 1979.

"The Catch-22 in any funding system is the inability of those not funded to complain — by definition, they are the unchosen, & hence their testimony is suspect." - FAS (Federation of American Scientists), Public Interest Report, v.33,n.1,p.4, Jan. 1980, (for last 2 paragraphs avove).

"Scientists & technologists are ordinary human beings. ...susceptible to...herd instinct, following the leader, & falling for fashions. .... Fashions rage among scientists. ...Big instruments make us force-fit our problems to the solution. .... As our instruments push us toward picoseconds, & 1Å, & ppb, we get ultimately reductionist in a sense, while the real problems go far beyond our data & papers, to the survival of local industry, & international trade, & nuclear annihilation."
 - Rustum Roy, Dir. Materials Research Lab., Penn. State U., (in American Lab., Sept. 1982, p.4, 6).

B.Q.3.4 FAMOUS BIOMEDICS, ANCIENTS:

"...The Chinese in the 9th century AD utilized a book entitled The Thousand Golden Prescriptions, which described how rice polish could be used to cure beri-beri, as well as other nutritional approaches to the prevention & treatment of disease. It was not until 12 centuries later that the cure for beri-beri was discovered in the West & it was acknowledged to be a vitamin B-1 deficiency disease." - Jeffrey Bland, PhD, Your Health Under Siege: Using Nutrition to Fight Back, p.43.

"Vesalius, a...layman, was born in 1514 (AD).... He...found things different from Galen's ideas. He found also that a man has just as many ribs as a woman, despite the fact that God used one of Adam's ribs to create Eve. He...prepar(ed) a new book on anatomy. .... It was not from the Church that he suffered persecution.... His fiercest opposition came from his colleagues, & he had to abandon his position as an anatomy instructor. In disgust, he burned his books & gave up the study of anatomy altogether. Later he was made a court physician. It is fortunate that he was not able to burn all his books & many remained in other hands. In due time, these books proved that Vesalius was far ahead of his day."

"...Father Philip. He is even credited with healing Pope Clement VII. .... After his miraculous cure, the pope spoke about it often.... There was the case of a woman who had a cancer of the breast. ....He prayed to the Lord in her behalf, reached forth his hand & touched the cancer. .... When the physician came to cauterize the cancer, he was amazed to find her perfectly healthy."
 - Carl J. Scherzer, The Church & Healing, c.1950, p.78-80.

"...In 1540...Ambroise Paré...persuaded doctors to stop the horrid practice of pouring boiling oil on wounds (&)...required all doctors to wash thoroughly before delivering babies or performing surgery.... ...(In) 1844...Ignaz Semmelweis in Vienna proved...that clean, well-scrubbed doctors would not infect & kill mothers at childbirth. For his efforts Semmelweis was dismissed from his hospital...(&) despite publication, his work was totally ignored. As a result, he became insane & died in an asylum, & his son committed suicide." (p.17-18).

"As a chemist working for the US govt. in 1916 on the island of Luzon (Philippines), (R.R.) Williams, over the opposition of orthodox medicine, had managed to eradicate beriberi...by persuading the population to drink rice bran tea. In 1917, Williams was recalled to the US, & thereafter orthodox medicine discouraged anyone from drinking rice bran tea, so by 1920 there were more beriberi deaths on Luzon than in 1915. .... In 1934, R.R.Williams (now) at Bell Telephone Labs., discovered thiamine (Vitamin B-1). (&) that thiamine in rice bran both prevented & cured beriberi." (Introduction).

"Christiaan Eijkman in Holland...shared the Nobel Prize for Medicine in 1929 for proving in 1892 ("37 years before!") that beriberi was not an infectious disease...."
 - Wayne Martin, BS, Purdue Univ.; Sr. Metallurgist, Sperry Gyro., & 3 large aluminum firms; (author, Medical Heroes & Heretics; &, "The Beri-beri Analogy to Myocardial Infarction", Medical Hypothesis, v.10, p.185-198, 1983; &, Lancet, n.8346, p.407, Aug. 13, 1983); We Can Do Without Heart Attacks, p.8-10, 17-18.

"In 1593, Sir Richard Hawkins noted & later published, in observations on his voyage into the South Seas, references that natives of the area used sour oranges & lemons as a cure for scurvy, & a similar result was noted among his crew. .... In 1804, regulations were introduced into the British Navy requiring use of lime juice.... ...(&) into law by the British Board of Trade in 1865.... ...It took 2 centuries to translate empirical observation into action...." - Maureen Salaman, MSc, Nutrition: the Cancer Answer, p.34.

"Scurvy is nearly allied to the Plague, as it occasions carbuncles, buboes (as in Bubonic; enlarged & inflamed lymph nodes), & cancer." - Martini, 1609 AD.

"In some, (with scurvy)...on each motion of their joints, a noise was heard as (, in arthritis,)...crackling...." - Sennerti, 1624 AD.

"I took 12 patients in scurvy on board.... They lay together in one place ...& had one common diet.... 2 (patients) had each 2 oranges & 1 lemon given them every day; these they eat with greediness.... The consequence was that most sudden & visible good effects..., one ... being at the end of 6 days fit for duty...." - James Lind, (1716-1794 AD), (also citing the last 2 paragraphs above this one).

"Scurvy is wont to occasion a consumption of the lungs." - Richard Morton, Phthisiologia, 1689 AD.

"Acute Lymphatic Leukemia (:)...The most striking clinical symptoms...are the hemorrhages.... The teeth sit loosely.... ...making a condition completely identical with that of scurvy." - Dr. Felix Pincus, (in Nothnagel's Encyclopedia of Practical Medicine, c.1905 AD, p.552).

- last 5 paragraphs above in W. J. McCormick, MD, "Have We Forgotten the Lesson of Scurvy?", Journal of Applied Nutrition, v.15, n.1&2, p.4, 1962 (reprint n.5H, by the Lee Foundation for Nutritional Research).

"Cotton Mather...asked (his slave) if he had ever had the pox. The slave... answered, 'Yes & no,' ...(&) explained that his tribe in Africa had the custom of (innoculation). Mather seized the idea as his own & today is credited with ... introducing innoculation to the New World." - Hugh Drummond, MD, (in Mother Jones, Found'n for National Progress, A Sourcebook on Health & Survival, p.38).

"'...This large & expensive stock in drugs will be unnecessary. By...doses of ...medicines...multiplying...combining them properly, 20 to 30 articles, aided by the common resources of the lancet, a garden, a kitchen, fresh air, cool water, & exercise, will be sufficient to cure all the diseases that are at present under the power of medicine.'" - Dr. Benjamin Rush, Signer, Declaration of Independence; Member, Continental Congress; BS, Princeton U.; 16 Introductory Lectures, p.288.

"'We have no discoveries in the materia medica to hope for from the Indians in North America. It would be a reproach to our schools of physic if modern physicians were not more successful than the Indians, even in the treatment of their own diseases.'" - Dr. Benjamin Rush, Medical Inquiries & Observations, v.1, p.46; & Appendix p.36-37, paraphrased next:

"In another essay, Rush states precisely the opposite - that the indigenous medicines of America...are useful, & that the doctor should not hesitate to find out from old women, midwives, nurses, 'even Indians & negroes', what they know." - Harris Coulter, PhD, Divided Legacy: the Conflict Between Homoeopathy & the AMA, p.38, 40, 79, (for last 3 paragraphs above).

"In the 1850's, Ignaz P. Semmelweiss, a Hungarian doctor, discovered that childbed fever, which then killed about 12 mothers out of every 100, was contagious ...& that doctors themselves were spreading the disease by not cleaning their hands. He was ridiculed.... Opponents of his idea attacked him fiercely. ...(&) brought on (his) mental illness. ...(He) died a broken man." - Salem Kirban, Health Guide for Survival, p.18.

"Marshall Hall...was rejected, reviled, & ridiculed, but his work concerning the reflex actions of the spinal cord was finally recognized. ....Bodington ...taught that tubercular patients needed fresh, clean air as part of their cure. His medical colleagues execrated him & called him a charlatan, but were later forced to admit that his work was logical & correct." - Donald Law, PhD, DBM, Psy.D., A Guide to Alternative Medicine, p.10.

"In Boston, somewhat later (than 1842), medics ask for - & get - a law permitting bathtubbing only on possession of a prized medical prescription."

"(In) 1844...Dr. William T. G. Morton, 2 years out of...dental college... runs into sulphuric ether. ...the birth of anesthesia. ...Physicians & surgeons...label him a 'quack', even while they hurry to capitalize on (it). (Morton) died a pauper."

"Sister Elizabeth Kenny, an Australian nurse...showed...how to cure... infantile paralysis.... ...(by) apply(ing) hot packs to the paralyzed limbs.... (She was) ordered...to leave the country." - Morris A. Bealle, The Drug Story, c.1949 & 1976, p.225-6, 233-4.

"Dr. Carlos Finlay knew the cause of yellow fever, but because he had not carried out experiments to 'prove' it, he was laughed off the rostrum at a medical meeting. 20 years later, Dr. Walter Reed found that Finlay had been right all along. How many died in the interim while the establishment waited for what they would accept as 'proof'?" - Herald of Health, v.82, n.12, p.10, Dec. 1977.

"What if Major Walter Reed had not listened & learned from an old Scotch - Cuban physician, Carlos Finlay, that yellow fever was due to a mosquito & not from the dank marsh air? Or contaminated feces? The great medicoes at Washington & elsewhere thought Reed was crazy & had done everything in their power to discourage him & his human-volunteer experiment - which finally scientifically proved the cause of the fatal 'Yellow Jack'."

"What of the mob howling & throwing stones outside the house of Dr. Crawford W. Long, the discoverer of ether anesthesia?" ....

"What of Frederic Gibbs, the brain researcher, who demonstrated one of the first electro-encephalographs in America ("now famous as the 'brain-wave' machine"..."EEG")? At an AMA meeting in 1934, the machine was publically called a 'fake'. By...'eminent physicians'...." - Herbert Bailey, A Matter of Life or Death: the Incredible Story of Krebiozen, p.177-8.

"...Until 1954, great & wonderful discoveries were based on what is now called ("disparaging"-ly) anecdotal evidence. .... In 1921, 29-year-old Frederick Banting in Canada, on no one's payroll & with $500, discovered insulin. .... A controlled study on insulin for diabetics would have been a legal form of murder....(:)...50 patients in one group.... ...would have been given no insulin. They would have died. .... In 1923.... ...Banting shared the Nobel prize for medicine for his anecdotal discovery of insulin."

"It took orthodox medicine 57 years to understand & accept Sir William Osler's teaching that a heart attack involved a blood clot in a coronary artery, followed by a myocardial infarction." - Wayne Martin, We Can Do Without Heart Attacks, p.175-6, 203.

"'Penicillin sat on a shelf for ten years while I was called a quack.'" - Sir Alexander Fleming.

"...Ramifications of those discoveries...threatened to obviate the establishment which embraced the conventional wisdom.... ...Those who expound new ideas...are ignored by the establishment.... They can't find teaching jobs, or research funds, & they can't find a forum in the journals of the day." - "The Laetrile Controversy - & the Cancer Racket", Los Angeles Examiner, Oct. 15, 1978, (in CCS, Cancer Control Journal, v.6, n.1, p.69, Jan. 1978, 1982).

"'But how long prevention will be avoided depends on how long the prophets of unbelief will succeed in obstructing the application of scientific knowledge in the cancer field. In the meantime, millions must die of cancer unnecessarily.'" - Dr. Otto Warburg; Nobel Laureate in Medicine twice; Director, Max Planck Inst. of Cell Physiology; "Lindau Lecture: The Prime Cause & Prevention of Cancer". (p.33).

"'The intolerance & fanaticism of official science toward Eijkman's observations (that refined rice caused beri beri) brought about the death of some half million people on the American continent in our own century between 1900 & 1910.'" - Josue de Castro, The Geography of Hunger, p.54.(p.75).

"'From about 1850 until the late 1930's, one of the standing jokes in the medical profession, was about a few idiots who called themselves doctors, who claimed that they could cure pneumonia by feeding their patients moldy bread. ...Until...they discovered penicillin...In moldy bread!'" - P.E. Binzel, MD.(p.70).

- Thomas H. Mansell, Cancer Simplified, c.1976 & 1977, p.33, 70, 75, (for last 3 paragraphs above).

"The English surgeon John Abernathy proposed in 1816 that cancer is a constitutional disease not confined to local growths, & that it should be regarded & treated accordingly."

"(In) 1829, two French investigators, Lobstein & Racamier, attributed the origin of tumors to embryo-nical cell proliferation which persisted into adulthood."

- Dr. Lynn Dallin, Cancer Causes & Natural Controls, p.11 & 32.

B.Q.3.5 NOBEL LAUREATES:

"...It would be possible to make much more progress than has been made if the NCI knew its job better, knew how to make discoveries. ...The NCI really does not know how to make discoveries. ....So long as the NCI is not willing to follow up ideas that seem to be good to people who have had experience in making discoveries, the work of the NCI is going to be pedestrian." - Linus Pauling, PhD; Nobel Laureate twice; Pres., Amer. Chemical Society;(& its Priestley Medalist); author; No More War ; &, Cancer & Vitamin C; L. Pauling Inst. of Sci. & Med.

"...What kills science in this country now, (is) that you must tell in advance what you will find, & what you will do exactly, & what you will spend your money on. And if you know it all, then you needn't do it. .... And so you cannot have (any) new discoveries." - Albert Szent-Gyorgyi, MD, PhD; Nobel Laureate; discoveror of vitamins C & P; Scientific Dir., National Found'n for Cancer Research.

- Non Fiction Television, WNET / Thirteen, PBS, The Cancer War, by Ralph Moss, PhD, et. al., May-July, 1983, (for last 2 paragraphs above).

B.Q.4.0 PRIVATE MEDICAL UNIONS & GROUPS:

B.Q.4.1 ACS:

"'The proponents of new or unproven methods of cancer management(:)....A few hold PhD or MD degrees.... They may have multiple unusual degrees...from correspondence school.'" - ACS, Unproven Methods ..., 1971.

"...60 advocates of unorthodox therapies whose credentials are given in the ACS book (above).(:)...Of these 60, thirty nine or almost 2/3, hold...medical degrees from such universities as Harvard, Illinois, Northwestern, Yale, Dublin, Oxford, or Toronto. 2 are osteopaths. 3...also hold...("PhD's")...scientific...reputable.... 8 other(s) received PhD's in such fields as chemistry, physiology, bacteriology, parasitology, or medical physics, from...Yale, Johns Hopkins, UC Berkeley, Columbia, & NYU. Thus, over 75% ... are medical doctors or doctors of philosophy in scientific areas." - Ralph Moss, The Cancer Syndrome, c.1980, p.80-81.

"'Radium will not cure cancer. It only destroys cancer tissue within a certain radius, but does not drive the disease from the blood.'" - Dr. Francis Carter Wood; V. Pres., ASCC (American Society for the Control of Cancer, which changed into ACS in 1944); Prof. Emeritus, St. Luke's Hosp., NY.

"'...Doctors' investments in radium...the price of radium increased 1,000% when they began to use it on cancer victims....'" - E. Josephson, MD.

"'"Now that you (the ASCC) have given us (the Clement Cleveland) medal, put us to work"'" - National Assoc. of Science Writers spokesman.

- last 2 paragraphs above in Emanuel M. Josephson,MD, Your Life Is Their Toy.
- (last 3 quotations above in Morris A. Bealle, The Drug Story, c.1949 & 1976, p.84, 85, 88.

"'Research in the US has been seriously affected by restrictions imposed by foreign cartel members. .... It has attempted to suppress the publication of scientific research data which were at variance with its monopoly interest. ....The hostility of cartel members toward a new product which endangers their control of the market(:)....In the field of synthetic hormones, the cartel control has been...detrimental to our national interest.'" - US Assistant Attorney General, Wendell Berge, Cartels, Challenge to a Free World, p.58, 81, 84.

"In...Berge('s book)...Elmer H. Bobst ("Chairman of the Board...of the ACS... (&) owner of" a major drug co., was) prosecuted by the Dept. of Justice for violation of the anti-trust laws. .... On Dec. 17, 1941, Bobst was found guilty by the Court, & fined $6,000." - David Kasson, "The ACS", The Independent, n.65, April 1957, (in Eleanor McBean, The Poisoned Needle, p.208, (for last 2 paragraphs above)).

"Indeed, dietary regimens are among the cruel & deceptive practices used by 'quacks' in attracting healthy people as well as cancer patients to follow their approaches & dangerous philosophy." - Dr. Vernon R. Young, Dept. Nutrition & Food Science, MIT; & Dr. Paul M. Newberne; "Vitamins...", ACS, Proceedings of the National Conference on Cancer Prevention & Detection - 1980, (Cancer Supplement,v.47,n.5,p.1227,March 1, 1981).

"...The ACS raised over $180 million last year through its network of 58 Divisions & 3,000 local Chapters. The Society's major public campaign is aimed at reducing smoking & the cancers related to it. Yet...the ACS has but a single (lobbyist) in Wash. (DC). The industry-supported Tobacco Inst., on the other hand, has a ten million $ budget which supports dozens of Washington staff." - Michael Jacobson, Dir., CSPI (Center for Science in the Public Interest, including, Health Charities Reform Project), (in Heartland, n.9, p.27, Win./Spring 1982).

"Questions arise with respect to ACS's accumulation of assets beyond the amount required for its next year's budget." ....

"...For many years, the primary focus of the (ACS's) promotional & fund-raising materials has been on the need for funds for research, for which (research) the percentile allocation (by ACS) has actually declined over this ten year period." ....

"...The percentage of...research to total expenses has ranged from a high of 36.8% in fiscal 1967, to a low of 27.1% in fiscal 1975. During the same ten year period, total assets have increased about $110,300,000, from about $76,500,000 to about $186,800,000; & total expenses have increased...to about $113,900,000."
- NIB (National Information Bureau), "ACS", n.1100, p.1 & 4, Oct. 27, 1978.

"'We are guilty of pussyfooting in a number of areas like this (diet & prevention).'" - AHA (Amer. Heart Assoc.) Deputy Exec. V. Pres. John T. Connoly.

"'Question arises whether if AHA received more in contributions, the additional money would go to research. .... AHA's assertion that it was 'forced to decline many (research) applicants deserving of funding because the money was not available to fund them' is misleading to contributors.'" - NIB (National Information Bureau) Report, April 19, 1979.

"...The NIB (is) an independent charity watchdog organization...."

"...The AHA (is) the second largest private charity in the US. (First is ACS -Ed.)" - Peter Barry Chowka, "Laying Bare the Heart Disease Industry: the 25 Billion-$-a-Year Dead End", East West Journal, v.10, n.11, p.52, Nov. 1980.

"Last year Americans gave over $6 billion to public health charities. But where are those charities when the Congress moves to dismantle OSHA or to weaken standards over substances linked to birth defects?" - Belita Cowan, Exec. Dir., NWHN (National Women's Health Network), NWHN Newsletter, v.7, n.2, p.1, March 1982).

"'Reach for a (cigarette) instead of a sweet' - ...advertising...slogan...(of) Albert...Lasker, (with) Mary Lasker, health philantrophists, & originators of the Lasker Awards, an American version of the Nobel Prize. ...(& MSKCC) Memorial Sloan Kettering trustees." - Ralph Moss, Cancer Syndrome, p.263.

B.Q.4.3 AMA, (ETHICS, OATHS):

"No satisfactory evidence has been produced to indicate any significant cyto-toxic (cell - poison) effect of Laetrile on the cancer cell." (Conclusions).

"All of the physicians whose patients were reviewed spoke of increase in the sense of well-being & appetite, gain in weight, & decrease in pain...." (Text).

"...Hemorrhagic necrosis of tumor is extensive.... .... Two cases...showed moderate changes...which might be considered as chemotherapeutic toxic cellular changes (caused by Laetrile)." (Appendix 3; by: J. Budd, MD, & J. L. Zundell, autopsy).
- Dr. Ian MacDonald, Chairman, & Dr. Henry Garland, Secretary, Cancer Commission, California Medical Assoc., Report (in Cal. Med., April 1953).

"A...Hypothesis(:) cigarette smoking is causally related to...cancer (&) coronary arterio-sclerosis. After studying the question for several years, notably in... bronchial cancer, it is my considered opinion that the hypothesis is not proven...."
- Dr. Henry Garland, (at Public Health Section, Commonwealth Club, San Francisco).

"(Smoking is) a harmless pastime up to 24 cigarettes per day. .... A pack a day keeps lung cancer away." - Dr. Ian MacDonald, (in "Here's Another View: Tobacco May Be Harmless", US News & World Reports, Aug. 2, 1957, p.85-86).
- last 5 paragraphs above, in G. Edward Griffin, World Without Cancer, c.1974 (Dec. 1976), p.24-36.

"'I will hand on...learning...to those pupils duly apprenticed & sworn, & to none others.'" - Hippocratic Oath. (p.220).

"'...Before the introduction of paramedics, less than 1% of the patients that suffered a cardiac arrest...lived through.... With...paramedics...23% (of same)... go back to productive work in society. We think that's pretty amazing. .... However, relating that to the medical community is sometimes very difficult.'" - J. Dolphin, paramedic. (p.230)

"...Only physicians are likely to be regarded as competent to judge the qualifications of potential physicians, so licensing boards in the various states...are typically composed...of physicians, ...members of the AMA. The boards, or the state legistlatures, ...give the AMA the power to influence the number of persons admitted to practice.(by:)lengthy training, ...(&) the list of 'approved' schools & hospitals (which) is generally identical with the list issued by the Council on Medical Education & Hospitals of the AMA." - Milton & Rose Friedman, Free To Choose, p.220, 228, 230.

"'...The physician may continue to enjoy his title & pursue his practice, although he may have violated every rule of professional honor & every principle of morality. It is surely time that this anomaly were rectified.'" - AMA President Alfred Stille, Transactions of the AMA, v.22, p.97, 1871.

"'...To mix yourselves up with an organization (e.g. homoeopathy) for which every member of the regular profession has a sovereign & immitigable contempt(:)... the AMA & all our colleges would unquestionably place the medical department of your university under the ban, & cease to recognize your pupils.'" - AMA President Samuel Gross; Proceedings of the Michigan Inst. of Homoeopathy, 1867, p.511 & 637; &, Peninsular Journal of Medicine, v.11, p.588, 1875.

"... Any such unnatural union as the mingling of an exclusive system, such as homoeopathy, with scientific medicine in a school, ...(will) render every school adopting such a policy unworthy the support of the profession." - AMA, Transactions AMA, v.8, p.55, 1855.

- Harris L. Coulter, PhD, The Conflict Between Homoeopathy & the AMA, (v.3, of Divided Legacy: a History of Schism in Medical Thought; (with v.2, Progress & Regress)), p.207, 208, & 211, (for last 3 paragraphs above).

"Our reasons for being in political action are exactly the same as the AFL-CIO's. Exactly." - AMA Vice Pres. James Sammons, on Phil Donahue Show, TV, Nov. 22, 1982.

"...The House of Representatives...voted...to exempt the business practices of state-licensed professionals ("including doctors & dentists") from (FTC) Federal Trade Commission jurisdiction. .... The 208 Representatives who voted for the AMA/ADA backed position received more than twice as much (on average) from those (AMA/ADA political action committees) PACs as the 195 Members who voted for the compromise." - Common Cause, "$3.3 million in PAC Money Pays Off In Key Legistlative Victory for AMA & ADA, Common Cause Study Shows", press release, Dec.3, 1982. (Bill killed in Senate.)

"Even Hitler could not control his physicians, as seen from the report of Dr. Karl Gebhardt, who was called in to treat R. Heydrich, the Chief of the Security Service... , who had been shot:

'...By daily personal telephone calls from Hitler & Himmler in person, asking for information, very many suggestions were naturally made.... I did not hesitate to take personal responsibility & state my own view.... ...I refused, in reply to direct demands, to call in any other doctor, not even Morell ('Hitler's personal physician') or (Ferdinand) Sauerbruch. Heydrick died in 14 days.'"

- Thomas Preston, MD, Prof., The Clay Pedestal: a Re-examination of the Doctor-Patient Relationship, c.1981, p.172.

B.Q.4.4 ADA, (FLUORIDE):

(As of 1983) "Belgium, West Germany, & Sweden have abandoned their pilot fluoridation experiments on human populations, & are not fluoridating any public water supplies. Sweden, Denmark, & Holland have banned it completely. Many other countries, such as France, Italy, & Norway have never fluoridated their drinking water. Only about 2% of the total population of Europe is living in a fluoridated area." - John Yiamouyiannis, PhD, bio-chem.; BS, U. Chicago; Pres., Safe Water Foundation; Dir., NHAC (National Health Action Committee); Fluoride: The Aging Factor, c.1983, p.112.

"'The fluoride ion exerts its toxic effect by inhibiting the action of many enzyme systems.'" Dr. L.P.Sumner, Cornell U.&Dr.H.Theorell, Uppsala U., Sweden; both Nobel Laureates, enzyme chemistry.

"'Thus some of the serious charges thet are being laid at fluoride's door,—genetic damage, cancer, birth defects, & allergy response—may arise from fluoride interference after all.'" - J. Amer. Chem. Soc., &, New Scientist, both Jan. 1981.
- (last 2 quotes above in:) NFA (Natural Food Assoc.), Natural Food & Farming, v.28, n.12, p.8 & 13, June 1982.

"'...An incongruity exists between the training of the dental health team & the influence of diet & nutrition upon oral health. Little or no time has been allocated in the dental curriculum to this subject.'" - Herman Corn, Pres., Amer. Soc. Preventive Dentistry.

"Though few dentists let it out that dentin is continuously growing inside the tooth throughout our lives, the dental research literature leaves no doubt about this fact. ...It is the body's repair response...." - Soaring Bear, Natural Dental Wellness, p.5, & 21 (for last 2 paragraphs above).

B.Q.4.6 AMER. DIETETIC ASSOC.:

"Although the stated purpose of licensure is to benefit the public.... Consumers...have learned that licensing may add to the cost of services, while not assuring quality. .... Charges...the legal sector that licensure restricts competition,& therefore unnecessarily increases costs to consumers. .... Like other professionals, dietiticians can justify the enactment of licensure laws because licensing affords the opportunity to protect dietitians from interference in their field by other practitioners.... This protection provides a competitive advantage, & therefore is economically beneficial for dietitians." - ADA (American Dietetic Assoc.) Pres., Marilyn Haschske, JADA, April 1984, (in East West J., v.14, n.11, p.42, Nov. 1984).

B.Q.5.0 MASS MEDIA:
B.Q.5.1 PRESS:

"The chief of the Dept. of Agriculture's Bureau of Chemistry (FDA now), Dr. Harvey W. Wiley.... ...wrote a book telling...how those ("Pure Food & Drug Laws") had been scuttled from within government. .... Wiley...turned his precious manuscript over to a printer. That manuscript mysteriously 'disappeared'.... ... Dr. Wiley valiantly returned to work, rewriting his book from scratch. This chore occupied him totally for ten years. ...His volume, The History of a Crime Against the Food Law was a primer on govt. corruption.... When distribution began in 1929, ... Books disappeared rapidly from bookstore shelves. Yet no letters were received from readers, ...& virtually no reviews. ...Copies could not be found anywhere. In desperation, Dr. Wiley put the few remaining books in libraries around the country - they disappeared from libraries as quickly as they had vanished from the stores." - William Dufty, Sugar Blues, c.1975, p.163, 173-4.

"...In 1963.... I had the audacity...to publish a list of beneficial cancer treatments, where to obtain them, & what doctors were using them. Not long after (this was) published by my friend, an arsonist set fire to (his building's) first floor & completely gutted it. Firemen (stopped) the fire just (before) his apartment. .... After the firemen told my friend that he could return to his apartment, the police stepped in & said no he couldn't, whereupon the police ransacked the apartment & even took the man's money which they never returned to him." - Arlin J. Brown, Health Victory Bulletin, v.8,n.11,p.1,Nov. 1982.

"...My first book K - Krebiozen — Key to Cancer?(:)... An ad. for the book was placed in the ___ ___ Times...the freest of the large circulation newspapers.... The Times categorically refused a 2nd ad.... ...The Times' medical counselors had advised against accepting an ad...."

"'...I went to the Main Branch of the New York Public Library, the largest in the world. The librarian-in-charge advised me that...the author 'went against' the AMA (&) it was decided that this book (K-Krebiozen...) was to be 'taboo'.'"

"Dr. Ivy (co-author of 1,500 articles).... sent his article (on Krebiozen) to one medical journal after another. ...The journals accepted his article for publication, only to return it with apologies. .... Dr. Ivy was informed that the publi-(-shers) were told by the AMA Headquarters they would lose all their revenue from pharmaceutical advertising if they published Ivy's article. .... Finally, in desperation, Dr. Ivy turned to a small general publisher ("Henry Regnery, Chicago") & arranged for publication of his medical work." - Herbert Bailey, A Matter of Life or Death: the Incredible Story of Krebiozen, p.270, 272, 283, 284.

"The ...Times...headlined the Ass't US Attorney...grand jury investigation of myself, 6 months before the grand jury was even selected. ....Soon after Bantam printed 200,000 copies of our book, ...Times bought the serial rights to it. ....After sitting on the serial rights for a suitable period, the...Times ...unctiously begged Bantam to be released from their gentlemen's agreement, & the serial market had been destroyed. ....Most libraries will not accept a book that has not been reviewed by the...Times or its affiliate...." - John Richardson, MD, Richardson Newsletter, v.1, n.5, p.3, 1979.

"Dr. Ernst T. Krebs, Jr., (& his secretary)...began serving a six-month prison term in May (1983 AD) in the San Francisco County Jail. (They) were found guilty of continuing to promote the merits of laetrile in cancer therapy in violation of terms of the probation they had originally secured following their 1973 conviction." - Committee for Freedom of Choice in Cancer Therapy, Choice, v.9,n.1,p.5, Spring 1983.

"...About Laetrile...we submitted two articles. The editor turned the article over to his medical advisor & received the same advice that had been given to (another magazine): Don't touch it."(p.74).

"...We were told that owners of drugstores, a vital outlet for paperbacks, had been notified that any druggist who displayed my book on his paperback racks, would not receive any more prescriptions from members of the AMA."(p.85).

"...After years of paying my income tax without any problems, in 1964, after my Laetrile book came out, I was summoned by the IRS for an audit...It took 3 years.... ...Again (in) 1974. The year before, I had (written) a book about corruption in Congress. I was summoned for another (IRS) audit, & there went another 3 years."(p.111).

"...The Salk polio vaccine (:).... ...When the final report of the (Salk) tests was ready for publication, there were no takers in the scientific field. The report was handed out at a press conference...."(p.35-6). - Glenn D. Kittler, (author: 40 books; articles in Reader's Digest, The Saturday Evening Post, Pageant, Catholic Digest, etc.; editor, Coronet, Guideposts) Laetrile: Nutritional Control for Cancer with Vitamin B-17, p.35-36, 74, 85, 111.

"The (MSKCC) Memorial Sloan-Kettering Cancer Center report on amygdalin, or Laetrile(:) It is incomplete because at least half a dozen experiments with amygdalin performed at the (MSKCC) between 1972 & 1976 have been omitted from the report. (These,) the positive experiments (showing effectivity against cancer) with amygdalin, carried out by veteran researcher Kanematsu Sugiura appear to be valid & are not successfully challenged by the report. (In contrast,) there are numerous errors in many of these (reported) experiments which allegedly prove amygdalin's ineffectiveness as a palliative or cure of cancer." - Second Opinion, Special Report: Laetrile at Sloan-Kettering, 1977 (Jan. 1978), p.1.

"'In cancer, the fertilization of the cell-nucleus is produced by the virus phase of the microbe - of a streptothrix in sarcoma - of commonly a staphylococcus in carcinoma(;) ...the cell invaded...& the nature of the microbe...determines the particular form of tumor.'" - William M. Crofton, MD, Lecturer in Special Pathology, U. College, Dublin, Ireland, The True Nature of Viruses, c.1936.

"Crofton's work was bitterly attacked, & he found it impossible to publish articles, although others confirmed his techniques & results."(p.42).

"A quick survey of the cancer papers in many medical journals will convince any reader who can plow through them that much research is trivial or of no consequence."(p.107)

- Dr. Robert Netterberg, & Prof. Robert Taylor, The Cancer Conspiracy, c.1981, p.42, 107.

"She reported that 'Dusty' Rhoads, head of Sloan-Kettering, told her he would use the Gerson Therapy if he had cancer, & explained the reasons he was blocked from using it at the hospital." - Norman Fritz.

"...An editorial of the Journal AMA, Jan. 8, 1949, discussed the Gerson Therapy under the heading 'Frauds & Fables'. At that time, Dr. Gerson's lawyer wrote a letter to the JAMA, threatening a suit for libel.... The editorial was withdrawn...(leaving) columns which were blank." - Charlotte Gerson.

- Healing, Journal of the Gerson Inst. & ... Therapy, v.2,n.1,p.5, 28, (for last 2 paragraphs above).

"...George Crile, Jr., a Cleveland (Clinic) surgeon, was rebuked by the Ethics Committee of the Cleveland Academy of Medicine for expressing in a newspaper interview his opinion that radical mastectomy was archaic & no longer necessary."

- Thomas Preston, MD; Prof. of Medicine, Univ. of Washington; Dir. of Cardiol., USPHS Hosp., Seattle; Fellow, Amer. College of Cardiol.; Fellow, AHA Council on Clin. Cardiol.; The Clay Pedestal, c.1981, p.174.

"In 1977, when the laetrile bill was first introduced to the North Dakota Legistlature, I was the only MD to testify for it. .... After that, my successful tenure...was ended & I was called before the State Medical Examiners Board in ND, for using vitamins & laetrile. ...I travelled...to work...with Dr. Davis, Dr. Cole, & Dr. Manner.... When I returned...I was refused re-instatement to the medical staff.... ...We are being investigated by the (state) Attorney General's office because our methods are not 'usual & customary'."

"...The doctors at M.D.Anderson (Hosp.) in Houston...were recently developing a cancer prevention program for Texas, the money & direction for which were appropriated by the Texas legistlature 40 years ago." - Brian Briggs, MD, U. Minn. Med.; Amer. Brd. Family Practice; (letter to Dick Ericson,BS,JD; June 1981).

"...The incidence of cancer among the ... nurse-anesthetists was three times the expected rate. ....When I presented the data at the annual meeting of the ... Anesthesiologists.... Several of the anesthesiologists present even went so far as to call the editor of the IARS Journal ..., & ask him to withhold publication of the paper. .... I was dropped without explanation from the ASA Committee of Effects of Trace Anesthetics on Health." - Thomas H. Corbett, MD, U. Michigan Medical School; USPHS; Prof. Anesthesiology, U. Mich. Med. Ctr.; Clinical Investigator, USVA Hosp.; USEPA Award; Cancer & Chemicals, p.178, 190, & 194.

"...If any patient had...hopelessly advanced cancer, & if he asked for laetrile, I should like to be able to give the substance to him to assuage his mental anguish ...." - Dr. Franz Ingelfinger, Editor, NEJM (New England Journal of Medicine), Editorial, May 20, 1977, (in Michael Culbert, Save Your Life, p.45).

"...The woman...had been relieved of her cancer by Laetrile. .... In the hospital they would not inject Laetrile as it was illegal. She died. This so incensed the editors of the Santa Ana Register (Dean & Martinez) that they wrote ("Laetrile Story",) a series of articles on cancer & the true story for the first time was sent by UPI to (almost) every country in the world." (p.3).

"When a person is found innocent of a crime.... He can never be tried on the same charge again. But in these cancer cases...a given doctor can be yanked into (administrative) court again & again on any charge. It's a crime that a professional doctor is not given the same privileges as a criminal." - Howard H. Beard, ScD, PhD, Yale U., The Anthrone Test..., p.3 & 4.

"Dr. Anthony Verlangieri, ...Rutgers U. ..., was refused funds for...reducing athero-sclerosis with vitamin C. .... Dr. Jorgen Schlegel (is) combating cancer with vitamin C at Tulane Med. .... & Dr. Eli Seifter (discovered) that vitamin A (fights) cancer tumors of viral origin. Yet both distinguished scientist have been refused funds.... Dr. Linus Pauling, ...2-time Nobel Prize winner... , has found it impossible to get federal funds for his research in treating cancer with ...vitamin C." - Jack Anderson, "Tired Blood in Federal Health Research", Rocky Mtn. News, Dec. 22, 1975, (in (Dr. Andrew C.) Ivy Cancer Research Found'n, Ivy Cancer News, v.12, n.1, p.2, Spring 1976).

"...Our paper's...article...(:) The research on which it is based has taken us no less than four years. Two of our chief writers have followed the treatments & checked up on patients' records for months on end. We have made journeys to America.... Our firm, at our request, has spent thousands of pounds on investigations.... ...Certain kinds of cancer have been...treated with success by a man (Harry Hoxsey) who is not a qualified medical practitioner, & who has in the past been bitterly attacked in public for the treatment he has given."
- Man's Magazine, Aug. 1953.

(This issue) "for some strange reason disappeared from the news stands."
- Health Research, Is Cancer Curable?, p.111, (for last 2 paragraphs above).

"...One of the few growth industries in contemporary Britain is...alternative medicine. ....A survey of the attitude of 100 young trainees in family practice revealed that 86 had a positive attitude toward alternative medicine. Of these, ...12 had made referals to non-medically qualified practitioners — a step that only a few years ago would have led to disciplinary action by the General Medical Council...."

"...The debate has gathered momentum since the Brit. Holistic Med. Assoc. was formed & since the Times published 3 major articles on various aspects of alter-native medicine by Ruth West & Brian Inglis...."

"The president of the Royal College of Physicians of London, Prof. Raymond Hoffenberg....could understand why patients with cancer seek alternative methods of treatment, & why any physician would welcome an unequivocal demonstration that a malignant tumor could be cured by any form of alternative medicine." ....

"...The Prince of Wales is immediate past-president of the British Medical Assoc. .... The British Royal Family has long had a high regard for homeo-pathic medicine, & ...the Prince made a plea to doctors to remember old-fashioned, traditional methods of healing." - John Lister, MD, "Current Controversy on Alternative Medicine", NEJM (New England J. of Med.), v.309, n.24, p.1524, Dec. 15, 1983.

"...Paul Crowther...herbalist in the British Isles....could recall at least 6 old cancer remedies which were withdrawn from service about 100 years ago because they were also powerful abortifacients, & the then medico-legal set up made inadvisable to be caught with them on your shelf." ....

"British herbalists have for centuries used complex infusions which include Periwinkle against cancer. The Periwinkle is also the source of the Vinca Alkaloids used in orthodox treatment. Why are the isolated Alkaloids so poisonous in marginally effective doses, whereas the herbal infusions are effective without giving any signs of toxicity?" ....

"(Ernst T.) Krebs (Jr., co-discoveror of vitamin B-15, & B-17), once wrote a book called The Biochemical Basis of Cancer, un-published, 700+ pages, 16,000 references. Probably a gold mine." ....

"...Some of the most valuable items of information have come by private communication." - Frank Hourigan; author, Shape of the Elephant (in press); England; letter to Ralph Hovnanian, Dec. 1984.

"...In most of the affluent populations I have considered, the prevalence of coronary disease is associated with the consumption of sugar. Since sugar consumption is only one of a number of indices of wealth, the same sort of association (to coronary disease) exists with fat consumption, cigarette smoking, cars...."

"Prof. Ian Macdonald of Guy's Hosp. in London....has found that, in young men, sugar raises the level of cholesterol in the blood, & especially...tri-glycerides."

"I did not agree...to having my article censored. .... The published report of the conference gives my name as a participant, but you will not find in it the paper I read. ....Scientists as a group are no more, & no less, influenced by emotional & irrational reactions than other people are."

"...Directors of a large food-manufacturing firm(:).... At one extreme(: one) said it was not his job to protect people from themselves; he was not forcing people to eat his products, & if they chose to do so at the risk of harming themselves, it was of their own free choice." - John Yudkin, MD, PhD; Prof.: Physiology, &, Nutrition & Dietetics, Queen Elizabeth College, London U.; Sweet & Dangerous, (lauded by Morris Fishbein, & Jean Mayer), p.96, 107, 108, 171, 172, 196).

"What is the explanation for the blind eye that has been turned on the flood of medical reports on the causative role of carbohydrates in overweight, ever since the publication in 1864 of William Banting's famous "Letter on Corpulence"? Could it be related, in part, to the vast financial endowments poured into the various departments of nutritional education by the manufacturers of our refined carbohydrate foodstuff?" - Robert C. Atkins, MD, Dr. Atkins' Diet Revolution, c.1972, p.4, 5.

"'Freedom of the press is reserved for those who own one.'" - A. J. Liebling.

"'(Whenever) a bill...proposed...investigating the deadly ("drug") industry, telegrams from the Proprietary (drug) Assoc. (of America) immediately blackmailed the...press into defeating the general welfare of the public.'" - George Seldes.

"...Business spends annually...$500 million to $1 billion (1977 $'s) to promote its editorial & institutional point of view."

"A p.r. firm for the Tobacco Inst....paid...reporters $1,000 a week...." - Mark Green, "How Business Is Misusing the Media", The New York Times, Dec. 18, 1977, (for last 4 paragraphs above).

"...The sympto-thermal method (of birth control, a "combination of ("basal body temperature"), signs & symptoms (mucous) of ovulation, & a math. calculation" ...:) .... For the 307 women...who confined intercourse to the post-ovulatory period, the (practical) use effectiveness rate...equals the (maximum) theoretical effectiveness of the (birth control) Pill."

(Continued)

"...Several issues of the American Journal of Obstetrics & Gynecology in 1977 & 1978 showed that contraceptive ads alone comprised anywhere from 18 to 43% of pages devoted to advertising." - Mary Shivanandan, Cambridge U.; BBC & CBS radio writer; Sex Education Coalition; Natural Sex, p.193 & 220.

"It took almost 6 months to persuade the public library in ... to include the book, The American Fluoridation Experiment, by F.B.Exner, MD, & G.L.Walbott, MD. Then, 1 year later it was found in the waste disposal container, stamped 'Discarded ...'." - Eden Ranch, Organic Consumer Report, v.58, n.19, May 9, 1978.

"Within weeks after Dr. Yiamouyiannis next spoke out against fluoridation, he was put on probation, was told that he would never receive a raise again, & was advised to find another job. Dr. Y. was ultimately forced to resign." - John Yiamouyiannis, PhD; bio-chem. editor, Chem. Abstracts Service, Amer. Chem. Soc.; Fluoride: The Aging Factor, p.129.

"The IRS...proposes to end the threat that Mother Jones poses (as a whistle-blower on corruption in many places), by putting it out of business.... The IRS has decided to deny us our tax exemption, asserting that Mother Jones magazine is a commercial enterprise 'unrelated' to the goals of its tax-exempt parent, the Foundation for National Progress." - Mother Jones, Jan. 1983, (in Libertarian Party News, Jan. 1983, p.20).

B.Q.5.2 TELEVISION:

"(In) 1970, in Camp Hill, Penna. ...Bruce Butt...convened a meeting at which he showed...Nature's Answer to Cancer. The film was made by the IACVF.... (The) attorney...defending Mr. Butt (said): Mr. Butt is criminally charged with 'unlawfully procuring & showing the film, Nature's Answer to Cancer', which the state of Pennsylvania claims '...constitutes dissemination of false or misleading advertisement, concerning the efficacy of Laetrile, as a cure or treatment for cancer'.(&) this constitutes the misbranding of a drug, ...although...all parties ("stipulate") that no drug ("Laetrile...") was sold,or offered for sale! Present at the preliminary hearing were...the USDHEW, & the FTC, ...& FDA.... Again when the film was advertised for showing in a public theatre in San Jose, the owner was threatened by the DA's office with a criminal charge, arrest,& seizure of the film." - IACVF, Cancer News Journal,v.5,n.9,p.22-23,Sept. 1970.

"...All the TV stations in the NY-Phila. Metro. area refused to sell time to Timex to permit public showing of a documentary it had produced on Krebiozen. ....Where the AMA previewed the documentary...." - "TV Censors Krebiozen", American Jewish Ledger, May 31, 1964, (ref. by Kitty Schumacher).

"Research into the cause & cure of cancer is in the hands of a great medical establishment. People who go to each other's meetings are not only published in the same prestigious medical journals, but decide who else is published.... And if these insiders, sizing up an outsider, conclude there's no promise in his theories, he becomes an 'un-person'. Funds dry up, journals reject his papers...."

"(Dr. Lawrence) Burton is on the ACS...blacklist, which effectively cuts him off from research money & from cooperation from doctors, hospitals, & research institutions. The ACS has not itself ever studied Burton or his research, & their objection is largely that he has not published his results.... Burton feels that's a Catch-22." .... In 1971 (he) tried one last time to get his research published in a medical journal. It was rejected." - Harry Reasoner, "The Establishment vs. Dr. Burton", (Produced by Philip Scheffler), CBS, 60 Minutes, v.12, n.36, p.1, May 18, 1980.

"DMSO...60 Minutes reported on...March 23 (, 1980).... The result: one of the largest outpourings of viewer response in 60 Minutes' 12-year history, possibly the largest. ...An estimated 37 million viewers.... After the broadcast, ...Dr. (Stanley) Jacob (focal researcher on DMSO) reported an average of 10,000 letter & phone contacts per week."

"(Dr. Jacob) says a drug company executive told him of DMSO: 'I don't care if it is the major drug of our century — & we all know it is — it isn't worth it to us.'."

- "The Strange Saga of a Pain Killer", TV Guide, July 26, 1980, p.3-6.

"To...Congressmen, doctors, &, ... cancer patients, ...(:) vested interests in conventional treatment ... are so strong that they often closed the door to scientifically valid new approaches." - Hugh Downs.

"...One of (ACS's) finest skills is in the area of public relations & work with the press, who are just putty in its hands." ....

"Dr. Stanislaw Burzynski. ....came to the US...following 5 unsuccessful attempts to leave his native Poland. .... His (discovery,) anti-neoplastons were...tested against human cancer tissue cultures. ...: malignant growth was impaired by 96% (&) healthy tissue was not harmed. ...The NCI postponed his funding.... ...With just $5,000 ... (he) started treating terminal patients. ....(Next,) a local hospital withdrew his staff privileges. ...the Texas prison system('s)...fresh urine...supply was cut off. .... (&, he) was regularly summoned before the Board of Ethics, of the Harris County Medical Society." ....

(ACS)"sent 400,000 doctors nationwide the news: that hydrazine sulfate had made its 'Unproven Methods' list.... Because of that article, a clinical trial planned by a major pharmaceutical company was effectively killed, due, as the company said, '...to the unfortunate, but nevertheless real, bias against these compounds that exists in certain influential quarters.'." - Geraldo Rivera.

- "The War on Cancer: Cure, Profit, or Politics?", 20/20 Special Report, ABC News, show n.137, Oct. 22, 1981.

"My estimate is that about 94,000 cancer fatalities for the future are being induced with each year of medical diagnostic X-rays (in US)." - John Gofman, MD, PhD, co-discoveror of 4 isotopes & 4 nuclear processes; Prof. Emeritus, Med. Physics Div., UC Berkeley; lecturer, Med. Dept., UCSF; Founder (for AEC (Atomic Energy Com.) & Dir., Biomed. Res. Div., & Assoc. Dir., Lawrence Livermore Lab.; Med. Dir., Lawrence Radiation Lab.; Physician, Radio-isotope Therapy, Donner Clinic, UC Berkeley; consultant, 3 cos.; co-inventor, pocket-worn heart monitor; awards from Amer. Heart Assoc., & Amer. College Cardiology & 3 others; author, 150 articles, & 6 books (Dietary Prevention & Treatment of Heart Attacks, & Population Control Through Nuclear Pollution, & Radiation & Human Health).

"...Radiation...the biggest lobby...in the world. It's involved in university research. ...industries.... ...the whole medical profession, ...the whole military establishment, & the economic & military policy of the country depends on people being willing to handle radio-active materials."

"The NCI sent(,)...to review our funding(,)....people connected with the nuclear establishment.... ...It was a pretty much foregone conclusion, that if you send people in to review the funding,who stand most to be hurt by this research, the funding will be denied." - Dr. Rosalie Bertell, Bio-statistician.

- Non Fiction Television, WNET / Thirteen, PBS, The Cancer War, by Ralph Moss,PhD, J.Praeger, S.Fischler, J.Sucher, P.Neshamkin, T.Manning, May-July, 1983, (for last 3 paragraphs above).

"Every family break-up means a doubling of the purchases of TV sets & washing machines. ...A corporate investment in the destruction of the family. ...Our mad agony of loneliness which makes the telephone co.'s (ads) so cruel. .... American education(:)....Cooperative work is considered cheating."

"'I Love NY' bumperstickers, ...drawing a pacemaker on the heart." - Hugh Drummond, MD, "The Lonely Ranger: Can Social Solidarity Protect Us From Stress-Induced Disease?". (p.37-41).

"...Poetic injustice...having made over Japan in our own image. The Japanese, ...are now, next to us, the greatest consumers of meat in the world."

"...Air pollution. ....Along major traffic arteries, it is about ten times higher than the pollution in the general community air. ....Joggers & cyclists are hyper-ventilating & thereby inhaling greater quantities of carbon monoxide...." - Hugh Drummond, MD, "A Telltale Heart". (p.29-30)

- Mother Jones, Found'n for National Progress, A Sourcebook On Health & Survival, p.29-30, 37-41, (for last 4 paragraphs above).

"...The connection between TV & real-life violence.... .... NCTV has found 15 reviews of the scientific literature since 1976 & every one concludes that a causal connection exists. (ie, TV influences behaviour, as advertisers well know, -Ed.) .... NCTV has now found 700 scientific studies & reports from the US & 15 other nations.... The overwhelming consensus of this research is that a significant & important connection exists. ...All age levels, social classes, ethnic backgrounds, & IQ levels are negatively affected in a variety of ways."

(Other)"'Clean Up TV' (groups) make no mention of trying to decrease violence, only sex."

"The average family now has the TV on for 48 hours...each week." - NCTV (National Coalition on Television Violence), NCTV News, v.2,n.4,p.1,2, July 1981.

"What is disturbing — & I have never had an adequate answer to this — is whether a corporation, simply by making a contribution, has a subliminal impact on the kinds of programs public broadcasting (TV) will undertake." - US Congressman Henry Waxman, (in TV Guide, June 20, 1981, p.8).

"...Based on (1400) energy-crisis stories seen on.... ...CBS, NBC, & ABC(,) correspondents relied on govt. sources more than 55% of the time. .... Outside sources — independent experts... — were consulted less than 3% of the time. (On) possible solutions to the crisis, the govt. was consulted a whopping 77% of the time." - "A New Study of Network Coverage Reveals Disturbing Omissions", TV Guide, Mar.6, 1982, p.6

"(The) Military - Industrial - Religious Oligarchy...business buccaneers... trogolodytes...company police...(:) their GREEN($)CURTAIN...." - Riley H. Crabb, Dir., Borderland Sciences Research Found'n; DMP, Soc. St. Luke the Physician; letter letter to Ed., (MDAC 1984, this book), Aug. 13, 1982.

"Day & night the telescreens bruised your ears with statistics proving that people today had more food...lived longer, worked shorter hours, were bigger, healthier, stronger, happier, more intelligent, better educated, than the people of 50 years ago. Not a word of it could ever be proved or disproved. .... The past was erased, the erasure was forgotten, the lie became truth. .... A Party member is required to have...the right instincts. ...Attitudes demanded of him are never plainly stated.... ...He is a person naturally orthodox.... ...In Newspeak, the expression of unorthodox opinions, above a very low level, was well-nigh impossible."

- George Orwell, 1984, (1948 writing), c.1949. (1961, Signet), p.64, 174, 254.

B.Q.6.0 <u>LAW</u> <u>vs.</u> <u>JUSTICE</u>:
B.Q.6.1 <u>FREEDOM</u> of <u>SPEECH</u> <u>&</u> <u>PRESS</u>, <u>(OFFENDED)</u>; <u>USPO</u>, <u>IRS</u>:

"On Feb. 11, 1984, the ACS released dietary guidelines recommending...fruits, vegetables, & whole grains (&) foods rich in vitamins A & C." ....
"No diet cures cancer...." (p.64).
"The Gerson Diet...has failed to withstand scientific scrutiny...." (p.65).
"...The Subcommittee identified about a dozen foundations involved in the dissemination of information encouraging the use of unproven remedies.... ... These foundations...have...been referred to the IRS & the Dept. of Justice for review. .... The IRS should exercise extreme vigilance in reviewing the activities of these & similar organizations, to insure the purpose of tax exemption is achieved & the self-aggrandizement of individuals eliminated."(p.157-9).
- <u>Quackery</u>, <u>a</u> <u>$10</u> <u>Billion</u> <u>Scandal</u>, Report, US Congressman Claude Pepper, Chairman, Subcom. on Health & Long-Term Care, Select Committee on Aging, US House, May 31, 1984, p.64, 65, 157, & 159.

"'The role & weight to be accorded medical testimony in Administrative hearings before the Post Office Dept. was established.... These decisions enunciate a rule that informed medical consensus & the 'universality of scientific belief' may be established through the testimony of a (one, single - Ed.) medical doctor.'"
"'If the fraud charges are proven, a fraud order...is issued, a promoter can receive no funds through the mail... , shut off. All mail sent to him is returned to the sender marked 'Fraudulent'....'" - J. Edward Day, Postmaster General, USPO.

"'Although I found that the booklet (<u>Stale</u> <u>Food</u> <u>vs.</u> <u>Fresh</u> <u>Food</u>) contained some helpful suggestions & its author, Mr. Robert Ford is a knowledgeable & sincere person (ie, no intent of fraud), I found the representations in the Respondent's booklet to be unproven & contrary to the weight of informed medical & scientific opinion. As indicated by Dr. ___, (the only USPO medical witness,) a danger of this publication is that it will deceive people who have arterio-sclerotic problems into believing that they can cure these problems by diet alone instead of seeking medical (AMA) help. Because the ads. & this booklet contain materially false representations, they violate the provisions of 39 US Code Sec. 3005. Therefore...a mail stop order ...should be issued....'" - E. S. Bernstein, Administrateve Law Judge, (1982).

"The USPS has prosecuted a disproportionate number of health book authors & publishers. (&) Chiropractors. The PO has refused to respond to our Freedom of Information Request for a copy of its policy manual which sets out the basis by which cases are selected for prosecution. The (PO) will not open their consumer complaint files to the public or to the Congress so you can see if it is going after the real criminals. ...or...if anyone complained...except the AMA." - Clinton Miller, Exec. Dir. & Legistlative Advocate, NHF.
- last 4 paragraphs above in "Statement of Clinton Ray Miller...before the Subcommittee on Postal Personnel & Modernization, (Committee on Post Office & Civil Service, US House,) on H.R.3973, & S.1407, July 15, 1982.

"The Postal Service may require...that any officer or employee designated by the Postal Service be given access at reasonable times, to inspect or copy any books, records, documents, or other objects that the Postal Service has reason to believe relate to any matter under investigation...."(#413, p.10) (Continued)

"Any person...who fails to comply...or...engages in conduct which assists any such person to...fail to comply...shall be liable to the US for a civil penalty in an amount not to exceed $10,000 for each day.... ...Separate penalties may be assessed ($20,000/day).... The resumption through use of any instrumentality of interstate commerce of any activity with respect to which a cease & desist order has been issued ...shall...be a failure to comply...."(#3012, p.15-16).

- A Bill, S.1407, with amendments, US Senate, June 22,1981, & April 29,1982, (unanimous resolution); (300 co-sponsors in US House, H.R.3973).

"Welcome to the new Dark Ages. Get ready for 1984. .... The (bill) would: ... Authorize...600,000 post office employees to 'demand' 'access' without search warrant to any home, business, private library...'to inspect...' (; &) Forbid the shipment... not only by mail, but any other 'instrumentality of interstate commerce' including airlines, parcel service, buses, trucks, or your own auto." .....

"The history of medicine & health care shows that nearly all progress has started with unorthodox ideas which were opposed to the 'weight of informed medical & scientific opinion'." - Maureen Salaman; Pres., NHF; Assoc. Ed., NHF, Health Freedom News; Hostess, Totally Yours radio talk show; author, Nutrition: the Cancer Answer; US Vice Presidential Candidate, Populist Party; in "Statement...before the Subcommittee on Postal Personnel & Modernization, (Com. on Post Office..., US House,) on H.R.3973 & S.1407, July 15, 1982"...

"It is especially imperative for Congress to exercise careful judgment in this area, because of the difficulty under existing laws, in obtaining judicial review of Postal Service abuses. ...We strongly oppose the legistlation's infringement of rights guaranteed under the First, Fourth, & Fifth Amendments to the Constitution." - John Shattuck, Dir., ACLU (American Civil Liberties Union), Washington Office.

B.Q.6.2 FREEDOM of CHOICE in HEALTH CARE, (DEFENDED):

"'...The charges concern medical practices in fields where knowledge has not yet been crystallized in the crucible of experience. For in the science of medicine, as in other sciences, experimentation is the spur of progress. It would amount to condemnation of new ideas without a trial, to give the Postmaster General power to condemn new ideas as fraudulent, solely because some cling to traditional opinions with unquestioning tenacity.'" - US Supreme Court, Reilly v. Pinkus, 339 U.S. 269 (1949).

- last 2 paragraphs above in "Statement of John Shattuck...on H.R.3973/S.1407... before the Subcom. on Postal Personnel & Modern., ...US House, July 20, 1982".

"A decision to obtain or reject medical treatment is not only a personal decision, but is one which profoundly affects one's development or one's life, &, as such, is a constitutional right encompassed by the right of privacy, (US Const.) Amendment 14." - US District Court, Houston, Const. Law 82 (7), Ruling, July 9, 1980, (in Marie Steinmeyer, Georgia Women's Coalition for Medical Rights, "Letters ...", NHF, Health Freedom News, v.3, n.1, p.14, Jan. 1984).

"Individuals for whom no orthodox cure is available surely are entitled to select a health care approach.... .... This right (is) specifically within...the 1st, 4th, 5th, 9th, & 14th Amendments to the (US) Constitution.... .... To be insensitive to the very fundamental civil liberties...(:) the choice...of the person whose body is being ravaged (by disease), is to display slight understanding of the essence of our free society & its constitutional underpinnings." - Judge Luther Bohanon, US District Court, Oklahoma City, Dec. 5, 1977, Rutherford v. US, (in Maureen Salaman, MSc, Nutrition: the Cancer Answer, p.247-249).

"According to 45 C.F.R. (Code of Federal Regulations) #46.103(c), the information to be disclosed to prospective (clinical research) subjects had to include:...'A description of any attendant discomforts & risks reasonably to be expected; (&) A disclosure of any appropriate alternative procedures that might be advantageous for the subject; ....'"

"The approved ('informed' patient) consent form...in use at M.D. Anderson for Phase I antitumor therapy. ...actually failed to list the potential side effects of the drug though promising a 'detailed explanation of the therapy procedures & the purpose of this therapy' ("emphasis added"). .... Moreover, the major objective of this Phase I study was to determine the maximum tolerated dose...before...'...heart failure, ...coma...'. (Yet) the consent form asserts that 'the amount of drug...will be free of toxic effects'." - Alexander M. Capron, Executive Director, President's Commission for the Study of Ethical Problems in Medicine & Biomedical & Behavioral Research, -in Oversight of the NCI, 1981, Hearings, Subcom. on Investigations..., Com. on Labor..., US Senate, Nov. 3 & 6, 1981, p.444, 447, & 448.

"The freedom of the individual to select his preferred system of medical care & free competition among physicians & alternative systems of medical care are prequisites of ethical practice & optimal medical care."(p.29).

"A physician should expose, without fear or favor, incompetent or corrupt, dishonest or unethical conduct on the part of members of the profession."(p.28). - AMA, Current Opinions of the Judicial Council of the AMA, 1981, p.28,29.

"Where medically significant alternatives for care or treatment exist, or when the patient requests information concerning medical alternatives, the patient has the right to such information." - AHA (American Hospital Assoc.), A Patient's Bill of Rights, c.1972, #3.

"Congress did not intend to empower the FDA to interfere with medical practice by limiting the ability of physicians to prescribe according to their best judgement." - US District Court Judge Robert E. Varner, decision, June 28, 1978.

"...The 4th Amendment (to the US Constitution:) The governing principle...is that 'except in certain carefully defined classes of cases, a search of private property without proper consent is unreasonable unless it has been authorized by a valid search warrant....' ...The manufacture & distribution of food & drugs has not yet been specifically held to be among these exceptionally regulated industries.... ...The inspection of any place thought by FDA agents to contain the regulated articles.... (is) ...an unconstitutional authorization of unlimited exploratory searches...." - US District Court Judge Robert M. Duncan, Eastern Div., So. Dist. of Ohio, ruling, on July 14, 1977 FDA search & seizure, (in Michael Culbert, Save Your Life, p.79, & 275).

"The Supreme Court...last summer(:).... In the Pireno decision...ruled that local medical societies & insurance companies could not refuse reimbursement for treatments ("in this case, chiropractic") deemed by American medical orthodoxy not to be 'reasonable or necessary', & that such actions are conspiratorial & violate the Anti-Trust Act. In the McCready decision (it) held that the plaintiff, who protested because her Blue Shield insurance coverage would not pay for her consultations with a psychologist ("orthodoxy argued she should have seen a psychiatrist — that is, an MD"), was in the right." - Michael Culbert (author, Medical Revolution in America, etc.), &, Robert Bradford (Knight of Malta, etc.), Choice, v.8, n.4, p.5, Fall 1982.

"At least one member of the (Medical Grievance Committee, Board of Regents, Univ., State of NY) which conducted the hearing evidenced a wholly unfair & partial attitude. .... This doctor effected a cure (of cancer) when the so-called orthodox methods of treatment had failed, & now he has been punished for it. It is not fraud or deceit for one already skilled in the medical art, with the consent of the patient, to attempt new methods, when all other known methods of treatment had proved futile, & least of all when the patient's very life had been despaired of. Initiative & originality should not be thus effectively stifled...." - Appellate Division, NY State Supreme Court, Stammer v. Board of Regents of Univ. of State of NY, 262 App. Div. 372, 29 N.Y.S. 2d 38, (in Howard H. Beard, ScD, PhD, Yale Univ.; Member, John Beard Research Inst.; A New Approach to the Etiology, Diagnosis, Treatment & Prevention of Some of the Degenerative Diseases Including Therapeutic Biochemistry, c.1965, Appendix, p.99).

"'...Each man is considered to be master of his own body, & he may, if he be of sound mind, expressly prohibit the performance of lifesaving surgery, or other medical treatment.'" - In Re Quinlan, 70 NJ 10, cert. denied, 429 US 922 (1976).

"Law suits against (vaccine) manufacturers have been based on 4 theories of liability: negligence; strict liability in tort; breach of warranty; or misrepresentation." - Tom Finn, Attorney, Freedom of Choice Law Ctr., Dangers of Compulsory Immunizations: How to Avoid Them Legally, p.11, 25, & 26, (for last 2 paragraphs above).

"In 1975, Judy Hall, the famous...singer from Alaska, was successfully treated far cancer at...Mexico's finest alternative therapy clinic. ...She joint-drafted a bill with Andrew McNaughton to legalize laetrile in Alaska. ...Judy gave the bill to (Alaska) Governor J.S.Hammond, whose wife was a cancer victim & later opted for laetrile treatment. Gov. Hammond agreed to support the legistlation. Thus, the first laetrile bill became law, setting the pattern for the 27 other states which ...have followed." - Maureen Salaman, MSc; Pres., NHF (National Health Federation); nutrition talk show hostess, KEST radio, San Francisco; lecturer; Nutrition: the Cancer Answer, p.246.

"The legistlation...of...fluoridation...is unreasonable & a violation of the due process clause of the Illinois Constitution...."

"This record is barren of any credible & reputable, scientific epidemiological studies &/or analysis of statistical data, which would support the Ill. Legislature's determination that fluoridation of public water supplies is both a safe & effective means of promoting public health." ....

"(Fluoridation) is unconstitutional.... (&)...an unreasonable exercise of police power...." - Judge Ronald Niemann, Circuit Court, Ill., Decree, Ill. Pure Water Comm. & Ruby Hale, vs. Dir. Dept. Public Health & Dir. EPA, State of Ill., n. 68-E-128, (in NHAC (National Health Action Committee), Health Action, v.3, n.2, p.3, Feb. 1982).

"...The evidence that the fluoridation of the public water supply at the rate of (1ppm) 1 part per million is carcinogenic is irrefutable."

"...Say someone shot somebody.... ...We...are so concerned about whether the evidence was admitted properly.... ...(&) not recognize the intrusion into our sacred individuality that is being caused every time people turn on the faucet? ....I am also astounded by how much untruth has been officially promulgated (pro fluoridation)." - Justice John Flaherty, Supreme Court of Penn., address, June 7, 1981, (in NHAC, Health Action, v.2, n.7, p.2, July 1981).

"The Assoc. for Childbirth at Home, International (ACHI) trains teachers.... ...The Ill. Attorney General....subpoena of....ACHI...listed 71 demands(:)....that ACHI should present to the State a complete list of all ACHI leaders in the world, a tabulation of every childbirth class taught by any ACHI leader anywhere — including...all parents...who have ever taken the ACHI series in...the world." ....

"Ill. District IV Appellate Court....concluded: (1) That based on the 1958 US Supreme Court ruling in Alabama vs. NAACP, the State could not require ACHI to submit the names...; (2) That ACHI's right to teach medical info. was covered by the First Amendment of the US Constitution...(4) That an organization engaged in education was not covered by the Ill. Consumer Fraud Act. ...Susan Dewitt, Chief ...Dept. of Consumer Affairs, stated...there were no consumer complaints on record against ACHI & they had broken no laws. ...The Ill. Attorney General...has now appealed the case to the Ill. Supreme Court." ....

"Ill. is the home of the AMA, AHA (Amer. Hospital Assoc.), Amer. Acad. of Pediatrics, ACOG (Amer. College of Obstetricians & Gynecologists), & NAACOG (Nurses' Assoc. ...) — all of whom are against home birth." - "Attack on ACHI...", NAPSAC (InterNational Assoc. of Parents & Professionals for Safe Alternatives in Childbirth), NAPSAC News, v.5, n.3, p.9, Fall 1980.

"A...couple has filed a class action suit against Blue Cross/Blue Shield (BC/BS) (Moscow v. BC/BS of Greater NY, Supreme Ct. NY, filed Aug. 18, 1980) challenging the insurance co.'s refusal to reimburse for midwifery services.(&)... asking damages for themselves(&)other...parents who did not even request reimbursement because they were told that (it was) not covered by their policy." - Health Law Project, Library Bulletin, v.6, n.1, p.18, Jan. 1981.

"...Nov. 19, 1982. ...a juvenile court judge in Virginia Beach, VA.... Judge Frederick Aucamp granted the exemption (from compulsory vaccination), citing a body of medical opinion that there are inherent risks to vaccinations, which outweigh the supposed benefits." - Grace Girdwain, Healthful Living, (T.C.Fry,Ed.), v.1,n.3, p.39,May 1982.

"Any person suffering legal wrong because of agency action, or adversely affected or aggrieved by agency action within the meaning of a relevant statute, is entitled to judicial review thereof." - Title 5, US Code, #702(a), (in Norman J. Landau & Paul D. Rheingold, The Environmental Law Handbook, (Foreword by Ralph Nader), FoE (Friends of the Earth), c.1971, p.382).

"(With) private right of action (one can) sue under the Administrative Procedure Act (APA) to force the Fed. Govt. to comply with the law. .... The APA allows suits by anyone 'adversely affected' by a federal agency's action." - EDF (Environmental Defense Fund; Janet Welsh Brown, PhD, Exec. Dir.), EDF Letter, Jan. 1982, p.4.

"...Equal Access to Justice Act ("EAJA"), 5 USC section 504 & 28 USC section 2412 (:).... The act provides for the award of 'fees & other expenses', including 'reasonable expenses of expert witnesses (or) analysis...necessary for the preparation of the party's case,& reasonable attorney fees...'. .... The key to winning fees under EAJA is to prevail against the govt. by obtaining either a final judgement, a favorable settlememt, or a voluntary dismissal of a groundless complaint. ....The act is relatively new & unknown." - "Law Provides Protection From Govt. Frivolty", Consulting Engineer, v.61, n.4, p.82, Oct. 1983.

B.Q.6.3 MEDICAL INQUISITION; CANCER:

"One doctor...J.W. Kannel, saved a young girl.... She had hopeless cancer of the spleen. ...One shot of Glyoxylide, & she became well (in 1943; still alive in 1983) ... For (this), Kannel was barred from all hospitals in Fort Wayne. ....The FDA had (Glyoxylide inventor, Dr. William Frederick) Koch arrested & thrown into an incredibly filthy jail cell in Florida in 1942." (p.168).

"In 1926...the AMA...attempt(ed) to send a doctor using Koch shots to prison. .... (In) Massachusetts....Justice Pierce....berated the District Attorney, calling the opposition to Koch 'a moral crime of the very worst kind'." (footnote,p.169-170).

– Wayne Martin, BS, Purdue Univ.; Sr. Metallurgist, Sperry Gyroscope Co., & 3 large aluminum firms; (author, Medical Heroes & Heretics); We Can Do Without Heart Attacks, c.1983, p.168-170.

"...Medical mankind in particular, were supposed to be waiting the advent of some new scientific discovery concerning the nature of cancer.... .... The physical martyrdom was lacking; but there are, as I can testify from experience, many more ways than one of burning a scientific man at the stake." – John Beard, D.Sc., The Enzyme Treatment of Cancer & Its Scientific Basis, c.1911 AD, p.ix.

"'...H. H. Beard has perfected...3 excellent (urine) cancer tests, all of a proven accuracy of 95% or better.... ...in 1942 & onwards.'"

"'...The enzyme beta-glucoronidase is necessary to...'trigger off'...laetrile ....After the laetrile injection, we injected directly into the tumor...beta-glucoronidase. The result was a white slough which encompassed...the (tumor) growth. ...The slough resorbed & was replaced by normal (tissue).'" – Arthur T. Harris, MD,U. Edinburgh,(under John Beard); PhD, Med.; DSc, Biochem.; Litt. D.

"Early one morning in 1946, our lab. was mysteriously destroyed by fire.... We then established a lab. at...our present location. Then again one morning in ...1947, this lab. was set on fire & completely destroyed." – Howard H. Beard, ScD; PhD, Yale U., Porter Fellow, Physiol.; MA, Columbia U.; Prof. & Dir., Biochem. Dept., LSU Med.; Prof., Biochem.: Chicago Med. School, &, Western Reserve U.; Chair., 1940 New Orleans Meeting, Federation of Societies for Experimental Biology; Member, AACR (Amer. Assoc. for Cancer Research); Dir., John Beard Lab. of Clin. Biochem.; A New Approach to the Conquest of Cancer, Rheumatic & Heart Diseases, p.96,208,222.

"Arthur Harris(MD,PhD)...was soon forbidden to use Laetrile on hospitalized patients. .... In...1953, Harris reported: 'Of the total number of cases (82) treated with Laetrile, 43 have been pay-patients, & 39 free-patients. Of the 43 pay-patients, many have paid only a part of their bills....' ...Dr. Harris.... received a summons from the LA Co. Medical Assoc. to appear for trial...for unethical conduct in overcharging 3 patients for Laetrile.... Files showed that the (3 patients) had not paid a cent of the bills.... ...Harris received notice that he had been expelled from the county medical society." – Glenn D. Kittler, Laetrile: Nutritional Control for Cancer with Vitamin B-17, c.1963, 1978, p.61-63.

"'I had to stand 3 expensive trials in California courts, where in all 3 actions against me, the charges were dismissed. Then I had to stand an even longer & more expensive trial in Federal Court in San Diego, where I was convicted of 'conspiring to smuggle Laetrile' & was fined $30,000. ...Cal. then revoked my license....'"

– John Richardson, MD, (in Wayne Martin, We Can Do Without Heart Attacks, p.220).

"Dr. (William D.) Kelly has been harassed by agents from the IRS, FDA, HEW, CIA, CDC, Texas medical & dental boards, controllers, US Postal authorities, US Chamber of Commerce, Consumer Protection Agency, ...local & county...police.... Dr. Kelley was told by the Texas State Board of Dental Examiners that if he would stop distributing his book to cancer patients, they would drop all charges. ...Blue Cross will pay for cancer surgery, for chemotherapy, for cobalt (radiation..."for a terminal cancer patient...of $30,000") but...refuses to pay for unorthodox treatments. .... My (5) visit(s) to Dr. Kelly cost...$150 per visit." - FACT (Foundation for Alternative Cancer Therapies), Cancer Forum, v.3,n.5,p.4 & 5,

"A little after 7 am...25 officers...(&) Cal. FDA, raided Halstead's residence.... .... The LA County DA's office charged (Bruce) Halstead (consultant to WHO (World Health Org'n.; Commander, US Navy; Dir., World Life Res. Inst.) with some 24 counts including 'conspiracy', 'grand theft', 'unlawfully selling drugs for cancer treatment', & 'fraudently providing a treatment to arrest cancer'. ....The DA took all of his cancer patients' records & refused to give him either a list or receipt for them...." - Choice, v.10, n.1, p.4, Win. 1984.

"The Committee for Freedom of Choice in Medicine.... ...has filed a complaint with the UN Center for Human Rights. ...charg(ing)...'medical genocide' & accus(ing) the AMA &...FDA.... (This) complaint...was spurred by...the recent raid on the home & offices of...Bruce Halstead, MD...." - "Med. Freedom Group Takes Complaint to UN", Spotlight, May 21, 1984, p.12 & 13.

"The Rev. Edward Stone, an...English clergyman...sought new drugs according to a rule. God (is) placing the cures for diseases in close proximity to their causes. .... In 1763...Stone...learned that the countryfolk...treated fevers with...bark of the willow, a tree common in marshy locations. ...Willow bark... had the same 'extra-ordinary bitterness' as quinine.... Stone...treated some 50 fever-stricken patients (&)...it reduced the fever & relieved pain in every case. ....Chemists later (were) isolating the bark's active principle &... synthesizing...salicylates....acetyl-salicylic acid...aspirin.... ...Stone's... re-discovery...of salicylate-containing plants had been known in antiquity...."

"...Dr. Bruce W. Halstead, Dir., World Life Research Inst. ....recalls ...Indian snakeroot...was 'laughed out of the office' of one important drug-co. official. Another co., with fewer prejudices, took the trouble to investigate it — & ultimately marketed millions of $'s worth of reserpine (,toxic)." - Dr. W. Modell, Prof. Pharm., Cornell U. Med.; Board Member, US Pharmacopoeia; Editor: Drugs of Choice, &, Pharm. for Physicians, &, Clinical Pharm. & Therap.; consultant to US Surgeon General; Author: Relief of Symptoms, &, Drugs; & Rene Dubos, Prof. Emeritus, Rockefeller U.; Pulitzer Prize; Arches of Sci. Award; &, Henry Morgenau, Prof. Emeritus, Yale; &, C. P. Snow, Author: The Affair, &, Corridors of Power; Consulting Editors, Drugs, Time-Life Books, p.121, 124.

"Gerson was treating 9 out of 10 (cancer) patients without cost."

"The AMA, of which (Dr. Max) Gerson was a member, promptly saw to it that he was no longer allowed to use the facilities of any NY hospital." - Health Research, Is Cancer Curable?, c.1954,(1969), p.74.

"A contributary factor to the increase in cancer might be the widespread use of anti-biotics since 1940. 'The antibiotics may absolve the body of the need to bring the normal immunological mechanisms into use....'"

"In Japan, the daily use of the hot full bath may destroy incipient cancers...."

(Continued)

"...Thousands more cancer patients were not given the benefit of such (fever/immuno-/(heat)) therapy since it was first initiated by (Dr. William Bradley) Coley 90 years ago.... ...The incredible barriers created by the FDA since 1963. (:) To rule Coley's MBV (mixed bacterial vaccine) as a 'new drug' when it had been used for 70 years in nearly 900 patients was incredible. The red tape involved in securing (IND) Investigational New Drug licenses.... Progress will now have to come from clinical trials in...countries which do not have such paralyzing restrictions."
- Helen Coley Nauts, Exec. Dir., Cancer Research Inst., "Bacterial Products in the Treatment of Cancer: Past, Present, & Future", read at Internat'l Colloquium on Bacteria & Cancer, (Cologne, 1982), in Bacteria & Cancer, Jeljaszewicz et. al., eds., c.1982, p.1-25.

"Dr. (Donald R.) Cole (formerly of "Sloan-Kettering & St. Vincent's Hosp. in NY") was charged on 3 counts: giving false hope to the terminally ill, using experimental drugs illegally,& practicing medicine in an unlawful & dishonest manner. .... The illegal drug charge was defined as the use of vitamins, enzymes, & laetrile. ...Dr. Cole administered laetrile...at the request of patients in the legally prescribed manner with a signed affidavit. ....An oncologist from Roswell Park (Memorial Inst.) who was brought in by the Hearing Panel...could not substantiate a single case of incompetence or negligence. ...Dr. Cole's license was revoked." - CCS, Cancer Control Journal, Betty Lee Morales & Lorraine Rosenthal, Eds., v.6,n.1,p.96,Jan.'78,'82.

"Dr. Emory Thurston, PhD, ScD, (lecturer, College of Pharmacy, USC; Member, APA (Amer. Pharmaceutical Assoc.), Exec. Sec'y, Inst. of Nutritional Research (had) ....inspectors from the Cal. Food & Drug office armed with a search warrant, (who) raided his business office. They confiscated several bottles of Laetrile...& every piece of literature that contained the word 'cancer'. (They) serve(d) a warrant for the arrest of Dr. Thurston on the charge of selling Laetrile & practicing medicine without a license. He was taken to county jail...." - IACVF, Cancer News Journal, v.8,n.3,p.28, 1973, Convention issue.

"Mrs. Joseph (Kitty) Schumacher...fought against the govt.'s ruling which bans the shipment of Krebiozen from the State of Ill. ...As a result of her efforts, she was indicted in federal court in Chicago. ...She criticized the judge..., ... govt., ...(&) prosecuting attorney. Yet, a jury found her not guilty." - Butcher Workman, Sept. 1968.

"Adolph Hohensee...operated a health farm near Scranton, Pa. But, the FDA were on his back for many years, hoping to find a violation, etc. Well, they did. They found he mislabeled a vitamin, & they took him out at 2 AM in his pajamas & imprisoned him...."

"...The Durovics (of Krebiozen:)...how costly (their) 9 month trial was,& no government paid their legal fees as was done for the FDA."
- Kitty Schumacher, Cancer Information Crusade, in letters on Sept. 14, & Oct. 6, 1982, to Ralph Hovnanian.

"'There is a strong possibility...that selenium may prevent &/or cure cancer. .... As a scientist, you have to consider the possibility that (Dr. Revici) has something to offer.'" - NCI selenium committeeman, Dr. Marc Micozzi.

"'...After a (NBC TV) Today Show report...on Revici & his unorthodox treatment using...selenium, ...officials suspended his license.'" - Miami Herald (for last 2 quotes above).

"...Dr. Emanuel Revici.... ...directs the Inst. of Applied Biology. .... (&) is a veteran of over 50 years of research in biochemistry & holds over 100 patents. The NYS Health Dept. charged Dr. Revici with fraudulent practice, gross incompetence, & gross negligence." - NHF, Health Freedom News, v.3, n.4, p.38, 39, April 1984, (for last 3 paragraphs above).

"'There is not one, but many cures for cancer available. But they are all being systematically suppressed by the ACS, the NCI, & the major oncology centers. They have too much of a vested interest in the status quo.'" - Robert C. Atkins, MD, Cornell Univ. Medical College; Bach., Univ. of Michigan; postgrad. med., Columbia & Rochester Univ.s; Member, IAPM (International Academy of Preventive Medicine); FICAN (Fellow, International College of Applied Nutrition); (author, Dr. Atkins' Diet Revolution, & Dr. Atkins' Nutrition Breakthrough); in NY Star, (in CCS, Cancer Control Journal, v.6,n.1,p.89, Jan. 1978,(1982)).

B.Q.6.4 MEDICAL INQUISITION; OTHER DISEASES:

"...The plaintiff's lawyers have already filed & won a case allegedly proving that I have abandoned my homestead. ...My beautiful homestead will be sold at auction by the Sheriff...." - V. V. Vetrano, Natural Hygienist,(by fasting).

"The suit charged Dr.(Herbert) Shelton (author of 12 books on fasting) & Dr. Vetrano with starving the guest (suffering side effects from "ethical pharmaceuticals") to death. Despite ample evidence produced to show that the guest did not die of starvation...." - T. C. Fry, College of Life Science, Healthful Living, v.2, n.7, p.24-5, Dec. 1983, (for last 2 paragraphs above).

"...For appeal purposes were several hostile rulings by the presiding Federal Judge on questions of admissable evidence. ...." - ANHS, Health Sci.,v.5,n.6,p.18, Nov. 1982.

"The Chicago Women's Health Center was struck by arsonists on the evening of (1983). .... Damage is estimated at $10,000. The damages are not covered by insurance. ....Clinic health workers take time to explain procedures & options to each patient they see...." - Heartland, n.14, p.32, Sum. 1983.

"...Mark Baum....MD....(adopted) living healthfully. ...(&) started advising healthful regimes for his clients. Dr. Baum's local medical society objected to his practices & invoked powers of state to close him down." - Healthful Living, (Life Science / Natural Hygiene), v.2,n.2,p.29, May 1983.

"Our attorney...then filed a running complaint with the Hearing Officer that the panel of doctors on this District Review Committee...could not possibly give Dr. (Alan H.) Nittler (MD, author, A New Breed of Doctor) a fair hearing, in that they were totally unaware of nutritional metabolic therapy...(&) prejudiced against him. ....The District Court of Appeals also denied Dr. Nittler's request for a stay.... ...The hearing...had to totally disregard all of the evidence presented by Dr. Nittler, & his witnesses, ...to revoke his license, the maximum penalty allowed." - FACT Journal, v.2,n.3,p.5.

"A person is a quack if: ... He claims he is being persecuted by the 'medical establishment'. (& or) He uses letters of testimonials...from patients in support of his treatment." - NY State Ed. Dept., Curriculum Dev't. Ctr., Bur. of School Health Ed. Services, Health Ed.: Cancer ..., c.1976, p.17.

"Doctors who have been doing home births, in many instances have lost hospital privileges, been threatened with loss of insurance, &...threatened with criminal prosecution. ...There certainly isn't criminal prosecution when something goes wrong in the hospital. .... I know horrendous stories of women...just really being abused within the hospital because they tried to have their babies at home.... Practitioners are threatened with loss of license...." - Michelle Harrison, MD, (author, A Woman in Residence), (in "Behind the Mask of Women's Medicine", East-West Journal, v.12, n.10,p.30, Oct. 1982).

"...Their (hospital's) annual application for renewal of their license to operate would not be granted unless the ortho-molecular (nutrition) program was closed." - M. Artery, attorney for Forest Hospital, (in NOHA (Nutrition for Optimal Health Assoc.), NOHA News, v.6, n.1, p.1-2, Win. 1981).

"...Incarceration & deprivation of the rights of mental patients, as if they were criminals rather than sick people(:)... In less than ½ of the states is a patient's right to communicate with the outside world protected by law; in less than ½ is his right to receive visitors protected by law; in less than 1/10 is he guaranteed the right to correspond with his attorney; the use of physical restraints is restricted in less than ½ of the states; & less than ½ of the states assure that he will receive a periodic examination for consideration for discharge." - Arthur Frank, MD, & Stuart Frank, MD, The People's Handbook of Medical Care, p.31.

B.Q.6.6 JUDICIARY, INTOXICANTS, COSTS:

"Utopians have no lawyers among them, for they consider them as a sort of people whose profession it is to disguise matters." - Sir Thomas More,(1478-1535).

"When this country was originally formed ... the first rule that was passed by every single body in the 13 original states said (that) two people shall be banned from this colony: felons & lawyers." - Rosemary Furman, (on Phil Donahue Show (tv), Donahue Transcript #12161, p.13).

"...If American bureaucracy turns its attention on you(:).... ...The men who sit in judgement on you will be the men who originally complained against you. ... You may...be ordered to stop doing something which is right. Perhaps you will be saved the burden of defending yourself by being tried in absentia. ...At a trial where all the witnesses testified in your favor, ...the courts will nevertheless uphold your conviction.... ...Final arguments were made in front of Commissioners, but the decisions were written in a secret back room by an entirely separate group of men." - Lowell B. Mason, Commissioner, FTC (Federal Trade Commission), The Language of Dissent, (in Suzanne Caum, Cancer Cures Crucified, p.52).

"...Whole plants differ in their effects from refined drugs(:) .... Plants are dilute preparations (of) the active principles.... ...Plants usually go into the body through the mouth & stomach, whereas purified chemicals can be put ...by snorting or injecting...directly into...bloodstreams without giving...bodies a chance to process them. ...Other compounds in drug plants...may modify the active principles, making them safer...."

"...Society's blunders in trying to control the abuse of drugs(:) .... Prohibition of opiates (& other drugs & plants) has directly spawned an ugly criminal underworld.... Addicts with habits costing $100's a day...resort to daily criminal activity...to avoid the unpleasant symptoms of withdrawal. .... Heroin maintenance...supplying addicts with pure (un-contaminated) legal heroin in (a) supervised setting (no: driving, firearms, health insurance, -Ed.) has been proposed..., but our society (is) unwilling to abandon its prohibitionist mentality. ....Major traffickers...are...powerful enough to stay in business. Instead, drug law enforcement falls disproportionately on small-scale dealers & users. .... In some states, people convicted for small-scale dealing of drugs...are treated more harshly by the law than rapists, armed robbers, & even murderers." - Andrew Weil, MD, Harvard Med.; BA, cum laude, Harvard U.; Res. Assoc., Ethno-pharmacology, Harvard Botanical Museum; Adj. Prof., Addiction Studies, U. Ariz.; & Winifred Rosen, (author, Cruisin for a Bruisin, etc.), Newbery Award nominee; Chocolate to Morphine: Understanding Mind Active Drugs, p.31, 32, 86, 88, 164, 166.

"Judges & the courts are by far the most often blamed & complained about part of the drunk driver control system. Often the complaints are well founded & the criticism well deserved. .... Chronic repeat offenders are not viewed by many judges as the dangerous criminals they really are.... Judges...give a break.... In some court systems, it is literally possible to buy your way out of an alcohol related charge. ....Mistakes & mishandling of drunk drivers by well-meaning but unknowledgeable judges often cost innocent people their lives or health." - Sandy Golden, How to Save Lives & Reduce Injuries: a Citizen Activist Guide to Effectively Fight Drunk Driving, NHTSA (National Highway Traffic & Safety Adm.), of USDoT (Dept. of Transportation), DOT HS 806 250, Nov. 1982, p.39, (also author, Driving the Drunk Off the Road).

"...A juvenile detention home(:).... ...Neither the boys nor the staff of the home were told that the aim of the menu changes was to reduce sugar intake, or that the boys' behavior was being studied. .... The 24 boys on the reduced-sugar diet showed a 45% lower incidence of formal disciplinary actions than the boys on the earlier diet." ....

"With the repeated successes of nutritional methods, one would think that ortho-molecular treatment would be revolutionizing our criminal justice system. Unfortunately, it is not. Ignoring scientific evidence & thousands of clinical reports, many in the psychiatric, law enforcement, & rehabilitation communities, still dismiss dietary treatment as quackery. The ortho-molecular approach isn't 'high-tech' enough; it isn't complicated & expensive, it doesn't require powerful drugs & armies of MD's — how could it possibly be effective?" - Barbara Reed, Chief Probation Officer, Cuyahoga Falls Municipal Probation Dept.; (testifier at US Senate Select Com. on Nutrition & Human Needs); Nutritional Guidelines for the Counselor, p.44 & 46.

"Dollar Cost of the Vietnam War...(Billions of $'s):

Past budgetry costs:	$128-171 (billion)
Future budgetry costs (veterans' benefits):	$ 304 "
Extra-budgetry costs (sacrificed earnings):	$ 70 "
Indirect costs (recession, inflation, balance of trade, (gross estimates)):	$ 378 "
Total:	$882-925 "

- Robert Warren Stevens, Prof., Vain Hopes, Grim Realities: The Economic Consequences of the Vietnam War, c.1976, p.187.

"Additional Tobacco Costs, (Yearly):

$: 29,400,000:	Gov't. appropriation to fight smoking, 1979.
750,000,000:	Gov't. purchase of tobacco to keep price up.
300,000,000:	Gov't. loan to tobacco farmers to raise tobacco.
100,000,000:	Gov't. direct support for tobacco, i.e. grading of tobacco, tobacco in "Food for Peace" (foreign aid), tobacco research, tobacco crop land adjustment, tobacco export, etc.
800,000,000:	Write-off by tobacco companies as advertising, tax credit....
9,000,000,000:	Medical care caused by smoking.
18,000,000,000:	Lost production, absenteeism, & lost wages, caused by smoking.
?:	Lost taxes on lost income & lost production....
	(Per Decade):
Lives: 3,460,000:	Premature deaths that will be caused by smoking in 1980's.
1,050,000:	Cancer deaths that will be caused by smoking in 1980's."

-ACS(?), (handwritten photocopied sheet, found in 1982, on distribution shelf of a local unit of a state division of ACS).

"'Waste, fraud, abuse, & mis-management'.... ...cost the federal govt. $51 billion to $77 billion (yearly; 1980), hundreds of new federal investigations & audits show. Yet...Elmer Staats (Comptroller General, USGAO) caution(s) that only a fraction of the fraud & waste has been uncovered." - Chicago Tribune, Jan. 18, 1981, City Ed., p.1.

"...For every dollar paid out of the (Michigan) state's welfare fund to...the poor, still another dollar is paid out to push a medical professional into the next higher income tax bracket." - "White Collar Welfare Fraud", Michigan Voice, v.7, n.9, p.12, Dec. 1983.

"...San Jose Mercury(:) US companies paid out over $77 billion in 1983 for health insurance premiums. That was more than those firms paid out in dividends." - Quality, v.24, n.1, p.134, Jan. 1985.

"Since I have been associated with the NCI Advisory Committee for the Diet, Nutrition, & Cancer Program, I feel very strongly that nutrition research has been consciously ignored...by the NCI. The Advisory Committee's final resolution, before it was abolished, was that a minimum of $15 million should be spent on new research programs. ...No such action was ever taken, even though the Congress subsequently recommended that the NCI spend a minimum of $7.5 million.... .... At the time our committee was terminated, there was a backlog of 119 projects needing a total of $26 million.... .... I think people who have training in clinical human nutrition are oftentimes not individuals who are medical doctors, but people who have a training in nutrition by quite another, different route."

"...The juice of a lemon(:)....consider the tremendous beneficial effects that this single dietary modification has had upon the seafaring nations.... ... Uncomplicated solutions to seeming complex problems of the past are often ignored...."

- Peggy C. Fry, PhD, Ass't Prof., & Chief, Nutrition Service, Children & Youth Project, Univ. of Texas Health Sciences Center, (in Nutrition & Cancer Research, Hearings, Subcommittee on Nutrition (Hon. George McGovern, Chair.), Committee on Agriculture, Nutrition, & Forestry, US Senate, June 12 & 13, 1978, p.30, 34, 35, 94).

B.Q.7.0 RELATED FIELDS:

B.Q.7.1 OLIGARCHY of MULTI-NATIONAL CORPORATIONS:

"The AMA protects the image of the food processors by its constant propaganda that the American food supply is the finest in the world, & that (those) who question this are simply practicing quackery. The food processors, in turn, protect the image of the AMA & of the drug mfrs. by arranging for the USDA & its dietetic cronies to blacklist throughout the country & in every public library, all nutrition books written for the layman, which(:)preach simple, wholesome nutrition, & attack ... both (:) the emasculation of natural foods; & orthodox American medical care, which ignores subtle malnutrition, & stresses drug therapy, ("as distinct from vitamin therapy"), for innumerable conditions. The drug mfrs. vigorously support the AMA since only MD's can prescribe their products." - Miles H. Robinson, MD; Prof., U. Penn. Medical School; Prof., Vanderbilt U. Med. School; exhibit in Vitamin, Mineral, & Diet Supplements, Hearings, Subcom. on Public Health & Environment, Com. on Interstate & Foreign Commerce, US House of Rep., Oct. 29,30, & 31, 1973, (p.490).

"The experience with the ICC & CAB, in which cartels are being protected from the public should not be confused with consumer protection statutes such as the F,D, & C Act, OSHA, CPS Act, & other legistlation which more clearly intends to prevent harm to the public." (Continued)

"In considering this legistlation, then, the question needs to be asked, will it significantly reduce the mounting toll of medical device-caused injuries & deaths, or will it simply further the cartel status of the largest companies which control this multi-billion dollar per year industry?" - Sydney M. Wolfe, Director, Health Research Group, Public Citizen, attachment to (prepared) statement, in: FDA Oversight: Medical Devices, Hearing, Subcom. on Oversight & Investigations, Committee on Energy & Commerce, US House, July 16, 1982, Serial No. 97-144, p.183.

"During the early years of Hitler's regime, the government's medical program was looked upon by many observers as one of the greatest props of the totalitarian state." - Canadian House of Commons committee report on health insurance, March 16, 1943, (in Melchior Palyi, Compulsory Medical Care & the Welfare State, "From Bismarck to Lenin...", p.24).

"...The German govt. health insurance plan is obligated by law to pay for a special 4 week treatment with nutritional therapy in post-intensive care hospitals every year for up to 5 years after the intensive care of every cancer patient...." - IACVF, Dade County Chapter, (Wm. Cleare Filer, member), Holy Cancer, p.9.

"We found that medical expenses for people who had been paying at least an average of $10,000 a year decrease approximately 80% over the 2 years spent in our ((w)holistic) program. ...Blue (Cross &) Shield is not likely to pay for what we do." - C. Norman Shealy, MD, PhD; Pres., AHMA (Amer. Holistic Medical Assoc.); Self Help for Patients, ICRF (Independent Citizens Research Found'n), p.18.

"Dr. Nathaniel W. Boyd...was an invited guest speaker at the recent annual national convention of the American Osteopathic Assoc. ....He has treated more than 8,000 patients.... Boyd's method(:)...injection of sclerosing agents to promote fibrous tissue growth in weakened areas that cause hernias & hemorrhoids. .... His success rate with hernias is an incredible 95%. .... In 1974, Boyd's license was suspended for six months because he had advertised...." ....

"As the Medicare program edges toward bankruptcy, it refuses...to pay $600 for non-surgical treatment of hernias, preferring instead to pay for the surgical methods, which today cost a minimum of $3,000." - Liberty Lobby, Spotlight, Feb. 11, 1985, p.14.

"50% of Blue Cross board members throughout the country are hospital administrators & trustees. Other Blue Cross directors are businessmen & doctors with hospital ties. .... Only 1/5 of Blue Cross plans make audits of hospital accounts. .... About 2/3 of all Blue Shield board members are doctors."

"Shortly after the V. Pres. of (a major bank) became chairman of (that state's) Blue Cross, Blue Cross' deposit in the bank jumped...with not one cent of interest for Blue Cross. ....The bank profited...by not paying interest to Blue Cross."

"For Medicare Part A, hospitals & nursing homes choose the intermediaries. Blue Cross handles 93% of Medicare payments to hospitals, & 53% to extended care facilities ("only 7 commercial insurance cos. are involved"). Under Part B, the fed. govt. chooses the intermediaries, 60% going to Blue Shield. Under Medicaid, the state govt. picks the intermediaries, which are also largely the Blues."

(Some) "profits on sub-contracts average a staggering 40%."

"...Group policies pay out in benefits 96% of the premiums collected, whereas individual policies pay out only 51%."

- Medical Committee for Human Rights, (S.F.Bay Chapter: Elizabeth Harding, Tom Bodenheimer, Steve Cummings, Ed.), Billions for Band-Aids, c.1972, "Capitalizing on Illness...", p.55-67.

"For every $ we collectively deposit in:	This is how much, roughly, we collectively get to withdraw:
A Savings Bank	$ 1.05 ...
Blue Cross	$ 0.93 ...
Group Health Insurance	$ 0.87
Individual Health Insurance	$ 0.50 ...
Auto Insurance	$ 0.62 ...
Cancer Insurance	$ 0.41 ...
Medical Malpractice Insurance	$ 0.18 ...."

- Andrew Tobias, (author: The Funny Money Game; 5 books tot.), The Invisible Bankers, p.74.

"Between 16 & 20% of every $ paid in malpractice insurance went to compensate the victim; the rest was paid to lawyers & medical experts. In (malpractice) cases, doctors are vulnerable only to the charge of having acted against the medical code, of the incompetent performance of prescribed treatment, or of dereliction out of greed or laziness. The problem, however, is that most of the damage inflicted by the modern doctor does not fall into any of these categories. It occurs in the ordinary practice of well trained men & women who have learned to bow to prevailing judgement & procedure, even though they know ("or could & should know") what damage they do."(p.22).

"The USDHEW calculates that 7% of all patients suffer compensable injuries while hospitalized......One out of every 5 patients admitted to a typical research hospital acquires an iatrogenic disease, ...1 case in 30 leading to death. Half of these episodes result from complications of drug therapy; amazingly, 1 in 10 comes from diagnostic procedures."(p.23).

- Ivan Illich, (author of Deschooling Society), Medical Nemesis, c.1975, (1977, Bantam), p.22, 23.

"...Patients in cancer wards being fed a hospital diet of syrup-stewed fruits, custard, ice-cream, pastries, pies, & adulterated, preserved vegetables, is demonstration of the most infamous professional negligence."(p.99).

"The doctor (treating cancer:) No one expects more of him than that he goes through the standard rigmarole. .... If he tried an unorthodox method &, even after a period of success, it failed, he could find himself the object of litigation. As long as he sticks to orthodox methods of certain failure, he is totally safe."(p.48).

"...Alternative medicine has grown from(:) 'old wives tales'...common sense ...experience & observations...."(p.4).

"If a researcher, working in a well recognized field, makes a small discovery, it is likely to be published in a learned journal. ...a tiny step into the still unknown. .... However, let someone take an unexpected leap forward, ... & his action will tend to engender surprise, criticism, perhaps ostracism, &...lack of acceptance."(p.2). - Dick Richards, MD, The Topic of Cancer: When the Killing Has to Stop, (c.1982, Pergamon Press Ltd.), p.2, 4, 48, 99.

"...The Senate Aging Committee termed pacemaker fraud & abuse a billion dollar scandal, alleging that 30-50% of all pacemakers prescribed were not medically necessary." - AARP (Amer. Assoc. of Retired Persons), 1983 Federal & State Legistlative Policy, p.62.

"...31% of all hospitalized patients on the medical wards suffered adverse effects that were probably or definitely drug related. .... At least 1% of all admitted patients...died of an apparent drug reaction. ...2 to 8% of all drug doses given in hospitals are in error: wrong drug, wrong dose, wrong route of administration, wrong patient, or failure to give the prescribed drug. .... (Calculate) this...%...applied to all patients admitted to all hospitals in the US: ...32 million admissions per year...." - Milton Silverman, PhD; biochem. & pharm., Stanford U. & U. Cal. Med.; Pres., National Assoc. of Science Writers; Lasker Award; Lecturer, UCSF Pharm.& Med.; Sci. Ed., SF Chronicle; sci. writer: Saturday Eve. Post, &, Collier's, &, Reader's Digest; &, Philip R. Lee, MD; Stanford U.; NYU Med.; Mayo Clinic; Palo Alto Med. Clinic; Health Dir., AID (Agency for International Development); Dir., UCSF Health Policy Program; Prof.& Chancellor, UCSF; Assistant Secretary for Health, USDHEW; Pills, Profits, & Politics, p.262-4.

".... The willingness of the representatives of both international & local capital to allow malaria to spread in some areas of the world is part of the repressive underdevelopment of those areas.... .... Only mosquito & parasite resistance (to pesticides) appears to be a 'purely technical' problem. ....Bureaucratic ineptitude could explain only the initial period (before).... widespread publicity & criticism of the programs...."

"...Capital tries to undercut...through shortages, especially in energy & food. ....Education in the US....(:)...the campus upheavals of the late 60's, have now been replaced by underdevelopment in the form of fiscal crisis, budget cuts, accountability, & restructuring." - Harry Cleaver, Dept. Econ., U. Texas, Austin, "Malaria, the Politics of Public Health & the International Crisis", The Review of Radical Political Economics, special issue on "The Political Economy of Health", v.9, n.1, p.81, Spring, 1977.

"...Americans...automatically equate dissension with disloyalty. They view any criticism of our existing social, economic, & political forms, as sedition & subversion. .... ("The growing reluctance of Americans to criticize, & their increasing tendency to condemn those who, in ever dwindling numbers, will still voice dissent") "is disturbing, deplorable, & truly dangerous."

"Today's dissenters mainly focus their attention & expend their energies on the most inconsequential of trivia. .... Allegedly serious intellectuals quibble endlessly over such ridiculous trivialities.... In the meantime, the public is lulled into a perilous somnolence, spoon-fed pap, & palpable untruths, many of which are turned out by special-interest & pressure groups & well-organized propaganda machines."

"Some of our newspapers & magazines are more concerned with the welfare of their advertisers than they are with the dissemination of news & the discussion of matters of lasting importance. .... Radio, television, motion pictures, popular books — all contribute...to...the stifling of dissent on all but the most banal levels. ...a renunciation of the most basic & precious of democratic principles." - J. Paul Getty, ("the richest man in the world"-Fortune, Oct. 1957), How to be Rich, p.120-123.

"Loans have been extended to dictators on many occasions in our history.... Money from the US, as reported by various sources, subsidized Nazi Germany as well as Lenin's Russia. But today it's much worse...." - US Congressman Ron Paul, Freedom Report, FREE (Found'n for Rational Econ. & Educ.), v.9, n.4, p.2.

"...Xerography & Polaroid film were developed by small innovator-entrepreneurs only after larger firms turned down the ideas." ....

"The 1969 increase in capital gains taxes from 25% to 49% dried up venture money, especially for small companies. From 1969 to 1975, the amount of new capital acquired annually by small firms sank from $1.5 billion to $15 million."
- "The Sad State of Innovation", Time, Oct. 22, 1979, p.71.

"'Styling cars sells cars & safety does not.'" - Lee Iococca, General Mgr., Ford Div., Ford Motors; CEO (Chief Executive Officer), Chrysler Corp. (p.5).

"'Automobile injuries reached epidemic proportions a generation ago.... Yet our efforts to control the problem are still largely based on a hodgepodge of supposition & inference derived from assumptions we have never verified (&) never seriously tried to verify.'" - US Senator Pat Moynihan. (p.43).

"'After I published ("How to Cut the Traffic (Death) Toll in Half..."), I got very bitter calls from Detroit. They were indignant. .... They even went to... my boss. .... They (Dr. Bross's Ivy League U. employers) get very nervous, especially around grant-renewal time.'" (p.105).

"'The language that will reach the auto. cos. (on auto safety) is simple...$'s. ....Successful lawsuits.'" - Irwin DJ Bross, PhD; Statistician, Aeronautical Labs, &, Med. College, Cornell U.; Prof., Biostatistics, U. Buffalo; Dir., Biostat. Dept., Roswell Park Memorial Inst. for Cancer Research; (for last 2 paragraphs above).(p.170).

"The 'amateur experts'...play a role in auto. design for safety. The real experts, the auto. engineers, have abdicated their responsibility." (p.16).

"...The safety engineer...recommendations...get lost...up the corporate ladder. (At) the dizzying height...of the v.-pres. for styling, they are treated like crank letters." (p.17).

"'(A very major auto co.) is a bureaucracy. It has leadership, but no values.... .... The guy who says too much about safety doesn't get the juicy job.'"-H.Wakeland.(p.29).
- Jeffrey O'Connell (grad.: Phillips Exeter, Dartmouth, Harvard Law; Prof. Law, U. Ill.; Assoc. Dir., Auto. Claims Study, Harvard Law), &, Arthur Myers (of Washington Post; published in 6 major journals), Safety Last, p.5, 16, 17, 29, 43, 105, 170.

"'If the compression ratio of an engine...were raised to...10...to 1, little gain...should be expected....'" - Charles Kettering, V. Pres., GM (General Motors); contributor to Mem. Sloan-Kettering Cancer Ctr.; in SAE (Society of Automotive Engineers), More Efficient Utilization of Fuels, June 1-6, 1947.

"30 years after his remark, Detroit was spewing out engines with 10.5 to 1 compression ratios.... If Charles Kettering can be wrong, so can the skeptic down the street." - Michael H. Brown, Brown's Alcohol Motor Fuel Cookbook, p.43-7, (for last 2 paragraphs above).

"...Francis W. Davis...developed power steering for autos....during the early 1920's.... ...Major auto manufacturers....figured their engineering staffs could come up with something similar that would get around his patent. After all, their available engineering talent & resources went far beyond those of a lone inventor. .... The manufacturers tried to invent their way around Davis but without success. 26 years later, in 1952, Chrysler introduced power steering...using Davis' early, expired patents." - D. Dial, "The Creative Spark vs. The Status Quo; or, Why Big Companies Aren't Interested in New Ideas", (in Michael H. Brown, Suppressed Inventions & How They Work, p.77).

B.Q.7.1.1 UFO's:

"Only about 40 years ago, Prof. Herman Oberth, the teacher of Dr. Wernher von Braun, offered his book, By Rocket to Interplanetary Space to about 10 different publishers. Each sent it back to him." ....

"In his day, Prof. Goddard was called 'moon-mad Goddard'. But...the (US) House passed a bill to establish...(a) National Goddard Day."

"Franklin was the subject of laughter at the English Academy of Science when he reported his discovery of the lightning rod. They refused to print his report." ....

"Finsen, discoveror of the curative powers of ultra-violet rays, was persecuted too...yet after his death, a monument was erected in his honor." (Continued)

"...Prof. Biefeld of Denison U. (&) Townsend Brown (made) the discovery of... electro-gravitational energy.... ...The behaviour of a condenser (capacitor) when charged with electricity....(:) The startling revelation was that, if placed in free suspension with the poles horizontal, the condenser, when charged, exhibited a forward thrust toward a positive pole! .... If the positive pole is up, the condenser moves up ("ie, becomes 'lighter'").... The greater the mass of the material between the plates (dielectric) the greater the effect. ...A 'space car' (or) 'saucer'.... They act as a surfboard on a wave; the electrostatic activity apparently creating a local distortion of the gravitational field, down which the vehicle 'slides'." - Rho Sigma, Ether - Technology: a Rational Approach to Gravity-Control, c.1977, p.15, 16, 27-31.

"...I did have occasion in 1951 to have 2 days of observation of many flights of them (UFO's).... They were at a higher altitude than we could reach with our jet fighters of that time. .... Those few astronauts who have continued...in the UFO field...do so very cautiously. There are several of us who do believe in UFO's & who have had occasion to see a UFO on the ground or from an airplane." - US Astronaut Gordon Cooper, UN Conference on Flying Saucers, Nov. 28, 1978, (in UFO Review)

"Our President Jimmy Carter has stated that he believes in UFO's because he has seen one. ...in 1973 (at) the Thomaston, Georgia Lions Club. About 20 other people also...watched it for ten minutes. .... Pres. Carter was quoted as saying it was the darndest thing he had ever seen, & that he would never again make fun of people who say they have seen UFO's." - Winfield S. Brownell, UFO's: Key to Earth's Destiny, p.1, 9, (for last 2 paragraphs above).

B.Q.7.1.2 WAR / PEACE:

"People in the long run are going to do more to promote peace than our government. .... One of these days government had better get out of their way & let them have it." - Dwight D. Eisenhower, US Pres. (in Common Cause, v.8, n.4, p.57, Aug. 1982).

"Every gun that is made, every warship launched, every rocket fired, signifies in the final sense a theft from those who hunger & are not fed, those who are cold & are not clothed." - Dwight Eisenhower; US Pres.; Supreme Commander, Anglo-American troops, WWII; (in The Hunger Project, A Shift in the Wind, n.16, p.2, Aug. 1983).

"...Senate Doc. No. 259. The 65th Congress(:).... ...The coal companies made between 100% & 7,856% on their capital stock during the war (to end all wars, WWI). ....The leather people sold your Uncle Sam (100,000's) of ... saddles for the cavalry. But there wasn't any American cavalry overseas!"

"...The war (WWI) cost your Uncle Sam $52 (billion). ...$39 (billion) was expended in the actual war period. This expenditure yielded $16 (billion) in profits."

"No one told these American soldiers that they might be shot down by bullets made by their own brothers here. No one told them that the ships on which they were going to cross might be torpedoed by submarines built with US Patents."

"It is dressed into speeches about patriotism, love of country...but the profits...skyrocket...."

"...We can all make more money out of peace than we can out of war...."

- US Marine Corps Maj. Gen. (Ret.) Smedley Butler, Distinguished Service Medal,.. 4th Officer to receive 2 Congressional Medals of Honor before WWI, War Is a Racket, (1935;&,1984, Noontide Press), p.20, 24-7, 31, 43, 62.

"Since the end of WW II, 25 million people have died in war somewhere in the world. War has been fought in as many as 12 countries at one time. .... In 1981 the world spent about $22 for military purposes for every $1 it spent on development aid to poor countries." - "War vs. Development", Oxfam America News, Winter 1983, Special Report, p.1.

"Every year, 20 million people die from hunger or related diseases; at least 450 million go hungry every day. US military aid...to the third world....(:) Some 57 countries in the third world are under military control, & 80% of them are flagrant human rights violators." - "Action Alert", Food First: Inst. for Food & Dev't Policy, 1984.

"...An Israeli jet raid on the outskirts of Baghdad....(:) Nuclear reactors are strategic targets. .... A disturbing conspiracy of silence seems to surround any recognition of this pervasive danger. .... In 1979, the...(OTA) Office of Technology Assessment published...The Effects of Nuclear War....nuclear power facilities were not mentioned. .... Each new reactor (has) a 40-to-1 payoff in death for any incoming missile that triggers it. ....With a single 100-kilo ton bomb (or even a conventional bomb(?), not missile delivered - Ed.) aimed at a reactor, (terrorists) 'can, by waiting for the proper weather conditions, devastate a substantial fraction of the industrial capacity of an opponent.'(MIT)." - FoE (Friends of the Earth), Not Man Apart, v.13,n.5,p.12 & 21, June 1983.

"The idea of constructing shields of any material at all, for protection against uranium & plutonium is only a temporary expedient. The time will come when the shields will be as dangerous as the cores."(p.17).

"...The atom bomb tests' distribution of strontium in the atmosphere(:) ... our primary danger is in thet stratosphere 'hold up' .... (which) will blanket the atmosphere layer & eat into it slowly, but irrevocably, & thus thin our life giving & life protecting blue envelope." - Walter Russell (PhD, Amer. Acad. of Science; lauded by Nicola Tesla as 1,000 years ahead of times), & Lao Russell, Atomic Suicide?, c.1957, p.17, 76.

"...The power to decide whether or not doomsday has arrived is in the process of passing from statesmen & politicians to lower level officers & technicians &, eventually to machines." - Herbert York, "The Ultimate Absurdity", Race to Oblivion.

"On Nov. 9, (1979), a (NORAD) North American Air Defense Command computer decided that the US was under attack.... ...The error was caught in 6 minutes, before more than a few airplanes were launched — & no missiles. .... The computer...was fed a 'test tape' in which simulated signals of an incoming attack had been recorded." - FAS (Federation of American Scientists), Public Interest Report, v.32,n.10,p.6, Dec. 1979, (for last 2 paragraphs above).

"From Jan. 1979 to June 1980, America's early warning computers made the same mistake 147 times: sending out a serious false alarm that the Russians had sent their missiles flying!"

"...The commander of a nuclear submarine. If he loses contact with command (it happens all the time), he can order his crew to wage a nuclear war all by themselves! One Poseidon sub can wreak havoc on every Soviet city over 150,000 people, & a Trident (can) destroy 400 Russian missile silos within 15 minutes of launch!"

"In 1973, when Major Harold Hering was learning to launch a missile from its underground silo, he asked: 'If I get an order to fire, how can I be sure its real?' Instead of an answer, the Air Force gave him his walking papers for having "A defective mental attitude toward his duties'." - "Nuclear Believe It or Else!", Citizens Against Nuclear Power, No Nukes News, v.5,n.3,p.5, mid-Oct. 1982.

"Peace is our Profession" - SAC (Strategic Air Command), USAF (US Air Force), letterhead, motto.

"If the Air Force is truly sincere about their commitment to peace, they would develop peace corps, peace academies, & dialogues with the peace movement." ....

"I should not be on trial, but the policy makers & strategists should be. .... Deployment of even 1% of the nuclear weapons would disrupt the planet for human habitation. If your 'best' weapons are un-usable, they are obsolete. ....It is time for a new philosophy. Mankind could have never reached the moon by an aircraft with propellers. Peace tactics are the only alternative. Peacefare...." - Kim C. Gates, A1C, USAF, "Rebuttal to Letter of Reprimand", (followed by Honorable Discharge).

"One of the signs (you) displayed (said): **QUESTION AUTHORITY.** Comments or slogans of this nature cannot & will not be condoned." - C.L.Wilson, 1st Lt., USAF, Commander, Hq. Sq. Section; 93 CSG/CCQ; "Letter of Reprimand", Jan. 5, 1984.

B.Q.7.2 ENVIRONMENT, NATURE; EPA:

"Did you know that...sperm whales have the largest brains of any animal? Their brains weigh over 9 kg. (20 lbs.)!" - CEE (Center for Environmental Education), The Whale Report, v.6,n.2,p.8,Spring 1982.

"...Over 100 million animals will die this year in our nation's hospitals, universities, & government & commercial labs....most of them for no scientific or medical reason. ...scalded, suffocated, frozen, electrocuted, mutilated, or starved.... .... Last year, ...American taxpayers spent 4 billion $'s on govt.-funded animal torment. ...encourag(ed by) the powerful animal supply industry... pushing many species ("primates") to the brink of extinction." - leaflet, People for the Ethical Treatment of Animals.

"...Chemicals(:).... We not only don't know whether what's going out there is dangerous — we don't even know what's going out there. It's what we don't know that can really hurt us — kill us. .... It is time we started putting chemicals to the test — not people. It is time we gave the people of this country some reason to believe that every time they take a breath, or eat, or drink, or touch, they are not taking their life into their hands. It is time that, down here on earth, we took a couple of small sensible steps on behalf of human health & life...." - EPA Administrator Russell Train, speech at National Press Club, Feb. 1976, (in Ida Honorof, A Report to the Consumer, v.13, n.289-290, p.1, March 1983).

B.Q.7.3 AGRI-BUSINESS; USDA:

"...Mechanical & chemical technology can exact a high price in terms of erosion & human health. ...I have become increasingly uneasy about the state of agriculture & what it portends for the future of rural America." - Secretary of Agriculture, Bob Bergland, (in Heartland, (Michael James, Ed.), n.7, p.5, Sum.1981.

"The chief fault of many American diets is that they provide too little of the essential minerals & vitamins. This fault is due in large measure to the fact that refined foods are consumed in such amounts that the intake of mineral & vitamin-rich natural foods is lower than it should be." - Food & Life, USDA Yearbook for 1939, p.104, (reprint n.22, by the Lee Foundation for Nutritional Research).

"Others are urging farmers to follow the lead of the cigarette companies which have been going into non-tobacco businesses & could survive without their tobacco profits. ...The Piedmont Vegetable Marketing Coop. (is) to encourage farmers to grow & market vegetables that can prosper in the sandy soil...." - Caveat Emptor, v.12, n.1,p.3, Jan. 1982.

"Today, despite the tremendous amounts of pesticides being used, approx. 1/3 of the crops planted in the US fail to reach harvest due to pest damage. .... Ironically, these problems are caused by the very chemicals formulated to control pests. (:)increasing...resistant insects(,) loss of...beneficial insects...."

"An estimated 40,000 people were treated for pesticide poisoning in 1978.(US?). The actual number of poisonings may be even larger since many cases are not reported or are misdiagnosed. ...The symptoms of pesticide poisoning often mimic those of common illnesses (flu - Ed.)."

"Integrated Pest Management is an inter-disciplinary approach(:)...Crop-Pest Eco-systems.... In...single plant communities, natural ecological balances are altered, leaving crops highly susceptible.... Biological Controls....(:) Preservation of natural enemies (& their) habitats....Predators...introduced from other countries. .... Disease causing...micro-organisms (attacking pests).... Phero-mones.... Pest-resistant plant (varieties).... Cultural Controls ...(:) crop rotation, & removal of crop residues which shelter pests after harvest. .... Proper timing of crop...life-cycle.... ...'Trap crops'.... Urban(:) ....Pesticide treatments were reduced 99%...." - USEPA, Integrated Pest Management, EPA-600/8-80-044, Sept. 1980.

"A decade ago the WHO (World Health Organization) estimated every year at least 500,000 people were poisoned — & 10,000 killed — by pesticides in the third world. ...Since then...Dr. P. Deemar, toxicology director of Thailand's Ministry of Agriculture, estimates that 500,000 people are poisoned by pesticides every year in Thailand alone. .... Citizens of the industrialized countries are also victims when we eat pesticides in the food we import." ....

"This circle of poison (from the industrialized's) chemical corps. ...led the (IFDP) & activist groups from 16 countries to form PAN, the Pesticide Action Network." - Food First, (Frances Moore Lappe, Founder), IFDP (Inst. for Food & Development Policy), Food First News, n.12, Fall 1982.

"...The export of banned pesticides (in, made by, &) from the industrial countries (US) to the third world. ....(is) later returning to us in the food we import (from) ...the third world." - David Weir & Mark Schapiro; Center for Investigative Reporting; &, Food First - Inst. for Food & Development Policy; Circle of Poison, p.3.

"The Pesticide Conspiracy by Robert van den Bosch(:)....(Bosch) has been mercilessly harassed because of his beliefs & actions — by colleagues & administrators at his university, by the professional societies to which he belongs, by government contracting agencies, by editors & referees of journals in his field." - Paul de Forest, Prof., Center for the Study of Ethics in the Professions, (Prof. Mark Frankel, Dir.), IIT (Illinois Inst. of Tech.), (in The Bulletin of the Atomic Scientists, v.35, p.41, May 1979).

"Anyone who speaks up against food adulteration in any of the many forms, is subject to 'name calling'. The most common epithets are 'food faddist' or 'food fakir'. If...you are offending...some of our largest & most influential corporations....We can be certain that the public relations counsellors will go to work...-even if that requires a bit of character assassination...." - Dr. Edward J. Ryan, Editor, Dental Digest.

"Our agricultural colleges continue to graduate specialists who become vocational agricultural teachers in the schools, & county agents, who go forth to extol the virtues of poison insecticides, herbicides, & commercial fertilizers." - Joe Nichols, MD; Pres., NFA (Natural Food Assoc.); Board Chair., Atlanta National Bank; "Please, Doctor, Do Something"!, p.159, 160, (for last 2 quotes above).

B.Q.8.0 <u>PEOPLE</u>:
B.Q.8.1 <u>UNDERMINED MINORITIES</u>:

"Description of the NIH Peer Review System(:).... Criteria for Scientific Review Group Membership(:).... Assessment of...competence is based on... publications in refereed scientific journals.... Usually a doctoral degree or its equivalent is required. Service also requires mature judgement, balanced perspective, objectivity...." - Committee Management Office, NIH, NIH Public Advisory Groups: Authority, Structure, Functions, Members, Jan. 1984, NIH Pub. No. 84-11, p.v, vii.

"'Why is it that the US Supreme Court says physicians may perform abortions, on the ground that the physician - patient relationship is inviolable; but that the same physician is not permitted to prescribe Laetrile for his patients...not to destroy life but to save it? Why are we told that a patient has the "right to die with dignity", but may not take Laetrile in an attempt to live?'" - Alan Stang, American Opinion, (in Robert F. Rich, Ass't Prof., Woodrow Wilson School, Princeton University, "The Political Implications of Laetrile..."). (p.74).

"'The average citizen in this country does not have...the background that will enable him to make enlightened decisions concerning the selection & use of therapeutic agents.'" - Acting Director, NCI. (p.162).

"In a study of 252 people who attended a Laetrile symposium sponsored by the (CCS) Cancer Control Society, we found that those attending were predominantly white, female, rural, & highly educated." (p.3).

- Gerald E. Markle & James C. Petersen, Profs. of Sociology, Western Mich. U.; Eds., Politics, Science, & Cancer: the Laetrile Phenomenon, AAAS Selected Symposium 46, p.3, 74, 162.

"...Nearly 8 out of 10 persons agree that 'since we don't know how to cure cancer, if Laetrile is harmless, people ought to be able to buy it if they want to use it.'. Reinforcing this view are public doubts about the FDA & other government health agencies." - Lou Harris Poll of 1,600 Americans, July 1977, (in Michael Culbert, Save Your Life, p.43).

"My position is that radical mastectomy is archaic. For some strange reason, in the US, surgeons continue to mutilate women by removing muscles & excessive tissue even though modern knowledge & cancer therapies have outmoded this form of crippling surgery." - George Crile, Jr., Emeritus Consultant in Surgery, Cleveland Clinic, (in (Dr, Andrew C.) Ivy Cancer Research Found'n, Ivy Cancer News, v.11, n.3, p.3, Nov. 1974).

"...Obstetrical...invention of forceps in 1588. ....(:)...Peter Chamberlen, ... designed the first forceps but kept the secret of his invention...for 3 generations. .... Eventually, the design of the invention leaked out, but by that time, the wonder & mystery of forceps had become so legendary, that doctors used the device on all but the speediest births, often harming rather than helping the process, by their lack of training." ....

"...In 1847, Sir James Young Simpson...discovered the anesthetic properties of chloroform.... Ministers, priests, scientists, philosophers, & politicians, all (said) that woman's condition was to suffer in childbirth.... Simpson eventually won his fight by convincing Queen Victoria to take chloroform for the birth of her child in 1853." - Suzanne Arms, Immaculate Deception, p.23 & 24.

"In the 20th century, the cluster of metaphors & attitudes formerly attached to TB split up & are parcelled out to two diseases. Some features of TB go to insanity: ...passionate extremes.... Other features of TB go to cancer - the agonies that can't be romanticized. ....(Yet,) the ancient metaphoric connection between cancer & a pregnancy. ...Descriptions of cancer...from...military terminology.(include:)... 'invasive'...'colonize'...'defenses'...'radical'.... Radiotherapy(:)...'bombard(s)'... with toxic rays. & chemotherapy is chemical warfare, using poisons. ...'the war on cancer'...(!) It enormously ups the ante. ...An officer...besieging the...refugee camp...called the camp 'a cancer in the Lebanese body'. .... The people who have the real disease are also hardly helped by hearing their disease's name constantly being dropped as the epitome of evil." - Susan Sontag, Illness as Metaphor, c.1977, (1979, Vintage), p.35, 43, 63-65, 80, 82.

"Mae West & V.E.Irons speak warmly of the value of periodic coffee colon irrigation." - Dr. Richard Passwater, (author: Supernutrition: Megavitamin Revolution; & Supernutrition for Healthy Hearts; & many articles on cancer in American Lab.), Cancer & Its Nutritional Therapies, c.1978, p.154.

"There are almost no 'minority' groups found in the dental profession & here's why (:)....It costs about $45,000 to $55,000 to finish 4 years of dental school, not including the cost of college. ....Only 1½% of the dentists are women." - Thomas L. McGuire, DDS, The Tooth Trip, c.1972, p.225.

B.Q.8.2 **PATIENT, PRACTITIONER, RESEARCHER:**

"The USPHS recognizes a mere 3,400,000 of our 230,000,000 people as being healthy! This is only 1½%. .... The number of physicians on so-called hard drugs is about 19 times greater than...among the general population (per) NY Times in mid-1975." - College of Life Science (Herbert M. Shelton, T. C. Fry), Careers in Health, p.5-8.

"My father died an almost classic death from cancer. &, as author of the best book on cancer ever written, The Savage Cell, ("published in 1964"; &, The Persecuted Drug: the Story of DMSO) & for 26 years science editor of the ACS, he should have known better." ....

"With nothing but vitamin C (&) A (&) enzyme..., the Janker Clinic regressed his lung metastases...by 20%." ....

"Then he fell into bad company, his old friends in the field. .... 'Oh.' said the surgeon looking at his watch & excusing himself. What he (the surgeon) had cut away (by error) was my father's power of speech. .... They...put guards at the door to keep me from (my father's) bedside...." ....

"...Abolish the ACS.... That institution is a disgrace." ....

"...NCI (should) follow up on every single cancer patient in the nation, whether he's treated with (orthodoxy) or laetrile or hypnosis...." - Pat McGrady, Jr.; Moscow Bureau Chief, Newsweek; Pres., Amer. Soc. of Journalists & Authors; "The Cancer Patient's Quandary", Newsday, Sept. 30, 1984.

"Though it is a great frustration to realize that less than 10% of all cancer patients are willing to make the necessary life-style changes, required by most alternative cancer therapies, all we can really do is to inform the patient as thoroughly as possible & then let him or her make the final decision. ....(:) To undergo the Orwellian nightmare of conventional cancer treatments or...(the) non-toxic alternative, the Utopian choice of Earth as a beautiful place.... ... Pro-Life Freedom of Choice...." - Hellfried Sartori,MD,MPH,MS,U.Graz Med., Austria; Pres., Life Sciences Universal (1200 Med. Centers in world); Cancer 1984, p.1,8,title.

"For many decades, isolated physicians & scientists have worked on individual treatment programs, all of which may be classed as parts of metabolic therapy; only now are these separate programs & modalities being brought together in an orderly way to provide a 'total' treatment program for cancer patients. (That) is the goal of this presentation...."

"...There is no single 'cookbook recipe' or single protocol..., & ... individualized protocols must be designed by the practitioner on a per-patient basis. .... Any such individualized program is of necessity an integrated one...." - Robert Bradford (Knight of Malta, Sovereign Order of St. John of Jerusalem; Founder & Pres., CFCCT (Committee for Freedom of Choice in Cancer Therapy), & Bradford Research Found'n), Michael Culbert (Editor, The Choice (of CFCCT); author: Save Your Life?; &, Medical Revolution in America; &, Freedom from Cancer; ...), & Henry Allen, International Protocols for IIMP (Individualized, Integrated, Metabolic Programs) in Cancer Management, p.2.

"...Some 3,000 letters from doctors in about a dozen countries....were in response to (my) article "Anatomy of an Illness..."....(,)...evidence of an open attitude by doctors to new or unconventional approaches...." - Norman Cousins; Adjunct Prof., Dept. Psych. & Bio-Behav. Sci., UCLA Med.; hon. degrees, 42 colleges & U.'s; author, 14 books (Anat. of an Ill.); Editor, Saturday Review; Hon. Chair., Planetary Citizens; many awards; emissary for 3 US Pres.'s; "What I Learned From 3,000 Doctors", National J. Nutritional Acad., v.1, n.2, p.11, Fall 1978.

"'The group on placebo who thought they were on (treatment, modality), had fewer (disease morbidity), than the group on (treatment, modality) who thought they were on placebo.'" - Dr. Thomas Chalmers, Mt. Sinai Med., NY.

"...Paracelsus, Holmes, & Osler, have suggested that the history of medication is far more the history of the placebo effect.... Such modalities as bleeding ("in a single year, 1827, France imported 33 million leeches...")...."

"Living in the 2nd half of the 20th century...confers no automatic protection against...dangerous drugs & methods."

"... ...Minutes of genuine belly laughter had an anesthetic effect & would give me at least...hours of pain-free sleep." - Norman Cousins, "Anatomy of an Illness ("as Perceived by the Patient")" NEJM (New England J. Med.), Dec. 23, 1976; &, (reprinted by special arrangement with the Editor of NEJM, in) Saturday Review, May 28, 1977.

"That cactus went right through my eye. It left my eye flat. They took me to a doctor & he said, 'We'll have to take the eye out.' ...I fought like a tiger. I said, 'No! Leave the eye alone. I am sure it will grow back.' The doctor said, 'You're too young to know.' .... But in a year's time that fluid came back, & that eye is just as good as the other one today." - Bernard Jensen, DC, ND, (author, The Science & Practice of Iridology), FACT Journal, v.2,n.5,p.6.

"Some doctors blame the patients for demanding treatment....(which is too) powerful & dangerous...for mild (illness).... Patients demand (also:)...more considerate care, more natural healing techniques, & discussion of alternatives - & doctors rarely give in on these issues." - Robert Mendelsohn, MD, (lecturer on "Who Are the Real Cancer Quacks?"; Chair., Med. Licensing Comm., St. of Ill.;etc.), Confessions of a Medical Heretic, p.42.

"We are not at all sure that the state is serving the public interest by enforcing a professional monopoly." - Florence Stroud, RN, Member, Calif. BMQA (Board of Medical Quality Assurance); Ass't Dir. Health, San Francisco; (in Amer. Med. News, (in NHF, Health Freedom News,v.2,n.2,p.35,Feb. 1983)).

"Robert DeBragga...was diagnosed with terminal lung cancer. ...metastasized ....He began to research all aspects of the medical literature (on cancer), including alternative treatments.... ...He amassed a data bank of various therapies.... He collected, correlated, & analyzed approx. 1,700 documents.... He worked closely with ABC(TV)'s 20/20 on its 1981 program, 'The War on Cancer: Cure, Profit, or Politics?' (He was) testifying...before (US) Senator Paula Hawkins' oversight committee.... ...until the investigative committee was disbanded....(;) there is still no reason as to why (it) was dispersed." - Project CURE, Impact, (Robert DeBragga, Pres.), v.1, n.1, p.5, Sum. 1984.

"Cancer is a chronic, metabolic, systemic nutritional deficiency...."
"...Man in his arrogance & ignorance has had the audacity to flaunt the laws of the Bible & the laws of nutrition & the laws of common sense." - Glen L. Rutherford, cancer patient; Plaintiff, Rutherford v. US (n.77-2049; n.CIV 75-0218-B; 10th Dist. Ct., OK); (in Acres USA, Feb. 1979, p.22).

"...The FDA was ordered by Congress ("Agricultural Act of 1938") to stop two years of experiments designed to learn the dangers of poisoning from lead & arsenic, commonly used as insecticides until largely replaced by DDT, & the test animals were ordered killed - a procedure Consumers' Research compared to the Nazi book burnings."(p.203).
"Many 'health stores' sell naturally grown products. ...but they also have much junk. There are quacks & frauds in their ranks, just as there are among chemical growers & processors who enjoy the favors of the Government."(p.219).
- William Longgood, Pulitzer Prize winner in journalism, The Poisons in Your Food, c.1960, 1976, p.203, 219.

"Don't rely on product labels for accurate ingredient info...because most of those labels are incorrect. So says Charlie Kellenberger, who heads up the (NNFA) National Nutritional Foods Assoc. Standards Committee. Only (30%) were labeled correctly.... The rest of the labels were so fraudulent...." - Natural Foods Merchandiser, v.5, n.3, p.14, March 1983.
"Extensive lab. testing...began...to verify suspicions that preservatives are routinely added to products but not to product labels, Kellenberger explains(,) despite label claims such as 'all natural' & 'no preservatives added'." - Natural Foods Merchandiser, v.4, n.12, p.1, Dec. 1982.
"Counterfeit lab testing reports on organic produce items were ciculated recently by a...wholesaler." - Natural Foods Merchandiser, v.4, n.11, p.31, Nov. 1982.

"Many of the plants familiar to the 'wise woman' or the 'witch doctor' really do have the healing powers that tradition attaches to them! There is no doubt that the judicious use of such herbs, flowers, & other plants for palliative purposes in primary health care can make a major contribution towards reducing a developing country's drug bill." - Dr. Halfdan Mahler, Director-General, (WHO) World Health Organization, "The Staff of Aesculapius", World Health, Nov.1977, p.3.(p.42).
"I think that herbs should be a regular part of any prospective study done by NCI." - Bernard Statland, MD, PhD; Dir., Clin. Chem., & Assoc. Prof. Path., Medical School, U. of Cal., Davis; oral interview with J. Heinerman, June 17, 1980.(p.106).
"The data...support the conclusion that folklore is a useful tool in predicting sources of anti-tumor activity. ....plants with toxicity to an infesting organism, but minimal toxicity to the human host." - Medicinal Plant Resources Lab., Plant Genetics & Germplasm Inst., USDA, (in Cancer Treatment Reports, "Plants & Cancer" issue, v.60, p.984, Aug. 1976). (p.123). (Continued)

"...The empirical application of plants to the ailing human body over thousands of years has...culminated in the development of many useful drugs.... ...It is easy to make fun of mediaeval recipes; it is more difficult & may be wiser to investigate them."- Dr. Jonathan Hartwell, NCI, "Plant Remedies for Cancer", Cancer Chemotherapy Reports, v.7,p.19-24,May 1960). (p.123-128).
- John Heinerman, The Treatment of Cancer With Herbs, c.1980, p.42, 106, 123-8, (for last 4 paragraphs above).

"The Indians had no scurvy & neither did the few daring (Pilgrim) Colonists who followed the Indian custom of drinking hemlock tea. (They) were accused of being protected by the devil from the illness. .... Those free of (scurvy) were put under surveillance & suspected of hemlock tea drinking. Amazingly, most people chose to have scurvy, rather than be ridiculed or burned at the stake as witches."
- Thelma Arthur, MD, (author, "Morph. ... Leukocytes as a Detection Test for Early Cancer", J. Am. Path. & Bact.,v.78,n.1,p.65a, 1975), (in ICRF, Facts ... Nutrition, c.1965, p.4).

"The white plague is upon us. .... White sugar & salt (& flour & 'lightening' (alcohol) - Ed.).... ...Our 'evolved' society have prostituted...(us with) the pornographic food of vested interests...." - "The White Plague", Newsletter, Natural Hygiene, Inc.,(Jo Willard, Pres.), May 1984, p.1.

"The dogma of the West...is that our dietary habits are based on reason; it is only remote foreign tribes which believe in taboos. We deceive ourselves...(:) certain articles of diet - particularly meat - are considered to be masculine, & others (salad? -Ed.) feminine.... Yet another...is the use of special foods as badges of social status. ...(:) cow heel & tripe are attributes of the lower castes.... As food supplies became more plentiful & more certain, one after another, the nuts & roots, small wild game, wild leaves of diverse kinds - & insects as well - were, first of all, less highly prized, & then, not being customarily eaten, became taboo." - Magnus Pyke, Food & Society, 1958, p.10, 11, 40, 41, (in Deborah Katz, & Mary Goodwin, MPH, Food: Where Nutrition, Politics, & Culture Meet, CSPI, c.1976, p.14, 16).

"Societies that eat unrefined foods produce large stools & build small hospitals; societies that eat fiber-depleted foods produce small stools & build large hospitals." - Denis Burkitt, MD, FRCS, FRS, (of Burkitt's Lymphoma; author, Eat Right to Stay Healthy & Enjoy Life More), (in Nutrition for Optimal Health Assoc., NOHA News, v.6,n.4,p.2,Fall 1981).

"...One health study comparing poor to non-poor areas of Chicago found that the poor areas had a 60% higher infant mortality rate, a 200% higher incidence of premature births, 200% more new cases of tuberculosis, & a 100% higher death rate from cancer of the cervix. In the country as a whole, the maternal death rate for non-whites is four times that of whites. In the city slums there is three times as much heart disease, five times as much mental disease, four times as much high blood pressure, & four times as many deaths before age 35 as compared to the national averages. ...In 1969, at least 400,000 children were found to be suffering from lead poisoning - most of them in the older ghetto(s)...." - R. Feldberg, in Science for the People, Issues of Health Care, Sci. & Soc. Series n.1, p.2.

"800 million individuals remain caught up in absolute poverty: a condition of life so limited by malnutrition, disease, illiteracy, low life expectancy, & high infant mortality as to be beneath any rational definition of human decency." - Robert McNamara; US Secretary of Defense; Pres., World Bank, (in Mrs. John Steinbeck, Meals for Millions/Freedom from Hunger Foundation, open letter).

"What people eat is affected not only by what scientists know, or by what doctors tell them, or even by what they themselves understand. It is affected by Govt. decisions in the area of agricultural policy, economic & tax policy, export & import policy, & involves questions of good production, transportation, processing, marketing, consumer choice, income & education, as well as food availability & palatability. .... People learn the patterns of their diet not only from the family & its sociocultural background, but from what is available in the marketplace, & what is promoted both formally through advertising, & informally through general availability...." - Dr. Beverly Winikoff, Rockefeller Foundation. (p.5).

"...Degenerative diseases.... ...to their causation. Our genetic makeup contributes.... Diet is one of the things that we can change if we want to. ....The diet we eat today was not planned or developed for any particular purpose. It is a happenstance...." - Dr. D. Mark Hegsted, Prof. of Nutrition, School of Public Health, Harvard U. (p.3).

"...There is an important balance between sodium & potassium, required for the proper flow of fluids among & through cells. (There are) connections between high salt intake & ... stomach cancer, & cerebrovascular disease, ... hypertension .... migraine headaches...." (p.48-49).

- US Senate, Select Committee on Nutrition & Human Needs, Hon. George McGovern, Chairman, Dietary Goals for the US, Feb., 1977, p.3, 5, 48-49.

"What...water is to thirst, so normal metabolism is to cancer." - John Richardson, MD, Richardson Newsletter, v.1, n.4, p.3, 1978.

"We are still debating approaches, devising alternate plans, & finding ways to motivate refractory (obstinate) organizations to take the lead, to initiate what clearly should be done in human nutrition & disease prevention. .... The main impediments, I believe, are cultural, social, & economic." ....

"...Work is needed in the identification of individual dietary requirements under different genetic, somatic, behavioral, & environmental conditions(,) .... nutrition & exercise...pregnancy, childhood, & old age." - Theodore Cooper, MD, Dean, Cornell University Medical College, (in Nutrition & Cancer Research, Hearings, Subcommittee on Nutrition (Hon. George McGovern, Chair.), Committee on Agriculture, Nutrition, & Forestry, US Senate, June 12 & 13, 1978, p.82, 86, 87).

"In a noted 1943 Harvard study, there were no cases of toxemia, congenital anomalies, or neonatal deaths among a group of well-fed women. In contrast, 2/3 of the children born to women who were on poor prenatal diets had congenital abnormalities, died...or (had) neurological dysfunction. (&) 44% of the mothers developed toxemia...." ....

"...Restrictive diets(:) weight control, salt restriction, & drugs ("especially diuretics..."), cause(:) intra-uterine growth retardation.... ...maternal...metabolic toxemia of late pregnancy, abruption of the placenta, severe maternal-fetal infection, & anemias. ...(&) brain damage in children...." - SPUN (Society for the Protection of the Unborn Through Nutrition), c.1978, 1 pager, (Jay Hodin, Robert Mendelsohn, MD,... on Board).

"Unfortunately, most obstetricians in the US are more concerned with monitoring external signs...than in...nutritional stress of pregnancy. ...Nutritional nonchalance.... For the last 10 years, SPUN has tried to encourage the application of preventive, scientific...principles in...prenatal care.... The establishment of such standards is not yet in sight. ...Spread the message to the American people: Prevention Now!" - Tom Brewer, MD, Tulane U. Med. School; Pres., SPUN; "Dark Ages...: 1982", The Pregnant Issue: Medicate or Educate?, SPUN, v.6, n.3, p.4, May 1982.

"Animals (fed) on raw milk & raw meat reproduce homogeneous litters & the usual causes of death are old age & injuries.... The cats fed pasteurized milk... show skeletal changes, lessened reproductive efficiency, & their kittens present progressive constitutional & respiratory problems. ....Cooked meat (fed) cats ...commonly (have)....heart problems, ...infections of the (organs), inflammation.... ....parasites....abortions...." - Francis M. Pottenger, Jr., MD, author of 55 articles, Pottenger's Cats: a Study in Nutrition, (Elaine Pottenger & R.T. Pottenger, Jr., MD, Editors), c.1983, Price-Pottenger Nutrition Foundation, p.10-11, 15.

"Emotions play a role in determining the amounts of enzymes that are produced, the quality & quantity of bile, the activity of the intestine, & the mucous secretion of its walls. For this reason, the emotional state of the person also has an almost direct effect on the kind of bacteria that grow in the gut."(p.344).

"...The 'culture medium' that we create inside the large intestine determines to a great extent the strain of bacteria which will grow there. ....the bacteria of the colon produce vitamins(;)...in man...B vitamins...."(p.335).

"Since it is the gastric juice that is primarily responsible for maintaining the relative asepsis of the bowel, it is very important that gastric acid not be exceeded by the amount of food taken in."(p.343).

"...Psychotic episodes...is...a 'cerebral allergy'...an allergic reaction which is thought to affect the tissues of the brain primarily."(p.526).

"...When institutionalized adolescents with behavioral & emotional problems were tested for food & other allergies, & were kept away from those substances to which they reacted, average time before discharge was reduced from 26 months to 9 months."(p.528).

"...We may have some capacity for manufacturing some of the very nutrients that are usually regarded as essential. ...Man...to synthesize vitamin C....(:) ...Women who were breast feeding their infants regularly put out in their milk & in their urine quantities of vitamin C that far exceeded their dietary intake."(p.533).

- Rudolph Ballentine, MD, Duke Univ.; Prof. Psychiatry, Louisianna State U.; Dir. of Bio-feedback,... , Himalayan International Institute; Diet & Nutrition, a Holistic Approach, c.1978,(1979), p.335, 343, 344, 526, 528, 533.

"If...the supply of oxygen, glucose, water, vitamins, minerals, & amino acids is inadequate for even a short period of time, important social, cognitive, & perceptive areas of the brain will not function optimally & the lower centers will take over."

"Over 60% of prisoners have abnormal glucose tolerance tests." - Lendon Smith, MD, Foods for Healthy Kids, c.1981, p.145, 147.

"Accident Causation. ...traffic (Automobile)... : *Human factors caused between 83 & 96% of the accidents. Environmental factors...between 16 & 33%. Vehicle factors ...4 to 13%.... *The 4 leading human factors were: (1) improper lookout (22-25%); (2) excessive speed (10-20%); (3) inattention (13-19%); & (4) improper evasive action (9-18%). *The leading environmental factors were: (1) view obstruction (6-12%); (2) slick roads (5-8%); & (3) roadway design problems (2-5%). *...Vehicular factors were: ...brake failure...tire underinflation...(&) tread depth...." - NHTSA, DoT, Traffic Safety '74, p.17.

"...During the summer of 1978 in Rhode Island, 300 advanced...members of TM (Transcendental Meditation) split up into small groups to meditate.... The entire state of Rhode Island benefitted. Statistics revealed: the state murder rate dropped 50%; traffic deaths decreased 48%; suicides dropped 45%; total deaths decreased 11%. Statisticians, state officials, psychiatrists...attested to the...success of the experiment. Dr. Charles Hill, Pres., RI Medical Society, admitted...we can...."
- Linda Clark, MA, Editor, Linda Clark's Good Health Keeping Newsletter, PPNF (Price - Pottenger Nutrition Found'n), v.2,n.1,p.5.

B.Q.9.0 <u>AUDITS & ANALYSES, OFFICIAL:</u>
B.Q.9.1 <u>HEW, NIH:</u>

"'...That the certificate of (JCAH (Joint Commission on the Accreditation of Hospitals))...is taken as a guarantee that the quality of the care...will be excellent. That isn't true at all.... When we accredit, we really are saying that there is nothing to prevent good medical care in this place....'" - John D. Porterfield, MD, Director, JCAH.

"The JCAH is a Chicago-based, non-profit agency controlled jointly by the AMA, the AHA (Amer. Hospital Assoc.), the Amer. College of Physicians, & the Amer. College of Surgeons. ....Congress...wrote the JCAH into (Medicare) legistlation...."

"...HEW decided to do a nationwide spot check on a sample group of 105 JCAH-accredited hospitals. ...68 were declared to be substandard.... ...Shortcomings included incomplete drug records (&)...lack of controls in the dietary depts., so that patients were not necessarily being given prescribed foods (..."malnutrition")."

"...<u>Neither</u> public nor private entities monitor the actual quality of health care provided by hospitals...."

"The 'confidentiality' of JCAH survey findings means that a veil is thrown over the whole issue of hospital quality." - Don Rubin, Pres., Consumer Commission on the Accreditation of Health Services, (in Health Law Project, <u>Library Bulletin</u>, v.5, n.4, p.90-98, (for last 5 paragraphs above)).

"...Congress...created PSRO's (Professional Standards Review Organizations) to review the utilization & quality of Medicare & Medicaid services. .... The public has no access to data about PSRO review decisions. ....Both HEW & Congress have consistently ignored the substantial benefits which would flow from disclosure of PSRO data. .... What consumers need is objective, accurate, meaningful information on the 'track record' of individual doctors & hospitals. ...What is their complications or mortality rate as compared to other providers treating comparable patients? ...Organized medicine....(has) create(d) a secret review system with no accountability to consumers." - T. Bogue, Health Research Group, Public Citizen, "PSRO's: a Magical Medical Mystery Tour", Health Law Project, <u>Library Bulletin</u>, v.4, n.6, p.180, June 1979.

B.Q.9.3 <u>SELF ANALYSIS:</u>

"...Mismanagement (causes NCI virus program procedures which) are apparently attuned to the benefit of staff personnel & are full of conflicts of interest. .... Because the direct targets have become fuzzy, although the available funds for the program continue to grow, the program seems to have become an end in itself, its existence, justifying its further existence." - "Zinder Report", by 11-member committee, chosen by NCI Dir. Dr. Frank Rauscher, & headed by Dr. Norton Zinder of Rockefeller University.

"The first time I went for (an NCI grant), they told me the idea was too radical. (The second time:) too conservative. .... The nature of peer review criticism is to drive you into an accepted mode of thought. They behave as though they had the answer, that's what's wrong." - Eli Seifter, PhD, Prof., Biochem. & Surgery, Albert Einstein College of Medicine.

- last 2 paragraphs above in <u>Newsday</u>, Jan. 10, 1977, article submitted by US Senator Robert Dole, into <u>Nutrition & Cancer Research</u>, Hearings, Subcom. on Nutrition, (US Senator George McGovern, Chairman), US Senate, June 12 & 13, 1978, p.122-123.

B.Q.9.4 <u>OFFICIAL</u> <u>NUTRITION</u> <u>RENAISSANCE</u>:

"In...1980, the NCI commissioned the NRC to...study of the scientific information (on) the relationship of diet & nutrition to cancer. .... Summary & Conclusions: ....Less attention has been paid to the B vitamins & others such as vitamin K. .... The epidemiological evidence is sufficient to suggest that foods rich in carotenes or vitamin A are associated with a reduced risk of cancer. .... The results of several case-control studies & a few correlation studies suggest that the consumption of vitamin-C-containing foods is associated with a lower risk of certain cancers, particularly gastric & esophageal cancer. .... Limited evidence from studies in animals suggests that vitamin E may also inhibit the induction of tumorigenesis by other chemicals. .... The assessment was severely limited by a paucity of relevant studies on all but two minerals - selenium & iron. ....Both the epidemiological & laboratory studies suggest that selenium may offer some protection against the risk of cancer. .... Iron deficiency has been related to an increase in the risk of Plummer-Vinson syndrome, which is associated with cancer of the upper alimentary tract. .... Different levels of dietary zinc either enhance or retard tumor growth, depending on the specific test design (& organ site). There is some epidemiological evidence that a deficiency of molybdenum & other trace elements is associated with an increased risk of esophageal cancer. ...Iodine deficiency, &...excess...may increase the risk of thyroid carcinoma. ....There is sufficient epidemiological evidence ...that consumption of certain vegetables, especially carotene - rich ("i.e., dark green & deep yellow") vegetables, & cruciferous vegetables ("e.g., cabbage, broccoli, cauliflower, & brussels sprouts"), is associated with a reduction in the incidence of cancer at several sites in humans." ....

"Interim Dietary Guidelines: .... The committee recommends that the consumption of both saturated & unsaturated fats be reduced.... (&) food preserved by salt - curing ("including salt - pickling") or smoking be minimized. The committee emphasizes the importance of including fruits, vegetables, & whole grain cereal products in the daily diet." - Committee on Diet, Nutrition, & Cancer, of the Assembly of Life Sciences, of the NRC (National Research Council), of the NAS (National Academy of Sciences), <u>Diet</u>, <u>Nutrition</u>, <u>&</u> <u>Cancer</u>, Executive Summary, (in <u>Nutrition</u> <u>Today</u>, <u>v.17</u>, n.4, p.20, July 1982).

"The NCI has developed a new program, called the Chemoprevention Program, ...Studies have identified...potential chemopreventive agents: ... protease inhibitors, ..., indoles, & uric acid. ....Beta-carotene, vitamins A, C, & E, & the trace element selenium may prevent, inhibit, or reverse carcinogenesis.... ... Beta-carotene......In animal & limited Phase I human studies, it has shown no toxicity. Dietary questionnaires designed for more general purposes happened to ask about the main beta-carotene source.... ...Cancer of the esophagus(:) low intake of ...thiamin, or riboflavin is a risk factor...." - OCC (Office of Cancer Communication), NCI, <u>Backgrounder</u>, "NCI's Chemoprevention Program", Nov. 1982.

"The report of the <u>Ad</u> <u>Hoc</u> Subcommittee on Diet, Nutrition, & Cancer Research, recommending support of 'a special research emphasis in nutrition & cancer', was adopted by the NCAB.... ...to investigate the role of nutrition in causation, prevention, & treatment of cancer.... .... Dr. (Maureen) Henderson explained that her subcommittee's report differed from the Diet & Cancer Report of (NAS - NRC).... Dr. Henderson said the NRC report 'is based only on published literature. It does not take into account ongoing research & it particularly has not ranged widely in the medical field looking at issues related to nutrition.' ....The subcommittee feels present research objectives in the area of chemopreventives are too 'narrowly focused to serve as the major NCI thrust in this area'. .... There is need 'to bring new sciences...(for) multi-disciplinary research approaches....'"
- NCAB, <u>Annual</u> <u>Report</u>, Oct. 1981- Sept. 1982, NIH Pub. No. 83-2605, "Nutrition",p.1.

"...In the history of medicine & science, no chronic or metabolic disease has been cured or prevented by factors foreign to the diet, (or) to biological experience."

"The agent that cures prevents, & the agent that prevents cures." - Dr. Ernst T. Krebs, Jr., DSc; International Medical Society for Blood & Tumor Diseases Award: John Beard Memorial Foundation; (in Spotlight, Oct. 23, 1978, (in CCS, Cancer Control Journal,v.6,n.1,p.67,Jan. 1978, 1982)).

"Cancerous lesions may be partially excised through surgery, just as in the Middle Ages, small pox pustules were removed by surgery." ....

"One of the many reasons that I am condemnatory toward the scientifically frivolous & utterly nonsensical nostrums that fall too frequently into the non-toxic 'alternative cancer therapy' category, is that these further bleed the already exanguinated cancer victim of health & money." ....

"What we need are several carefully run clinical centers. .... (for) the catalogued, systematized, correlated, & quantified corpus of the science.... ... (of) physiological oncotherapy...." ....

"The report on Diet, Nutrition, & Cancer, of the NRC of the NAS, ...1982.... lists the Cruciferae as containing anti-neoplastic factors comprising the thio-cyanogenetic glyco-sides.... The a-glycone or non-sugar portion of such molecules contain - in some cases - indole. ...anti-neoplastic (?).... (These) 'thio-cyano-phoric glyco-sides', in my terminology are called 'thio-nitrilo-sides' or sulfur-containing nitrilo-sides, that are hydrolyzed to HCN, sugar, etc., through the same glycosidases that so hydrolyze the non-sulfur-containing nitrilo-sides ("Laetrile")...."

"The ...transparency of some...latter day nutritionists is expressed in their caveat that the cancer victim must not overdose on ordinary vitamin A, but rely on the physician - prescribed, synthetic, 'vitamin A's' - the retinoids of (a drug co.)."

"Diagnostically...the detection...of the trophic hormones exclusive to trophoblast. (:)...cancer is trophoblast in spatial &/or temporal anomaly ("hybridized or un-hybridized, with contiguous hostal or somatic tissue")." - Dr. Ernst Krebs, Jr., co-discoveror of Vitamins B-17, & B-15, (in letter to Ralph Hovnanian, Dec. 4, 1982).

"According to recent ACS reports, the discovery of the anti-tumor properties of beta-carotene (nutrient "from which the body makes vitamin A") is one of the most important developments in cancer research of the past ten years, ie, since the passage of the National Cancer Act. ....The NCI & the NIH...did not participate in the initial development or funding of the beta-carotene studies! ....The NCI has promoted...retinoic acid & retinoids, chemically related peripherally to vitamin A.... The chemicals...were known by the NCI to be dangerous to...animals even before the NCI tests with the retinoids were initiated; however, these chemicals (retinoids & acid) were inaccurately represented as being less toxic or more efficacious than (Vit. A & beta-carotene).... ...We have been applying to the NIH for grant support on (beta-catotene) since 1974. However, the NCI had consistently rejected both (the) grant requests & the concept of using beta-carotene, until the collapse of the retinoic acid studies. ....We found that beta-carotene increased the effectiveness of tumor therapeutic agents, whereas retinoic acid only served to increase the toxicity of the chemotherapeutic agents. .... When novel studies were proposed, the NCI seemed determined to stamp them out. They were so restrictive as to discourage the development of even one concept that did not conform to their dogma. ....

(Continued)

The NCI & the NIH are...creating unnecessary confusion among scientific workers who were misdirected by the distortions.... .... I fear that some members of important sections of the NCI may have been more concerned with service to themselves & their associates than to the public or the extramural scientific community, & repeatedly have made grevious errors.... ...Your (legistlative) committee might determine if these errors can be rectified, & procedures altered to prevent repetitions of grievous errors by the NCI & NIH." - Eli Seifter, PhD, Prof., Surgery & Biochemistry, Albert Einstein College of Medicine, (in letters to US Senators Orrin Hatch & Harrison Schmitt, on July 16 & Aug. 4, 1982, resp.).

"Wherever possible, the nutrients required should be obtained from natural foods rather than synthetic preparations. This is particularly true of the vitamins. Synthetic vitamin concentrates, tablets & pills, may not contain all of the known nutrients, either as such, or in optimal proportions. Furthermore, they obviously may not contain lesser known or unknown nutrients, which are, however, provided by natural foods." - US Army Nutritional Manual, 1949, (in Beatrice Trum Hunter, The Great Nutrition Robbery, c.1978, p.133).

"Recent studies have uncovered a shocking degree of overt undernutrition among hospitalized patients. ....Nutritional management('s)...inclusion in patient care may largely pay for itself by tradeoffs in other areas." - OTA (Office of Technology Assessment, US Congress), Nutrition Research Alternatives, OTA-F-74, Sept., 1978, p.55.

"...Nutritional science is interdisciplinary & complex.... ...Malnutrition in the hospitalized patient...has been reported to occur by a number of nutrition surveys. ....Several surveys have uncovered certain vitamin deficiencies among the elderly." - Artemis P. Simopoulos, MD; Chair, Nutrition Coordinating Committee, NIH; "Overview of Nutritional Status in the US", Nutrition in the 1980's: Constraints on Our Knowledge, c.1981 Alan R. Liss, NY, p.237-247.

"Nutritional Support of the Cancer Patient: The patient can be fed intravenously or by stomach tube. ....the form of nutrient being determined more by the manufacturing requirements than by the needs of the patient. .... If the patient is hospitalized, the immediate problem is how to deal with the mediocre food served.... Unless...the staff...knows how to prepare nourishing meals, we strongly recommend that members of the family prepare food at home & take it to the patient."

"Cancer Politics: To suggest people eat less meat infuriates the cattleman's assoc. To suggest people eat less candy angers the confectioner's assoc. To suggest people eat more fresh vegetables throws the canner's assoc. into fits." - Ross Hume Hall, PhD; principal cancer researcher, Roswell Park Memorial Institute; Prof., McMaster Univ., Canada; Director, ETI (En-Trophy Institute); (author, Food for Naught); "Cancer & Nutrition", En-Trophy Review, v.3, n.3, p.9 & 12.

"The hospital that feeds you refined sugar, white bread, canned soup, bouillon cubes, & frozen vegetables should be closed by the health dept. as a menace to the public health." - Dr. David Reuben, Everything You Always Wanted To Know About Nutrition, c.1978, (in John Heinerman, The Treatment of Cancer With Herbs, c.1980, p.146).

"...The introduction of trans-trans-linoleic acid in the 1920's in margarines & refined vegetable oils was a main cause of the pandemic of myocardial infarction (coronary heart disease), & ... since 1960, orthodox medicine has been fostering (promoting) a cause of this disease as the cure." - Wayne Martin, "Margarine ("Not Butter") the Culprit?", Lancet, v.2, n.8346, p. 407, August 13, 1983.

"Avoid foods that don't interest you (:)...cauliflower, corn, broccoli, beans...."(p.4).
"Hints (:)...Add milk powder...."(p.18). "...Choose from: ...Angel food cake, Popsicles, ... Hard & jelly candies."(p.21). "Use mixes, frozen ready to eat main dishes, & take out foods whenever possible."(p.30). "...fry...."(p.31). "Microwave oven...."(p.32).
"Recipes....high in nutritional value(p.33)(:) ...non-dairy creamer (p.54).... ...ice-cream (p.59).... ...condensed milk (p.65).... ...soft shortening...chocolate chips (p.67).... ...sugar...oil...baking soda...baking powder...salt (p.77) ...." - OCC (office of Cancer Communications), NCI, Eating Hints ..., (by Yale-New Haven Med. Ctr.: M.Morra; N.Suski, dietician; B.L.Johnson), NIH Pub. No. 80-2079; Jan. 1980; p.4, 18, 21, 30, 31, 32, 33, 54, 59, 65, 67, 77.

"...Recipes...selected (p.iii)(:) ...ice cream...carbonated beverages (p.16) ....processed sharp cheese spread (p.24).... ...sausage or hot dog (p.28).... ...lard or shortening...sugar...soda...baking powder...all purpose flour (p.38).... ... ...baking soda...salt (p.42).... ...cooked or canned vegetables (p.48).... ...chocolate...malted...ice cream, jello (p.50).... ...coffee, coffee substitute, carbonate beverages (p.56).... ...bread(,)enriched white (p.57).... ...pureed, baby, or whole cooked (...canned or frozen) (p.58).... ...sweets as desired, hard candy,..jellies, jams (p.59)...." - ACS, Nutrition, for Patients Receiving Chemotherapy & Radiation Treatment, c.1974, p.iii, 16, 24, 28, 38, 42, 48, 50, 56, 57, 58.

"Rinse the child's mouth with a mixture of hydrogen peroxide & warm water when mouth & gums are sore. This Mouthwash Should Not Be Swallowed."(NCI's emphasis).
"Have your child use a good fluoride toothpaste & mouthwash." (No warning from NCI). (p.27).
"Allowed Foods: Carbonated beverages...fruit-flavored drinks...sugar candy... salt...ice cream...chocolate...cereals, refined...oils...pork...fudge...lollypops ...crisp bacon...." (p.40-44).
- DNCP (Diet, Nutrition, & Cancer Program), NCI, Diet & Nutrition: a Resource for Parents of Children With Cancer, NIH Pub. No. 82-2038, May 1982, p.27, 40-44.

B.Q.10.0 RESEARCH of RESEARCH:
B.Q.10.1 STATISTICS, (SURVIVAL, DELAYED TREATMENT, DETECTION):

"In...categories which make up about... eight % of the incidence, 5-year survival rates have actually fallen — those are cancers of the lip, penis, esophagus, vulva, & bone, & invasive cancer of the cervix (all where prognosis is worse now than in 1950's)."
- Newsday, Jan. 10, 1977, article submitted by US Senator Robert Dole, into Nutrition & Cancer Research, Hearings, Subcom. on Nutrition, (US Senator George McGovern, Chair.), US Senate, June 12 & 13, 1978, p.116.

"After approx. 2 decades & several billion dollars.... Among the various types of cancer that account for 78% of the incidence...the upward trend in survival rates has not exceeded a few %.... ...a far gloomier picture than has been generally conveyed to a hopeful public by our leading cancer research institutions....A generally passive lay press has been the means of transmission."
"Papanicolaou published for 15 years before anyone would listen to him, but now you find ACS extolling the virtue of the Pap test." - Daniel S. Greenberg, (Editor, Science & Govt. Report; columnist, NEJM), "Cancer: Bad News", Washington Post, Jan. 19, 1975, (in ICRF Newsletter, v.4,n.4, p.1, Winter 1975).

"'In many quarters, the superiority of combination therapy ("surgery & radio-therapy") is accepted as established dogma,& re-examination of treatment policies as heretical. Despite the confident air of this position, a life-sparing effect, specifically attributable to the radio-therapeutic component of combination regimens, has not been proved.'" - Morrow & Di Sala, "The Role of Post - Operative Irradiation ...", American Journal of Roentgen-ology, Aug., 1976, (in Leon Chaitow, An End to Cancer?, p.119).

"...This issue...will explore...all forms of cancer therapies, even those frowned upon, &, in some cases, actively thwarted, by organized medicine." ....

"The medical establishment would have us believe that before all treatment procedures become acceptable for general use, they are subjected to exhaustive studies which have proven both safety & effectiveness. This belief is reinforced by (medics') criticism of the non-medical cancer treatments, the most damning of which is: 'They are unscientific.'" ....

"...Surgical & radiation treatments....do not lend themselves to double-blinding or use of placebo." ....

"According to...JAMA, over 30 different surgical procedures have been introduced over the years for the relief of angina & myocardial blood supply, yet only 2 were subjected to the appropriate controlled studies." - Maryann Napoli, Ed., & Arthur Levin,MPH,Dir., Center for Medical Consumers, & Health Care Info., Inc., Health Facts, "Cancer...", v.3,n.13,p.1-3, Jan. 1979.

"...Whereas spontaneous cure (of cancer) remains a scientific curiosity with a rate of 0.000,01%, the administration of Krebiozen has given a recovery rate of 12.5%, or a 1,250,000 fold increase." - Stevan Durovic, MD; post-graduate at U. Vienna, & Pasteur Inst.; "Cancer & Krebiozen...", Today's Japan Orient / West, v.6,n.5,p.51, May, 1961.

"'It is often necessary to make a decision on the basis of knowledge sufficient for action but insufficient to satisfy the intellect.'" - Immanuel Kant, (1724-1804).

"...Epidemi-ologic(:) Comparison of mortality & incidence rates between countries & within a country, surveys of migrants, & retro-spective & prospect-ive case-control studies have established that cancer is not an inevitable consequence of aging." - Ernst L. Wynder, MD; Pres., Amer. Health Found'n; Chief of Epidemiology, MSKCC (Memorial Sloan-Kettering Cancer Ctr.); "Cancer & the Dietary Environment", J. Nutritional Acad., v.2, n.1, p.28, (for last 2 paragraphs above).

"...I am distressed that relatively few inquiries are under way. We urgently need more case-control studies &, in particular, more large-scale, long-term, prospective studies. ...(&) to speed up the use of such longitudinal data as are available(:)...sera obtained...since the 1940's in the Framingham pop. & other cohort studies...done...." - Dr. Saxon Graham, Dept. Social & Preventive Med., SUNY, "Results of Case-Control Studies of Diet & Cancer...", ACS, Workshop Conf. on Nutrition in Cancer Causation & Prevention, AACR (Amer. Assoc. for Cancer Research), Cancer Research, v.43, n.5, Suppl., p.2412s, May 1983.

"(The) Percent Distribution of Persons with...Limit in Major Activity...Due to Chronic Conditions, Under 17 (years old, in:) 1967 (was) 1.1(%)
(& in:) 1976 (was) 1.9(%)."
- NCHS (National Center for Health Statistics), Vital & Health Statistics, Series 10, n.119, 52, Tables 9 & 14.

"...Increased proportions of younger persons are suffering from chronic disease." - "The Rise of Chronic Disease In Young People", J. Nutritional Acad., v.2, n.3, p.15, (for last 2 paragraphs above).

"...Pathological states are the consequence of several determinant factors acting simultaneously.... The manifestations of any given agent differ profoundly from one person to another. ....Each noxious agent can express itself by a great variety of different pathological states. ....Different agents can elicit similar reactions. .... The total environment & the (interior medium) constitute a multifactorial system...." - Rene Dubos, MD; Prof., Rockefeller Inst.; Prof., Harvard Med.; (Mary) Lasker Award; Ways of Health.

"...Most diseases can be detected only after symptoms appear.... Repetitous annual exams of healthy individuals seem to be profitable only for the physician." - Dr. Richard Spark, Harvard Med., (in George Berkley, PhD, Cancer..., p.132).

"...One-third of the cancers found in the (HIP) Health Insurance Plan study were not felt by the clinician. ...Two-fifths of the cancers were noted by the surgeon, but not detected by the radiologist. In only one-fifth of the cases were the cancers found by both physicians." - Philip Strax, MD, Early Detection, p.13.

"The fact that a patient survives for 5 years after an operation does not imply that he is cured. .... The number of recurrences drops after 5 years only because the total number of survivors has dropped.... In reality, the curves show that between 1 month & 10 years, the rate of death remains constant." - Lucien Israel, MD; NCI consultant; French hospital director; Conquering Cancer, p.6 & 7.
- (last 4 paragraphs above in:) Cameron Stauth, (co-author: Starch Blocker Diet/ Cookbook;&Folk Med. for Today; chief ed.: J. Nutr. Acad.; & J. Health Sci.; & Internat'l Health Inst. Ltr.; tv health host; Founder, Cancer Prev. Soc.), The New Approach to Cancer, p.68-70, 258-9, 283-4.

"'There isn't one shred of evidence that early diagnosis does any good, except perhaps in the cancer of breast, cervix, & bladder.'" - Dr. James Peters, NCI Division of Cancer Cause & Prevention Director. (p.126).

"Doctors...from the Office of Info. Tech. at Harvard U.(:).... Their appraisal of 46 surgical or anasthesia breakthroughs...suggested...only 13% were highly preferred (&)...in nearly half the cases the new therapy was no better than the therapy it replaced. ...About 12% of the innovations increased complications ...." (p.187).

"In 1971, the Joint Task Force of the USDA, in...An Evaluation of Research in the US on Human Nutrition ...(concluded) that.... ...(in the US) a more fundamental (less "convenience-food") diet.... ...would result in 1.2 million fewer cases of heart & vascular disease each year, 64,000 fewer cancer deaths & 120,000 fewer cases of cancer each year, 49 million fewer cases of respiratory infections, 3 million fewer cases of birth defects, 8 million fewer cases of arthritis, 2 million cases of diabetes either avoided or improved, 3 million fewer cases of osteo-porosis, 16,200 fewer cases of blindness, 3 million fewer cases of allergies, & 2½ million fewer mental health problems necessitating hospitalization." (p.41).
- Jeffrey Bland, PhD, Biochem., U. Oregon; Assoc. Prof. Clinical Chem., U. Puget Sound; Dir., Bellvue-Redmond Medical Lab.; Dir., Lab. Nutritional Supplement Analysis, & Research Assoc., Linus Pauling Inst.; (author: Medical Applications of Clinical Nutrition; &, Recent Progress in Nutrition); Your Health Under Siege, p. 41, 126, 187, (for last 3 paragraphs above).

"...Cancer patients are constantly being urged to go to their doctors as soon as the 'danger signals' appear.... The implication is always that patients...with the shortest possible duration of symptoms, will have the best prognosis. The results of this study certainly do not support this." - G. H. Green, Assoc. Prof., Postgrad. School of Obstetrics & Gynecology, U. Auckland, New Zealand, "Duration of Symptoms & Survival Rates for Invasive Cervical Cancer", Aust. & NZ J. Ob. Gyn., v.10, n.4, p.242, Nov. 1970.

"Taking a biopsy often aggravates & stimulates malignant growth - & does not indicate how many secondary tumors have developed." - Dr. Charles Mayo, (in Dr. Lynn Dallin, Cancer Causes & Natural Controls, p.54).

"...The resort to a biopsy is a confession of failure, due to clinical inexperience or lack of data from other methods of diagnosis." - Dr. Ewing, Beaumont Foundation Lecture, (in Boyd, Textbook of Pathology, 2nd ed., p.337, (in Health Research, Is Cancer Curable?, c.1954,(1969), p.13)).

"There seems to be little doubt that cancer can be spread from the primary site to distant tissues through ... the numerous ways that surgical manipulations (e.g. biopsy, therapy) could be responsible for this phenomenon." - Vincent De Vita, MD, Dir., NCI; &, Steven Rosenberg, MD, PhD, Chief Surg., NCI; &, S. Hellman, MD, Dir. Radiation, Harvard Med.; (Eds.), Cancer: Principles & Practice of Oncology, (ref. in Judith Glassman, The Cancer Survivors, p.43).

"Biopsies...should be undertaken with the greatest caution. .... Even needle biopsy does not appear to be safe. .... It...gives credence to what our patients already think & tell us — that cutting into cancer spreads it & makes it grow." - George Crile, Jr., MD; Emeritus Surgeon, Cleveland Clinic; (author, What Women Should Know About the Breast Cancer Controversy); "Is Biopsy Safe?", Amer. Surgeon, v.21,p.733, 1957, (in H.H.Beard, A New Approach to the Conquest of Cancer ...,p.90).

"...Establishing a diagnosis...'benign' or 'malignant' is not an exact science. In spite of the aura of infallibility....pathologists are human....(:)the super specialist (with) 'tunnel vision'.... Histo-techs....make grevious errors....(:) proper patient....sample...injuries to the tissues.... Pathologists are not omniscient...(; some) afflicted with such delusions. ....Trapped by semantics. ...A 'guessing game' when patients' lives are at stake." - Roger Terry, MD, "Pathology of Ca.", Clinical Oncology: a Multi-disciplinary Approach, ACS, p.37-42.

B.Q.10.2 PROOF:

"...All too many...scientists...have forgotten that not everything that counts can be counted, & not everything counted, counts." - Denis Burkitt, MD, FRCS, FRS; of Burkitt's Lymphoma), (in Judith Glassman, The Cancer Survivors, p.368).

"...Half or more of the numerical data published by scientists in their journal articles is unuseable because there is no evidence that the researcher accurately measured what he thought he was measuring, or no evidence that possible sources of error were eliminated or accounted for." - Dr. Richard W. Roberts, Dir., NBS (National Bureau of Standards), (in Robert Mendelsohn, MD, Confessions of a Medical Heretic, p.205).

"It is not enough to show that drug A is better than drug B on the average. One is invited to ask, 'For which people ("'& why'") is drug A better than drug B, & vice-versa? If drug A cures 40% & drug B cures 60%, perhaps the right choice of drug for each person would result in 100% cures." - Lancelot Hogben; MA,(Sr. Schol. & Smart Prize, Trinity Col., Cambridge; SSc, U. London; DSc, U. Wales; MSc & LLD, U.Birmingham; Regius Prof., U. Aberdeen; Prof., Med. Statistics, Birmingham U.; Fellow, Royal Soc. (& of Edinburgh, Gold Medal); Hon. Member, Soc. Exp'l Biol.; author, Nature & Nurture, etc.; Assoc. Ed., Brit. J. Exp'l Biol.; Deputy Dir., Med. Statistics, Brit. War Office; (paraphrased in Annual Review of Medicine, v.9, p.349, 1958, (in Harris Coulter, Divided Legacy: the Conflict Between Homoeopathy & the AMA, p.483)).

B.Q.10.3 EXPERIMENTAL TECHNIQUE CRITIQUE:

"...To test new materials... ,it was reasoned that the primary mouse cancer used should...respond the best to the then existing anti-cancer drugs. Accordingly, ...leukemia has become the standard for testing.... ...This has resulted in the development of several drugs that are highly effective clinically against (A.L.L.) leukemia, chorio-carcinoma... , but of only limited effectiveness against the commoner (solid) cancers. ...There are anti-cancer agents with a high degree of effectiveness against a solid tumor ("melanoma") although totally ineffective against the leukemias. ...We suggest...each material...be tested on...solid tumor regardless of its effectiveness...against the leukemias (during initial "primary screen")." - Dr. Roy O. Asplund, "Isolation of Anti-tumor Poly-saccharide Fractions from Yucca ...", Growth, v.42,p.223, 1978, (in John Heinerman, The Treatment of Cancer With Herbs, c.1980, p.133-4).

"'...I am told that I cannot discover anything more because I had discovered other concepts in the past & those are now regulations. ...I am the senior author of the randomized clinical trial. Now, I am told by the FDA that, if I don't do a randomized clinical trial, I can't do research. .... When I ask them where they got that dumb idea, they cite my publications.'" - Dr. Emil J. Freirich, head, Developmental Therapeutics, MD Anderson Hosp. & Tumor Inst., (in Pat McGrady, Jr., "The Cancer Patient's Quandary", Newsday, Sept. 30, 1984).

"...The NCI...retrospective analysis...of Laetrile(:).... Among 67 case records that were all submitted...the NCI...could find...complete response in only 2 patients...."

"...The NCI...prospective trial.... ...of....Laetrile....could be neither controlled & randomized nor blinded. .... The lack of concurrent controls was partially offset by the fact that all patients were in the advanced stages of a disease known to be almost uniformly & rapidly fatal. Any objective responses in tumor size or apparent prolongation of survival could be identified by comparison with historical controls." - Arnold Relman, Editor, NEJM, "Closing the Books on Laetrile", NEJM, v.306, n.4, p.236, Jan. 28, 1982.

"The (Laetrile) efficacy tests...clinically in humans...(by) the US NCI...were obviously conducted so that a negative result could be formulated. The limited number & types of human cancer cases selected...the omission of necessary additional measures ("eg, dietary"), the far too short observation periods, & the undefined chemical properties of the (Laetrile)...all contributed to devaluation of...conclusions...."

"...The oral (Laetrile) had been 'toxified' by adding cyano-urea in the NCI.... (NCI's) Mayo (Clinic) dismissed well responding patients to discard them from statistic evaluation. ....This kind of fraud which I expressed...& which was openly published...has...not resulted in any denial." - Hans Nieper, MD; Pres., IAPM (Internat'l Acad. of Preventive Med.); Dir., German Soc. for Med. Tumor Treat.; Member, German Cancer Soc.; Member, German Soc. Circulation Res.; author, 200 articles, & Conversion of Gravity Field Energy Resolution in Technology, Medicine, & Society, & Mineral Transporters; in Who's Who of World Science, & Two Thousand Men of Achievement; life member, Deutsche Ges. fur Naturforscher und Arzte; head, Aschaffenburg Hosp. Lab.; Med. Dir., Silbersee Hosp.; co-developer of cyclo-phosph-amide (chemo-therapy); in IACVF, Cancer News Journal,v.16,n.3,p.20,Fall 1981, & v.17,n.2,p.8,Summer 1982.

"The slight variations in extracting procedure cause many of the amygdalin (Vitamin B-17, laetrile) molecules to change to a form unknown to nature(:) isomers..... There are...purveyors who label their 'iso-amygdalin' products 'amygdalin' contrary to all of the recognized specs..... ...For commercial or political purposes, they certainly cannot justify such fallacy.... This scientific heresy & commercial fraud...(is) tremendously reducing the effectiveness of amygdalin therapy. .... To mislabel iso-amygdalin as amygdalin is scientifically, medically, & morally indefensible." - Dr. Ernst T. Krebs, Jr., discoveror of vitamins B-15 & B-17, "The Extraction, Identification, & Packaging of Therapeutically Effective Amygdalin", (in Maureen Salaman, Nutrition: the Cancer Answer, p.294-5, 299).

"...Adequate dosage by the most effective & least toxic route. ...("Laetrile") is about 44 times more toxic when given by mouth than by intra-muscular injection, & 21 times more toxic than intra-venous injection. .... When the patient is on high dosages of vitamin A, alcoholic beverages are absolutely prohibited."

"An excellent example of what not to eat is the nutritional program as recommended in the booklet published in 1974 by the ACS, Inc., under the misnomer of 'Nutrition'." - Bruce W. Halstead, MD, (author: Laetrile Poisoning & Cancer Politics; &, The Scientific Basis of EDTA Chelation Therapy; &, Gerovital ("Procaine") Therapy; &, Hyper-baric Oxygen Therapy), Metabolic Cancer Therapy, p. 13, 15, & 18.

"Amygdalin ("laetrile...")...has been employed medically for many centuries. Ancient herbal pharmacopeias recommended the bitter almond for the treatment of a variety of ilnesses...."

"Six patients with advanced cancer were treated with amygdalin ("laetrile") at dosages similar to those employed by laetrile practitioners. ...intravenously ...(&) orally.... No clinical or lab. evidence of toxic reaction was seen (by us)."

"One patient had severe pre-treatment pain resulting from skeletal meta-stases .... At...5 weeks after the onset of (laetrile & metabolic) therapy, she claimed complete relief...." - Charles Moertel, MD, (& 3 MD's & 2 PhD's), Dept. Oncology, &, Comprehensive Cancer Ctr., Mayo Clinic / Foundation, "A Pharmaco-logic & Toxico-logical Study of Amygdalin", JAMA (Journal, AMA), v.245, n.6, p.591, Feb. 13, 1981.

"A nationwide Harris Poll showed that the public favoured the use of Laetrile in treating cancer by a 30% margin. .... In over 250 cases of cancer with which I have been associated, all of whom have used (Laetrile, vitamin) B-17, not a single one had side-effects as a result...." - Leon Chaitow, ND, DO; Member, British Naturopathic & Osteopathic Assoc.; An End to Cancer?, p.144.

"If a useful (therapy) became available...it would be difficult to find an adequate number of experienced investigators to test it. The great danger might be not that a useless material was judged useful, but rather that a worthwhile one was rejected by inexperienced investigation." - Ernest Herrman, PhD, (in Postgraduate Medicine, May, 1964, p.50, (in ICRF (Independent Citizens Research Foundation for Study of Degenerative Diseases), Is the Answer to Cancer Just Around the Corner?, c.1964, p.4.

"In the early 1700's, two physicians ... learned about pinkroot's efficacy from the Indians. The word soon spread to the general public, who praised this worm treatment, particularly against roundworms, for the next 200 years. Pink-root fell into disuse in the early 1900's, simply because greedy herb dealers adulterated or even substituted shipments of true pinkroot with quantities of other plants...." - Michael A. Weiner, PhD, nutritional ethno-medicine, Univ. of Cal., Berkeley, Earth Medicine - Earth Food: Plant Remedies, Drugs & Natural Foods of the North American Indians, c.1972, 1980, p.140.

"Conclusions (by the Food Protection Committee of the NAS), of the (original) studies, are included without proper regard for the quality of methodology originally used. Studies lacking adequate statistical design are given equal weight with sounder studies; many clinical & epidemiological studies yielding questionable conclusions are given uncritical acceptance. ...Possibly erroneous results gain added stature & interpretive errors are perpetuated." **- FDA: Bureau of Medicine, Dr. John J. Schrogie; & Bureau of Science, Dr. Herman F. Kraybill; (in Beatrice Trum Hunter, The Sugar Trap, c.1982, p.101).**

B.Q.10.4 BIOMEDICAL INFORMATION EXPLOSION:

"The field of immunology is expanding at an exponential rate. This growth is such that it is difficult for even the professional immunologist to keep up with all the latest discoveries. It is estimated that there is a flood of immunological literature of about 7,000 articles appearing in 800 technical journals throughout the world each year." - Bruce W. Halsted, MD; Dir., World Life Research Inst.; consultant to WHO (World Health Org.); Commander, US Navy; (in Anabolism, v.1, n.3, p.7, Oct. 1982).

"The notion that physicians know what's contained in the literature is bizarre. .... It's estimated that there are 3,300 established medical journals."

"The work of 1000's of physicians has given us a rich literature on (one drug). This literature, international in scope, covers a wide variety of medical disciplines. Published in many languages over a period of years, it is spread far & wide. But intermingled with millions of other studies, this literature is almost lost unless someone seeks it out." - Jack Dreyfus, head, Dreyfus Medical Foundation, A Remarkable Medicine Has Been Overlooked, c.1970 (1982), p.110-111.

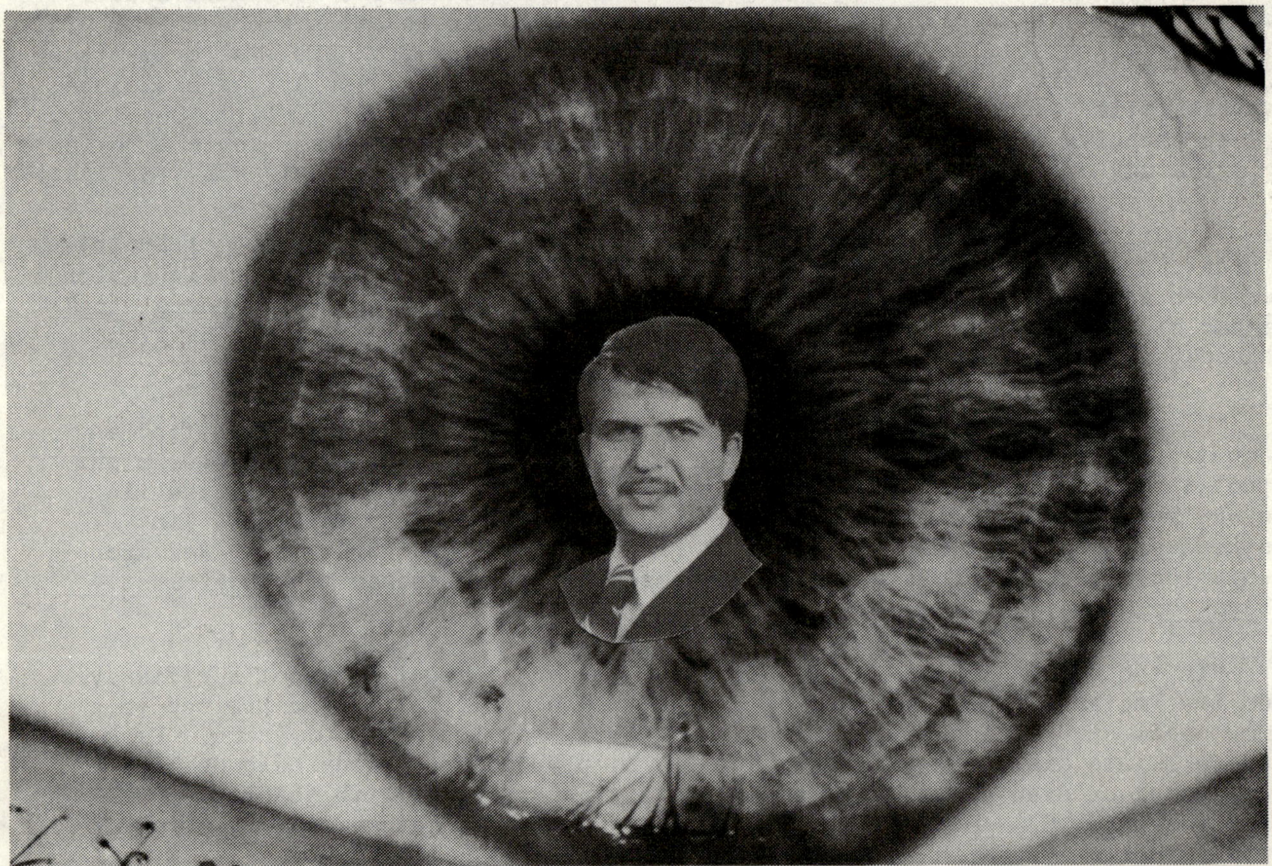

Reflection / Insight, of Mind's Eye. (Author's portrait in his iridology photo.)

2ND EDITION to READINGS RECOMMENDED, BOOKS: (Continued from p.124)

SURVEYS of Alternative Therapies of Cancer & Their Politics:

- Leon Chaitow, An End to Cancer?, (Thorsons, Britain; 1978, 1983).
- Dore Deverell, How I Healed My Cancer Holistically, (1978).
- John Heinerman, The Treatment of Cancer with Herbs, (Bi-World, 671 N. State St., Orem, UT; 1980).
- Thomas Mansell, Cancer Simplified, (Woodlawn, 604 Briarcliff, Aliquippa, PA 15001; 1976).
- Nutrition & Cancer Research, Hearings, Subcom. on Nutrition, US Senate, (Hon. George McGovern, Chairman), June 12 & 13, 1978.
- Dick Richards, MD, The Topic of Cancer, (Pergamon; 1982).
- J. Gordon Roberts, Cancer: How & Why It May Be Wiped Out, (Roberts Ca. Res. Pub., POBox 1662, Clearwater, FL 33517; 1977).
- Maureen Salaman, Nutrition: the Cancer Answer,(NHF; &,Liberty Lobby; &,Statford; 1983).
- Cameron Stauth, The New Approach to Cancer, (English Bro.; 1982).

SINGLE Alternative Therapy of Cancer & Its Politics:

- Herbert Bailey, A Matter of Life or Death: the Incredible Story of Krebiozen.
- Howard H. Beard, A New Approach to the Conquest of Cancer, Rheumatic & Heart Diseases, (Cancer Book House).
- Glenn Kittler, Laetrile: Nutritional Control for Cancer with Vitamin B-17, (Royal Pub., Nutri-Books; 1963, 1978).
- Robert Netterberg & Robert Taylor, The Cancer Conspiracy, (Pinnacle, NY,NY; 1981).

MISC.:

- Robert Bradford & Michael Culbert, International Protocols for IIMP (Individualized, Integrated, Metabolic Programs) in Cancer Management, (survey; no politics), (CFCCT; &,Bradford Found'n, POBox 1003, Los Altos, CA 94022; 1983).
- Lynn Dallin, Cancer Causes & Natural Controls, (survey;few politics), (IACVF; &, Ashley Books; 1983).
- Walter Ermer, A Program for the Prevention & Early Detection of Cancer ....
- Judith Glassman, The Cancer Survivors & How They Did It, (Dial; 1983).
- Linus Pauling & Ewan Cameron, Cancer & Vitamin C, (few politics), (Linus Pauling Inst.; 1979, 1981).
- Hellfried E. Sartori, Cancer 1984, (Life Science Universal, Wash., DC; 1984).
- John Tobe, Cancer: How to Prevent & Gain Remission from Cancer, (Provoker Press).

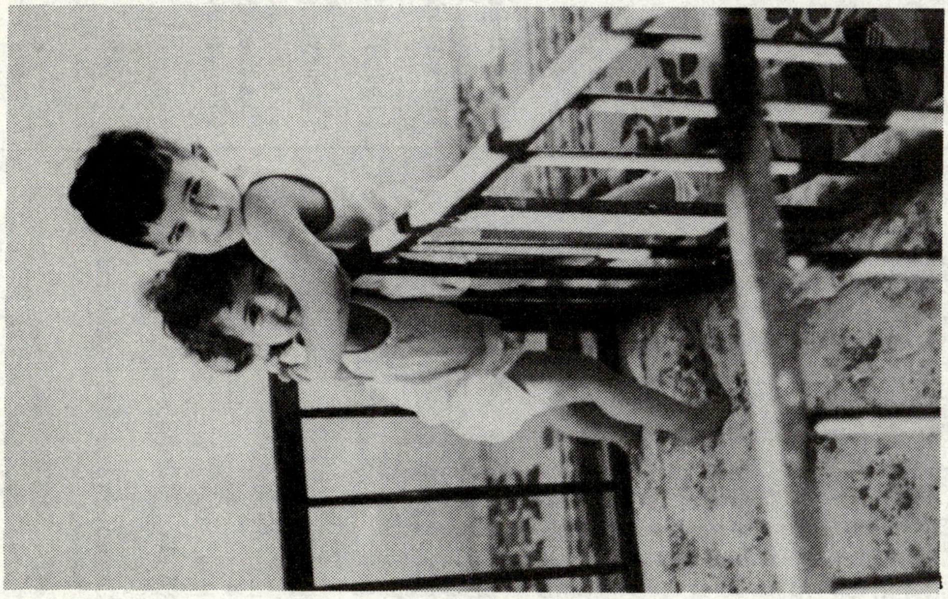

Author, freshly hatched, behind bars of playpen, hugged by big brother, circa 1948.

PUBLIC INTEREST HEALTH GROUPS; JOURNALS & ADDRESSES; (Continued from p.125–129):

● **CANCER / ACTIVIST / FREEDOM OF CHOICE / ALTERNATIVE THERAPY**

Project Cure
2020 K St., NW; Suite 350
Wash., DC 20070-2008

Nutrition Health Review
143 Madison Ave.
NY, NY 10016
(Tel. 212-679-3590)

People's Doctor
(Newsletter)
POBox 982
Evanston, IL 60204

Center for Health Action
(Update)
POBox 1004
Delaware, OH 43015

Project 100,000
(Robert McNellis)
507 South Oakes St.
Helena, MT 59601
(Tel.: 406-442-4596)

National Council on Wholistic Therapeutics & Medicine
271 Fifth Ave.
New York, NY 10016
(Tel. 212-683-4793)

Homeopathic Educational Services
2124 Kittredge St.
Berkeley, CA 94704
(Tel.415-658-4325)

John Beard Memorial Found'n
POBox 685
San Francisco, CA 94101
(Tel. 415-824-1067)

Dean Burk Found'n
4719 44th St.
Wash., DC 20016
(Tel. 202-363-6279)

McNaughton Found'n
POBox B17
San Ysidro, CA 92073
(Tel.: 714—428-6114)

Irwin DJ Bross
109 Maynard Dr.
Eggertsville
Buffalo, NY 14226
(Tel.: 716-832-4200)

Cancer Research Inst.
Helen Coley Nauts, Dir.
1225 Park Ave.
NY, NY 10028
(Tel.: 212-722-8547)

IAT (Immune Augment. Therapy)
101 W. Park
Olathe, KS 66061
(Tel.: 800-IAT-HELP)

A. Keith Brewer Library
Richland Center, WI 53581
(Tel. 608-647-6513)

Thomas Mansell
NHF, CCS, CFCCT
604 Briarcliff Dr.
Aliquippa, Pa. 15001

Kent Private Clinic
Sandwich, Kent, CT13 9DL
ENGLAND
(Tel. 0304-612910)

Newsday, Inc.
235 Pine Long Road
Mellville, Long Island
New York 11747

Patrick McGrady, Jr.
Route 1, Box 450-H
Port Ludlow, WA 98365
(Tel.: 206-437-2291)

Wayne Martin
25 Orchard Drive
POBox 1133
Fairhope, AL 36532
(Tel.: 205-928-3975)

Ga. Women's Coalition for Medical Rights
3985 Lynfield Court
College Park, GA 30334

Ms. Judith Glassman
Cancer Counselling & Research C
6060 North Central Expressway
Dallas, TX 75206
(Tel.: 214 373-7744)

Cancer Prevention & Control
POBox 387
Tomball, TX 77375
(Tel. 713-376-8079)

Institute of Applied Biology
164 East 91st St.
NY, NY 10028
(Tel.: 212-876-9669)

International Academy of Biological Medicine (IABM)
POBox 31313
Phoenix, AZ 85046

International Academy of Preventive Medicine (IAPM)
Suite 200
10409 Town & Country Way
Houston, TX 77024

American Academy of Medical Preventics, Suite 922
8383 Wilshire Blvd.
Beverly Hills, CA 90211
(Tel. 213-878-1234)

American Holistic Medical Assoc./Inst. (AHMA/AHMI)
(Journal)
6932 Little River Turnpike
Annandale, VA 22003
(Tel. 703-642-5880)

Society of Ultra-molecular Medicine (Journal)
6125 W. Tropicana, Suite C
Las Vegas, NV 89103
(Tel. 702-367-0206)

Dr. John Richardson
American Biologics
Condominio Gallego, Suite 607
3401 Blvd. Agua Caliente
Tijuana, Baja California
MEXICO
(Tel.: 800-227-4458)

Commonweal
POBox 316
Bolinas, CA 94924
(Tel. 415-868-0970)

...FREEDOM OF CHOICE... (continued)

Federation of Homemakers
5610 16th St., NW
Arlington, VA 22205

College of Life Science, Healthful Living
6600-D Burleson Rd.
Austin, TX 78744
(Tel.: 512-385-2781)

Natural Hygiene, Inc.
POBox 2132
Huntington, CT 06484
(Tel. 203-929-1557)

Total Life Ministries
POBox 1411
Brevard, NC 28712

JURY
POBox 70
Evanston, IL 60204
(Tel. 312-764-1264)

Health Happenings Hotline
3370 Sunset Trail
Northbrook, IL 60062
(Tel. 312-272-5887)

Keating Found'n for Cancer Research
715 South 25th Ave.
Bellwood, IL 60104
(Tel.: 312-544-6500)

(See list in: Leon Chaitow, An End to Cancer.)

● NUTRITION

Nutrition & Cancer: an International Journal
(Franklin Inst. Press)
POBox 710
Rockville, MD 20853

Center for Research on Vitamins & Cancer
Box C 278
Health Sciences Center
University of Colorado
Denver, CO 80262

Maureen M. Henderson, MD
(Chair, NCAB Ad Hoc Subcom. on Diet, Nutrition, & Cancer)
Prof., Medicine & Epidemiology
School of Medicine
University of Washington
Seattle, WA 98195

American Health Found'n
Hammond House Road
Valhalla, NY 10595
(Tel: 914-592-2600)

ETI (En-Trophy Inst.)
(Review)
Box 984, Station "A"
Hamilton, Ontario L8N 3R1
CANADA
(Tel. 416-525-9140, x2783)

Pritikin Longevity Center
1910 Ocean Front Walk
Santa Monica, CA 90405
(Tel. 213-450-5433)

Anabolic Found'n, (Anabolism)
POBox 1763
La Jolla, CA 92038

Vegetarian Society, Inc.
POBox 5688
Santa Monica, CA 90405
(Tel. 213-396-5164)

Vegetarian Assoc. of America
POBox 547
South Orange, NJ 07079

Orthomolecular Medical Society
2698 Pacific Ave.
San Francisco, CA 94115
(Tel.: 415-346-5692)

Institute of Nutritional Research (defunct)
5175 Hollywood Blvd.
Hollywood, CA 90027

FRAC (Food Research & Action Center)
2011 Eye (I) St., NW
Wash., DC 20006
(Tel. 202-452-8250)

Community Nutrition Inst. (CNI)
1146 19th St., NW
Wash., DC 20036
(Tel.: 202-833-1730)

(See lists in CSPI, From the Ground Up: Building a Grass Roots Food Policy.)

● HEALTH / ACTIVIST / CONSUMERISM

People's Medical Society
(Newsletter)
14 E. Minor St.
Emmaus, PA 18049
(Tel. 215-967-2136)

Center for Medical Consumers
237 Thompson St.
NY, NY 10012
(Tel. 212-674-7105)

Health & Medicine Policy Research Group
Health & Medicine
220 So. State St., Suite 300
Chicago, IL 60604
(Tel. 312-922-8057)

The Hastings Center: Inst. of Society, Ethics, & the Life Sciences
360 Broadway
Hastings on Hudson
NY 10706
(Tel. 914-478-0500)

National Emergency Medicine Assoc.
2025 I St.
Wash., DC 20070

PUBLIC INTEREST HEALTH GROUPS; JOURNALS & ADDRESSES; (continued):

● PSYCHIATRY

Association for Humanistic Psychology
325 9th St.
San Francisco, CA 94103
(Tel. 415-626-2375)

● DENTAL

Amer.Assoc. of Dental Victims (AADV)
3320 E. 7th St.
Long Beach, CA 90804

Soaring Bear, Ninos del Sol
Academy of Barefoot Dentists
2509 North Campbell, #262
Tucson, AZ 85719

● MULTI-DISCIPLINARY SCIENCE

Leading Edge Bulletin
POBox 42211
LA, CA 90042
(Tel. 213-258-7333)

Advanced Sciences R & D Corp. (... Advisory)
POBox 109
Lakemont, GA 30552
(Tel. 404-782-5347)

Heartland Journal
7000 N. Glenwood Ave.
Chicago, IL 60626
(Tel. 312-465-8005)

(See list by: Science for the People.)

● ENVIRONMENT / POLLUTION

Irving J. Selikoff, MD
Director, Environmental Research Lab.;(Member, NCAB);
Mount Sinai School of Medicine
1212 Fifth Ave.
New York, NY 10029

Human Ecology Action League (HEAL)
(The Human Ecologist)
POBox 1369
Evanston, IL 60204
(Tel. 312-864- 1995)
&
Suite 6506
505 No. Lake Shore Dr.
Chicago, IL 60611
(Tel. 312-836-0422)

Action on Smoking & Health (ASH)
2013 H St., NW
Wash., DC 20006
(Tel. 202-659-4310)

Friends of the Earth (FOE)
(Not Man Apart)
1045 Sansome St.
San Francisco, CA 94111
(Tel.: 415-433-7373)

Environmental Task Force
Suite 918
1346 Connecticut Ave., NW
Wash., DC 20036
(Tel. 202-296-0798)

Illinois Pure Water Comm.
606 Washington Ave.
Alton, IL 62002

Carcinogen Information Program, POBox 6057
Webster College
470 E. Lockwood Ave.
St. Louis, MO 63119

● ENVIRONMENT / ECOLOGY

Greenpeace, USA
2007 "R" St., NW
Wash., DC 20009
(Tel.: 202-462-1177)

Animal Protection Inst. of America
POBox 22505
5894 So. Land Park Dr.
Sacramento, CA 95822
(Tel.: 916-422-1921)

Amer. Veterinary Holistic Medical Assoc. (AVHMA)
2214 Old Emmorton Rd.
Bel Air, MD 21024

● POLITICAL / ECONOMIC / LEGAL

Robert White, Inc.,
The Duck Book Digest
POBox 1928
Cocoa, FL 32922

● PEACE

Federation of American Scientists (FAS)
307 Mass. Ave., NE
Wash., DC 20002
(Tel. 202-546-3300)

Campaign Against Nuclear War
122 Maryland Ave., NE
Wash., DC 20002
(Tel.: 800-528-6050, ext.47)

Nuclear Weapons Freeze Campaign
4144 Lindell Blvd., Suite 404
St. Louis, MO 63108

(See lists by last 2 above, esp.: "Stop Nuclear War", by Camp. Against " " .)

● NETWORKING

NIB (National Information Bureau)
419 Park Ave. South
NY, NY 10016
(Tel. 212-532-8595)

Self-Help Center
Suite S-122
1600 Dodge Ave.
Evanston, IL 60201
(Tel. 312-328-0470)

(See lists from: NIB; Self-Help Inst.; East West Journal (esp.: Nov. 1977, p.13; &, Dec. 1980, p.64-5); Oxfam, "Educational Resources Catalogue"; &, Joshua, Journeys of an Aquarian Age Networker.)

AFTERWORD:

"The list goes on." - "Medicine, Morality, & Money", Evanston Hosp. Corp., Pilot, Sum. 1983, p.4.

"...Lack of knowledge...has made of the people of the US a nation of sheep... endorsing any solutions...which come from a source apparently better informed than themselves." (p.8).

"We...clamor for leisure time without knowing how to use it...." (p.11).

"...Most immoral of all — the government & press have not been honest with us." (p.30).

"There are twice as many governmental public-relations men in Washington as there are journalists." (p.119).

"We are being treated as bored customers...not as citizens whose independent opinions mold the destiny of our democracy." (p.124).

"The press is dependent on the two wire services...." (p.163).

"The great mistakes...are repeated in this book to remind you that you did not know about them until late in the game, & then you neither grasped their significance nor did anything to correct them. You exhibited no indignation, no citizen's interest. You passively kept chewing your cud, feeling secure in a nation of sheep." (p.184).

- William Lederer, (co-author, The Ugly American), A Nation of Sheep, p.8, 11, 30, 119, 124, 163, 184.

"This book was not printed to waste paper & sit on a shelf." (p.6).

"If this copy...is gathering dust...please pass it on (loan it - Ed.) to someone who can make use of it. ....I would appreciate if you would send comments, ...new experimental info., & printed reviews." (p.2).

"What you can offer...: Establishing a local...program. .... Translating this into other (major) languages.... Transporting books...in your travels." (p.i).

"(&) Distribution...(to:) Library, info. service, &...conference(,)...course... ...study in depth(,)...clinic in poor neighborhoods & countries." (p.ii).

- Soaring Bear, Natural Dental Wellness, p.i, ii, 2, & 6.

"Use Don't Let Cancer Throw You as a Christmas greeting, birthday remembrance, or thank you, to: postman, barber, pastor, doctor, relative, or neighbor. Encourage your club or church to order 100 for sale at cost, or free distribution to members. Let your corporation spend P/R or adv. funds for 1,000 as a civic endeavor. .... A copy should be in every church, hospital, & public library in America.... One concerned citizen has already donated a copy to the Library of the 7,000 churches of his denomination."

"This book is not copyrighted & may be reproduced in whole, or in part, for the good of humanity — but not for profit."

"Man's inhumanity to mankind is only exceeded by man's inhumanity to himself."

"Prayer is a force as real as terrestrial gravity." - Bill W. H. M. Stover, Don't Let Cancer Throw You, inside front cover, p.2, 81, & 87.

EPILOGUE:

"...Nowhere is a systematic approach being taken that incorporates a number of reforms at once. ...The matrix ("An Urban Food System Matrix: Strategies for Reform") is organized by scale of implementation — at the level of the consumer, neighborhoods, citywide, county, & state (& national & global? -Ed.) — & by the type of strategy — lifestyle, economic, technological, & public policy. Different actors are required to initiate & implement different strategies, but we must all work together to bring them to fruition." - Paige Chapel & Kent Peterson, "Menu for Reforming...", Heartland, a Free American Journal ..., (Michael James, Ed.), n.14, p.11 & 33, Sum. 1983.

"...At all levels - national, regional, & local. These enlightened & courageous individuals will form the vanguard of the movement, the pioneers, the trail blazers... in the wilderness of a politically entrenched & recalcitrant medical system. They will approach their local newspapers, radio & television stations, health depts., community hospitals, health systems agencies, regional health planning committees, professional societies, private health care concerns, community officials, legistlators, governors, & political leaders at all levels." - David Stewart, PhD, Pres., NAPSAC Internat'l, The Five Standards of Safe Childbearing, p.12.

GLANCES:

"...Surgery.... Unfortunately, it is true that there a few charlatans in the profession as in any other profession. ...These 'spiritual dwarfs'....are unfit to decide rightly when confronted with momentous events in the lives of other persons."

"Surgery is still an art. The 'exact sciences' have been our allies & helpers." - August P. Hovnanian, (father of Editor), MD, Assist. Prof. Surg., AUB (American Univ. of Beirut) Med.; FACS (Fellow, Amer. College of Surgeons); Diplomate, Amer. Board Surg.; Scholar in Surg.: Rockefeller, &, Brit. Council; Specialty Ed., International Surg.: Surg. Oncology, &, Surg. Res.: Member: BMA (Brit. Med. Assoc.), &, Internat'l Soc. Surg., &, NYAS (NY Acad. Sci.), &, College Amer. Pathol., &, Pan-Pacific Surg. Assoc.; Instructor, Pathol., Albany Med.; Assoc. Prof. Surg.: AUB, &, Chicago Med.; Dir., Surg. Res. & Ed., St. Francis Hosp., Evanston, Ill., &, Huron Rd. Hosp., Cleveland; Surg., Kaiser Found'n Clinic; Dir., Lemmon Hosp., So. Dakota; & etc.; Grantee: NIH, &, ACS, &, Damon Runyon Cancer Fund; Author: 34 articles, & book on ureter surg. (draft); "The Making of a Surgeon", Lebanese Med. J., v.4, n.6, p.309, Nov. 1951.

"Dr. Phillip Hovnanian (...grandfather of Editor). .... After graduating from college, he attended the American University of Beirut & completed Medical School in 1909. .... During the death marches (the genocide of 1½ million Armenians by some violents of the Turks), many were the times when he saved families & individuals from certain death, torture, rape, & many from being forced to convert (religion). ...He was accused of aiding & abetting Armenian Guerrillas, & taken...for trial. This was a charge that, guilty or not, would certainly result in the death penalty. ...The presiding officer visited Dr. Phillip in jail. (The officer said:) '...One of your workers found a Turkish woman lying at the doorstep of the hospital. The doctor in charge gave orders to admit her for a thorough checkup. ...She was suffering from typhus.... After 3 weeks of excellent care, she was healed. .... The doctor was kind enough to make...sure she had her travelling expenses covered. ...That woman was my wife, & you were the physician. Furthermore, she made me swear that if ever possible, I return the favor.' The next day, Dr. Hovnanian was set free."

"On another occasion, a worker was brought...seriously wounded.... Dr. Phillip discovered the patient to be the murderer of his brother.... ("During the 1909 atrocities, the doctor's father & 2 brothers...were killed. (His father) was among the 39 martyred in the...Church...on his way to the Armenian...Church Convention....") Dr. Phillip had the opportunity to avenge his brother's death without arousing suspicion. But he recalled Christ's words...(Mat. 6:14) So he ordered the nurses to care for the man.... Dr. Phillip said (to the patient): 'I treated you knowing that you are my brother's murderer.... ...to show you that the Spirit of Christ can love & forgive an enemy, & return good for evil. .... Go in peace....'."

"Dr. Phillip died...from an infected thumb wound suffered while performing surgery." - The Herald, (Armenian Presby. Church, Paramus, NJ), "Heroes of the Faith", n.8, Sept. 1982.

"The Hippocrates Oath is most often replaced by insurance forms, in the doctor's office."

"Most doctors have forgotten, or do not practice, their foremost basic education: Sterile Technique."

"If your patient expires, it is relatively excusable if you have an MD degree." - Arpine Hovnanian, (mother of Editor), BS, Northwestern U.; Lab. Tech., Amer. U. B. Hosp., &, Albany Med. Ctr.

"I find your suggestions very much to the point, & if you would like to detail them further, ... I will try to put the information to work. .... There is a problem which I may wish to have your assistance on dealing with...." - Ralph Nader, letter to Ralph Hovnanian, March 3, 1969.

"It's amazing the kinds of free fun facts found far from mainstream mass media. Check these quotes out for instance: ...." - Ralph Hovnanian, "Censor Sense" (column), The North Shore Examiner, v.13, n.8, p.6, Aug. 19, 1983.

Ralph Hovnanian: "Russian peasants have a joke they tell Americans. They say, in the Supreme Soviet we have one candidate for office, in America, you have two, what's the difference? With our voting machines, 95% of them being taken care of by one company, in California, that maintains them & counts the votes electronically, with nobody looking over their shoulder as to whether they're counted correctly...."

Phil Donahue: "You believe we need an audit on the votes then?"

Hovnanian: "There's a lot of computer crime. 200 million ($) theft in New York & nobody.... ...Everybody goes to watch it (, the election totals)."

Donahue: "So, when you see the totals this November, you're not going to be sure that those are accurate. Ayy! I'm getting on the boat! I'm leaving here! I'm getting out of here!"

- Ralph Hovnanian, audience, Phil Donahue Show, WBBM-CBS-TV, Sept. 25, 1984, ("live" air date, Chi. & NY).

Ralph Hovnanian: "...If people chose the most important thing they could be doing at the moment, then they'll want to do that over anything else, & they won't feel lonely! Choose real problems, not fake problems! ...& do it at any time you feel like it - (when) you feel lonely!"

Phil Donahue: "Yeah! That assumes that all of us are healthy enough to make the distinction between the two!"

- Ralph Hovnanian, audience, Phil Donahue Show, WBBM-CBS-TV, Nov. 21, 1984, (pre-recording date, Chicago).

REVIEWS OF THIS BOOK'S FIRST EDITION:

Having self-published to avoid trepidation, delays, or censorship, this author/editor is trying to establish credibility & reader interest by reviews of this work. Certainly, one is entitled to apply the evidence herein (on how some publishers, distributors, & retailers are swayed by allegiances to major customers, advertisers, stockholders, & creditors), & opt for self publishing. These generous reviews of this self-published work are submitted humbly & dutifully to the Reader, the ultimate jury. All these reviews are from letters to Ralph Hovnanian, (unless otherwise noted); dates & copies of any are available on request.

REVIEWS OF THIS BOOK'S FIRST EDITION; (continued):

"To the Evaluators of this book:

Every public, private, & medical library should take the opportunity to include Medical Dark Ages Circa 1984 or Cancer Alternative Therapies' Cure Rates in their collection. Of very broad scope, it is supported by a highly organized, concise, & relevant presentation. Well over 70,000 pages of literature have been condensed into this compact compilation of under 200 pages. It is filled with valuable, often overlooked information, that can save the entry level reader, or patient, months of full time research. It will similarly be useful to the professional in health, politics, & alternative therapy, of medicine generally, & of cancer in particular."

- Dean Burk, (PhD; US NCI (National Cancer Institute), 1939-1974, Ret.; chief, Cyto-chemistry dept., NCI; USDA; Prof., Cornell U.; Harvard U.; U. C. Berkely; U. London; Kaiser Willhelm Inst. of Bio.; USSR Acad. of Sci.; Domagk Prize for Cancer Research; Knight Commander, Medical Order of Bethlehem; Knight, Mark Twain.

"You have made an especially valuable contribution through the brilliantly compiled tables (pp.13-64) in MDAC 1984 (Med. Dark Ages C. 1984). They afford a level of utility & quick reference, heretofore not generally accessible, in so-called 'alternative cancer therapy', nor, for that matter, in standard so-called 'conventional oncotherapy'. As you are undoubtedly aware, there is a remarkable confluence into an organized or unified pattern, among virtually all of the listings that you've made. .... Again, many thanks for...your brilliant contributions." - Ernst T. Krebs, Jr., (DSc; AB, U.Illinois; student: Hahnemann Medical College, & U. of Cal. Berkeley; International Medical Society for Blood & Tumor Disease Award; discoveror of Vitamin B-15, & B-17 (with father, Ernst T. Krebs, Sr., MD); Founder & Pres., John Beard Memorial Found'n).

"...Medical Dark Ages C. 1984. The title is appropriate & the lists of various things in the book are unique & show that a great deal of organization & thought went into this work. The quotations are not the usual banalities on cancer. Some are quite stimulating. .... It is ironic that even in times when orthodox religions were in power, it was often possible for unorthodox scholars to find a niche. Nowadays, in an era of free speech, such niches are few & far between." - Irwin D.J. Bross, (PhD; Director of Biostatistics, Roswell Park Memorial Inst.; Prof., Biostatistics, U. Buffalo; Statistician, Medical College, &, Aeronautical Labs, Cornell U.).

"I will review (Med. Dark Ages C. 1984), & appreciate the vast amount of work you've done & the diligent concern that forms its background." - Irving J. Selikoff, (MD; Member, NCAB (National Cancer Advisory Board); Prof., Environmental Sciences Lab., Mount Sinai School of Medicine, NY).

"I would like to thank you for the kind words & your appreciation of the work of the NCAB Subcommittee on Diet, Nutrition & Cancer. I am pleased to learn about your extensive interest in the subject & am most appreciative of the annotated bibliography obviously put together with a great deal of care.... ...I am sure they will both be valuable & thought provoking." - Maureen M. Henderson, (MD; Chair, Subcom. on Diet, Nutrition, & Cancer, NCAB (National Cancer Advisory Board); Prof., Epidemiology & Medicine, Univ. of Washington).

"...Your interesting book (Med. Dark Ages C. 1984:) .... You have done an enormous amount of research.... Thank you for letting me see what you are working on." - George Crile, Jr., MD; (Emeritus Consultant in Surgery, Cleveland Clinic; author, What Women Should Know About the Breast Cancer Controversy).

"...I...found (Med. Dark Ages C. 1984) to be first class. .... It's good to know...people whose work stands out like a shining beacon in different parts of the world."

"...Med. Dark Ages C. 1984...: One of the most remarkable things about this altogether remarkable work, is that it took 'till 1984 to be published & circulated to a readership, which must have thirsted for it & would certainly have benefited from it, decades ago."

"It is clearly the work of a man both learned in his field, & utterly courageous in his attitudes. He is fearless of the criticism of the orthodox world, &, as medical practitioner & author myself, I cannot compliment him too highly on providing a shining beacon & focus, for the thoughts & efforts, of both professional workers &, above all, patients."

"Ralph Hovnanian will never have better fortune than I wish him for his self-less devotion & continuing humanitarian efforts." - Dr. Brian "Dick" Richards, Bachelors of: Med., Surg., &, Sci.; Fellow of Royal: Acad., &, Soc. of Med.; Member, NY Acad. Sci.; Major, RAMC; Consulting Panelist, Brit. J. of Sexual Med.; Editor, Alternative Med.; contributor, 100's of publications, radio & TV, many countries; Author: The Topic of Cancer (Pergamon; 1982), &, Live to Be a Hundred; Kent Private Clinic, Sandwich, Kent, England.

"I have read, with absorbing interest, Med. Dark Ages C. 1984 ... , consisting of many reports, from numerous journals, & compiled into an assimilable monograph. The author's aim of bringing (together) the various aspects of newer knowledge in the alternative therapies of cancer, for the benefit of the unknowing ones, is very laudable! He takes to task the Establishment's double standard on research: strict on small researchers, lax on those working with products of big drug companies & institutions; (&,) the (Establishment -Ed.) opposition to freedom of choice in cancer therapy, since, this (Establishment -Ed.) stand contradicts the right of the cancer patient to...use a...drug of his own choice, (& not) to use the accepted drugs with very serious side effects, ...immuno-depressant, etc., which hasten the patient's death. This book cites the innumerable medical heretics, whose works were first condemned or disparaged, but were later proven to be correct, after so many years, with the loss of so many lives, caused by this opposition to new ideas or knowledge. Truly, Quintillan was correct when he stated that(:) they condemn what they do not understand." - Manuel Navarro, MD; Prof., Biochem. & Therapeutics, Faculty of Med. & Surg., U. Santo Tomas, Manila, Philippines; member, 10 med. groups; author, 130 articles & 2 books: lecturer, International Cancer Congresses.

"...Med. Dark Ages C. 1984. You have certainly compiled a considerable amount of important & useful information. If I can get it reviewed, I shall be glad to do so...." - Albert Schatz, PhD; discoveror of Strepto-mycin; 6 hon. degrees (DSc.); 6 medals; FRSH(Fellow, Royal Society of Health); Human. Extra-ordinaire, Amer. Acad. Holistic Pioneers; author, 3 books, &, 500 articles (some, lay press); guest, 250 radio/tv shows.

"...Your book...on alternative therapies for cancer(:) I am frequently asked about the alternative therapies & your material will provide excellent background for this. .... I wish you well in your enterprise & research in this area." - Ross Hume Hall, (PhD; Prof., Biochem. Dept., McMaster Univ.; Dir., En-Trophy Inst.; Principal cancer researcher, Roswell Park Mem. Inst.; author, Food for Nought.

"...Med. Dark Ages C. 1984. I appreciate very much...reading through the most interesting information. Your efforts in trying to put this information together in a cogent, readable style is most important, & I hope you will receive general readership." - Jeffrey Bland, (PhD, biochemistry, U. Oregon; author, Your Health Under Siege: Using Nutrition to Fight Back, & Medical Applications of Clinical Nutrition; Prof., Nutritional Biochem., Univ. Puget Sound; Dir., Bellvue-Redmond Med. Lab.; Research Assoc., & Dir., Lab. for Nutritional Supplement Analysis, Linus Pauling Inst. of Sci. & Med.).

"...Ralph Hovnanian...has collected in this volume the most comprehensive listing & comments ("pro & con") on alternative cancer therapies. I think you & your staff will find it interesting & helpful." - Robert S. Mendelsohn; COO (Chief Operating Officer), People's Doctor (Newsletter); sole guest, twice +, Phil Donahue Show (tv); guest, 700 Club (tv); letter to Phil Donahue, WBBM-TV, July 8, 1982.

"...I now want to call attention to a publication which is not written by anyone in the health field & which is not available in bookstores. Ralph R. Hovnanian.... ...he lives in my home town of Evanston, Illinois.... Calling himself a 'Member of Laity' & 'Curator of Cure Rates', Hov....entitles his publication Med. Dark Ages C. 1984. This 146-page volume (1st ed.) contains the most complete up-to-date statistics on every kind of cancer therapy ("including sham surgery") you can think of. In addition, the author has compiled hundreds of quotations about cancer, doctors, nutrition, & immunizations, from a broad spectrum of authorities, both recognized & otherwise. While this is hardly an elegant publication ("the typewritten copy is crowded & difficult to read"), I nevertheless recommend it to anyone who is seeking a kaleidoscopic view of cancer therapy, both alternative & orthodox." - Robert S. Mendelsohn, (MD, U. of Chicago; Chair, Medical Licensing Comm., State of Ill.(Illinois); Assoc. Prof., School of Medicine, U. of Ill.; Adjunct Prof., College of Urban Sci., U. of Ill.; Chicago area Med. Dir., Project Head Start; Pres., NHF; Board Member: SPUN, & NAPSAC, & ABCC; syndicated columnist, People's Doctor; author: Confessions of a Medical Heretic, & MALe Practice...; lecturer, "Who Are the Real Cancer Quacks?"), in People's Doctor, "Cancer Book Up-To-Date", Summer & Fall, 1982.

"Your many hours of study have given you very substantial information, but I think that in your effort (in Med. Dark Ages C. 1984) to be fair to all sides, you haven't established your own point of view." - Nathan Pritikin, (Founder & Dir.: Pritikin Longevity Center, & Pritikin Research Found'n; co-author: Live Longer Now, & The Pritikin Program for Diet & Exercise (with Pat McGrady, Jr.), & The Permanent Weight Loss Manual; Guest Editorial, Preventive Medicine, v.11,p.733, 1982).

"...Medical Dark Ages Circa 1984. I've glanced through the first part, a catalogue of treatments & their categorical data, & then enjoyed the 'Cancer Quotations Collage'. You have put this together expertly. It will be very useful." - John Richardson,(MD, Univ. Rochester Medical School; Fellow, Kaiser Hosp.; author, Laetrile Case Histories, & Richardson Newsletter).

"Upon reviewing your excellent compendium of data regarding alternative cancer therapies, I'm deeply impressed by the great amount of research & organization of references that obviously were required. You have done an outstanding job of bringing together information that should be of vital interest to cancer therapists & patients alike." - G. Edward Griffin, (BA, U. Mich., Regent's Alumni Scholarship; first prize, Hearst national oratrical contest; m.c., CBS network radio show; Chairman: AMF (Americans/(Californians) for Medical Freedom);&, VOCAL (Victory Over Cancer Action League); Editor, Health World News/Voice of Medical Freedom; Author: The Fearful Master - a 2nd Look at the UN; &, World Without Cancer).

"...How impressed I was with your work, Medical Dark Ages C. 1984. A tremendous amount of work went into it, & it seems quite a definitive compilation on the extent of unproven methods. I wish you a great deal of success with it." - Ralph W. Moss, (PhD; author, The Cancer Syndrome; Assist. Dir. Public Affairs, MSKCC (Memorial Sloan-Kettering Cancer Center); articles on cancer in Science Digest, & The Progressive, & Science & Society; co-author, An Alternative Approach to Allergies; major contributor, to: Second Opinion ("Laetrile at Sloan-Kettering"); &, The Cancer War, Non Fiction Television, WNET/Thirteen, PBS, May 11, 1983).

"The prized copy of Med. Dark Ages C. 1984(:)... I cannot express in a few words how impressed I am with the monumental research you have done in organizing it. What you have done is the most needed condensation, of the greatest area, in the field that embraces(:) nutrition, degenerative conditions in general, & the 'cancer of politics', that is prohibiting the realistic conquest of cancer, in our time! Only public opinion can muster the kind of pressure & force, that may, hopefully, combat this crime. Your book should be the fulcrum towards this goal. Indeed, I was so impressed with reading it, skipping here & there, then going back to miss not a word...." ....

"Congratulations, & my personal & grateful thanks, for this wonderful contribution to education, on the nitty-gritty essence of the cancer problem; which doesn't stop there, by any means. .... We are not big in books, but do handle a few selected ones we feel we want to lend some energy to circulating, & yours, for myself, is #1. .... I treasure the book...." (on Nov. 22, 1982, letter to R.H.)

- Betty Morales, (PhD; Pres., CCS (Cancer Control Society); V. Pres., NHF (National Health Federation); Ed. & Pub., Organic Consumer Report & Cancer Control Journal); former Pres., IACVF (International Association of Cancer Victims & Friends)).

"Ralph R. Hovnanian is the author of a remarkable book, the title of which is the subject of this report. The book is about cancer, & in 146 pages (1st ed.;it) condenses & simplifies the essence of almost every book, report, claim, research, result of experiment, etc., on the subject. .... For openers, Hovnanian has brilliantly condensed a review of some 500 cancer treatments, modes & theories, categorizing the % benefited, total number treated, measure of benefit, disease severity, researcher credentials, & reference publication(s). Should any doubt exist regarding the conspiracy to suppress any but orthodox cancer treatment, no matter how well documented or successful, & particularly if non-toxic, look no further! This publication is a wealth of information & 'ammunition'. No cancer patient, & no doctor treating cancer patients, should be unfamiliar with the facts & implications in this book. .... 'Who are the real quacks?', is a spontaneous reaction to the subjects covered. (It is) a permanent reference to 100's of published works on the subjects."

- Betty Morales, (PhD; Pres., CCS; V.Pres., NHF; Ed. & Pub., Organic Consumer Rep., & Ca. Control J.; former Pres., IACVF), "Medical Dark Ages - Circa 1984", Organic Consumer Report, Eden Ranch, v.62,n.49,p.1,Dec.7,1982.

"...Med. Dark Ages c. 1984. It is a scholarly work which will help us & millions of others. A (state) Representative, Hon. ... asked me to provide him with a rebuttal to the NCI claim.... We have sent him today your...work.... Please send us your rebuttal to the NCI tests if you ever have time to prepare one." - Clinton Miller, (Exec. Director, NHF (National Health Federation), & its Legistlative Advocate).

"...Med. Dark Ages C. 1984. You have obviously put a lot of work into this publication which I hope will be widely read. Your work is important & I'm just hoping that it can be read without difficulty to the average reader. .... Perhaps we should do a review in the Journal. .... I can see it...as a patient's reference book. ...I am proud...that you have used the Cancer News Journal as a constant referral document. .... Your book...addresses itself to the professional community so... , I think it will serve a good purpose. .... I think your work is great! .... Stay with the good work." - Ann Cinquina, (Exec. Director / Editor, IACVF (International Association of Cancer Victims & Friends) / Cancer News Journal).

"Med. Dark Ages C. 1984(:).... This extensively researched book was written by Ralph Hovnanian. In it, (he) condenses over 20 categories & 100's of experiments ("or clinical trials") of alternative cancer therapies. He shows that the alternative therapies are much less expensive, less harmful, & more effective, than the orthodox therapies of surgery, radiation, & chemotherapy. He also includes a book list of recommended reading, a list of public interest health groups, & (their) journals & addresses, & a list of organizations supplying directories of doctors & (their) addresses. There are numerous mentions to March of Truth on Cancer, by Arlin J. Brown." - The Arlin J. Brown Information Center, Health Victory Bulletin, v.10, n.8, p.1, Aug. 1984.

"Mr. Hovnanian's book is an outstanding & valid attempt to collect & present information on alternative cancer therapies & the dismal record of conventional medicine. I highly recommend it as an objective, valuable resource." - Peter Barry Chowka, (author, radio, & television spokesperson, on politics of therapy; Contributing Editor, East - West Journal).

"On behalf of Michio Kushi (author: The Cancer Prevention Diet, & Cancer & Heart Disease, & The Book of Macro-biotics; about) your new book, Med. Dark Ages C. 1984(:) We...hope your book will be well received & contribute to improving the health & well-being of thousands of people. .... Along with your efforts & those of many others, we hope to contribute to a more enlightened approach to medicine & healing...." - Alex Jack, (Editor, East-West Journal).

"I will review (Med. Dark Ages C. 1984) in my Herb Report. ...God bless you in the work you're doing." - John Heinerman, (author, The Treatment of Cancer with Herbs; medical anthropoligst).

"Med. Dark Ages C. 1984 ...: This rather curious, somewhat angrily written & jumbled up book.... The first few pages of his curiosity are in & of themselves quite singular, if not peculiar. Over half of the first page goes into the legalities of his copyright.... ...His sporadic academic background.... One wonders how correct he is, for there are a lot of puzzling aspects to this work waiting to be discovered by the reader. Mr. Hovnanian's book is rather like wandering through a maze of tunnels & corridors never really knowing just where you might come out in the end. .... The work itself, believe it or not, has a lot of useful information, brought together in one volume, but in such disarray, that it takes some time to try to sort it all out, if you can. ("I'm still trying myself.") Mr. Hovnanian seems to be a good fellow, with a kind heart, who means well, & wants to help people, as much as he can. He is to be complimented for his efforts as a humanitarian. But, — an author & publisher he is not, from the appearance of what he has put together. Still, it is one of those one-of-a-kind things, which ought to be purchased by those who collect the strange & very unusual." - John Heinerman, "A Strange Publication", "Book Reviews", Herb Report, March 1984.

"I reviewed Mr. (Richard) Ericson's book (Cancer Treatment: Why So Many Failures? What You Can Do About It) along with yours (Med. Dark Ages C. 1984 ...), but gave his a little longer review, because I felt it was laid out better, & a lot easier to read. This is no reflection on the content of your book, which I felt was maybe more thorough, but the style was too jumbled up for even someone like myself to follow. You may wish to consider this when reprinting a 2nd edition. I...could not answer your letter until now, ...25 minutes to midnight, Jan. 1st, 1984. .... This year I've given 94 lectures around the country, made 51 TV-radio appearances, & spoken at about 9 large conventions. ...God bless... your righteous endeavors." - John Heinerman, (Medical Anthropologist; Author, 16 books, including: The Treatment of Cancer with Herbs, &, The Science of Herbal Medicine, &, The Complete Book of Spices (Forward by Henry Heimlich, MD, of Heimlich Maneuver against choking), &, Herbal Research Manual ... (Forword by Arthur Kaslow, MD, of Kaslow Stomach Tube), &, Understanding Herbal Medicine (... Studies in Med. Anthropology); &, "The Roots of Herbal Med.", Whole Life Times, n.26, p.17-31, April 1983; Editor, The Herb Report).

"Ralph Hovnanian has performed a Herculean task in tracking down the 'alternative' cancer treatments & summarizing the claims made for them. In dissipating much of the murkiness that has beclouded the less toxic options, he has performed a valuable service for researchers, authors, physicians, patients, & their families." - Patrick McGrady, Jr., (co-author, The Pritikin Program for Diet & Disease; author, The Janker Clinic, &, The Youth/Love Drs., &, "...Cancer...", Newsday, Sept. 30, 1984; Pres., Amer. Soc. of Journalists & Authors; Moscow Bureau Chief, Newsweek).

"Your book (Med. Dark Ages C. 1984) shows a tremendous amount of work & is a valuable source of information." - Thomas Mansell, (author, Cancer Simplified; Chapter Chairperson, CFCCT (Committee for Freedom of Choice in Cancer Therapy)).

"Thank you for sharing the fruits of your...assiduous labors with our office. (e.g. Med. Dark Ages C. 1984) They include much valuable & important information & will become a permanent part of our library." - Susan M. Silberstein, (PhD; Exec. Dir., (Chapter of) FACT (Foundation for Alternative Cancer Therapy)).

"Many thanks for your most interesting book on Medical Dark Ages. .... You must really have put in a lot of effort to collect the material." ....

"I can understand your problem. I have encountered all kinds of criticisms for my work,because the average biologist has no understanding whatsoever of Bio-Physics on which my theory & (high pH; cesium, rubidium, potassium) therapy is based."

"...The A. Keith Brewer Library...of Richland Center, WI 53581 is disseminating cancer papers all over the world.... ...I have about a ($) million invested in it (as a charity)." - A.Keith Brewer, (PhD, Univ. Wisconsin; National Research Fellow, Cal. Tech.; Chief, Mass Spec. & Isotope Sect., NBS (National Bureau of Standards); Chief, Scientific Sect., Naval Operations; Distinguished Civilian Award, US Navy; Wisc. St. Legistlature Award), (in letter to R. Hovnanian, March 28, 1983).

"...Med. Dark Ages C. 1984 is a great inspiration to all cancer victims looking for an alternative. It started my spiritual friendship with its author. For the new edition, we will see an even more in-depth coverage of the field(:) complemental & empirical cancer treatments. .... Thanks to Ralph R. Hovnanian, these alternatives are now made public...(:) choose...Orwellian...or...Eu-topian.... May this book be the torch in the Darkness of our Age of Modern Medicine." - Hellfried Sartori,MD,MPH,MS,U. Graz Med.,Austria;Pres., Life Sciences Universal (3 teaching hosp., 1200 Med. Centers,in world); Cert.,Am.Brd. Family Practice; author, Cancer 1984.

"I studied your opus (Med. Dark Ages C. 1984); it is a treasure chest.... I find it quite useful. You are doing a service to many with that. .... Scientific work is a continuous struggle. It would of course be nice...to separate the wheat from the chaff, but that is nearly impossible today. It is not known in many cases what the wheat really is here." - Georg F. Springer, (MD; Dir., Immunochemistry Research, & Prof., Microbiology - Immunochemistry,& of Surgery, Evanston Hosp., Northwestern Univ.).

"Today I started reading the (Med. Dark Ages C. 1984) books you sent me & must say they look fascinating. .... I am the Secretary of a doctors' group who treat cancer in alternative ways. Though it was my plan to give my time to study, much of it is taken up in fighting the authorities, which is a shame & a pity. Must sound familiar to you." - Hans Moolenburgh, (MD; "The Gentle Method"; Haarlem, Holland).

"Thank you so much for your kind gifts (Med. Dark Ages C. 1984) & the complimentary remarks on our research work. I shall circulate them within the Unit as you requested." - K. W. Pettingale, (MD, FRCP; Consultant Physician/Sr. Lecturer, Human Studies in Cancer, Faith Courtauld Unit, King's College Hosp. Medical School, England).

"I did distribute the (Medical Dark Ages C. 1984) books among the members of the Staff, ... Wishing you all success in your enterprise...." - Ernesto Contreras, (MD; post-doc., Harvard U. Medical School, Children's Hosp.; Prof., Histology & Pathology, Mexican Army Med. School; Chief Pathologist, Mexican Army Hosp.; General Dir., Centro Medico del Mar).

"I...am sure that (Med. Dark Ages C. 1984) is beneficial material. I will keep in touch & let you know if any of this can be incorporated into my practice." - H. Ray Evers, (MD, Vanderbilt U.; Knight, Order of Malta; many awards).

"...I was reeling from the termination of my NCI-sponsored program.... Ironically, interest in plants I collected in China, & in the mayapple, for lung cancer, has increased since our program was terminated. .... While I believe that Nature has already developed several undiscovered cures for cancer, I fear we're being lured away from those natural cures in our ("US") rather unnatural search for synthetics. Perhaps the natural medicines will be discovered in countries more interested in people than profit."

"I'm afraid since I am no longer officially associated with the cancer screening program, that it would be inappropriate for me to comment officially on your book. But thanks for your books & your kind words & for carrying the 'baton' I have been passively forced to drop." - James A. Duke, (PhD; Chief, Germ-plasm Resources Lab., & Economic Botany Lab., Agri. Research Serv., USDA (Dept. of Agriculture)).

"Thank you very much for the interesting material on cancer therapy you recently sent. (including Med. Dark Ages C. 1984.) Our committee's charge relates only to prevention of cancer, & we have therefore not considered therapy. I appreciate your helpfulness." - Clifford Grobstein, (PhD; Chair, Committee on Diet, Nutrition, & Cancer, of Assembly of Life Sciences, of NRC (National Research Council); Prof., Biol. Sci. & Public Policy, Program in Sci., Tech., & Public Affairs, U. of Cal., San Diego).

"...Thank you for dropping by my office.... I enjoyed our conversation; it is evident from your remarks & your monograph on alternative cancer therapies that you have devoted a great deal of time & energy to researching the field." ....

"Scientists & physicians (are) as human & fallible as anyone else.... The ancients...would be astounded by the technical accomplishments of our society.(&) .... They...would ("as we do") also find reason to be dismayed, ("& amused") since human nature has not changed that drastically." ....

"The world of medicine & medical research needs its critics & certainly has an abundant supply. However, the real trick is not to create an all white or all black tapestry, but rather to compose a portrait in which black, white, & grays are assembled in patterns which come close to representing reality." ....

"...What your monograph lacks is any sense of balance. .... The measures of benefit used range from unsubstantiated claims to controlled experiments." ....

"If 'alternative' approaches have made any contribution, it is because such ideas, methods, or materials, have become the subjects of conventional techniques of testing & development, & have yielded demonstrably useful results."

"You have done a monumental amount of work in researching & writing your monograph; I only wish you had dedicated your efforts to a constructive use, rather than to the destructive end of undermining public confidence...." - Bayard H. Morrison III, (MD, Assistant Director, NCI, (in letter to R.Hovnanian, July 21, 1983)).

"Thank you for making a copy of your book, Medical Dark Ages Circa 1984, available to Dr. Vincent T. Devita, Jr., Director of the National Cancer Institute (NCI). NCI scientists are glad to consider new theories about cancer. Your ideas, along with those obtained from many other sources, will be carefully considered by them."
- Robert M. Hadsell, PhD, Acting Chief, Public Inquiries Section, OCC (Office of Cancer Communications), NCI.

"We have reviewed your book, Med. Dark Ages C. 1984, & have decided to add it to the NLM (National Library of Medicine) collection." - Chief, Technical Services Div., NLM, NIH, PHS, letter, to R. Hovnanian, June 29,1983.

"Chairman (James) Miller has asked me to respond on his behalf, to your recent letter in support of the work of the (FTC) Federal Trade Commission in the health care field (on the AMA monopoly -Ed.). The Chairman appreciates your kind words & especially thanks you for the material (Med. Dark Ages C. 1984) that accompanied your letter. We, at the Commission, are always delighted to hear from individuals such as yourself, who study health care topics, & who help develop & support new ideas & approaches toward promotion of competition, efficiency, & quality of care in this industry. We have reviewed the book that you authored on alternative approaches to cancer treatment, ... & will keep (it) on hand for reference." - Arthur N. Lerner, (Assistant Director, FTC (Federal Trade Commission)).

"...Med. Dark Ages C. 1984.... This is a magnificent storehouse of information, & will undoubtedly be a great assistance in our legal efforts, when we have our non-toxic & alternative therapies (on trial)." - Kirkpatrick Dilling, (Esq. (Attorney), NHF General Counsel).

"...Med. Dark Ages C. 1984. You have spent eons of time & energy compiling this information, & it will stand as a reference & source document which will help a lot of us in our research. I have spent over ten years of research as shown by the attached documents. I congratulate you for having the intestinal fortitude to go ahead & put this information in one place. .... I have already referred to it several times, when I need to find the source of the thoughts that I am trying to put...on paper." - Glen L. Rutherford, (plaintiff initiating class action suit, Rutherford v. US; US District Court Judge Luther Bohanon allowing interstate trade of Laetrile for terminal cancer patients with affidavit; case to US Court of Appeals 5 times, & US Supreme Court once).

"... I wish you would send copies of the book (Med. Dark Ages c. 1984) to.... our Appeal lawyer & (the attorney) assisting him. .... Together Dr. Vetrano & I have a big struggle ahead, but with your loyal support, we should win. With best wishes to you...." - Dr. Herbert M. Shelton, (author of 12 books on Natural Hygiene, supervised 30,000 fasts).

"Ralph Hovnanian has catalogued the many references to research on alternative therapies for cancer. This book & the information within it should be made available to all cancer researchers & to anyone who has a serious interest in this important health concern. Ralph Hovnanian has clearly shown that skeptics of alternative health care can no longer say that there is no research on the effectiveness of alternative therapies in treating cancer. These skeptics simply are not familiar with the scientific literature." - Dana Ullman, (MPH, U. of Cal. Berkeley; author: Health Report, San Francisco Found'n; & "Beyond Medical Chauvinism", California Living, (Sunday S.F. Chronicle & S.F. Examiner mag.), Aug. 21, 1983; Exec. Dir., Homeopathic Educational Services).

"... (Med. Dark Ages C. 1984) will be most helpful — especially if a legal challenge of the policies of the ACS & NCI is implemented. .... I sincerely admire you for your dedication to getting the truth out about cancer. Hopefully, our joint efforts will soon bear fruit. .... Your comments about judicial recourse are quite interesting & I believe will be helpful...." - Robert F. McNellis, (Chairman, Project 100,000, petition for: "a Congressional Investigation of the 'Cancer Establishment'...that continues to reject overwhelming proof that they are on the wrong track").

"...Med. Dark Ages C. 1984.... I greatly appreciate it, & wish you every future success." - John F. Banzhaf, III, (Exec. Dir., ASH (Action on Smoking & Health)).

"I really appreciated receiving & reading (Medical Dark Ages C. 1984). Sincere best wishes." - Bernard Jensen, (DC, ND; author, The Science & Practice of Iridology, & 10 other books; Founder, Hidden Valley Health Ranch).

"Congratulations! Your Med. Dark Ages C. 1984 is an overwhelming opus. I am delighted to have this massive production & am studying it with care. Perhaps in a subsequent edition you will elect to give space to criticizing the research on which you have reported & cite references involving contrary findings." - Walter Heiby, (author, Live Your Life, & ...Dynamic Synthesis, & 1,000 page book(s) on nutrition to be published).

"I would like to persuade you to...borrow, if you like, any or all of my writing. I would like to talk you into passing up the scatter-gun attack, & concentrate on a few things that can be done. .... You have one reference out of order." - Wayne Martin, (BS, Purdue U.; Sr. Metallurgist, Sperry Gyroscope Co., & 3 others; author: Medical Heroes & Heretics; & We Can Do Without Heart Attacks; & "Treating Cancer Metastasis"; & IACVF, Cancer News Journal, many issues;&"The Beriberi Analogy to Myocardial Infarction", Medical Hypotheses,v.10,p.185, 1983;&"Margarine ("Not Butter") the Culprit?", Lancet, v.2 for 1983, n.8346, p.407, Aug. 13, 1983).

"When I get the time, I hope to read it from cover to cover. I may even publicize it in my journal, The Hygienist. .... People should...realize that plain living & high thinking will lead them to health & happiness. I remain yours in the fight for freedom for health maintenance." - Keki R. Sidhwa, (ND, DO; Pres., Brit. Natural Hygiene Soc.; author, 4 books, inc. Medical Drugs on Trial? Verdict "Guilty!").

"...Cancer Alternative Therapies' Cure Rates is being used in 3 different universities by...a sociologist...hygienist." ....

"Let me know more details of your book. Is it being marketed? How are you using this valuable information?" - Jo Willard,(Pres., Natural Hygiene, Inc.).

"...Med. Dark Ages C. 1984 — it is definitely a 'masterpiece' of work; it is both informative & inspiring to all concerned citizens who wish the best in health measures. I know key people who I'm sure would be delighted to know about this work.... (It) will be well received by the general public who are continually seeking remedies for their many ills..... I cannot compliment you enough on your book, Ralph. ...The faith you stir in others, God will make even stronger for you, & others who have been helped by your efforts."

"No matter how much knowledge you attain - never, never lose sight of God, without His grace & blessings we are nothing - for the good we do comes from God above."
- Grace Girdwain, (Volunteer for Special Human Rights Services).

"...Med. Dark Ages C. 1984 — it is the best source of data I have encountered bearing specifically on cancer alternative therapy. You have indeed produced a wonderful piece of work based on extensive research, (with) data quoting the findings of many medical doctors. Whoever reads this book will find it not only shockingly interesting, but (also) pointing the way toward a more effective approach to cancer control; as well as, presenting data which certainly poses a big question.... My compliments for your fine endeavors, Ralph Hovnanian, & may your readers carry on the word from there & keep spreading it until humanity is fully enlightened on the real truths of Natural Hygienic Health." - Grace Girdwain, (natural hygienist, & anti-(forced)-vaccination-ist),

"...Med. Dark Ages C. 1984. ...(is a) monumental work. It is one of the most informative documentations that I have ever put my hands on in this particular area. It confirms many of my thoughts, & it goes along with what the Church of Natural Hygienic Living espouses, that, 'God Heals Through Nature'." - Dr. R.M.Bramms,DD,MNHL.

"Wonderful things are happening in the health field. Your helpfulness is greatly appreciated (for Med. Dark Ages C. 1984)." - Ann Wigmore, (DD; ND: Founder & Pres., Hippocrates World Health Org'n; author, Why Suffer?...Wheat Grass God's Manna!; &, Garden Indoors; Recognition Award for Work in the Field of Youthfulness & for Efforts in Regeneration of Human Cells & Tissues, Nobel Prize Found., Royal Laplander Acad. Sci., Finland; over a dozen honorary degrees).

"...The wonderful book (Med. Dark Ages C. 1984; ... "you have done a great job putting all that info together!"). We may be reviewing it...in (an) issue of The Sproutletter. .... Keep up the good work!!" - Jeff Breakey, (Editor, Publisher, & co-Author, The Sproutletter).

"I just came across your book. I had to call you. I couldn't let this one go by. Say if there's anything I can do to sell it for you. I can sell it at conventions. .... It's been a long 50 years in medicine. .... Would you be interested in writing a book on my work in colon therapy?" - Dr. Robert A. Wood, Australian Health Inst., Gary, Indiana, (para-phrased telephone conversation to Editor).

"Dr. (Robert A.) Wood (Australian Health Inst.) wants to thank you very much for your efforts (Med. Dark Ages C. 1984).... If you can...with Dr. Wood...write...on colon therapy for your new (edition?)" - Judy, (Sec'y to Dr. Wood).

"Your book (Med. Dark Ages C. 1984) looks as though you put a tremendous amount of work into it. .... Is there any way we can work together? We all need more distribution to reach the public! .... Much that can be done — we have the facts!" - Blanche Leonardo, (PhD; Founder & Pres., Vegetarian Society, Inc.; author: Check That Chick; & Cancer & Other Diseases from Meat Consumption ...; & Natural Nutrition — Answer to Cancer).

"As a colleague & co-worker with Dr. John Scharffenberg (MD; MPH; Assoc. Prof. Appl. Nutrition, Loma Linda U.; author, Problems With Meat), I recently saw your publication, Med. Dark Ages C. 1984.... The work intrigued me, ...as I also am involved in disease prevention (including cancer).... I will examine (it) with great interest." - Jim Florence, (Dr.H.Sc.; MPH; Health Ed. Coordinator, San Joaquin Community Hosp.).

"I am writing from Commonweal, an environmental health center with a strong & open minded interest in alternative cancer therapies. (We) are working...on a survey of alternative cancer therapies. We are interested in reviewing your book, Med. Dark Ages C. 1984...." - Amy Lee; & Michael Lerner, PhD; Commonweal.

"I've looked through (Med. Dark Ages C. 1984, &) wish you success in getting them distributed. CSPI needs to focus very narrowly on governmental policies that are inconsistent with clear scientific evidence. So much of the cancer - treatment world does not fit into this region of action." - Michael Jacobson, PhD; Executive Director, CSPI (Center for Science in the Public Interest); author, Eater's Digest; co-editor, Food for People, Not for Profit.

"(Med. Dark Ages C. 1984 is) a monumental piece of work. My God, what a project. I'll never know how you did it. But I would like to! ....I wondered if you had considered seeking grants or other kind of funding, so that you could maximize public & professional awareness of this book & its invaluable contents. ...My favorite wish for all who are on the side of the angels: 'May you enjoy love, health, money, & the time to enjoy all three.'." - Myron Sylton, (Pres., People Against Cancer; auth., ed., & pub., International Directory of Alternative Cancer Tests & Therapies; Pres., Boston Evening Clinic; Litt.D.: Portia Law School, & also Calvin Coolidge College).

"...My good friend Ralph R. Hovnanian.... ...in a humanitarian effort to help with the cancer problem. As you can see, he did a terrific job in compiling information regarding all, & I mean all (in friendly jest), of the various treatments for cancer & their sponsors & innovators. .... Note he has a BS from Princeton U. & an MS from Stanford U. & hence is very capable of compiling the extensive review of all of the known alternative treatments for cancer listed in his book. .... I believe he has made an outstanding contribution to the treatment of cancer following alternative(s).... ....a very commendable effort.... I trust you will find it helpful. .... I am sure you will appreciate the very extensive work,(Med. Dark Ages C. 1984)." - Richard Ericson, (BS; JD; patent attorney; author, Cancer Treatment, Why So Many Failures?, What You Can Do About It; Exec. Dir., GE-PS Cancer Memorial; WWI veteran; architect; chem. engineer).

"Hovnanian did a terrific research job."(letter to Richard Ericson, July26,1982).
"Dick (Ericson) recently sent me a copy of your book. You certainly devoted a tremendous amount of time in the effort." - Walter Ermer, (Exec. Dir., International Health Council; author, A Program for the Prevention & Early Detection of Cancer ...; legistlative advocate for alternative therapies of cancer).

"Dick Ericson: Walter Ermer sent me a book that I have really marvelled at, since it has statements from reliable individuals: doctors, lawyers, scientists, etc. I am inquiring if you sent copies to Senators...Congressmen....as I feel it is dynamite to anyone who has concern in cancer, etc. ...the book is Medical Dark Ages Circa 1984...." - Kitty Schumacher,(head, Cancer Information Crusade; activist for Krebiozen; lawsuit against chlorination).

"I am pleased to send this letter as I pride myself for good judgement regarding your book,Med. Dark C. 1984. ....It is terrific to read! So much research. You are a genius. ...The book...(is) a treasure indeed.... If I had the means, I would send every Senator & Congressman a copy, as no where have we read such dynamic information. We realize the time devoted, & this makes it more valuable. ....Why...I just can't get over the information one can become involved in!" - Kitty Schumacher.

"Dear Kitty: Some of the material which crosses my desk absolutely startles me ***the reference of course is to Med. Dark Ages...by Ralph Hovnanian***it is absolutely super. You & I know that we both have put in thousands of hours in our lifetime, in our pursuits & endeavors, but this guy Hovnanian appears to have put us to shame with his effort with the book***the amount of time consuming detail scares me." - Gene Basalegas, (health farmer, co-worker & relative of Adolph Hohensee).

"Congratulations for your monumental Med. Dark Ages C. 1984.... What I have read, & know is there, still to be read, & useful for future reference, is evidence of your tremendous effort for a worthy cause &, yes, 'urgent topic'. Your selfless dedication & effort will not go unrecognized or unheralded I am sure! I shall do my bit to see that the world will hear of your work. Thus, I would like to order...more of the 'priceless collector's item'...one...to Ruth Desmond, Pres., Federation of Homemakers...."
"With your exposure to the orthodox in the medical, chemical, political, etc., etc., it is good to realize ("from your publication") that you have "survived" & have not come to that stage of education where one learns...no longer an awareness of the whole! Nor have you, apparently, been influenced by the $." ....
"I hope 'some generous, ample donations will result from' your initiative. If a fund of some kind is established for the purpose of distributing & further printing of your present work, & for continued research & writing as you indicated in 'scope', ..." - Pearl Thiessen, (U. Wisc.; Dir., Food Services Dept., Wisc. State Inst. for the Mentally Retarded).

"...Information Science(:) the general layout & style of your book (Med. Dark Ages C. 1984)..(&)the scrupulous way in which you present the references without intruding any hint of hypothesis...."

"...The best plan will be to complete my acquisition of a working familiarity with your book; this will stop short of memorization, which is the eventual goal, but will mean being able to work without a copy in my hand." ....

"Seriously, your book is rather monumental in the present edition, while it is certainly possible to expand it to advantage, it might be as well to remember that there is a law of diminishing returns. After all...it does need to be kept within the limits of easy transportability."

"...I am overwhelmed.... ...Please rest assured that you can rely on me for any aid in your efforts, which I can give." - Frank Hourigan, (cancer alternative therapy theoretician; mechanical engineer; England).

"...Your wonderful book has been my constant companion ever since I've had it. It's really excellent. .... I also visited a man...on the board of NHF, & heads the Santa Barbara IACVF chapter. He has seen your book & was very impressed by it. .... I did have the feeling you did not...search out original journal articles which had not been referenced elsewhere. Perhaps that will be my task. ...I'm indexing your book. It seems that it would be a good beginning to indexing pertinent facts & statistics on cancer treatments. .... Please try & get your book distributed. It's valuable. Hope we can work together sometime." - Phil Lipson, Dir., CCRP (Comprehensive Cancer Research Project).

"...Med. Dark Ages C. 1984. Your booklet is unique in offering so much information in such a concise format & without personal bias. .... We would that your self-less spirit could spill more over into the war against cancer." - Santa Barbara Chapter, IACVF (International Assoc. of Cancer Victims & Friends).

"...Your super book (Med. Dark Ages C. 1984). .... If all the groups & members that are of one mind band together, they'll have to listen to us. ...Best we start banding together before they destroy us...." - Jay Sherwood, (Chapter Pres., IACVF (Internat'l Assoc. of Cancer Victims & Friends)).

"You have some fine information in (Med. Dark Ages C. 1984). .... Excellent." - Alta Klier, (Northwest Cancer Association).

"...Med. Dark Ages C. 1984. It is a masterpiece! ...Can I become a distributor for (it)?" - Chester P. Yozwick, (ND; Pres., Nutritional Science Assoc.).

"I found (Med. Dark Ages C. 1984) interesting & was pleased...." - Eydie Mae Hunsberger, (author, How I Conquered Cancer Naturally).

"I have looked at your work (Med. Dark Ages C. 1984) carefully, & fully appreciate the amount of work necessary to accomplish what you have done. There are many needs for such a book. ....I wish you the best of luck." - Harry D. Williams, II, (Pres., Amer. Business Cancer Research Found'n,Inc.).

"I, personally, was most interested in your interest & background in searching through 'alternative' & 'unorthodox' therapies. ....You might have an interest in presenting...a...workshop on 'Unorthodox Alternative Therapies'....(at) our next Annual Meeting...." - Richard S. Shepard, (DDS; Secretary & Treasurer, HDA (Holistic Dental Assoc.).

"I can see you really did a lot of work (on Med. Dark Ages C. 1984); gathering material takes so much time." - Faye Willard, (Founder & CEO, AADV (Amer. Assoc. of Dental Victims)).

"I have just received your publication, Medical Dark Ages C. 1984...which at first glance seems to be very interesting. I will be reading the work much more thoroughly as time allows...to familiarize ourselves with the ideas you present. I am sure it will be 'well worn' before long." -

"Also, I am pleased to say that our membership has grown to 250,000." - Chris Cook, Director, Greenpeace.

"An effective cancer cure is another lost cause, as you should well know. Your opus is certainly well documented; & there is plenty of proof that several effective cancer cures have been developed & proven out in clinical practice...." - Riley H. Crabb, (Director, Borderland Sciences Research Found'n; Doctor of Meta-physics in the Society of St. Luke the Physician).

"(Med. Dark Ages C. 1984, or) Cancer Alternative Therapies' (Cure Rates),Hovnanian. About 1 person in 6 will get mutilated, burned, or poisoned in current treatments.... Here is a huge collection of the many alternative methods that are often so simple.... An absolute 'must' as survival education or insurance." - A. H. Fry, Incredible Inquiry Catalog, n.7, back page, n.8, p.3.

"...You have done a great job." - A. H. Fry, (of "The World's Most Unusual Publication Catalog").

"I think your book would go pretty well with ads.... Its a lot of work for little reward, but someone's got to do it." - Al Fry, (of Fry's).

"We consider the information concerning these books very interesting & useful. It is taken from a Book Review sent to us by our friend Al Fry.... .... Med. Dark Ages C. 1984.... This unique book briefly covers dozens of alternative cancer therapies, how effective the treatments were, & where the research information was found. Filled with information available no where else." - Cathleen Moore, Librarian, Advanced Sciences R&D Corp., Advanced Sciences Advisory, Jan. 1984, p.45.

"Ralph Hovnanian is a networker in the field of Health ("Nutrition, Natural Foods, Alternatives, Holistic Health, etc. ..."). He & I met in Chicago, through the Center for Appropriate Nutrition, a local group striving to educate others...."

"...Med. Dark Ages C. 1984.... ...contains results of over 200 experiments....(&) as Ralph calls it, a mozaic of quotes to try to give the Big Picture."

"If anyone would be interested in contacting Ralph on any questions on health, to find other individuals in the field ("a networking function"), or more information about his book, please feel free to write or call...my good friend, Mr. Hovnanian."

- Joshua, ("a seeker of Truth"), Journeys of an Aquarian Age Networker, "A Directory of Public Interest Health Groups ("Journals & Addresses, by Ralph Hovnanian")", c.1982, p.283.

"Your book (MDAC 1984) is fascinating & sure represents a lot of dedicated effort. I...plan to loan out the second copy to several people who've expressed an interest in the book. Hopefully, the medical society will sit up & take notice! ...The quotes in the book are excellent...!" - Emilie Cowan, BA, Vassar; pianist.

"(MDAC 1984:) It's mammoth, a work of art, terribly scholarly. ...I love how you excerpted parts of literature.... ...It's kind, beautiful, healing, caring, intelligent, chock full, optimistic...." - Susan Meyers, Russo-logist.

"(MDAC 1984:) It was interesting to read - in fact I hope that you can expand it into a sequel...." - Ruth Roberts, BS, Oberlin; MS, Harvard, Occupat. Therapy.

"(MDAC 1984:) I can tell much blood, sweat, & tears went to its production." - Thelma Bunce, Nurse.

"...Your interesting book (MDAC 1984; I) hope to read (it) soon...." - Mimi Kaplan, "Y-Me?" (breast cancer self-help group) co-founder.

"(MDAC 1984:) I...was mighty well impressed by the big job you did & especially taken with the beautiful 'Discussion of Experiments', p.5&6. .... There's some other info that should be in any update you write: ...J.H. Tilden, MD, ...in the 1920's...was subjected to similar 'Catch-22' 's then." - Ed Newman, Major USAF Ret., Okinawa, Japan.

"...Med. Dark Ages C. 1984 - a good title. .... So much required to restore one's health is free. Namely, air, water, sunshine, exercise, rest, diet, & religion (self esteem). .... One of the primary causes of problems in our society is a lack of communication." ....

"One part of your book intrigues me very much." ....

"If I published that which pleased me, (Allergy Today) would have been a statistical report, & this turns off 99%+ readers." ....

"This is a hard statement to make, but I feel that one of our major diseases may be represented by this symbol: $." - Stanley W. Mattoon, (author, Allergy Today).

"Keep up the good work (on Med. Dark Ages C. 1984)." - Richard Kearns, DVM.

"Thanks a million. I know you have already helped at least 2 people, & I'm sure many more you're not aware of." - George Catanzaro, (PE (Professional Engineer), health lobbyist (in NJ)).

"I really appreciate the work you've put into (Med. Dark Ages C. 1984)." - Lee Taylor, (author: "Medicine Men of the Cancer Industry" (article); Everychild's Christmas).

"...Med. Dark Ages C. 1984(:) I think the information would make a great live presentation by putting it onto film, slides, or video." - John-Michael Wenzel, (Editor, Transformations).

"Here I am, writing my last column, thinking back on the last 5 years.... The best part has been learning about all the exciting things you guys are up to. You are certainly a diverse lot, from Rolfers in India to ... , & each new piece of mail I get informs me of another new adventure one of you has embarked on."

"-- ran for Lt. Gov. of Vermont & won!" ....

"I recently got a postcard from Ralph ("Hootenanny") Hovnanian. Hoot reports that he has just finished a book entitled Med. Dark Ages C. 1984.... The book compiles the effectiveness of over 200 therapies & arranges over 400 quotes on why they are illegal to use & other medical politics." - Robert Mauterstock, Jr., (in "68", Princeton Alumni Weekly, v.83,n.15,p.53, April 6, 1983).

(Please start on p.242 for the above "Reviews".)

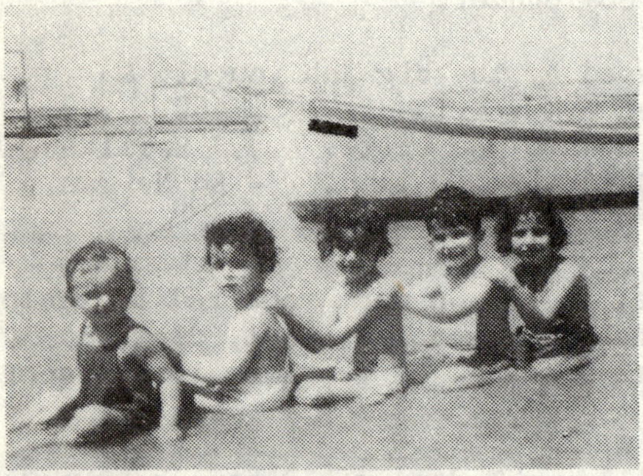

Friendly relatives, sun, fresh air, ocean water.

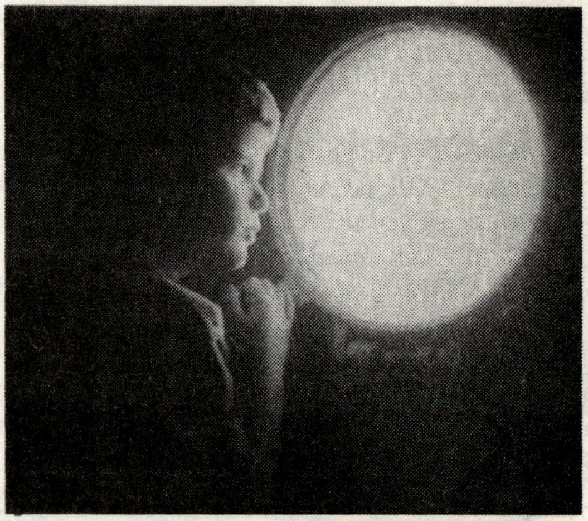

Author porthole (pier) peering, for pre-teen peers.
Dark Ages to Light Years.
(Photo by author's father,MD,FACS.)

TABLE of CONTENTS for DETECTION:

DETECTION: CANCER ALTERNATIVE DETECTION ACCURACY RATES:

DETECTION, Diagnosis, Evaluation, (Mode, Theory)	ACCURACY, % of total, or #	DIAGNOSED, total #	MEASURE of ACCURACY	DISEASE DIAGNOSED	RESEARCHER, Credentials	REFERENCE, Publication
D.1.0 CONTROLS for COMPARISON D.1.1 ORTHODOX DIAGNOSIS D.1.1.1 BIOPSY, HISTOLOGY, PATHOLOGY. Tissue cellular exam. Only 40% of breast tumors diagnosed as malignant are biologically malignant.	40%	all USA diagnoses	biological malignant (need no orthodox therapy)	diagnosed malignant: (breast)	Maurice Fox, PhD; Dept. Bio., MIT.	"On the Diagnosis & Treatment of Breast Ca.", JAMA, v.241, n.5, p.489, Feb.2, 1979. (L.V.Ackerman, MD, ... The Pathology of Tumors, ACS, 1972, p.10, 20, 29.)
D.1.1.2 X-RAY & RADIO-ISOTOPE IMAGING, misses 97-99% of "occult" metastases (from primary tumor).	97-99% 1-3%		false negatives accuracy	ca. & metastases (rarer ones)	A.R.Kagan, MD; &, H.A.Gilbert, MD; Dept. Radiotherapy, So. Cal. Permanente.	"The Detection of Occult Metastases with Imaging Studies", ACS, Metastases & Disseminated Ca., 1975, p.40.
D.1.1.3 General. Diagnosis of patient was in full agreement with autopsy in only 45% of 9,000 cases.	45%	patients: 9,000	full agreement on cause of death	mortality	Attending MD's vs. autopsy Pathologists, 75 hosp., Great Britain.	HMSO, Accuracy of Certification of Cause of Death, 1966; ref. in: Leon Chaitow, An End to Ca.?, p.116.
D.1.2 ORTHODOX DIAGNOSES "SIDE EFFECTS" D.1.2.1 Biopsy spreads ca. cells out of tumor, & along weakened tissue surfaces from surgery.						P.Rubin, MD, (Ed.) Clinical Oncology: a Multidisciplinary... in: Moss, Ca. Syn., p.40.
D.1.2.2 X-ray & radio-isotope detection cause ca.	94,000 in #	US pop.	ca. deaths per year	x-ray diagnosis caused	John Gofman, MD, PhD; Prof. Emeritus, UCBerkeley; AEC.	Radiation & Human Health. (R.Glasser, The Greatest Battle.)
ALTERNATIVE / ECLECTIC / UNORTHODOX, / WHOLISTIC / METABOLIC / NATURAL / ENVIRONMENTAL: DIAGNOSIS / DETECTION in HUMANS.						
D.2.0 SPIRITUAL, MENTAL ... D.2.7 PSYCHIC DIAGNOSIS D.2.7.1 Psychic acts as "intermediary between the people & the spirit of Dr. Fritz (great surgeon, deceased)".	518 in#	patients: tot.:1,000 545	diagnosis matched patient's own MD's	med. records: none "on hand	Jose Arigo; (tested by Andrija Puharich, MD, Northwestern U. Med.); (see 2.7.1).	Reader's Digest, Mysteries of the Unexplained, p.281.
D.2.7.3 Psi: Telepathy, Clairvoyance, Precognition, Psychokinesis.	80% 70% 60%	patients: 17 78 25	accuracy: site cause p=.05	pain	C.Norman Shealy, MD, PhD; Dir. Pain & Rehab. Ctr.; Pres., Am. Holistic Med. Assoc. 2 of 7 psychics	Arthur Hastings, PhD, Prof. Stanford U.; (&... Eds.), "Alternative ... Diagnosis", Health for the Whole Person, (NIMH; For. US Sen. T.Kennedy), p.471.
D.2.16 Neuro-Muscular coordination; test by HANDWRITING Analysis: ca. patient's (ink) pen stroke is segmented (microscopic) from twitch. Separates high from low risk groups.	90% 84% 72% 87%	patients: 10,000 700	accuracy: (10% false-) (16% false+)	many diseases & ca. ca. other dis.	Alfred Kanfer, consult.: Austrian Dept. Justice; &, Huntington Hartford; Strang Clinic; ACS grant. Dr. D. F. Casten, Hosp. Joint Dis., NYC. D. Miller, Med. Dir., Strang Clinic.	"Neuromuscular Aberrations with Developing Malignancies", Proc. Am. Assoc. Ca. Res., n.163, Abstracts, 1970; Bull. Hosp. Jt. Dis., v.19, p.1-19, 1958; ref. in: ACS, Unproven Methods ..., p.119.

DETECTION: CANCER ALTERNATIVE DETECTION ACCURACY RATE; (continued):

DETECTION, Diagnosis, Evaluation, (Mode, Theory)	ACCURACY, % of total, or #	DIAGNOSED, total #	MEASURE of ACCURACY	DISEASE DIAGNOSED	RESEARCHER, Credentials	REFERENCE, Publication
D.4.0 HEAT D.4.1 THERMO-GRAPHY. Detect more energy emitted from tumor than normal tissue metabolism. Micro-wave emitted by deep tumors escapes body, & is detectable; but heat wave is resorbed by body, so shows only external tumors.	80% 100%	women, pre-screen	accuracy	breast tumors: malignant benign	Graphic Stress Corp., LaJolla, Cal.	Dick Ericson, JD, (hosp. construction, WW I, France), Ca. Treat. ...?, p.29.
	70%			"	Alan Barrett, Astrophysics, MIT	"Medicine", Time, June 20, 1977.
D.5.0 ELECTRO-MAGNETIC RADIATION (E&M) D.5.9 Detect energy frequencies emitted from patient to indicate disease & its location.	95%	cows: 400	accuracy	disease mix	Thomas Colson, & a vet. State Inspector. (Fred Hart, Pres., Elect. Med. Found.; found., NHF.)(See 5.9).	Molecular Radiation, p.33.
D.5.14 Detect BIO-ELECTRONIC Potential at various points on body (skin): heat, pH, oxygen, conductivity.	80% 86% 72-93% 98%	patients: 160 227 of tot.: 1,000	accuracy: site	cancer spinal coccyx	H.A. Morton Whitby, Chief Urol. Ass't., West London Hosp.; Consult Surg., St. Marg. Clin. Tumors; Hon. Urol., St. Mary's, Natal; Ass't Colonial Surg., Falklands; Surg. Registrar, London Lock Hosp.	Bio-Electronic Detection of Ca. & Other Diseases, p.x, 21, 23, 146. (Proponents: Dr. Brümmer, Supt., Stranger Hosp.; Prof. Sir Bryan Matthews; Dr. Celia Culver-Evans; Dr. R. A. Holman; & 11 Dr.'s.)
D.5.15 NMR (Nuclear Magnetic Resonance). Ca. cells hold hydrogen of water in less ordered way than normal cells, so half life time of hydrogen's (nuclear spin state) return to equilibrium (in a steady external magnetic field) after being excited (by external radio waves) is longer.		patients	(tbd)		Raymond Damadian, MD, Downstate Med. Ctr., NYC; Freeman Cope, MD. Dr. Ling, grad. stud., U.Chi.; Dept. Molec. Biol., Penn. Hosp. Dr. Carleton Hazelwood, Internat'l Soc Supra-molecular Res. Dr. D. Sodi-Pallares, Pres., National Acad. Med., Mexico; author, 300 articles.	Dick Ericson, BS Chem. Eng.; JD (law); Cancer Treatment, Why ...?, 1979, p.28. "FONAR", Healing: J. Gerson Inst., v.2, n.1, p.14, 1982; (ref. to: R. Damadian, Nature, v.228, p.76, 1970AD; & Science, v.171, p.1151, 1971AD).
D.9.0 NUTRITION, GENERAL D.9.4 URINE / SALIVA Test. Urine pH shows stomach acidity; (hi pH if not digest minerals). Saliva pH shows bowels & pancreas; (lo pH if liver toxic; hi pH if too much sugar in blood). Urine sugar shows blood sugar; (hi sugar blocks oxygen, & need energy if low sugar, to brain).	(Note: Hi urine cellular debris shows body aging. Hi urine urea & ammonia shows excess protein eaten. Hi urine salt shows mineral crystals in body.)				Carey Reams, PhD; (see 9.4.2). Harry Metsker, Pres., Intern'l Col. Healthology. Robert Preston, author, How to Prepare for the Coming Crash.	Preston, Healthology.... (Nord Davis, Pardon Me, But ... 'The Curse Causeless Shall Not Come', ...Ca.... Salem Kirban, ...Vibrant Health.)

DETECTION: CANCER ALTERNATIVE DETECTION ACCURACY RATE; (continued):

DETECTION, Diagnosis, Evaluation, (Mode, Theory)		ACCURACY, % of total, or #	DIAGNOSED, total #	MEASURE of ACCURACY	DISEASE DIAGNOSED	RESEARCHER, Credentials	REFERENCE, Publication
D.10.0 NUTRITION, LAETRILE							
D.10.6.3 Beard Anthrone Test (BAT). HCG (Human Chorionic Gonadotropin) measured in urine indicates ca. Trophoblast of pregnancy or malignancy secretes HCG. More HCG detected as therapy busts ca. cells. Ectopic germ cell (outside uterus/embryo stage) changes to ectopic trophoblast cell (ca.) by meiosis. Chymo-trypsin of pancreas(es) digest tropho-blast. So, trophoblast, & chymotrypsin inhibitor, & somatic tissue, & female sex hormone, & carcinogen, cause ca. In pregnancy, trophoblast invades maternal tissue, & absorbs maternal blood nutrients. BAT detects ca. anywhere in body, not locally, & 6 months earlier, in contrast to biopsy. BAT is false (+) (falsely finding disease) for cancer, while really pregnancy or recent sex (male).	pregnancy (A-Z) test:	94.5%	patient tests:	accuracy: result (+)	ca.	H.H.Beard, author, 150 articles; (see C.10.6.3); (& ran tests for 500 Drs.)	(John Beard: Lancet, June 21, 1902AD, p.1758; & Feb.4, 1905; Med. Rec., Jan.5, 1907; ref.in:) Howard Beard, A New Approach to the Conquest of Cancer...., p.26, 59, 90, 188-197, 222; (ref. to: H. Beard & Terrell, So. Med. J., v.48, p.1352, Dec. 1955; &, Exp. Med. Surg., v.7, n.4, (3 articles), Nov. 1949; &, Science, v.105, p.2767, 1947; &, 4th Internat'l Ca. Congress, St. Louis, 1947;...)
		94 %	2,000	(−)	no ca.		
	milk (clot) assay:	95 %			ca.		
		95 %			ca.	" , & T.C.Terrell, MD.	
	Anthrone test (color):	95.8%	51	(+)	ca., biopsy, diagnosed terminal		
		100.0%	1,000	(+)	ca.	A.H.Roffo	
		100.0%	1,000	(−)	no ca.		
		92 %	287	(+)	ca.	S.Sakai	
	" , &	100.0%	50	(+)	ca.	J.A. Restifo, MD, PhD, (see C.10.6.2)	
	Navarro changes:	100.0%	50	(−)	no ca.		
		100.0%	405	(+)	ca., clin. diagnosis	Manuel Navarro, member, 10 med. societies; Prof. Biochem., U. Santo Tomas Med., Philippines. (See 10.7).	
		100.0%	50	(−)	no ca.		
		99.8%	1,115		no ca./ca. (& biopsy)		H. Beard, The Anthrone Test ..., p.8.
	biopsy:	63 %			ca./no ca.		(" ref. to: Navarro: International Ca. Congresses: 7th, London, 1958, & 9th, Tokyo, 1966 (n.50704); &, UNITAS, v.31, p.331, 1958; &, Phil. J. Ca.: v.1, p.131, 1957; &, v.2, p.123 & 285, 1958; &, Santo Tomas J. Med.: v.9, p.468, 1954; ...; &, ACTA, v.15, 1959).
D.11.0 NUTRITION, ENZYMES							
D.11.5 PANCREATIN pills (daily, 4 weeks); if: (feel worse, then cancer), (feel better, then pre-cancer), (no change, then normal); digests ca., frees toxins.		95%	patients		ca., 6-36 months after start, months before Clinic.	W.D.Kelley, founder, Nutritional Academy; (see 11.5; C.11.5.1)	One Answer to Cancer, p. 13-15, 61.
D.16.0 BLOOD EXTRACTS							
D.16.12 "B"-Protein found only in serum of ca. patients.		90%	patients	accuracy	ca. mix	Edsel Bucovas, PhD, Prof. Biochem., U. Tenn. Health Sci. Center.	3rd Internat'l Symp. Detect. & Prev. Ca., 1978, p.257-269; ref. in: Ericson, Ca. Treat. ...?, p.28.

DETECTION: CANCER ALTERNATIVE DETECTION ACCURACY RATE; (continued):

DETECTION, Diagnosis, Evaluation, (Mode, Theory)	ACCURACY, % of total, or #	DIAGNOSED, total #	MEASURE of ACCURACY	DISEASE DIAGNOSED	RESEARCHER, Credentials	REFERENCE, Publication
D.16.13 HLB Test of dried blood. ROTS (Reactive Oxygen Toxic Species (Super-oxides, Hydroxyl radical, Hydrogen Per-oxide)) causes markers (seen at 200x): fibrin net dis-integrity, color changes, translucent voids, small particles, flakes.	90-98%	patients	accuracy	ca., & other chronic diseases	HLB: Dr. Henry Heitan. Dr. Philippe LaGarde. Robert Bradford, Knight, Malta; Pres., CFCCT; Pax Mundi Dipl. Acad., Brussells; Stanford U. H. L. Bolen, MD, dept. head, 2 hosp. Mass.	Committee (CFCCT), Choice, v.6, n.2, p.13, Sum. 1980. ("A Practical & Inexpensive Screen Test for Ca", Am. J. Digestive Dis., v.17, n.2, Feb. 1950; ref. in: Arlin Brown, March of Truth on Cancer, p.112.)
	97%	350		ca.	N.P. Norman, MD. Anna Slicher	M. Culbert, Save Your Life, p.208; (& R. Bradford, Internat'l Protocols in Cancer Mgmt., p.151-6).
	83%			lung ca.	Tufts Med., USPHS grant	
D.16.14 Hema-Cytology Index (HCI). View (microscopic) changes in blood cells, to detect ca.	92%	patients: 151	accuracy	ca., histo-pathology	Thelma Arthur, MD, DO. Barbara Johnston, MD, NYU Med.; Dir., Cytol. Res. St. Luke's, NYC.	"Malignancy Related Changes in Peripheral Blood Smears", Acta Cytol., v.11, p.304, 1967; ref. in: ACS, Unproven Methods..., p.95, 98, & 103.
	94%	495				
	99%	340		other disease/ normal		
	92%	1,005				
	90%			ca. mix, no lung	O. Cameron Gruner, MD; Royal Col. Physicians; ACS, NIH, Damon Runyan grants; (see: 18.7; B.3.5)	(A. Brown, March... Ca., p.113.)
	75%			lung ca.		(R. Ericson, Ca. Treat...?, p.27.)
Immuno-Status Differential. Evaluate immunity to ca. in body.	89-98%			ca.	Harold Harper, MD, U. Tex.; Pres., IAPM (International Acad. Prev. Med.).	"The Immuno-status Differential Early Detect. of Ca....", JIAPM, v.6, n.1, p.1-48 (17&35), 1979.
Carcino-Embryonic Antigens (CEA)	14-79-98%				W. J. Clifford, MS, U. Ariz., Sigma Chi.	
D.16.15 Crenation of RBC (Red Blood Cells) of over 5% in # (in standard "blood count" (except 1% sodium chloride is dilutant)), indicates cancer.					Emerson B. Hartman	(Professional Secrets; ref. in: A. J. Brown, March of Truth on Cancer, p.113.) letter to Ed. (RH), Nov. 18, 1977.
D.16.16 SURFACE TENSION/ENERGY of blood. Does a drop of blood, on a flat surface, "ball up" (normal), or "lie flat" (acute angle edge, chronic cancer).						
D.17.0 IMMUNOLOGY						
D.17.1 Blood test, (see 17.1; A.17.1; C.17.1).		humans: tot.: 193	accuracy:		Lawrence Burton, (see 17.1); 3 PhD's & 2 MD's; offered ACS grant. Drs. Weinberg & Clement.	Judith Glassman, The Cancer Survivors, p.265.
	100%	10	(+)	ca.		
	100%	183	(-)	no ca.		

DETECTION: CANCER ALTERNATIVE DETECTION ACCURACY RATE; (continued):

DETECTION, Diagnosis, Evaluation, (Mode, Theory)	ACCURACY, % of total, or #	DIAGNOSED, total #	MEASURE of ACCURACY	DISEASE DIAGNOSED	RESEARCHER, Credentials	REFERENCE, Publication
D.17.15 Delayed Double Diffusion (3D-Lewis) test. See precipitin lines of reaction on immuno-diffusion (thru wells cut in agar; (i.e. modified Ouchterlony)) of reagents: human test sera vs. antibodies (against human ca.; made in, & extracted from, horse plasma).	91% 81% 99.7%	patients: 961 341 2,680	accuracy: (+) (-)	ca. mix, histo-path. disease mix healthy	H. James Rand, (see 17.15). Andrew Lewis, BA. J. Ernest Ayre, MD. Norman Daily, Lab. Dir., Found'n Oncologic. Res.	("A Sero-logical Test for Ca.", Medical Lab., v.2, 2, 22, July 1968; &, Ca. Cytol., v.6, p.55, July 1966; &, Internat'l J. Industrial Med. Surg., v.37, p.113, Feb. 1968; ref.in:) ACS, Unproven Methods..., p.145.
D.17.26 Skin reaction from T-antigens of RBC (red blood cells) indicates ca.	98%	patients, women: 150	accuracy	breast ca.	George Springer, MD, Prof. Microbiol.-Immuno. & Surg.; Dir., Immuno-Chem. Res.; Evanston Hosp., Northwestern U. Med.	Progress in Allergy, v.26, p.42-96; ref.in: R.Ericson, Ca. Treat. ...?, p.194.
D.22.0 MAPPINGS of BODY D.22.1 Auriculo-diagnosis. Acupuncture points on ears inspected visually, & tested electrically & mechanically for pain.	73%	patients: 34	accuracy ($p\leq.01$)	disease mix	Drs. David Bresler, Terrance Oleson, & Richard Kroening, Pain Control Clinic, UCLA	Arthur Hastings, PhD, Prof. Stanford U., "Alternative Diagnosis", Health for the Whole Person, p.469.
D.22.2 IRIDOLOGY. Site of disease shows in mapping on iris. Iris is connected to retina by projection thru eye's humours, & by nerves. Retina is connected to brain & thus rest of body by nerves. (Nerve fiber transmits color as in fiber optics?-Ed.)	95%	patients: 1,273	accuracy, site	disease mix	Dr. Evgeni Velkover, Head, Dept. Neuro., &, Dr. Fyodor Romashov, Patrice Lumumba U., Moscow.	(?). (Bernard Jenson, DC, ND, The Science & Practice of Iridology.)

TABLE of CONTENTS for RELATED ESSAYS:

* * * * * * * * * * * * *

*Note: Not a word in this book is intended to offend anyone; if it is inferred by the Reader, it is not implied by this Author/ Editor; who sends you Peace, Love, & Cheer.

* * * * * * * * * * * * *

RELATED ESSAYS:
RE.1 FACTORS in NUTRITION, (OUTLINE):

(For children 0 - 200 years. Object: You list these in order of importance:)

Additives (including "intentional" &"incidental" poisons), (exemptions from labelling)
Subtractives (e.g. refining), (white: sugar, flour, rice, salt, "lightning")
Changes (of temperature & pressure, e.g. state of matter)

Natural vs. Synthetic

Pleasure ?/? Stress see saw, cause/effect cycle
Stress;
Environmental (e.g. Pollution)
Emotional (causes poor digestion, or good!)...(boredom, habit)
Exercise (aids digestion, e.g. g.i. tract smooth muscle tone)
Lifestyle (~~smoke~~, ~~drink~~, ~~coffee~~ (nah! Mine is OK, yours isn't!)), Sex
Weather;

Inertia to change habits

Social
Economic
Political
Cultural
Personal
Familial (Family, Friends, & Relatives)

Variety (for emotional/nutrient needs & to prevent food allergies (Rotary Diet))
but vs. Mono Diet (to eat one species (e.g. grapes) per meal/day/month)

Nutrients
Micro-Nutrients
Vitamins
Minerals
Enzymes
Macro-Nutrients
Carbohydrates
Sugars
Starches
Fats
Protein

Water
Farming
Cooking (dilute out water soluble nutrients; change structure by heat)
Drinking (dilutes digestive juices; hot hurts gastro-intestinal lining, cold slows digestion)

Air (e.g. don't farm near an expressway)

Sunshine (full spectrum, over body; (e.g. helps body absorb minerals, & Vitamin D use))

Nutrition as:
Prevention
Detection (needs increase with disease, e.g. tolerate more synthetic Vit. C before diarrhea; monitor early signs, e.g. disease of teeth, gums, skin, hair, energy)
Therapy

Price to consumer
  Long term (savings on prevention...)
  Short term (energy loss, need extra hours of sleep, sick days, hospitalization)
  Seasonal (surplus / shortage)
  Monopolies
  Middlemen

Food Staple Commodities vs. Herbs & Spices vs. Food Supplements (price, concentration)

Genetic Strain of food (Inbred / Hybrid)

Biochemical Individuality of consumer (ancestral genes adapted to geography; biochemical lesions; alternate metabolic pathways; genetic requirements; susceptibility at conception, pregnancy)

Balance
  Yin - Yang (expand - contract) of Macro-biotics (e.g. fruits vs. root vegetables)
  Ratios of nutrients
  pH (net effect on whole body after digestion)

Raw vs. Cooked (damage to nutrients by cooking vs. ease of assimilation if cooked?) (enzymes damaged at 110°F approx.)

Vegetarianism vs. Lacto-Ovo- Vegetarianism vs. Omnivore (animal products cause mucous barrier to absorption of nutrients), ... Fruitarianism, Breatharianism

Eat Low on Protein Chain (eat plants over fish over fowl over cattle; less expense & pollutants; easier to digest & metabolize)

Food Combining (foods can help or hurt digestion of other foods; pH & reaction times in g.i. tract)

Synergism vs. Antagonism (of one nutrient aiding or blocking another nutrient)

Chrono-biology (organism is affected by time (of eating))
  Day (wet foods in morning, dry at night) (no high protein before bedtime: hard to digest)
  Month (Calcium rich foods for pre-menstrual syndrome)
  Year (fruits in summer, roots in winter)
  Eat when hungry (for availability of digestive juices)

Digestion
  Chewing (enzymes in saliva for carbohydrates; increased surface reaction area)
  Digestive Juices (of body) (decreased with age, emotional upset)
  Motility (tone of smooth muscles of g.i. tract affects transit time; as does food's enzymes, fiber, fluidity, warmth,& seasoning, speed digestion)

Bulk / Fiber
  Transit Time through colon is decreased,(so less build-up of toxic by-products of bugs in intestines)
  Dilutes toxic liver bile
  Many other benefits

Micro - Organisms (bugs, microbes) & their By-Products of metabolism, in:
  Intestines
    good bugs (provide host with the by-products of: B Vitamins, Vitamin K)
    bad bugs (poison host)
  Food
    good bugs make food richer in vitamins (yogurt), minerals, enzymes
    bad bugs cause food allergies (chocolate)

Hygiene / Good Manufacturing Practice
  Animal Contamination (worms, eggs, excrement)
  Botulism, Salmonella, ...

Bio-Physics-Chemistry
Atomic
Biological Transmutations, from one element to another, by a natural occuring nuclear reaction within the cell (whose structure concentrates stellar energy onto a target nucleus)
Molecular Isomers (unnatural replaces natural ineffectively)
Cis- vs. Trans- (group of atoms on same or opposite side of molecule)
Levo- vs. Dextro- (left or right handed spiral of atoms in molecule)
Secondary or Tertiary Superstructure (relating one molecule to another, by inter-molecular forces (e.g. hydrogen bond), in colloid, membrane transport, DNA)

Consumer Choice as Vote for Allocation of Resources to a cost center or system
World Hunger (exported commercial cash crops displace indigenous staples of peasants)
Poverty (processing, transport, & distribution increase profits to middle-man compared to farmer) (unions)
Grow your own (in winter: sprouts, hydroponics)
Soil
Synthetic
Pesticide (damages human cells too), (collects in seeds: peanuts crop rotated with cotton)
Fertilizer (plants form their Vitamins from Trace Minerals absorbed, NPK fertilizer causes depletion of other minerals)
Depletion of minerals due to erosion from poor farming practices (desertification from loss of root system that holds moisture)
Allelopathy (plant/species secretes selective biocide (to prevent crowding by others)).
Anti-nutrients
Phytates (in bread, prevent absorbtion of zinc)
Avidin (in egg white, causes depletion of biotin, a B Vitamin)
Starch blockers (in legumes), trypsin inhibitors (in soybeans)
Goiterogens
Pleasure of Eating (color arrangement, aroma, taste, texture) aids digestion
"Full stomach" "security" vs. indigestion of over-eating; Moderation

Young, Live foods to eat
Sprouts (increase Vitamin content many-fold)
Raw, fertilized eggs

Species of food particularly useful, for a certain nutritional goal, usually work in many pathways towards that goal (pineapples have both Vitamin A & enzymes to fight cancer)

Fasting
Organs shift from digestion to cleansing & repairing body
Breaking a Fast
Start with wet cleansing fruits (oranges, grapes); then cooked starchless vegetables (spinach);
Never start with: starchy (potatoes), very sugary (dates), flesh foods (meat)
Variations in nutrient content, within a species of food (due to its genetic strain, agriculture (soil minerals), processing)
MDR's, RDA's, Megadoses; Deficiency, Toxicity; (protective nutrient co-factors; population subgroups)
You are what you eat, digest, absorb, assimilate, metabolize, excrete.
Mind (regulates bodyweight; thinking / worry increases need for B Vitamins; vice-versa)
Hunger (eat only when hungry; finish meal while still hungry; mind over matter)
Fresh vs. Stale (rancid; vitamin loss)(inventory control)
Labels (definitions ("Organic" ... "Natural")

RE.2 DRINKING WATER DISTILLER EVALUATION:

April 6, 1980

The Honorable Douglas M. Costle
Administrator, Environmental Protection Agency
401 "M" St., N.W.
Wash., D.C. 20460

Dear Mr. Costle:

To minimize controversy and maximize benefit in environmental quality is understandably worth implementing. Since the resistance to cleaning all the water in our environment is hampering that effort immensely, on an interim basis the EPA should place a greater priority on cleaning water intended for drinking only. Presently the EPA has no program for this at the user (drinker's) end of the water cycle. Drinking water needs to be of the highest quality, and attaining that purity need not be hampered by the difficulties in water quality for other, larger scale, uses. The EPA needs to evaluate the various, best commercial means available to economically clean water for drinking exclusively, and publish reports, readily available to the consumer. These activities will only enhance other water quality efforts, necessary for our food chain, ecology, etc. This evaluation of commercial products would be within the scope of present EPA activities, considering the EPA evaluation of automobiles in the "Gas Mileage Guide".

Many doctors recommend pure water in both prevention and cure of chronic degenerative disease. Drinking purified water, with minerals mostly removed from it, can "sponge" or "erode" beneficial as well as harmful minerals out of the body. Thus, biologically active beneficial minerals are added back in.

Specifically, there are presently commercially available family size water purifiers whose test results indicate significant improvements in water quality. Laboratory analysis are submitted to the EPA herein. For the Distiller, note the decrease of TCE (tetra-chloro-ethylene) from 2103 ppb (parts per billion) (at the tap), down to 2 ppb (at $42^{\circ}C$ distillate). Also, note the decrease in chloroform from 110 ppb (at the tap) down to 1 ppb (at $80^{\circ}C$ distillate). Distillers consume much energy, most operating on electricity, some on solar heat. The container meterial in contact with the purified fluid should be non-contaminating (e.g. stainless steel, some glasses). For the Reverse Osmosis-Charcoal Filter unit, note the decrease in total solids from 342 ppm (parts per million) (at the tap), down to 3 ppm (after filtration). Some ion-exchange resins for reverse osmosis are made of bis-chloro-methyl-ether, itself a carcinogen. Traces of this are then to be removed by filtration of the water through activated charcoal, boiling, and aerating in the sun.

You are welcome to contact me for any further information on this. Your efforts are greatly appreciated.

Respectfully yours,

Ralph R. Hovnanian

RE.3 LOW AIR POLLUTION, HIGH MPG AUTO:

Auto - erotic Car - toons
by
a Rehabilitated Bureaucrat

Please don't take this or any other story as gospel, but investigate for yourself, using sufficient independent sources of proper motivation, from various places & times. My current opinions, biased (?), are based on these:

General Surveys:

(1) Gasolene Crisis Answers, by James "Ambassador" Jackson, (available from: NCDA (National Car Drivers Assoc.), POBox 1111, Tacoma, WA 98401);
(2) NCDA Report, & "Sixteen Myths of the Oil Crisis", (from NCDA);
(3) Suppressed & Incredible Inventions, by John Freeman, Ch.1 & 2, (from: Fry's, 22511 Markham, Perris, CA 92370; & Health Research, POBox 70, or 8349, or or 70 Lafayette St., Mokelumne Hill, CA 95245);
(4) The Spotlight, dozens of issues, (from Liberty Lobby, 300 Independence Ave., S.E., Wash., DC 20003);
(5) Newsreal, n.2, "Suppressed Inventions", & National Exchange; by Tom Valentine;

Specific Details:

(6) NEWsletter, v.1, n.1, May 1982, (from New Energy World, 14411 Vanowen St., Suite 102, Van Nuys, CA 91405);
(7) Suppressed Inventions, &, Brown's Alcohol Motor Fuel Cookbook, both by Michael H. Brown, (POBox 89, Draper, Utah 84020).

Informal conversations on others' experiences have added to these & many other documents.

There is widespread belief, among those who care for the environment, that very energy efficient, over 200mpg, gasolene powered, safe, non-polluting, autos will require at least 5-10 years before full scale production. This belief is a close relative of the dogma that we are still not sure that a certain carcinogen causes cancer & we must wait for more research. Leading to "paralysis by analysis", it is the main argument forwarded by those who quarterly, as their duty would have it, empathize for profits, for lack of loftier loves. It is used successfully & frequently by auto & oil cos., banks, press, & govt., interlocked via board memberships, loans, ads, & taxes. It is no stranger to "They are taking care of it!", & "Leave it to the experts!".

History is full of long lag times, between when an invention or discovery was initially made, & when it was accepted. In this century alone, the press in general refused to witness the Wright brothers for 5 years after their first flight. There is no evidence that the situation has changed.

Many, very efficient & clean energy, auto inventions are gathering dust. Example, illustrative: By allegedly only putting a different carbureter on some gas guzzler autos of the 1930's, 200mpg was attained, using gasolene processing of that era. This (Pogue) carbureter worked by channelling by-product heat from the engine, to evaporate all gasolene going through the carbureter. Fully evaporated gasolene burns totally (approx. 80% burnt in Pogue), while a mist burns only on the surface of the tiny liquid droplets (approx. 10-20% burnt in "modern" cars). This patented carbureter gave a 5-10 fold increase in mpg, & so, a 5-10 fold decrease in toxics (pollution) per mile (tpm).

I used the above example because it has been heavily advertised in "mass media" magazines since 1982. I'm sorry that I'm no longer surprised that I haven't seen news reports or editorials on it, in mainstream "mass media".

Certainly, there are hoaxes; some very crafty & cruel. But while dwelling on on these, auto journalists, proud recipients of new cars from Detroit yearly, neglect to remind their readers that all we need is one innovative, workable system, amongst the many claims.

Automakers have for so long been reciting the refrain, that such high mileage is un-feasible, that they now sincerely believe it. Can we expect the unexpected?

The most important criteria in evaluating an invention, is not how or why, but whether, it works. Verifying whether it works includes: first hand observation, interviewing witnesses, historical documentation, etc., weighed against any ulterior motives, hidden devices, sleight of hand, etc., or honest mistakes, zealous bias, etc. Many innovators have no formal training (& so are daring to attempt the "impossible" to the trained);their rustic explanation of the "how" or "why" might seem at first contradictory to the laws of nature as we know them; nevertheless, these apparent disparities may be resolved, as history has shown.

So, here is an opportunity, for academic, sophisticated, naturalists & environmentalists to talk & work with individualistic, self-taught, "seat-of-the-pants", engineers & inventors.

One needs no interest or personal experience in any of this, except the following. By full scale production of safe, 200mpg, gasolene cars in one year, the US can soothe its woes in:

(1) Energy;
(2) Environmental Pollution (50% of urban air pollution from vehicles; ... forests & coastlines scarred by oil drilling...);
(3) Health Care (respiratory & (w)holistic costs of air pollution, well over $25 billion/year (early 1970's EPA estimate));
(4) Balance of Payments (deficit import of oil at $70-100 billion/year);
(5) Unemployment (auto / supply / steel industry hiring & ripple effect);
(6) Inflation (lowered by higher hirings, & lesser imports of high mpg autos & oil);
(7) Nuclear War (over Persian Gulf oil).

A nation does not have to decline if it "resorts" (back) to a democracy; a plausible, God-respecting resort. (Time to take a "think break"!!)

Do we have the resolve? We don't need long lead times for R&D. All we need is tooling up for manufacture of a few new parts. Instead of re-tooling, for the 40-50mpg auto, by the mid-'80's target, the US should aim for the 200mpg auto by then. Otherwise, we will be left behind once again by foreign competition, & this time we might not recover.

Furthermore, we don't need to trade off safety for energy efficiency. (Accidents in smaller cars cause three times as much morbidity & mortality.) The NHTSA (National Highway Traffic & Safety Administration) has developed an energy & environmentally efficient ESV (Experimental Safety Vehicle) with Minicars, Inc.of Goleta, CA. This car is relatively "crashworthy", with "passenger compartment integrity", & "passenger restraints". (But, ironically, it is flammable. Proof that "Specialization is for Insects!".)

Yet another example: Hydrogen cracked from water by electricity from solar cells is stored under (low) pressure as a NON-flammable liquid hydride; (consider airplane, auto, lawn mower safety). By an inexpensive modification of the carbureter, the liquid hydride is converted to hydrogen gas just before entering the engine. The by-product of combustion (in the exhaust) is simply water (H_2O)! Clean! .... Hmmm! Warrants close SEC scrutiny!

One closing example, with hundreds more you can look up: Dr. W.D.Guentzler, Prof., Power Tech., San Diego State U., has used "off-the-shelf", commercially available parts, to modify a 1972 MG Midget. It now gets 106mpg, city driving, on diesel gas, bought in Mexico at 19¢ a gallon. I have only seen him on one TV show, That's Incredible, or is it?

Still, the lack of "mass media" attention.... Is it relinquishing its responsibility to inform the electorate, in exchange for its "Freedom of the Press"? Is it "guilty by omission" in its "tacit consent" of a "conspiracy of silence", the "Green($)Curtain"? Can it afford to "ruffle the feathers" or "step on the hoofs" of auto & oil advertisers, loaning banks, board members, parent companies, ...? Would its public audience appreciate the risks taken by the "mass media" to inform?

Understand, the top oil company had annual sales of over $100 billion (not million) in 1982. (Compare to $40 million to fund a US Presidential campaign.) Yet, 74% of the price of crude oil drilled in Alaska, at entry to the refinery, is for federal & state tax. And, admirers of the California coast might be relieved that tests show there is more oil around Duck & Gull Island (near Alaska's Prudhoe Bay), than in all of Saudi Arabia.

By shunning technological innovation, the finance, sales, & marketing leaders of large corporations avert yielding turf to upstart engineers & firms. But, auto-oil executives can learn from the union of medical professionals that fought bitterly against socialized medicine, only to profit immensely by its advent. Instead of "squabbling over deck chairs on the Titanic", or competing over a bigger portion of the economic pie, let's cooperate to bake a bigger pie.

RE.4 HEALTH, POLITICS, FOOD, (an OVERVIEW, CONDENSED & ABRIDGED):

CANCER, POLITICS, FOOD: THE HIDDEN VIETNAM

Cancer: 2/5 million manslaughters (negligence) in U.S. yearly. Patients swept by medical mysticism, rely on "closed shop" (unionized) doctor. Doctors rely on medical schools, colleagues' experiments, journals, and corporate salesman.

"Modern medicine" is allopathy, treating symptoms, not underlying systemic causes. Allopathy's dominance is from historical power alliances. Prevention and other therapies (naturopathy, herbalism, homeopathy, spiritualism,cosmic energies, etc.) are less harmful and more effective, yet neglected because unprofitable.

Of medical schools, only 1/10 teach nutrition, a result of the foundation sponsored Flexner report promoting drug research. Foundations are influenced by owners' interests.

Medical schools discourage poor from entering. Doctors' views of "female problems", mastectomy and hysterectomy, is sexist. These, tonsillectomies,& appendectomies, are well known abuses; but, consider also that other organ transplants or removals, amputations, arterial (coronary, brain) bypasses, artificial organs, are unnecessary with less "heroic" treatments. Yet, over half of deaths from car accident abdominal injuries are from improper emergency room diagnosis and treatment.

Surgery aside, 1/5 of teaching hospital patients are harmed during "health care", relating to diagnosis, drugs, or malnutrition. This remains uncorrected by the "malpractice crisis", artificially created by malpractice insurance companies and also benefiting lawyers and "expert witnesses". Rather, most infectious diseases have been eliminated by public health / environmental prevention.

Experiments are funded & controlled by NCI & FDA. NCI contracted chemical companies delaying finding chemicals causing cancer. NCI claims cure of cancer is unknown, necessitating increased research funding, diverted into radiation & drug development for industry, boycotting known preventions & cures.

Medical journals controlled by editors, ACS, PMA, AMA. Editors would ignore a Lister or Harvey; history repeats. ACS's Board has conflicts of interests, using donations for propaganda. AMA controlled by AMPAC, and investment/advertisement ties to profit oriented health care corporations.

Corporate salesman influence isolated, rural doctors. Corporations fund studies on their products, flooding medical journals.

FDA management dominated by segments of industry it "controls". The FDA requires $50-80 million in red tape to "approve" a new drug; only big firms can afford this, with each new drug costing less, due to savings from duplication. FDA maintains strict food standards unrelated to health,but partial to large corporations. Occasionally public "protection" is a result of a disaster, but usually of competition between rival food factions (sugar vs. artificial sweeteners, butter vs. margarine, wheat vs. fish meal, etc.) having no monopoly agreements. When a vertical monopoly's food subsidiary is competing with a small independent food firm, the monopoly's affiliates stop selling raw materials or maintenance parts to that independent firm, ignored by government. Lobbying and campaign contributions also buy exemptions from regulation (tobacco pesticides, including arsenic), labelling (dairy products- ice cream contains automobile antifreeze, lice killer),etc.

Agribusiness is monopolizing and centralizing. Longer transportation and "variety" inventory requires longer shelf life. So, food is embalmed, refined,and devitalized. To lower costs, food is grown synthetically, and its inferiority is masked; to raise prices, "junk foods" are invented.

Agribusiness dominates land grant universities, NAS/NRC, and USDA research studies, standards, or enforcements on food. Its advertising pressures a mass media blackout on criticism. Agribusiness spends only 12 million on research, including safety of 13,000 chemicals used in food; approximately 1/10 of synthetic chemicals cause cancer; in contrast, it spends 1.4 billion on advertising. The chemical industry promotes agribusiness' avalanching dependency on synthetics, killing beneficial earthworms, multiplying resistant pests, and weakening plants to plight.

Examples of these interrelationships are too many. Here are a few. Avoid all "whites"! "Whites" and other refined foods and drinks (coffee, alcohol) "sponge" nutrients from our bodies, causing deficiencies not recognizable early by "modern" doctors. White sugar has been a major economic product of black slavery, outside the U.S. South Africa has special trade privileges for white sugar into the U.S. Both cancer and cardiovascular disease might be prevented or cured in some, by Vitamin B6, but 98% of it is lost in "whitening" bread. Cancer causing food coloring is sometimes added to disguise white bread as "brown"; or synthetic Vitamin B1 & B2 are added, increasing bodily need for Vitamin B6.

Government regulation is used by dominant corporations in a market, to eliminate smaller, innovative competitors, rather than help consumers.

The present impact in billions of dollars sales annually in the U.S.(in 1977) is: cancer-18, health care total-150, agribusiness-150, chemicals-70, remainder mainly air and water pollutors. Other industries impact, in that aluminum baking powder or pots and pans are toxic, and that glass windows, TV, and maybe electrical wiring harm bodily electromagnetic environment.

Major international bankers, institutional bankers, and foundations, by owning 5% of a large corporation's stock, control many of them. The same group profits from both causing and curing cancer. They invest/ profit from both sides elsewhere; Republicans and Democrats, Arabs and Israelis, Pakistanis and Indians, Lenin and Hitler, etc. Our social system needs more concered humanism on the inside as well as outside. Hopefully by now, we ALL realize that radioactive gold is not worth a mushroom cloud. War never determines who is right, only who is left. We can ask GOD for Heaven on Earth.

RE.5 CALL for COALITION of GROUPS for HUMANITY:

March 21, 1981

Dear Executive Officers, Editors, Board Members:

All of you are idealists, otherwise you would be making much more money working in the profit centers, considering your leadership capabilities. Each of you has made tremendous advancements in your own areas of expertise. But, if you are to compete with the "Big Interests" at the federal or state level, you need to unite in the minimum areas of consensus. You all know that knowledge is power; so you can develop this knowledge/power by using the enclosed mailing list of "Public Interest Health Groups" for: communication with each other, including sending subscriptions of periodicals, and UNITING.

To be effective in helping our Republican Democracy arrive at the best decisions on the issues, we need to be as organized as our "Big Interest" competitors, (some of whom are in a separate list attached). Diverse sources (such as Barnet & Muller, Global Reach, p.50, and several U.S. govt. requirements (10 CFR 50. RDT F2-2, & MIL 9858)), agree in placing ORGANIZATION of groups and responsibilities as the most important quality for success in top management and activities. It is in the nature of members of "underdog" groups to be individualistic, but rather than this becoming our "Achilles heel", let us be an example of how to nurture individualism in unity and organization.

Will your group coordinate a union (of public interest health groups) based on some common goals? Attached is a sample questionnaire to send them, to determine common areas of consensus. In forming a union, please beware of infiltration at the very top by undercover representatives of our competitors. This has happened to some labor unions, and a few public interest groups not directly in the enclosed list. (Perhaps forming a loose federation, with checks and balances, like our U.S.Constitution, would prevent this. Each health group would be considered a "state", and each member of such a group, as a "citizen", etc.)

To aid a willing group in expediting this union, I have sent this letter to each of 102 (public interest health) groups listed, (p.125-128; p.129, & 236-238 added later). You might offer, (in a form letter to each group), to receive and tabulate the results of the survey, add up the number of individuals represented on each issue, and present the findings to the public, press, and govt. officials, etc. Photo-copies of the enclosed list may be used as address labels for communication/subscription; and this list may also be distributed to your individual membership (via newsletter). To be included in this list are many other groups I was not familiar with.

I apologize for having to mail this letter anonymously. As an individual, immersed in alternative health science, I have no time/resources to defend against counter-measures to weaken such an effective venture as unity. So as Ben Franklin said, "Let us all hang together, or we shall surely hang apart".

A 20th Century Person

Enclosures:
1) Public Interest Health Groups (8 p.)
2) Questions to Establish...Issues...for Unity (1½ p.)
3) "Big Interest" Organizations (½ p.)

(Note: re: RE.: 3, 4, 5, 6, 12, 16. The opinions (albeit one-sided) expressed herein are merely to balance the "Centrist" mass media & medical presses' partisan perspective, which (despite their image & pretense of impartiality) are coopted by advertisers, stockholders, owners, & lenders, individual & institutional. (See Hodding Carter & Phil D., Donahue Show, CBS-TV, Feb. 5, 1985.) No personal slight, innuendo, or offense is intended. (See: "Disclaimer"s, p.2, 147; "Note", p.261.))

QUESTIONS to ESTABLISH PUBLIC INTEREST HEALTH ISSUES of COMMON INTEREST for UNITY

Name of Group:______________________________, # of Members:__________

Address, # & Street:____________________, City:__________,State:________

Zip:________, Tel:____-____-_____, Officer Signature:____________________

Would your group support the following stance:(check "yes" or "no" or leave blank)

#1 ___ ___ yes no — Shift the federal funding of research, development, & other studies, from Universities (/Institutions) "accreditated" (/controlled) by "Big Interests", to funding independent public interest health groups, without "red tape".

#2 ___ ___ yes no — Restore "Freedom of Choice in Health/Medicine": diagnosis/therapy shall not be banned because of disagreement on its effectiveness (e.g. there are dozens of proven cancer therapies, banned from use, that are more effective, less harmful , and 80% less expensive).

#3 ___ ___ yes no — Stop all tobacco growing subsidies and advertisement tax deductions.

#4 ___ ___ yes no — Stop poisonous pesticide spraying (on farm, park, home?) and replace by proven natural controls (companionate; predator; breeding cycle; physical).

#5 ___ ___ yes no — Stop over-refining and poisonous additives in food (preserve by Vit. C, freeze dry, etc. FDA presently requires some poisons, bans healthy food ads.)

#6 ___ ___ yes no — Stop poisonous pollution of air and water (air: mass-produce proven 200mpg car; water: replace chlorine by air irradiation of uv light; fluorine is the only element more electro-negative than oxygen and replaces oxygen in body).

#7 ___ ___ yes no — Require auto co.s receiving public loans to mass produce 200mpg, non-polluting, much safer cars, based on proven technologies presently repressed.

#8 ___ ___ yes no — Stop arms race (laser, satellite, nuclear, chemical, biological, conventional) globally by negotiations and real guarantees (e.g. unannounced open site visits).

#9 ___ ___ yes no — Stop spread of nuclear technology globally (immediately; it may already be too late. Discourage sales by other nuclear countries to unstable 3rd world.)

#10 ___ ___ yes no — Prevent possibility of accidental nuclear war (by personnel, computer malfunction. False alarms on Nov. 9,'79, June 3&6,'80, had our jets scrambling for nuclear attack. See US Gen'l Acctg. Off., LCD-80-22.)

#11 ___ ___ yes no — Give natural birth control training to the overpopulated parts of the world. (e.g. Recognize infertile part of ovulation cycle, starting 4th day after end of wet mucous period, and ending at menstruating.)

#12 ___ ___ yes no — Stop tax incentives and govt. aid to multi-national agribusiness' replacing of 3rd world subsistence farming with cash crops for the rich;(worsens hunger).

#13 ___ ___ yes no — Give surplus food to starving people effectively;(prompt, nutritious).

#14 ___ ___ yes no — Stop monopoly control of TV air waves, originally owned by the public, with an alternative (e.g. lottery) to allocate air time democratically.

#15 ___ ___ yes no — Prevent crime by proper nutrition;(food allergy: nutrition deficiency; heavy metal poisoning removed by nutrition, bathing, and exercise).

#16 ___ ___ yes no — Prevent crime by restitution to the victim by the criminal.

(Cont'd next page)

QUESTIONS to...ISSUES...for UNITY (cont'd)

#17 ___ ___ yes no — Prevent crime by legalization of narcotics to certified users surrendering certain societal priveleges and responsibilities (e.g. driving, gun possession, insurance coverage for mental care. Ends need of crime to raise money for drugs : expensive (& profitable to supply monopoly) since illegal.

#18 ___ ___ yes no — Simplify laws to help those not wanting to wallow in jargon-ese rationalizations of decisions based on emotions, politics, and economics.

#19 ___ ___ yes no — Protect animals, endangered species, marine mammals (some whales have brains bigger than humans'; not due to body size, since dinosaurs'was nut sized);... elephants (anti-inflationary tusks).

#20 ___ ___ yes no — Recycle garbage/sewage, free of toxic pollutants.

#21 ___ ___ yes no — Eliminate fraud, error, and waste in government spending (federally, 34 (to 71) billion $'s, annually, per USGAO (of Congress) in Chicago Tribune, Jan. 18, 1981).

#22 ___ ___ yes no — Stop all foreign aid to oppressive, despotic, dictatorships, that practice violence & torture.

"BIG INTEREST" ORGANIZATIONS: Examples of Sometimes Competitors to Public Interest Health Groups; (nothing personal, friends, sorry for stereotyping).

Medicine:
- AMA(Amer. Medical Assoc.)
- AHA(" Hospital ")
- ADA(" Dental " or
- " Dietetic ")
- ACS(Amer. Cancer Soc. or
- " College of Surgeons)
- PMA(Pharmaceutical Mfr. Assoc.)
- Blue Cross/Shield

Agribusiness:
- Baltic Exchange
- GMA(Grocery Mfr. of Amer.)
- NAFC(National Assoc. of Food Chains)
- NCA(National Canners Assoc.)
- AFBF(Amer. Farm Bureau Fed.)
- Tobacco Inst.
- Amer. Meat "
- Nutrition Found.
- Sugar Info. "
- " Research "
- Fertilizer Inst.
- Cereal "

Energy:
- API(Amer. Petroleum Inst.)
- AMA(Automobile Mfr. Assoc.)
- Edison Electric Inst.
- ANS(Amer. Nuclear Soc.)

Industry:
- NAM(National Assoc. of Mfr.)
- Chamber of Commerce
- Business Roundtable

Law:
- ABA(Amer. Bar Assoc.)

Finance:
- CFR(Council on Foreign Relations)
- Trilateral Commission

Mass Media:
- NAB(National Assoc. of Broadcasters)
- AAAA(Amer. Assoc. of Advertising Agencies)

RE.6 (W)HOLISM for MASS MEDIA CENTRISM:

Medical Dark Ages
Circa 1984

Dear CEO of TV Programming; or Movie Producing; or News Reporting:

Democracy only works if the public is informed. TV has become our major teacher, the average US household having it turned "on" on the average for 40 hours per week, & only 1% of the public doing serious reading outside jobs or school. Yet, the major commercial networks have been coopted by advertizers working thru associations (AMA, GMA, NAM, etc.). Grants are used to control public TV also. So, the democratic responsibility rest on the shoulders of the few truly ethical leaders left in this "Brave New World"; leaders who value the health & "General Welfare" of American taxpayers, citizens, voters, workers, & audience, more than the vested interests (of the mis-allocators of concentrated capital as a vote for what is to be produced).

Alternative therapies, as a whole, are more effective, with much fewer "side effects", & approx. 80% less costly, than the dogmatic, high technology practices. Certainly, your advertising corporations, would prefer to pay only 20% of what they now do for employee health insurance. Why should corporate management subsidize the "closed shop" medical union, or pass on the expense as reduced real wages, unemployment, inflation (of consumer prices), & smaller stock dividends.

Will you rent & show the BBC documentary, "Go Climb a Mountain", (produced by Gordon Thomas, &), aired in England, (on Nov. 3, 1980), to a near record 14 million viewers?

Will you make a (made for TV) movie on the orphan of a book, You Don't Have to Die, by Harry Hoxsey? The narrative of this colorful autobiography, & its dialogue, lend themselves directly into a box-office attraction. The setting starts at the turn of century (ours, silly!), quite rural, of nostalgic popularity now. The theme, "Individual vs. Bureaucracy & The State", is almost Kafka-esque, or Orwellian. An attractively novel & personally involving arena for that theme, is its play on Medical Freedom. The autobiographer's attempts at curing (cancer) with an effective, non-toxic, & in-expensive mode are juxtaposed to a full spectrum of responses from the Medical Establishment. If it were only viewed as a documentary, the present concern with the sky rocketing expenses of "medical care", & the renewed interest in wholistic, non-aggressive therapy would guarantee its success. But, with its flashbacks, American heartland locale, family inheritances (of secrets) & betrayals, prison, & winning against great odds, it compares with: The Rievers; The Heartland; Chariots of Fire; Flashdance; Rocky; The Verdict; Injustice for All; The Hospital; ...Cookoo's Nest; Papillon; Ghandi; Reds; 1984;..., & bread & butter serials: Quincy; Medical Story;...; many great others. Too, the copyright has expired.

More remarkably: $12 billion per year (1981) is spent on TV ads on the premise that TV affects behavior, but we insist that the violence (& medicine...) in the programs between the ads has no influence on actions, let alone thoughts.

Is it healthy for a democracy, that Star Wars (defense) was reported by Randall Operation Survival (Oct. 1977; Oceanside, CA), & by Free for All (Dec. 7, 1977; Madison, WI), 3 years before the mass media disclosed it to the pampered public (BBC World;...; Time, Sept. 15, 1980)?

We are ready to obey, to be drafted to kill or die (in true bravery) for our country, but not to think freely, to live & love for it, our best hope for world freedom.

Sincerely,

Dismayed at the
"Green($)Curtain"

RE.7 <u>LAG</u> <u>in</u> <u>HIGH</u> <u>TECH</u>, (<u>KEYBOARD</u>):

Jan. 1984

Dear CEO of Typewriter / Computer Keyboard Company:

Cheers. Can you imagine the sales potential of a keyboard (for typewriting, or manual input to computers), whose letters are in alphabetical sequence, rather than the scrambled gibberish in vogue? The scrambled keyboard's utility is obsolete, since it was originally designed for mechanical typewriters. It was based on negative human engineering, to slow down a typist, from the speedier straight alphabetical keyboard, so the typist would not jam the mechanical keys. This, a far cry from the micro-second response of electronic keyboards, that we have had for decades; after decades... we finally have software to convert a keyboard, at unwarranted complexity & expense.

Here is highly visible & simply verifiable evidence to the white collar worker, of lag time in applying innovation, & rebuts the dogma that "If it is so good, we would be using it!". Witness that the most frequently used letter of our alphabet, "e", is not on the home row; nor are "o" & "i". Also, to type the the very common sequence, "ed", the past tense, etc., the same finger is used. This is slower than alternate fingers, which in turn is slower than fingers of alternate hands. Moreover, in manual typewriters, the most used letters were for our strongest fingers. But strength is not needed for electronic keyboards, where the limiting human factor is mental / nerveous ability, which can be greatly aided by a simpler layout of the letters. (Today, no one would venture to scramble the numbers, would they?)

Learning a keyboard for the first time, adults as well as children will appreciate the ease of your alphabetic, "user friendly" system, with no confusing "negative transfer" from the alphabet, one of the first inventions of civilization, to the wanton scrambled keyboard. Children weaned on your keyboard at school (a vast potential market), also adult beginners, will develop a "brand loyalty" in their later purchases. You can help the beleaguered user / consumer, while expanding your market (shares).

Ads targeted to feminist customers can sell your company as exposing a myth: the myth of male designer / engineers evaluating female job applicants on their typing speed, as if that only depended on the typist.

Sincerely,

Ralph Hovnanian

Ref.: (1) <u>Portable Computer</u>, Nov. 1983, p.52.
(2) <u>Personal Computing</u>, Jan. 1984, p.262.

RE.8 <u>RE-CYCLE PRODUCTS</u> <u>from</u> <u>ANIMALS</u> <u>KILLED</u> <u>by</u> <u>MOTORISTS</u>:

An open letter to the Honourable Hunters, Trappers, Fur Traders, Tanners:

Just by recycling the furs of millions of unfortunate animals accidentally killed by autos, large sectors of the fur industry would flourish without intentional slaughtering. A national toll-free hotline could help coordinate the collection of carcasses off roadsites by local public or private groups, & the shipment of these various carcasses to specialized furriers & tanners nationally. Its label would say that the final fur / hide product was made from animals killed only by real accidents or natural causes. (There would be severe, enforced penalties for fraud & abuse.) In essence, a new market would be created by expanding sales to the environmentally aware consumer. By cooperation, & novel solutions, all sides can gain!!!

Yours in good faith, ...RH.

RE.9 LAG in FAIR FEDERAL HIRING:

April 2, 1980

to: Allan K. Campbell, Director
OPM (Office of Personnel Management)
1900 "E" Street NW
Washington, D.C. 20415

Dear Mr. Campbell:

To comply with Civil Rights (Public Laws 92-261 & 93-259 and Executive Orders 11478 & 11590) in eliminating discrimination on the basis of National Origin, Age, and Sex, the application forms for Federal employment by the Agencies that utilize the OPM need revision.

The requested information that could lead to discrimination are in the application forms:

1.0 SF-171 (of Dec., 1977), requesting:

1.1 "Birthplace (...foreign country)" in Item #8.

1.2 "Birth date (Month, Day, Year)" in Item #9.

1.3 "Identify ...by...birthdate" in Instructions for Item #21.

1.4 Sex-"Preferred title...Mr., Mrs., Miss, Ms." in Item #5.

2.0 CSC Forms (of April 1978), requesting:

2.1 "Birth Date" in Form 1280, Question #11.

2.2 "Enter ... title ... Mr., Mrs., Miss, Ms." in CSC Form 1282, Form A-1 Instructions, Item #4.

There are no requests for National Origin in the CSC 1200's Forms, an improvement over SF-171.

Other Federal job application forms used by OPM, or by Federal Agencies exempt from OPM, need to be reviewed/revised for compliance with Civil Rights. Non-compliant questions, necessary for record keeping/verification, can be asked after employment. Similarly, non-compliant questions, necessary for Affirmative Action, can be optional to the applicant.

The most obvious is often overlooked , in our zeal for complexity. Even the EEOC (Equal Employment Opportunity Commission) is required to use the non-compliant SF-171.

Although we are the best country in the world, there is always room for improvement. Your continous efforts are greatly appreciated.

May I temporarily withhold my name to avoid quasi-legal, un-Constitutional harassment by several other Federal Agencies?

A Concerned Citizen

RE.10 CRITERIA for DEVELOPMENT of TECHNOLOGY:

Logistics Factors in Conceptual to Mid-Design Phase
Checklist for (Prelim.) Design Review
Technical Projects (...Biomedical Engineering...)

1. Reli-ability (Hi Rel/Redundancy/Design Out of (Safety,Mission) Critical Items; QA/QC (Quality Assurance / Quality Control))
2. Avail-ability, (Readiness)
3. Maintain-ability (Preventive/Preservation/Lubrication; Inspect/Test/ Adjust/Calibrate/Align/Service; Unscheduled/Corrective; Repair/Replace/ Overhaul; Parts (Inventory, Spare, Repair (Lowest Level), Consumables); Provision: Standard Tools; Diagnostic Fault Isolation; Test Equipment)
4. Dur-ability (Endurance)
5. Surviv-ability (Vulner-ability)
6. Safety (Passenger Compartment Integrity (, Protrusions), Crashworthiness)
7. Oper-ability
8. Train-ability, Skills (Level; Speciality)
9. Human Factors (Sensory, Reach, Fatigue, Attention, Boredom)

9.1 Access-ibility

10. Visibil-ity (from Inside Outward & vice-versa)
11. Inspect-ability, Test-ability (In-Service, Built-in Test Equipment, Fault Detection, False Alarms)

11.1 Calibration

12. Transport-ability (USA, "Foreign Nations"; Clearances; Packaging; Handling)
13. Install-ability, Deployment
14. Remove-ability (Tear-Down), Recover-ability, Restoration
15. Supply Support (Operation Consumable Supply, Long Lead Items...)
16. Support-ability (Facilities/Depot; Re-conditioning; Re-supply Time; De-bugging; Special Tools)
17. Stowage/Storage (Shelf Life, Corrosion, Stock Pile Reli-ability)
18. Design Simplicity

19.1. Compatibil-ity (Interface)
19.2. Inter Change-ability
19.3. Inter Oper-ability
19.4. Standardized: Tools
19.5 Compar-ability
19.6 Modular-ization
19.7. Strategic Material Substitutes
20.1. Labelling & Identification
20.2. Trace-ability

21. Manufactur-ability, Produce-ability (OSHA)
22. Engineering Disciplines, Coordination: (Nuclear, Bio-Medical, Chemical, (NBC); Mechanical, Aero-Nautic (Shockwaves), Civil (Gross Wt., Road Clearance), Electrical, Electronic (EMP(Electro-Magnetic Pulse)), Thermo-Dynamic, Materials, Geologic, Inter-disciplinary)

22.1 Technological Advancement Application, Innovative Concepts Identification

23. Performance, Capabil-ity, Depend-ability
24. Effectiveness, Mission (Multi-functional)
25. Modelling, (Scenario, Games, Simulation), Iteration Risks, Trade-Off, Viable Alternatives, Life Cycle, Drive Times, Thresholds, Interface, Partitioning, Baseline, Optimization, Goals)
26. Costs (Lines of Supply)
27. Time (for Failure & Repair; Critical Path (PERT))
28. Sensitivity (Secret)
29. Environment (Inter-action; Impact; Salvage-ability)

RE.11 <u>NEW CAR SELECTION AID</u> / <u>BUYING CHECKLIST</u>

This evaluation checklist is for criteria to purchase an existing auto design (make, model, year), not an "as built" specific unit (serial #), delivered to you, that may have individual idiosyncrasies in production & transport.

<u>CRITERIA</u>:

PRICE:	Basic Model:			
	Options:			
	Dealer Charges:	Prep.:		
		Ad.:		
		Surcharge:		
	Tax:			
	Transport:			
	Tariff:			
	Currency Exch. Rt.:			
	Interest Rt.:			
	Resale Value:			
MPG:	City:			
	Combined:			
	Country:			
	Trans-mission:	Auto.:		
		Manual:		
	Emission Control:	Cal.:		
		Other 49:		
	Engine:	Size:		
		Diesel:		
	Axle Ratio:			
	Tires:			
	Source:	EPA:		
		Other:		
SAFETY:	Visibil-ity:	By Driver:	Blind Spots:	
			Wind-shield: Tint:	
			Curve:	
			Glare Reflected:	
			Adjust-able: Seat:	
			Headrest:	
			Mirrors: Rear:	
			Sides:	
			Defrost.: Front:	
			Rear:	
			Controls: Panel:	
		By Other Driver:	Color: Night:	
			Snow:	
			Road:	
			Height:	
	Accident Avoid Handling:	FWD (Front Wheel Drive):		
		Rack & Pinion Steering:		
		Suspension:	Heavy Duty:	
			Independ.:	
		Roll-over:		

SAFETY: (Cont'd)	Brakes:	Independent:		
		Stop Distance, (OEM Tires),(Fade):		
Surviv-abil-ity:	Passenger Re-straints:	Effectivity:		
		Adjustability:		
		Ease of Use:	Belts:	
			Head Rest:	
			Air Bag:	
Crash-worthi-ness:		Padded:	Dash:	
			Steering Hub:	
			Roof:	
			Doors:	
		Prot-ruding:	Knobs: Door:	
			Dash:	
			Gearshift:	
			Steer.Shaft:	
	Passenger Compart-ment Integ-rity:	Front:	Engine:	
			Hood:	
		Side:	Doors:	
			Beams:	
		Roof:	Frame:	
	Vulner-ability:	Fuel:	Tank:	
			Remote Wall:	
			Filler:	
	Pedes-trian:	Gougers:	Front:	
			Side:	
		Flip up, not down:	Low Front Profile:	
	NHTSA Crash Test Results & Fatality Rates:		Driver:	
			Passenger:	
		Wind-shield:	Retention:	
			Intrusion:	
		Fuel Leak.:	Front:	
			Rear:	
	Recalls:			
	Tires, (OEM) (USDoT):	Traction:		
		Temp.:		
		Tread:		
		Puncture Material:		
		Ply:		

RELIABILITY/QUALITY:	Frequency of Repair:	Safety:	
		Mechan.:	
		Elect.:	
	Failure Effect:	Safety:	
		Performance:	
MAINTAINABILITY:	Availability:	Parts:	
		Service:	
	Dealer Record:		
	Accessibility: (Design Simplicity)	Preventive: (Tune-Up)	Dipsticks:
			Fillers:
			Filters:
			Plugs:
		Corrective:	
	Accident Repair Cost:		
INSURANCE COST:	" " "		
	Safety " :		
	Theft " :		
SPACE:	Passenger:	Driver:	Head:
			Seat:
		Other:	
	Trunk:		
	Clearance:		Entry:
			Exit:
POWER:	Torque/rpm:		
	Acceleration:		
	Hills:		
	Tow:		
PERFORMANCE:	Ride:	Noise:	
		Comfort:	Bumps:
	Handling:	Cornering:	Sway:
			Turn "0":
		Suspension:	
		Steering:	
	Availability:	Cold Start:	Battery Reserve:
			Diesel:
		Traction:	FWD
	Parking:	Clearance:	
		Visibility:	
	Visib. & Access.:	Instrument & Controls	
ENVIRONMENTAL POLLUTION:	Particulate: (Diesel)		
	Gaseous:	Other 49:	
		California:	
		MPG Inverse:	
AESTHETICS:	Status:		
	Style:		
	Color:		
	Interior:	Color: (Relaxing)	
		Material: (Out-gas)	

RE.12 <u>EPIGRAMS</u> / <u>ASIDES</u>:

Today is yesterday's "Tomorrow", & tomorrow's "Yesterday", so make it good.
- Mary Ann Kelly; Mgr., Food Serv., Dist. 65, Evanston, Ill.; RD (Registered Dietician) Intern.

Why waste dreams for only when I am asleep? (Careful!)

Meditation is easier than I think.

Rich are poor with money, poor are rich without money!?

"Ignorance of the law is no excuse", but, "He who is his own lawyer has a fool for a client"?

Mass Media: "OK boys, bring on the rape (/violence) scene."
Audience: "Monkey see, monkey do!"

Studies show, if mice see no sunlight, they prefer alcohol to water, so: "If no Sunshine, then Moonshine!".

A cartoon of a cannibal feast: Mother: "Junior, please hold your fork with your right hand, too, hold that right hand with your fork."

"God gave to you; will you give back to God?"- Mary Ann Kelly, transcont. cyclist.

<u>1984</u> was one of the first book titles I could easily read, I admit.

Look around you. Every man made thing you see was once an alternative, un-orthodox, un-proven, innovation.

Man is yet unable to communicate in another species' language, yet monkeys can communicate in man's.

Only 15% of what we learn from a new speaker is content, the rest is context (looks, tone),(per psychology). We only use 10% of our brain (per Einstein). So, 10% of 15% = 1½% = the part of our brain used for content of a new speaker. (Homoeopathic dosage?)

We reward the greedy (not needy), by conferring power to them. The process that gives the choice between "the lesser of two evils", (or of 1, in some judgeships), is the problem. We are shocked by bribery overseas, yet accept "campaign contributions". ....
- Santa Claus, Birthday Party, 1984.

RE.13 <u>MODEL MATRIX</u> for <u>NUTRIENT INTER-ACTIONS</u>:

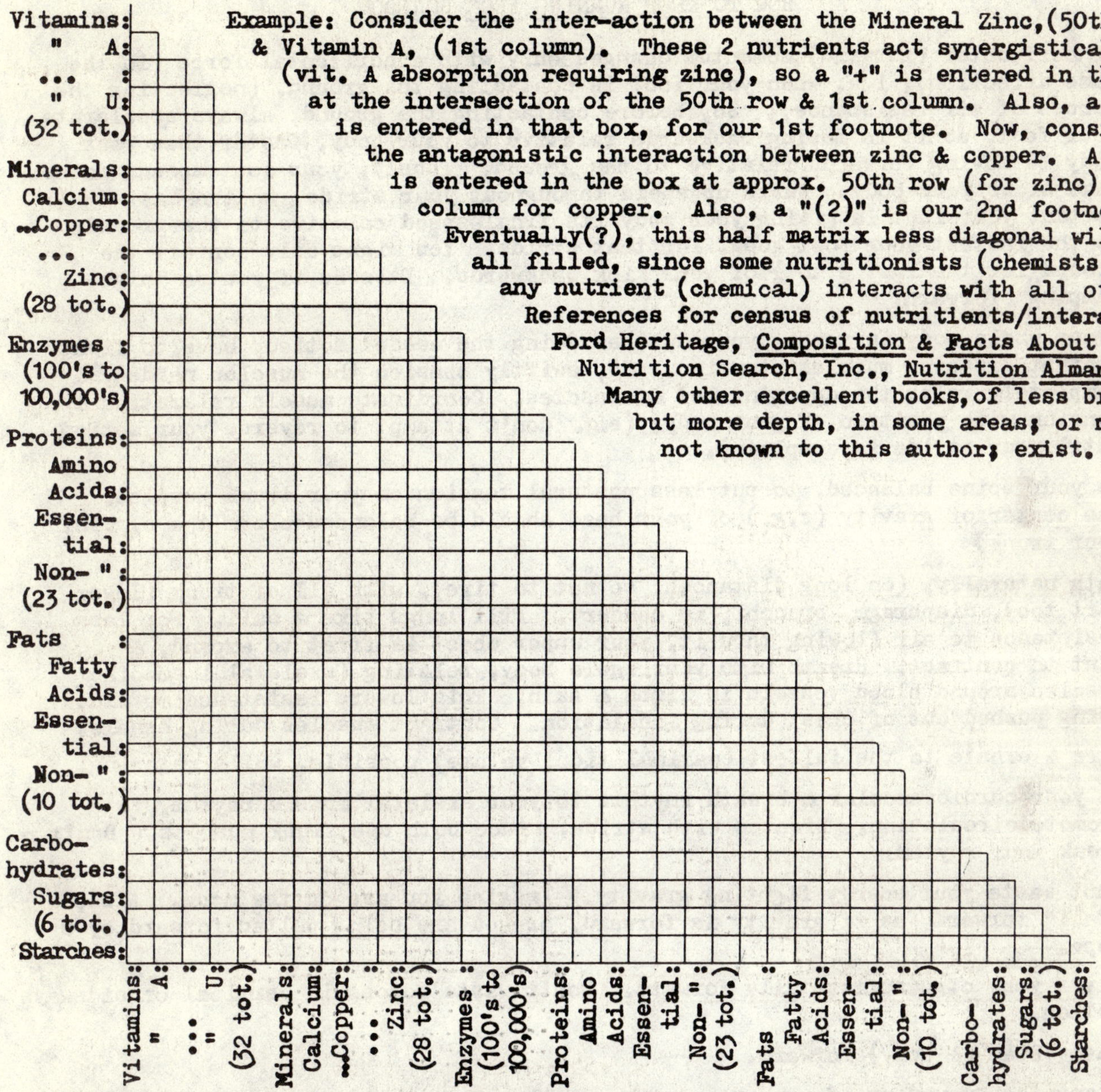

Example: Consider the inter-action between the Mineral Zinc,(50th row), & Vitamin A, (1st column). These 2 nutrients act synergistically, (vit. A absorption requiring zinc), so a "+" is entered in the box at the intersection of the 50th row & 1st column. Also, a #"(1)" is entered in that box, for our 1st footnote. Now, consider the antagonistic interaction between zinc & copper. A "-" is entered in the box at approx. 50th row (for zinc) & 30th column for copper. Also, a "(2)" is our 2nd footnote #. Eventually(?), this half matrix less diagonal will be all filled, since some nutritionists (chemists) feel any nutrient (chemical) interacts with all others. References for census of nutritients/interactions: Ford Heritage, <u>Composition & Facts About Food</u>; Nutrition Search, Inc., <u>Nutrition Almanac</u>. Many other excellent books, of less breadth, but more depth, in some areas; or mostly not known to this author; exist.

This suggested model, from matrix algebra, represents the inter-relationship between n nutrients, by a symmetrical matrix with n rows & n columns. Each element in the square matrix array represents the interaction between the nutrient in the i-th (horizontal) row & the nutrient in the j-th (vertical) column. By symmetry, only half the matrix need be drawn, (as a (isosceles right) triangle), the other half being a mirror image of it, reflecting off a diagonal. The elements comprising the diagonal can first be deleted, since they represent the (identity) interaction between the nutrient & itself. So, the number of elements sufficient, is = to: ((n x n)-n)/2. For approx. 100 nutrients, this ='s:((100 x 100)-100)/2 = 4,950 = approx. 5,000 elements in the array.

In the human body, if two nutrients i & j interact synergistically, (adding to the effect of each other), a "+" is entered in the element (box) at the intersection of the i-th row & j-th column. But, if two nutrients act antagonistically, a "-" is entered in that box. Supporting footnotes are referenced in the box in ( ).

RE.14 EXERCISE:
RE.14.1 PRINCIPLES of RUNNING:

HOW TO KEEP RUNNING FROM BOREDOM

Your horizontal (forward) momentum changes only with a horizontal force (in the same direction); i.e. when your foot is contacting the ground, (neglecting the forces of air resistance). So, before contacting the ground, always accelerate your foot, so it is moving backwards relative to your body, faster than your body is moving forwards relative to the ground. Thusly, your foot speeds rather than slows your body. Build up speed throughout your stride, so the last instant your foot is giving your body its final speed relative to the ground, is the fastest your foot goes, for that stride. You might only contact the ground for the last $\frac{1}{2}$ to $\frac{1}{4}$ of your kick backwards. It's as if you're "high jumping" forward.

If your whole body is tense, your muscles doing the needed motion, have to fight against opposing muscles' tension. So, swiftly tension the muscles needed, & completely relax the opposing set of muscles. Coordinate muscle relaxation &/ tension with position of your body; (e.g. don't attempt to reverse your motion until your stride is complete).

Keep your spine balanced, to put less postural tension on your trunk muscles. The center of gravity (c.g.) of your head should be balanced above the c.g. of your trunk.

Breath naturally, (on long distances, so not to tire), with all of trunk (lower part too), diaphragm, bronchi, in concert. Fill lungs like a sail. For less resistance to air flowing thru it, your upper chest is first to expand, & last to contract. Breath with your whole body, relaxing (skeletal & smooth) muscles around blood vessels in limbs & skin, This lowers resistance to blood being pushed out of chest during inhalation. Contract muscles during exhale.

Inhale & exhale to the fullest (maximal tidal volume) possible, while relaxing.

Link your cardiovascular & breath rhythms to your skeletal muscle rhythm, to promote circulation. Breathe with stride, since both use trunk muscles. Don't break your rhythm.

Do not waste your energy fighting gravity. Imagine you are on the moon. Also, "fall" forward, as if gravity is forward, or you are being pulled forward by a rope.

Deliver your c.g. horizontally forward. Don't waste forces in vertical or sideways motion.

Float! Head (& body) forward.

Contact the ground as if you are a rubber ball. Stretch & contract your body (leg stride) as if you are a rubber band.

Feel the flow of (muscle shake, or) longitudinal & transverse mechanical energy waves jiggling through your body, synchronize a stride for a wave, aimed for gaining distance; like a slinky (toy).

Use power of trunk muscles, especially lower back (arching spine at backwards kick) & hips (rotating, around c.g., backwards on same side as kicking leg).

Rotate your trunk around the vertical axis through your c.g. (Trunk to rotate more for distances, & arch more for sprints?)

Stay low, close to ground. (But don't fight gravity, for fear of falling.) So, lengthen stride, accordingly; & consequently, the distance over which your foot can pick up energy, for your jump forward.

Sprinting, go for longest stride with leg, foot, & toes, in that sequence, "jumping" you forward, so they are all pointed (fully extended) backward at the end of your stride(& contact with the ground). At which time too, your spine is at its maximum backward arch; & now lean spine forward & relax while floating thru air, reaching fully forward with other foot for the next kick back.

Initially contact the ground lightly, with the whole bottom of your foot, to not concentrate stresses on any part, (& for better traction). On contact, your foot points straight forward or slightly inward. Your footsteps are almost aligned in a straight line, & with a maximal stride. Always keep a light vertical contact with ground, with a harder horizontal push as the kick progresses in a stride.

Glide feet along ground to avoid wasted motion (& stresses) vertically.

Use whole body in concert, (even neck muscles, to rotate & arch trunk, by "push off" against inertia of head). If any part of body hurts, use other parts to take up load. For aching muscles, try breathing more to bring oxygen to normalize metabolism. Concentrate attention away from the pain, but use pain as a signal.

Mental: Use lower brain, as well as higher. Stay interested & excited; think fresh, not tired. Place running (balance, breath...) as much as possible on "automatic". Send messages to adrenals (above kidneys) to secrete. (Your centers of gravity & (proper) breathing are located between adrenals & navel, so don't neglect region.) Imagine just waking up, for pituitary to secrete (ACTH). Imagine tapping into the infinite energy of the universe thru the top of your head at each inhalation; the more energy you use, the more you can take in; you are as light as air; you move with the wind. So, think light, keep your body light, & it will be easier to move it. If tired, think of the present, don't think of how much more you have to run. Avoid worry; it will slow you down. Meditate on your c.g. during peak exhalation (contraction), & on the universe at peak inhalation (expansion). MEDITATE ON GOD.

Look forward: part way up the sky, for inspiration; straight ahead, for direction (vertical & lateral motions minimal); & at ground for speed, footing, & no tripping.

Imagine your body mechanics as if you are suspended by a string, only from the top of your head, like a puppet on a plumb line.

Avoid tripping, while feet glide along ground, by visual monitor, & practice. Snap back a leg imagined to be snagged, while jumping over the snag & lurching forward with the free leg, to regain balance. (To unsnag,) the direction of stride (of both legs) is immediately reversed at first feeling of a snag.

Environment: Avoid air pollution (from main roads, rush hour, specific sources). Avoid heat (from midday sun, heated ground by afternoon).

Learn from motion of fastest animals: Mammals: Snow leopard (jumps 40 feet straight up), cheetah (sprints 60mph), horse (race; only the best), greyhound (race); Birds: ostrich (45mph), hummingbird (1,000's of bpm(beats per minute); (for swimming, study sea mammals, fish).

Training: Breathing: inhale & exhale fully, rhythmically, from center of body, (as in Aikido). Weightlifting: deadlifts (to learn using lower back in kicking), & sit-ups; fast. Stretching: to lengthen stride & arch back, (as in Yoga, Karate).

Nutrition: General: Eat foods that oxygenate, vasodilate, metabolize, & are vitamin & mineral rich. Many hours before running: Eat fresh, raw, organic, whole fruits, vegetables, & herbs; nuts & seeds; legumes & grains; yoghurt; etc. (No solid food should be left in the stomach during a run.) Just before a run: Drink good water; freshly pressed fruit, vegetable, & sprout juices, chlorophyl rich; garlic, onion; bee pollen; .... Take fluids in anticipation to what you will lose in sweat; too much fluids (or food) does not leave room for deeper breathing.

Excretion: Before run, excrete urine & feces as much as possible, to make room for breathing (with whole trunk). During run, relax pores all over, for cooling sweat.

Equipment: Clothing: Hat: wide brimmed & air circulating, to prevent heat from sun, & promote air cooling. Shoes:...check for uneven wear on feet or shoes, to correct shoes or motions. Waistband: keep loose, to allow breathing. Shorts (& shirt): thin & low friction, between legs, & under arms; allow sun on more of body, to activate metabolism of minerals.

These secrets on highly competitive sports are offered in the spirit of cooperation & genuinely friendly competition, to promote world peace & love, as well as personal health.

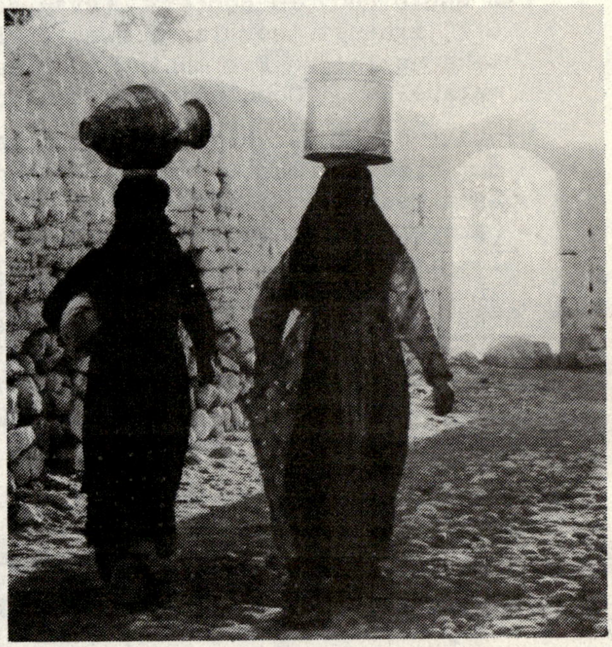

Balance:

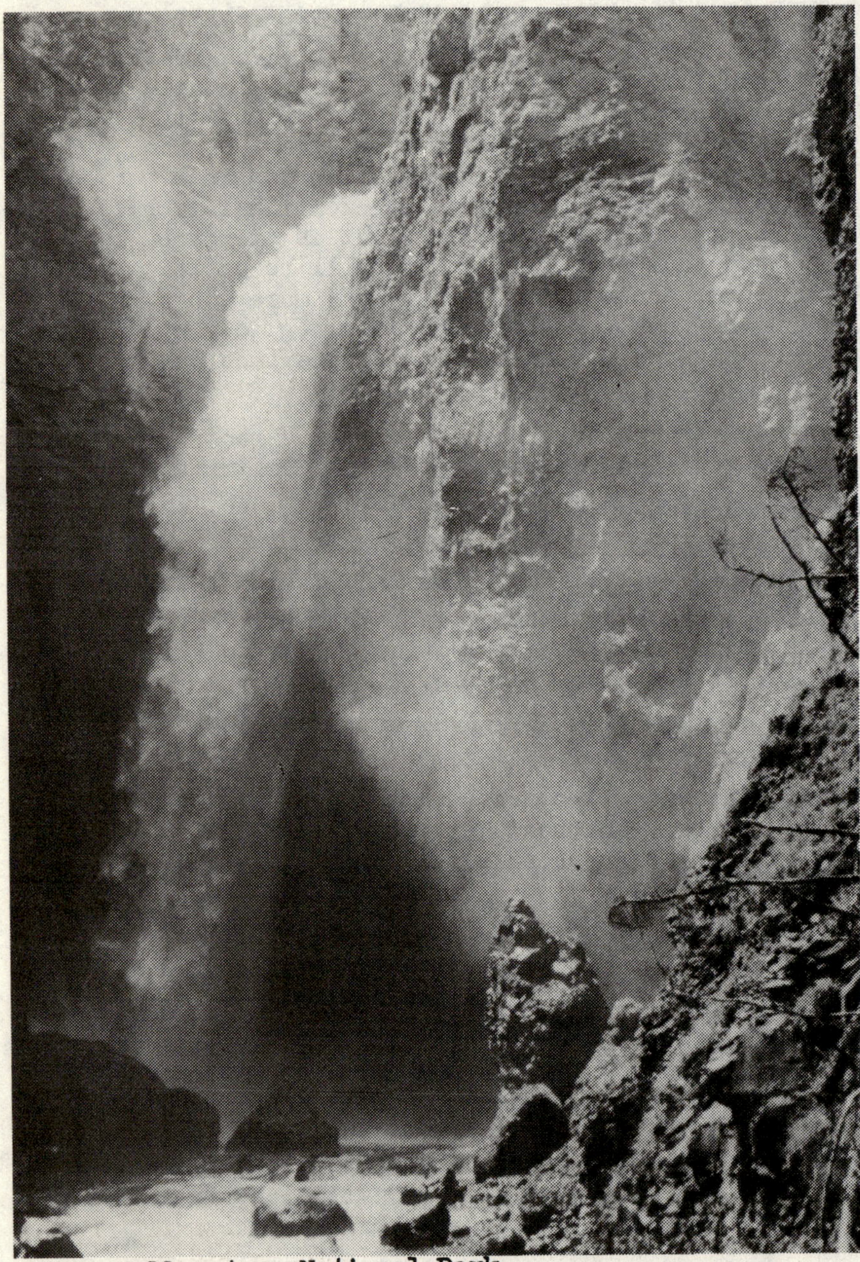

: Energy.

Momentum:

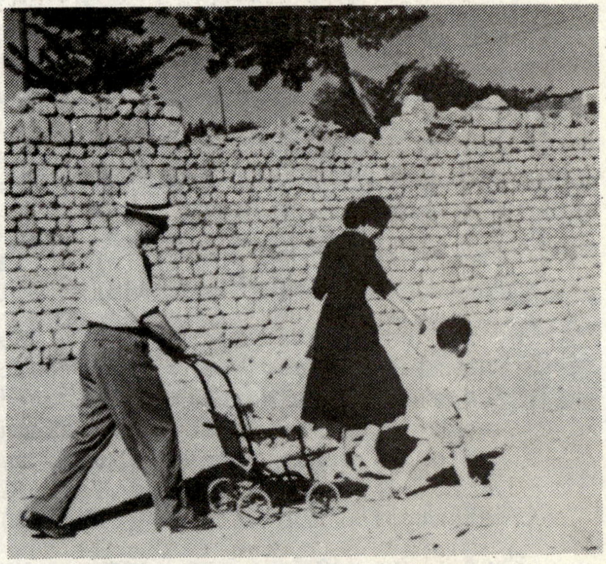

Yellowstone National Park.
Negative air ions. (Photo by R.H.)

Author (in stroller) & family.

Please do not misuse this info, or show it to anyone who would. It is submitted to women / children / potential "victims", to use in exercise, to peacefully defend themselves, to surmount the "victim" self image (indoctrinated by the mass media), & to deter a few forms of violence (supplanting an irresponsible criminal justice system).

Without any one of these basics, there is no martial arts (m. arts); concentrate on all of these general principles at the same time:

Only use m. arts as a last resort, for really good causes. Be always sure God would OK it. Never abuse the privilege of knowing m. arts.
Show your partner (who could (?) be your opponent) ways out of a fight, without hurting his ego. Point out his good qualities to him. Show he can ask his God for forgiveness, go in peace, & actively make up for his sins.
Defend yourself (& loved ones, ...) without harming partner, if you can.
Prevention: Skillfully avoid conflict as soon you recognize possibility. Avoid dangerous places & times.
Learn by: Correct Understanding, Exact Observation, Self Criticism, Practice, Discipline, Determination, Emulation (of Good Teachers), Purity of Spirit.
Keep One Point: (at your center; move your center as fast as needed; resist from your center; center your activities there).
Keep Weight Underside: (in stance, roll, focus, ...).
Extend Ki (Chi, Prana): (this Universal energy flows into your body through the top of your head, through your body center (adrenals, center of gravity), & out thru your body implements (hand, foot, elbow, knee), to inter-act with partner's energy).
Relax: (completely, yet be alert; use nerve energy to relax body).
Stay Calm: (in spirit & motion. Be good humored routinely; smile. Have no fear/ panic, or anger/enragement. Do not be disconcerted.)
Think not of distractions: (of self, time, place....) Master the instant, with empty mind, of karate, or moving zen meditation.
Concentrate in a trance of alertness in the here & now; in nothingness, to perceive partner's motion. Slow down partner's motion by your attentive perception, & speed up your motion. Think without language; it slows you. Notice how your mind can limit the speed of your body, or vice versa, & speed up your slowest.
Mind & Body connect as whole, inseparable; one helps the other; one is part of other. Act at thinking of it, just simultaneously.
Move to final position from stationary position, without thinking of continuum in between. Speed your whole motion, even beginning. Notice motions of partner immediately. On seeing attack on you in the midst of your motion, immediately defend by changing your motion midstream & moving into a new technique. Be able to stop (or change) your motion at any instant. Save time.
Having learned a mental picture of critical flashes, scenes, & positions in a technique, simultaneously (to the thought) & instantaneously do it, realizing which muscles to be used & which to relax. Snap quickly thru each position, with the least of either overlap or gap in timing between muscle groups used.
Have continuity of motion. Be consistently good.
Energy: Make & send energy to reach all of your body simultaneously. Use extra reservoirs of energy, ki. Use fullest power of all muscles contributing to a motion, keeping other, useless muscles totally relaxed. Contract useful muscles quickly & simultaneously. Largest muscles of body are to move as fast as smallest. On contacting (imaginary) target, tense all muscles (focus). Since energy, $E=\frac{1}{2}mv^2$, (=(.5)x(mass)x(velocity)x(velocity)), then one can make up in (speed) velocity, what he lacks in mass, producing more energy, for breaking target.
Momentum: (=mv, (=(mass)x(velocity), in same direction as velocity (velocity having both speed & direction). It is easier to change direction of partner's momentum, than its magnitude. Choose an energy or momentum intensive technique, depending on partner's energy or momentum.

Physiology: Large, postural, slow, (white) muscles can be made fast, (pink), & relaxed, by training. An average human has 20,000 lbs. of force in all his muscles combined. Maybe ½ of these muscles could be used simultaneously. This includes calf, thigh, hip, trunk, etc., muscles; so females can excel.

Time your cardiovascular & breathing rhythms to your muscle rhythm.

Mechanical Energy: Flow & rebound of waves through your body, is useful in going from one technique to the next. Action - reaction of opposite side of body aids motion of your implement (side of body). Whip action can be useful, sometimes.

Be flexible: (like rubber; stretch, bend, & twist; rebound, reach); feel light.

Distancing: Keep proper distance from partner. A long reach gives more distance for your body force to act (pick up speed, accelerate), creating more mechanical energy for your implement. (Energy, $E=Fd=$(Force)x(distance).) Choose the longest path for your implement, time permitting.

Center of Gravity (c.g.) of your body: Turn, twist, & bend your body around its c.g. Keep centered (when throwing partner, rolling,...). Move your body's c.g., & your implement, in straight lines, circles (in horizontal, vertical, & oblique planes), & spirals.

Balance: For non-acrobatic techniques, keep c.g. low without strain or stiffness. Keep c.g. within stable base formed by feet, except for short moments when balance can be recovered. Momentum lends balance; (rotation of gyroscope).

Stance: Keep a low stance for stability (balance), distance, & (esp. with a short partner,) visibility. Stance supports your body at contact with target / focus.

Focus: On contacting (imaginary) target, focus your energy / ki. First keep tense the muscle set used to move your body to that position, & right after, tense (& "lock") all muscles (like "rock"), to transmit shock of impact thru your feet to the hard ground, (not absorbing any shock in your body). (At other times, do not lose your energy from feet to ground.) During focus, while tensing muscles, relax head & exhale (with a "kiaii" yell), so blood pressure to brain is not too high.

Contact: Tense surface of your implement (fist, heel...), on contact with target. Contact target at right angle (perpendicular) to its surface; & towards the plumb line of the target to avoid a glancing blow, or away from the plumb line to twirl the target. For breaking, contact minimal area on target, for maximal concentration of force there. Use proper implement of your body, to not hurt self.

Breath: Exhale with relaxed, open, passages, while tensing (proper) body muscles during focus. Tense muscles protect your body, at places. (Inhale through your nose (time permitting), & exhale through your mouth. Use power from your diaphragm muscles, ki. Increase breathing before a (possible) contest, to increase your oxygen reserve. Regular breathing is best if smooth, deep, & relaxed.

Vision: Keep eyes wide open, eyeballs looking away from each other, for maximum field of vision. Face towards partner's center. Listen behind you. Do not be blinded by emotions, speed, or tricks (confusion, distraction, attack to eyes by dirt, chemicals...). Be wary of outstretched parts of your own body blocking the view of partner's body. Watch partner's eyes, to notice intent.

Technique: To be excellent in a few basic (widely applicable) techniques, is better than to be passable in many. Expect the unexpected. !@#$%¢&*()_+-=?/'". Glide feet along floor. Jump & land softly & lightly, like a cat. Keep your posture; your back is stretched (esp. on bending to balance an outstretched leg); your lower back (pelvis) is thrust forward & upward on contacting target/focus. Pivot lightly on the center of either foot. Drop your shoulders, for the larger muscles of your trunk to help your arms. Withdraw your kicking foot rapidly, to avoid its being grabbed. Maintain Stealth.

Partner: Anticipate attacks. Know partner's tactics. Respect partner's ability. The tip of the iceberg, is what one sees of others; know the movement of others' minds, that one cannot sense (see). Watch partner's eyes, for his readiness &

direction. Use m. arts at best time, distance, ..., distracting partner. Do not "tip off" partner via any defensive posture by you. Do not "telegraph" your technique from your stance; keep smiling, or a blank facial expression (& direction of eyes) revealing nothing. Watch partner's initial attack all the way, & counter-act at the latest moment you can. Join with partner's mental & physical energy / ki at start or at maximum momentum, of his attack. Observe gaps in partner's timing. Do not let partner know your technique, timing, breathing, kiaii, until used at last. Whoever attacks or throws, is vulnerable to partner's counter attack. Do not expose yourself, unless you want partner to attack there, (as bait). Induce partner to go off balance, or to create an opening in his defense. Attack when partner is exposed, at a proper distance. Enter partner's defense. Use partner's momentum to your own advantage. Blend into it, divert its direction without wasting your energy in slowing it down. (Divert it to other partner or wall...). Escape & enter, to counter-attack in direction opposite to partner's velocity, & so approaching the target at a faster closing velocity. Duck, dodge, weave, & bob, in all directions. Evade or block only as far as is necessary. Or, block hard to discourage partner.

Surprise: Act reflexively & intelligently to surprise attacks anywhere & anytime; especially just before & after a "contest", also, during. Always watch partner. Stay alert of surroundings & partner's actions, while yourself acting & focusing (at target). Instantly invent new actions for new situations; improvise; spontaneously counter any (surprise or unfamiliar) attack.

Contacted: Tense covering muscles to protect underlying body parts. Protect other sensitive parts instantaneously. (Keep teeth together.) If somehow partner makes contact with your body: immediately pull back & attack (preferably simultaneously). (e.g. Pull back your attacked head, while you kick, (going into a somersault or roll). Quickly retaliate, before you are too stunned or weak from injury.

Falls: Never roll on rough ground; land on all 4's. Falling horizontally onto smooth ground, keep head tucked in, & be at full spin (angular momentum), before contacting ground; or, at contact, immediately roll into a spin. Roll away from partner. Spread impact surface, to dilute impact forces; &, ..., to whittle impact forces, further, use centrifugal force, of spin.

Multiple Partners: While looking in one direction, focus technique to another; deceiving. If circled by partners, go between the 2 most advantageous, simultaneously contacting both; or, use (the slowest) one as a shield (blocking the way of faster ones). Re-direct momentum of a partner towards another partner who otherwise would be contacting you next. Hear partners from behind; (kiaii silently),....

Laser Beam & other Hardware: Prevention is utmost critical. Talk to partner: "You are a miracle, don't blow your chance!". Know uses of hardware. Against a a knife or sword, use any handy object to block or defend. Against a gun, only if you are sure it will be used: defend while partner is drawing or raising the weapon; feint, decoy, deceive, & then act; (plead for mercy, getting closer in distancing for disarmament); evade direction of gun at first, & then (by contact) control its aim.

Practice: Make ki a part of your personality & everyday life, giving energy. Learn mental images of initial & final positions in techniques. Build reflexes by noticing speedy actions (e.g. each frame of a movie or tv, droplets of water splattering on ground, notes of music), & by shooting nerve energy up & down body (e.g. nerve twitch). Do exercises faster. Learn balance by turning in smaller circles.

God: God is infinite & He/She has to be at an infinite number of places, so He/She leaves it up to us to make this world a better place. Let us work & pray for Heaven on Earth. - one person's idealistic belief.

RE.15 CROSS-INDEX of RESEARCHER to RESEARCH to SUPPRESSION; only includes Researcher, whose Research & its Suppression are both in this treatise: (Listed alphabetically: by Subject, under which Researchers are Grouped):

THERAPY / Subject: RESEARCHER:	Contribution to Medicine, esp. Cancer Therapy; TABLE/MATRIX (Section S.#.#):	Suppression & Harassment of Researcher as Reward by Society; CANCER QUOT. COLLAGE (page-paragraph #-#):
BOOKS:		
Is Cancer Curable?	many	94-5
March of Truth on Cancer	many	94-9, 189-7
Chelation: (EDTA)		
Evers, H. Ray	10.14	100-(1-5)
Chiropractic:	A.3.2	83-8, 85-8, 140-9
DMSO:	(A.)18.3	74-(9, 10)
DETECTION: J. Arigo, H. Beard, R. Bradford, L. Burton, H. J. Rand, C. Reams, shifted out.		
Hartman, Emerson	D.16.15	98-1
Electro-Magnetism:	5.0	
Reich, Willhelm	5.2	94-10, 97-10
Enzymes:		
Shively, Frank	11.3	70-9
Fasting:	(A.)8.1	
Shelton, Herbert	8.1	205-(2, 3)
Fluoridation:	(A.)7.1.1	173-(4-8)
Yiamouyiannis, John	7.1.1	194-3
Glyoxylide:	18.1	
Kannel, J. W.	18.1	202-(1, 2)
Koch, Will. Fred.	18.1	88-1, 97-(11-13)
GROUPS:		197-3
IACVF	many	140-6, 143-11, 194-5
NHF	many	143-11
HEART: H. R. Evers & Shutes shifted elsewhere.		
Pritikin, Nathan	C.9.5.10	95-5

(Note: A fractional paragraph at top of page is counted, references are not.)

Therapy: Researcher:	Table/Matrix (Section S.#.#):	Cancer Quot. Collage (page-paragraph #-#):
Herbs:		
Duke, James	(C.)14.4(.2)	176-3
Hoxsey, Harry	14.1	71-7, 72-4, 76-1, 95-(8, 9), 98-4, 192-4
Kloss, Jethro	14.1	94-5
McQueen-Williams, Morovith	14.4	96-(12-14)
Montagna, F. Joseph	14.10	94-7
Homoeopathy:	18.7, B.3.5	170-4, 188-1
Hydrazine:	A.18.4	195-6
Gold, Joseph	18.4	
Hyperthermia:	(A.,B.,C.,D.) 4	84-10
Cole, Donald	(B.)4.5	204-2
Immunology:		
Burton, Lawrence	(A.,C.,D.)17.1	171-4, 194-8
Burzynski, Stan.	16.9	195-5
Coley, Bill Bradley	(A.,C.)17.16	84-10, 204-1
Crofton, William	17.9	89-9, 191-(1, 2)
Jackson, Eleanor	(A.)17.10	143-10
Lincoln, Robert	17.8	84-10
Livingston, Virginia	(A.)17.10	
Rand, H. James	(C.)17.15	171-3
Krebiozen:	17.2	70-(7, 8), 76-13, 171-1, 190-(1-3), 194-6
Durovic, Stevan	17.2	204-(4-6)
Ivy, Andrew C.	17.2	72-(10, 14), 175-9
Laetrile:	(A.,B.,C.,D.)10	72-1, 73-3, 76-(4-7, 13) 95-(10-13), 98-3, 117-(11-14), 175-(2, 3, 6, 7), 190-6, 232-(5,6), 233-(1,4-6)
Beard, Howard H.	(C.&D.)10.6	94-4, 202-6
Beard, John	10.1, C.10.2.2	202-3
Bradford, Robert	D.16.13	99.6
Briggs, Brian	10.18	191-7
Burk, Dean	7.1.1	120-6, 178-8

RE.16 QUIPS & COMMENTS, Misc. YARNS: (Unfair Generalizations; would you agree that?:)

Catch 22 of Alternative Cancer Research: We won't institutionalize your findings unless you're published; we won't publish you unless you're from our institutions. Exception: Even if you're published, from our institutions, you were misled, so now we'll ignore you, not to misguide the public.

In America, we pride ourselves in not paying homage to titles, yet observe who will listen to you on health matters, without an "MD" after your name.

We are advertised & edited into substituting credentials for credibility, & credibility for evidence.

To defer to the professional doctor or lawyer on medicine or law, is like deferring to the prostitute on love; both are limited by the profit motive; at least, with the prostitute, this is understood. (eg: Planned Obsolescence, Defense)

Better to prostitute the body, than the soul.

Our biggest occupational disease is that altho theoretically we have a Constitutional republican democracy, we entertain a totalitarian dictatorship in most of the work world. (Vertical Hierarchies; Unions, too?)

In some "Regimes", the heinous are concentrated in the "Secret Police"; in "Free Nations", they are diluted throughout society.

Any system that has silently persisted in not allowing "terminal" cancer patients a choice of treatment, so long as it does not harm, is bancrupt of any ethics, in its "business as usual" attitude. Used car salesmen, farm weather forecasters, fortune tellers, campaign managers, & stock market analysts have (deservedly) protections, that alternative cancer therapists have dearth of succor in.

Surgeon: "If cancer, cut it out." Non-MD: "So, if a headache, cut off head?" Surgeon: "Only if a bad headache!" Anesthesiologist: "It's a gas!"

Nuclear Freeze/...Nuclear Winter? Tomahawk to Tokamak. Maginot (one) Line(rs).

RE.15 CROSS-INDEX of RESEARCHER to RESEARCH to SUPPRESSION (continued):

Therapy: Researcher:	Table/Matrix (Section S.#.#):	Cancer Quot. Collage (page-paragraph #-#):
Halsted, Bruce		203-5, 234-2
Harris, Arthur	C.10.4.4	202-7
Kowan, Maurice	10.4	98-(5-7)
Krebs, Ernst, Jr.	10.1	94-1, 190-5, 193-3, 226-(3-8)
Manner, Harold	10.19.1	88-10
McNaughton, Andrew	10.11, 10.13	71-11
Privetera, James		(98-7)-(99-2)
Richardson, John	(A.)10.5	99-(5, 9-12), 190-4, 202-8
Sugiura, Kanematsu	10.20.7, C.12.1.5.2	190-10
Mental:	(A.,B.,C.,D.)2	76-11
Arigo, Jose	(D.)2.7.1	180-8
Nutrition:	many	many
Brandt, Johanna	12.2.3	94-(5, 6)
Gerson, Max	(C.)9.2, A.3.1	88-1, 191-(4, 5), 197-3, 203-(6, 7)
Kelley, Wm. Donald	(C.)11.5	88-3, 95-2
Reams, Carey	(D.)9.4.2	93-(10-12)
Nutrition, Anti-biotic:		
Drosness, Phil		
Lazenby, Lilian	12.1.3	117-13
Vitamin A:	(A.,B.,C.) 9.7	
Seifter, Eli		224-8, 226-9
Vitamin C:	(A.,B.,C.)9.6	80-8, 192-3
Pauling, Linus	1.1.6, 1.2.2, 9.6	89-(1, 3)
Vitamin E:	(A.)9.9	
Shute, Evan & Wilford	9.9.1	100-7

RE.17 HEART ATTACK & STROKE, THERAPIES:

The following purported therapeutic modalities are submitted for further investigation. Time constraints prohibit investigating reports on these therapies' effectivity, by this compiler. These are very incomplete lists.

Heart Attack: cayenne, kiaii (loud yelling of martial artist), thumping chest, water,- for emergency (acute episodes); &, hawthorne berries, garlic (onion ...), cinnamon, vitamin E (natural; fresh wheat germ oil, safflower oil), (no heated, refined (vegetable) oils;...but do:) selenium, choline (grapefruit), yoghurt, evening primrose oil, vitamin C (natural), vitamin B-6 (brewer's yeast, whole wheat, bananas), potassium (figs, dates, green leafy veg., bananas), magnesium (nuts, seeds), chromium (grapes, cloves, cinnamon), vanadium (sea foods, olives), potassium magnesium orotate & aspartate, chelation (EDTA), avoid: smoking, sugar, charred food, antibiotics, alcohol, high protein, synthetic vitamin B,- to prevent / reverse chronic condition. Do also, relaxation, meditation, exercise, fasting, clean environment, etc.

Stroke: DMSO, HBO (HyperBaric Oxygen), lecithin, vitamin E, garlic, periwinkle, molasses, enema, etc.

Injuries: vitamins E, C, B-15,..., chlorophyll, herbs (camomille, comfrey, cayenne), clay, etc.

RE.18 HOW to GET PUBLISHED, (on E&M/GRAVITY/SOUND WAVES):

"Why did Mt. St. Helena repeatedly erupt a couple of days after the March 1982 date for the 'Jupiter Effect' planetary 'line-up'? Suppose gravity 'waves' travel much slower than light waves. Then, even though we (optically) see the planets 'lining up', we do not feel their gravitational effects until later, (by a couple of days?). Is this similar to the couple of days delay, proposed by some, between the visual appearance of a sunspot & its belated effect on Earth? As an anology, remember the delay between when a sprinter sees the starting gunfire, & when he hears it. Maybe gravity 'waves' travel as fast towards a gravitational 'source' as an object 'falls' through space towards that 'source'. One may picture the gravity 'waves' pushing along the object, just as an ocean wave pushes a surfer. This is just a hypothesis, a dream, yet worthy of publication, so others can test it. History reveals that many scientific 'truths' started as 'dreams'." - Ralph Hovnanian, (edited into:) "Grand (Planetary) Alignment Update: Mt. St. Helena Eruption", Aquarian Fellowship Newsletter, (Joseph November, Ed.), v.2, n.3, p.4, May 1982. (Ref.: Rodney Collins, The Theory of Celestial Influence; Rho Sigma, Ether-Tech.; George Lakhovsky, The Secret of Life.)

Is the ratio of the speed of sound, in a medium, to the speed of light, in that same medium, a dimensionless ratio for that medium, a clue towards a fundamental universal constant, or ?*#@!? i.e.: v(sound)/c = ? - Ralph Hovnanian.

RE.19 SONG: "LET'S WASH D.C.", (lyrics by Ralph Hovnanian).

Let's	get	the	Ache	out	of	Akron,	Let's	put	the	Boy!	back	in	Boise,
"	"	"	Brrr	"	"	Birmingham,	"	"	"	Beaut!	"	"	Butte
"	"	"	Boss	"	"	Boston,	"	"	"	Fair	"	"	Fairbanks,
"	"	"	Shy	"	"	Chicago,	"	"	"	My!	"	"	Miami,
"	"	"	Sin	"	"	Cincinatti,	"	"	"	Maxi	"	"	Minneapolis,
"	"	"	Fort	"	"	Lauderdale,	"	"	"	Can	"	"	Kansas City,
"	"	"	Little	"	"	Little Rock,	"	"	"	New	"	"	New Orleans,
"	"	"	Loss	"	"	Los Angeles,	"	"	"	Fill	"	"	Philadelphia,
"	"	"	Nor	"	"	Norfolk,	"	"	"	Rich	"	"	Richmond,
"	"	"	Fee	"	"	Phoenix,	"	"	"	Saint	"	"	Saint Louis,
"	"	"	Pit	"	"	Pittsburgh,	"	"	"	See	"	"	Seattle,
"	"	"	Sag	"	"	Saginaw,	"	"	"	Spring	"	"	Springfield,
"	"	"	Witch	"	"	Wichita;	"	"	"	Wash	"	"	Washington.

Idea Roulette:
a "Drop in the Bucket" & "Shot in the Dark"
or,
a Unified Field Theory of Gravity & Electro-Magnetism?

Gazing up at the starlight while pouring water down at my face from a vessel, I felt another "unified field theory", combining Gravity with Electro-Magnetism (E&M) coming.... Only later did I realize the inspiration came from watching someone giving Jesus (or, other Prophets &/ Disciples) water whilst (S/)He carried the cross. (Perhaps the Lord was taking pity on me.)

(The vessel I tipped vertically reminded me of a hollow (cylinderical; metal) resonance cavity that can set up a standing wave of E&M (akin to the notes of a pipe organ). This is irrelevant, except in turn reminding me that:) Starlight has an "averaged out", & (like Sunlight) a "brightest direction", from "straight above", as viewed from Earth. Yet water pours from "straight above" also; the direction of Gravity. This had to be my anticipated clue! Finally, a new overlap region between Gravity & E&M, & it was in "direction"! (Gravity & E&M are also alike in being (frictionless; Energy) Conservative Fields that "fall off with the reciprocal of the square of the distance ($1/r^2$)").

Could it be that the Steller/Cosmic/Ether waves from the whole Universe could push the water down at me? Gravity has a "Universal constant" factor, as well! (Aside: I would not have reflected underneath, if it were rocks, instead of water, coming at me. .... Newton's apple, maybe....)

Background: Light waves have also been considered as (Newton's) "corpuscles", having momentum, hence mass. (Light beams can move delicately balanced mirrors.) This supports the "ether" theory. (The oft touted Michelson-Morley experiment only proved the lack of <u>direction</u> (vector) of ether relative to the Earth's surface, but not the <u>magnitude</u> (scalar) existence of ether. (Ref.: Dr. Dirac (Nobel-ist; of Fermi-Diraq, & Dirac-Delta terms), etc., (in Rho-Sigma, <u>Ether-Tech</u>., p.62-63). Zounds! Shades of gravity as a force from "outside in" to a planet, (akin to Walter & Lao Russell, <u>Atomic Suicide</u>, p.14).

Meanwhile, back to our new theory: The "earth" of a planet would "lightly shade" or "filter out" (in proportion to its thickness (or diameter)) the "bottom half side" of the stellar waves that would otherwise reach an object on the planet's surface. The net effect would be to "push down" the test object, because the stellar waves from "below" would be weakened on travelling through the planet, compared to the waves from "above".

An already known overlap between Gravity & E&M is that the magnitude of both <u>F</u>orce <u>F</u>ields fall off with farther distance, (r; (between <u>c</u>enters of <u>m</u>ass (c.m.), etc.)) by the reciprocal of the square of the distance, ($1/r^2$). (You are now experiencing some math(!), & re-emphasis).

Our new hypo-thesis does not contradict perceived symmetries of Nature, for some boundary conditions & distances (r_{s-p} = distance between c.m.'s of <u>s</u>atellite & <u>p</u>lanet; & R_p = <u>R</u>adius of <u>p</u>lanet) (c.m.=<u>c</u>enter of <u>m</u>ass) (M_p=<u>M</u>ass of <u>p</u>lanet):

If r_{s-p} <u>is much larger than</u> R_p (i.e. $r_{s-p} \gg R_p$), the solid angle "shadow" (of stellar waves) subtended by the planet at the satellite is proportional to $1/(r_{s-p})^2$, the phantom "pull" on the satellite being proportional to both that (solid angle) & this (thickness times cross-sectional area of planet, proportional to R_p^3). (Let $\propto$ symbolize "proportional to".) Gravity $\propto M_p \times 1/(r_{s-p})^2 \propto R_p^3/(r_{s-p})^2$, too.

Going farther to outer space, infinitely, $1/r^2$ approaches zero; the "ether" pushing equally in all directions, there is no net force. Nor by gravity.

(Yikes, are we close to a jackpot?! No cheating, please.)

Another boundary condition to satisfy is right at the surface of the planet ($r_{s-p}=R_p$). There, the filtering of stellar waves by the planet, & gravity (g), are both proportional to R_p. ($M_p \propto R_p^3$, & $g_p \propto M_p/R_p^2 \propto R_p^3/R_p^2 = R_p$.)

At the center of a planet, $r_{s-p}=0$, but there is no net direction to the "ether wind" because the earth filters equally along all angles. Nor is there any net gravity because the planet pulls equally from all sides.

But now, (uh-oh!), for some intermediate range of r_{s-p} not extreme relative to R_p, the calculation is more complex, (requiring "your generous interest vs./ coopted attention", as well as, "calculus"), yet similar results are expected for stellar waves & gravity, reaffirming our hypothesis.

For all distances (r_{s-p}), in the "corpuscle" theory for E&M (stellar waves), the force vector is in the same direction (co-linear) with the distance vector, as it is for gravity. (A vector has both magnitude & direction. End of math!)

Can stellar waves have such momentum? Considering they travel at the speed of light, hmmm...! Just a hypo(not hyper)-thesis. Competing for Peace, on this Hiroshima Day, 1986: Ralph Hovnanian

author, Medical Dark Ages Circa 1984, or, Cancer Alternative Therapies' Cure Rates, from which is quoted (2nd. Ed., p.288):

"Why did Mt. St. Helena repeatedly erupt a couple of days after the March 1982 date for the 'Jupiter Effect' planetary 'line-up'? Suppose gravity 'waves' travel much slower than light waves. Then, even though we (optically) see the planets 'lining up', we do not feel their gravitational effects until later, (by a couple of days?). Is this similar to the couple of days delay, proposed by some, between the visual appearance of a sunspot & its belated effect on Earth? As an anology, remember the delay between when a sprinter sees the starting gunfire, & when he hears it. Maybe gravity 'waves' travel as fast towards a gravitational 'source' as an object 'falls' through space towards that 'source'. One may picture the gravity 'waves' pushing along the object, just as an ocean wave pushes a surfer. This is just a hypothesis, a dream, yet worthy of publication, so others can test it. History reveals that many scientific 'truths' started as 'dreams'." - Ralph Hovnanian, (edited into:) "Grand (Planetary) Alignment Update: Mt. St. Helena Eruption", Aquarian Fellowship Newsletter, (Joseph November, Ed.), v.2, n.3, p.4, May 1982. (Ref.: Rodney Collins, The Theory of Celestial Influence; Rho Sigma, Ether-Tech.; George Lakhovsky, The Secret of Life.)

Is the ratio of the speed of sound, in a medium, to the speed of light, in that same medium, a dimensionless ratio for that medium, a clue towards a fundamental universal constant, or ?*#@!? i.e.: v(sound)/c = ? - Ralph Hovnanian.

To protect against claim jumpers, please note to yourself the date you received this:

Signature:____________________

Date:____________________

You are encouraged to mediate entering these as articles, or for awards, if opportune; thanks!

Ralph Hovnanian
2128 Prospect Ave.
Evanston, IL 60201 USA
(Tel.: 312-869-4346)